# THE ROUTLEDGE HANDBOOK OF PHILOSOPHY OF DELUSION

Delusions play an important and fascinating role in philosophy and are a particularly fertile area of study in recent years, spanning philosophy of mind and psychology, epistemology, ethics, psychology, psychiatry, and cognitive science. *The Routledge Handbook of Philosophy of Delusion* explores the conceptual and philosophical issues in the study of delusion and is the first major reference source of its kind.

Comprising 38 chapters by an international team of contributors, the Handbook is divided into six clear parts:

- The Nature of Delusion
- Delusion in Disorders
- Epistemology of Delusion
- Delusion's Place in the Mind
- Delusion Formation
- Responsibility, Culture, and Society.

Within these sections, key topics are discussed including delusions and wellbeing, delusions as they occur in wider mental disorder, the epistemic profile of delusions (evidence, justification, rationality), how delusions are formed, delusions and folk psychology (how they relate to belief, self-deception, imagination, and so on), and delusions in the wider social and cultural context.

An outstanding resource for both students and researchers, *The Routledge Handbook of Philosophy of Delusion* is essential reading for those working on delusion in philosophy departments, and also suitable for those in related disciplines such as psychology, psychiatry, and cognitive science.

**Ema Sullivan-Bissett** is a Reader in Philosophy at the University of Birmingham, UK. She is the editor of the volume *Belief, Imagination, and Delusion* (2024) and the author of *Irrationality* (2024). Her book *How Belief Functions: A Philosophical Inquiry* is forthcoming from Routledge.

# ROUTLEDGE HANDBOOKS IN PHILOSOPHY

*Routledge Handbooks in Philosophy* are state-of-the-art surveys of emerging, newly refreshed, and important fields in philosophy, providing accessible yet thorough assessments of key problems, themes, thinkers, and recent developments in research.

All chapters for each volume are specially commissioned, and written by leading scholars in the field. Carefully edited and organized, *Routledge Handbooks in Philosophy* provide indispensable reference tools for students and researchers seeking a comprehensive overview of new and exciting topics in philosophy. They are also valuable teaching resources as accompaniments to textbooks, anthologies, and research-orientated publications.

## Also available:

### THE ROUTLEDGE HANDBOOK OF EMBODIED COGNITION, SECOND EDITION
*Edited by Lawrence Shapiro and Shannon Spaulding*

### THE ROUTLEDGE HANDBOOK OF THE PHILOSOPHY OF EVIDENCE
*Edited by Tarja Knuuttila, Natalia Carrillo, and Rami Koskinen*

### THE ROUTLEDGE HANDBOOK OF NON-IDEAL THEORY
*Edited by Hilkje C. Hänel and Johanna M. Müller*

### THE ROUTLEDGE HANDBOOK OF CAUSALITY AND CAUSAL METHODS
*Edited by Phyllis Illari and Federica Russo*

For more information about this series, please visit: https://www.routledge.com/Routledge-Handbooks-in-Philosophy/book-series/RHP

# THE ROUTLEDGE HANDBOOK OF PHILOSOPHY OF DELUSION

*Edited by Ema Sullivan-Bissett*

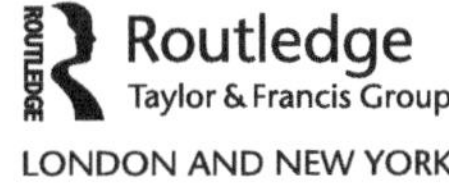

LONDON AND NEW YORK

Cover image: Simona Dumitru / Getty Images

First published 2025
by Routledge
4 Park Square, Milton Park, Abingdon, Oxon OX14 4RN

and by Routledge
605 Third Avenue, New York, NY 10158

*Routledge is an imprint of the Taylor & Francis Group, an informa business*




*British Library Cataloguing-in-Publication Data*
A catalogue record for this book is available from the British Library

*Library of Congress Cataloging-in-Publication Data*
Names: Sullivan-Bissett, Ema, editor.
Title: The Routledge handbook of philosophy of delusion /
edited by Ema Sullivan-Bissett.
Description: Abingdon, Oxon; New York, NY: Routledge, 2025. |
Includes bibliographical references and index.
Identifiers: LCCN 2024018962 (print) | LCCN 2024018963 (ebook) |
ISBN 9781032283388 (hbk) | ISBN 9781032283432 (pbk) |
ISBN 9781003296386 (ebk)
Subjects: LCSH: Delusions. | Psychology, Pathological—
Philosophy. | Philosophy of mind.
Classification: LCC RC553.D35 R68 2025 (print) |
LCC RC553.D35 (ebook) | DDC 616.89—dc23/eng/20240807
LC record available at https://lccn.loc.gov/2024018962
LC ebook record available at https://lccn.loc.gov/2024018963

ISBN: 978-1-032-28338-8 (hbk)
ISBN: 978-1-032-28343-2 (pbk)
ISBN: 978-1-003-29638-6 (ebk)

DOI: 10.4324/9781003296386

Typeset in Sabon
by codeMantra

# CONTENTS


*List of contributors*                                          *ix*
*Acknowledgements*                                              *xiv*

Introduction                                                    1
*Ema Sullivan-Bissett*


**PART 1**
**The nature of delusion**                                      **31**

1  Delusion and pathology                                       33
   *Valentina Petrolini*

2  Delusion and meaning                                         46
   *Rosa Ritunnano and Jeannette Littlemore*

3  Delusion and adaptiveness                                    62
   *Lisa Bortolotti and Martino Belvederi Murri*

4  Delusion and malfunction                                     73
   *Kengo Miyazono*

5  Delusion and natural kinds                                   87
   *Richard Samuels*

**PART 2**
**Delusion in disorders**                                                                103

  6  Delusional disorders                                                  105
     *Luigi Grassi and Federica Folesani*

  7  Delusions in psychosis                                               122
     *Marianne D. Broeker and Matthew Broome*

  8  Delusions in anorexia nervosa                                        135
     *Stephen Gadsby*

  9  Delusions in obsessive-compulsive disorder                           147
     *Judit Szalai*

10  Delusions in depression                                               158
     *Anna Bortolan*

11  Delusions in the disorders of old age                                 173
     *Julian C. Hughes*

**PART 3**
**Epistemology of delusion**                                                             187

12  Delusion and evidence                                                 189
     *Carolina Flores*

13  Delusion and double bookkeeping                                        202
     *José Eduardo Porcher*

14  Delusion and rationality                                              215
     *Quinn Hiroshi Gibson and Adam Bradley*

15  Delusion attribution                                                  228
     *Sam Wilkinson*

16  Delusion and introspection                                            245
     *Chiara Caporuscio*

17  Delusion and epistemic injustice                                      258
     *Eleanor Palafox-Harris*

**PART 4**
**Delusion's place in the mind**     275

18  Delusion and action     277
*Maura Tumulty*

19  Delusion and doxasticism     292
*Paul Noordhof*

20  Delusion and non-doxasticism     308
*Paul Noordhof*

21  Delusion and imagination     324
*Amy Kind*

22  Delusion and self-deception     336
*Jordi Fernández*

23  Delusion and memory     347
*Sarah Robins and Si-Won Song*

24  Delusion and dreaming     361
*Philip Gerrans*

25  Delusion and folk psychology     376
*Dominic Murphy*

**PART 5**
**Delusion formation**     387

26  Empiricism     389
*Federico Bongiorno and Matthew Parrott*

27  Rationalism     402
*Jakob Ohlhorst*

28  The one-factor theory     414
*Ema Sullivan-Bissett*

29  The two-factor theory     430
*Martin Davies and Max Coltheart*

30 The prediction error theory      450
*Philip Corlett*

31 Delusion and salience      463
*Peter McKenna*

32 Delusion and inference      477
*Urte Laukaityte and Matteo Colombo*

33 Delusion and hypnosis      491
*Michael H. Connors*

**PART 6**
**Responsibility, culture, and society**      503

34 Delusion and moral responsibility      505
*Matthé Scholten*

35 The social turn in delusions research      520
*Daniel Williams*

36 Delusion and culture      533
*Ian Gold and Joel Gold*

37 Delusion and conspiracy theories      544
*Joseph M. Pierre*

38 Delusion and the unrealistic comparator      557
*Richard Bentall*

*Index*      573

# CONTRIBUTORS

**Richard Bentall** is a Professor of Clinical Psychology at the University of Sheffield and a Fellow of the British Psychological Society and the British Academy. His research has focused on the cognitive and emotional processes involved in symptoms such as hallucinations and delusions, the influence of social risk factors (e.g., childhood adversity) on psychosis, and the effectiveness of psychological interventions for affected patients.

**Federico Bongiorno** is an FCT researcher at the Centre of Philosophy, University of Lisbon. Before this, he was a postdoc at the University of Oxford. His research lies at the interface of philosophy of mind, cognitive science, and the philosophy of psychiatry.

**Anna Bortolan** is a Senior Lecturer in the Department of Politics, Philosophy and International Relations at Swansea University (Wales, UK). Her main research interests are in phenomenology, philosophy of emotion, and philosophy of psychiatry.

**Lisa Bortolotti** is a Professor of Philosophy at the University of Birmingham and Editor-in-Chief of *Philosophical Psychology*. Her main research interests are in the philosophy of psychology and psychiatry.

**Adam Bradley** is currently an Assistant Professor in the Department of Philosophy and Fellow of the Hong Kong Catastrophic Risk Center at Lingnan University, Hong Kong.

**Marianne D. Broeker** is a DPhil student in Experimental Psychology at the University of Oxford, looking at alterations in consciousness in psychosis through phenomenology and psychophysics. Marianne is also getting trained as an existential-analytic psychotherapist and works with clinical patients.

**Matthew Broome** is a Chair in Psychiatry and Youth Mental Health, Director of the Institute for Mental Health at the University of Birmingham, Distinguished Research Fellow at Oxford Uehiro Centre for Practical Ethics, University of Oxford, and Visiting Professor at Suor Orsola Benincasa University of Naples.

**Chiara Caporuscio** is a Postdoctoral Researcher at Charite – Universitätsmedizin Berlin and Otto-von-Guericke Universität Magdeburg. She works at the intersection of philosophy, psychiatry, and cognitive science. Her research interests include altered states of consciousness, self-knowledge, and delusional belief.

**Matteo Colombo** is an Associate Professor at the Tilburg Center for Logic, Ethics and Philosophy of Science, Tilburg University, The Netherlands. He mainly works in the philosophy of mind and cognitive science. His current interests include issues in the foundations of theoretical neuroscience and computational approaches to psychiatric disorders.

**Max Coltheart** is an Emeritus Professor of Cognitive Science at Macquarie University. He is interested in cognitive neuropsychology (especially the study of acquired and developmental disorders of reading and spelling), cognitive neuropsychiatry (especially the study of delusional belief), and the methodology of cognitive neuroscience.

**Michael H. Connors** is a Senior Conjoint Lecturer at the Centre for Health Brain Ageing and the Department of Psychiatry and Mental Health, University of New South Wales, Sydney, Australia. He is also a psychiatry registrar at Prince of Wales Hospital, Sydney, Australia.

**Philip Corlett** received his Bachelor's degree in Natural Sciences (Experimental Psychology) from the University of Cambridge in 2002, and his PhD in Cognitive Neuroscience from the University of Cambridge in 2007. He came to Yale in 2010 on a one year Parke-Davis Exchange Fellowship, and never left! He joined the faculty and started the Belief, Learning, and Memory Lab in 2012.

**Martin Davies** is an Emeritus Wilde Professor of Mental Philosophy at the University of Oxford and an Adjunct Professor at Monash University, Australia, where he was an undergraduate. He is interested in anosognosia and other delusions, implicit knowledge, and the methodology of cognitive neuropsychology.

**Jordi Fernández** is an Associate Professor of Philosophy at the University of Adelaide. His research interests are in philosophy of mind, epistemology, and metaphysics. He is the author of *Transparent Minds: A Study of Self-Knowledge* (2013) and *Memory: A Self-Referential Account* (2019).

**Carolina Flores** is an Assistant Professor of Philosophy at the University of California, Santa Cruz. She works in philosophy of mind and social epistemology, focusing on evidence-resistance. Her work has appeared in *The Journal of Philosophy*, *Philosophical Studies*, and *Synthese*.

**Federica Folesani**, MD, is an Assistant Professor of Psychiatry in the Department of Neuroscience and Rehabilitation, and PhD student at the Doctorate Program in Translational Neuroscience and Neurotechnology, University of Ferrara, Italy.

**Stephen Gadsby** is a Fonds Wetenschappelijk Onderzoek (FWO) Postdoctoral Fellow at the Centre for Philosophical Psychology, University of Antwerp, Belgium. His research employs theoretical and empirical methods to explore a broad range of topics within philosophy, psychology, and psychiatry.

**Philip Gerrans** focuses on neurocomputational explanation of psychiatric disorder. His most recent work is a project on the relationship between interoception, emotion, and self-representation in psychiatric disorders characterized by altered self-awareness.

**Quinn Hiroshi Gibson** is currently an Assistant Professor of Philosophy and Director of the Medicine, Health, and Human Values programme at Clemson University, USA.

**Ian Gold** is a Professor of Philosophy and Psychiatry, and Chair of the Department of Philosophy at McGill University, Montreal. His research focuses on the study of delusions, the theory of mind, and reductionism in psychiatry and neuroscience.

**Joel Gold**, MD, is an Assistant Clinical Professor of Psychiatry at the Icahn School of Medicine, Mount Sinai, and the consulting psychiatrist to the National Hockey League Players' Association. He has a private practice in Manhattan.

**Luigi Grassi**, MD, is a Professor and Chair of Psychiatry and Chair of the Department of Neuroscience and Rehabilitation, University of Ferrara, Italy.

**Julian C. Hughes** has been both honorary professor of philosophy of ageing at Newcastle University, UK, and professor of old age psychiatry at the University of Bristol, UK. Mainly he was a NHS consultant in old age psychiatry.

**Amy Kind** is the Russell K. Pitzer Professor of Philosophy at Claremont McKenna College in Claremont, California. She has authored numerous articles and book chapters on imagination, consciousness, and other topics in the philosophy of mind. She has also authored two textbooks, *Persons and Personal Identity* (Polity 2016) and *Philosophy of Mind: The Basics* (Routledge 2020), and edited or co-edited several volumes, most recently *Epistemic Uses of Imagination* (Routledge 2021).

**Urte Laukaityte** is a PhD candidate at UC Berkeley, working within philosophy of psychiatry and cognitive science. She has research interests in the theoretical implications of recent empirical developments in the mind and life sciences, including basal cognition. Some of her focus areas include mind-body phenomena such as functional disorder ("hysteria"), cultural syndromes, placebo/nocebo, and hypnosis.

**Jeannette Littlemore**, BA, MA, PhD, PGCHE, FAcSS, is a Professor of English Language and Applied Linguistics in the Department of English Language and Linguistics, University of Birmingham, Birmingham, UK. Her research focuses on the role played by metaphor and metonymy in the understanding and expression of emotional experiences.

**Peter McKenna** is a psychiatrist who has worked at different times as a clinician and an academic, and for the last 15 years as a researcher in the FIDMAG Hermanas Hospitalarias Research Foundation in Barcelona. He works principally on the psychological and biological bases of schizophrenia.

**Kengo Miyazono** is an Associate Professor of Philosophy at Hokkaido University, Japan. His main research areas are philosophy of mind, philosophy of psychology, and philosophy of psychiatry. His recent publications include *Philosophy of Psychology: An Introduction* (Polity, 2021, with Lisa Bortolotti) and *Delusions and Beliefs: A Philosophical Inquiry* (Routledge, 2018).

**Dominic Murphy** is a Professor of History and Philosophy of Science at the University of Sydney. He is the author of *Philosophy in the Scientific Image* (MIT Press 2006) and has written articles in the philosophy of psychiatry, moral psychology, and philosophy of mind.

**Martino Belvederi Murri** is an Associate Professor of Psychiatry at the University of Ferrara, Italy. His main research interests are in clinical psychiatry, particularly on depressive and psychotic disorders.

**Paul Noordhof** is an Anniversary Professor of Philosophy at the University of York. His main research interests are in the philosophy of mind, action theory, and metaphysics. His work in the philosophy of mind mainly focuses upon the nature and explanatory character of consciousness.

**Jakob Ohlhorst** is a postdoc at Vrije Universiteit Amsterdam, with support from the Swiss National Science Foundation. His research specializes in philosophy of psychology, hinge epistemology, and virtue epistemology.

**Eleanor Palafox-Harris** is a PhD candidate in Philosophy at the University of Birmingham. Her current research focuses on delusion, epistemic injustice, and epistemic vigilance. Her research interests span philosophy of mental health, social epistemology and ethics.

**Matthew Parrott** is an Associate Professor at the University of Oxford and a Tutorial Fellow at St Hilda's College. His research focuses on questions in philosophy of mind, cognitive science, and philosophy of psychiatry.

**Valentina Petrolini** is a philosopher of psychology and psychiatry. She currently works as Juan de la Cierva Postdoctoral Researcher at the University of the Basque Country (UPV/EHU), where she is a member of the Language in Neurodiversity Lab (Lindy Lab).

**Joseph M. Pierre** is a Health Sciences Clinical Professor in the Department of Psychiatry and Behavioral Sciences at UCSF. His clinical work has focused on the treatment of psychosis, while his academic work addresses the "grey area" between psychosis and normality including voice-hearing and delusion-like beliefs.

**José Eduardo Porcher** is a Research Fellow at the Pontifical Catholic University of Rio de Janeiro, Brazil, working in the philosophies of religion and psychiatry. He is writing a book titled *Afro-Brazilian Religions and Philosophical Methodology* for Cambridge University Press.

**Rosa Ritunnano** is a consultant psychiatrist in early intervention for psychosis in the UK, where she moved after completion of her residency at the University of Verona (Italy) in

2016. Her joint doctoral research (University of Birmingham and Melbourne) spans philosophy, psychology, and linguistics, and employs phenomenological and narrative methods to address the question of meaning in delusions.

**Sarah Robins** is an Associate Professor of Philosophy at Purdue University. Her research is focused primarily on memory, through which she writes on a range of issues in philosophy of mind, psychology, and neuroscience.

**Richard Samuels** is a Professor of Philosophy at the Ohio State University, and previously held appointments at King's College London and the University of Pennsylvania. He is a co-editor of *Advances in Experimental Philosophy of Science* and *The Oxford Handbook of Philosophy of Cognitive Science*, and has published numerous papers on topics in the philosophy of psychology and foundations of cognitive science. His *Number Concepts: An Interdisciplinary Inquiry* (co-authored with Eric Snyder) is forthcoming with Cambridge University Press.

**Matthé Scholten** has a PhD in Philosophy from the University of Amsterdam and currently works at the Institute for Medical Ethics and History of Medicine of the Ruhr University Bochum, Germany. His research focus is on mental health ethics. He is co-coordinator of the SALUS project (www.bochum-salus-project.com) and currently co-edits a volume on mental health ethics for Oxford University Press.

**Si-Won Song** is a PhD candidate in the Philosophy Department at the University of Kansas. He is writing a dissertation about the role of ] in delusions.

**Ema Sullivan-Bissett** is a Reader in Philosophy at the University of Birmingham. Her research concerns the nature of belief and its connection to truth, as well as delusional belief formation and implicit bias. She is the editor of the volume *Belief, Imagination, and Delusion* (Oxford University Press, 2024), and the author of *Irrationality* (Cambridge University Press, 2024).

**Judit Szalai** is an Associate Professor of Philosophy at Eötvös Loránd University, Budapest. Her main interests are philosophical psychology and psychopathology, the philosophy of mind, the philosophy of technology, and the history of 17th-century thought.

**Maura Tumulty** is a Professor of Philosophy at Colgate University in Hamilton, New York. She works on issues at the intersection of philosophy of mind and moral psychology.

**Sam Wilkinson** is a Senior Lecturer in Philosophy at the University of Exeter. His interests are in the philosophy of mental health and wellbeing, with a specific focus on hallucinations, delusions, trauma, and brain injury. He is the author of the *Routledge Contemporary Introduction to Philosophy of Psychiatry*.

**Daniel Williams** is a Lecturer in Philosophy at the University of Sussex. He specializes in the philosophy of psychology and the social sciences, and has published extensively on topics such as belief, delusion, irrationality, and political epistemology.

# ACKNOWLEDGEMENTS

Many thanks to Tony Bruce at Routledge for inviting me to put together this Handbook, and to Adam Johnson for his brilliant support in moving it through to publication. I am grateful to Lisa Bortolotti for many things: her friendship, her inspiring work, and in this particular case, her advice on topics to include at proposal stage (although any omissions are mine). Thank you also to the contributors for their excellent work and their patience. I am grateful to Paul Noordhof for many years of collaboration on this topic, and for stepping in late in the process to write an additional chapter. Thanks also to the Arts and Humanities Research Council for funding my work on this project (*Deluded by Experience*, grant no. AH/T013486/1).

Finally, Tom Stoneham sat on my Thesis Advisory Panel at York where I completed my PhD on the nature of belief. In that role, he once asked me if I had ever thought about delusion. I had not. Here seems the right place to thank him for being the first to point me towards such a rich and fascinating topic.

# INTRODUCTION

*Ema Sullivan-Bissett*

Delusions are typically characterised as beliefs with bizarre contents, which are formed on the basis of evidence which does not properly support their content, and which are highly resistant to counterevidence. The nature of delusions, their role in our mental lives and the disorders in which they often occur, as well as their implications for theories in the philosophy of mind, epistemology, and ethics, are topics that have become more popular in philosophy in the last couple of decades. And, of course, delusion has for many years been a major topic of study in cognitive science and psychology. Recently, there has been a surge in interdisciplinary work carried out by researchers in these areas, providing a wealth of important insights into delusion, as well as prompting further questions.

The topic of delusion is a very wide ranging one, giving rise to questions concerning their etiology, pathological status, epistemology, whether they can be understood with the tools of folk psychology, how they compare to other attitudes with strange contents, their implications for moral responsibility, and more besides. These questions are of natural interest to philosophers of many stripes, as well as cognitive scientists and psychologists. I have tried to do justice to a broad range of such interests in this Handbook but naturally there are omissions.[1]

The introduction has the following shape: in Section 1, I try to get the phenomenon of delusion at least roughly in sight. I do this by offering some representative examples before drawing on clinical definitions. The examples will do two things. First, they will help demonstrate some commonly agreed upon features of delusions present in the diagnostic definitions, but second, they will illustrate the heterogeneity of delusions, and how criteria for them might be thought inadequate. In Section 2, I give some background for each of the parts and overview the chapters within them.

## 1. Introducing delusion

Let us begin then with some examples.

- Fred has the delusion that *his wife has been replaced by an imposter.* (Capgras delusion[2]) Fred reports that the woman in his home, wearing his wife's clothes, strongly resembling his wife (unless you know what to look for), is not his wife after all. He doesn't know



DOI: 10.4324/9781003296386-1

where his wife is, although he doesn't report her missing. He's a bit suspicious towards the imposter who seems to have replicated even the minor details, right down to the engraving on the wedding ring she wears.

- Mira has the delusion that *she has ceased existing*. (Cotard delusion)
  It's difficult to explain but Mira feels out of touch with the world around her. Although she recognises that she can walk and talk (rare occurrences for those who do not exist, she has to admit), she reasons that some non-existing people simply must retain these abilities.
- Sandeep has the delusion that *Taylor Swift is in love with her*. (Erotomania)
  An observer would note that there is no evidence for Sandeep's belief. Indeed, the two have never communicated, nor even been on the same continent at the same time. Nevertheless, Sandeep remains convinced of Taylor Swift's adoration.
- Alisha has the delusion that *MI6 are following her*. (Delusion of persecution)
  Alisha doesn't know why this is happening, and claims to be innocent of any crime, although she suspects that the interest from MI6 relates to her ability to read tea leaves and see people's auras, skills probably of a lot of value to security agencies.
- Amir has the delusion that *he retains full motor function following his stroke*. (Anasognosia)
  His doctors don't seem to believe him, and try to catch him out by asking him to clap or tie his shoelaces. Amir thinks he can do these things, but often simply doesn't feel like it when he is requested to do so.
- Freya has the delusion that *her arm is being moved by alien forces*. (Delusion of control)
  It seems to move in a way which surprises her, and which doesn't result from her intentions.

In the cases of Fred, Mira, and Freya, the contents of these delusions are sufficiently bizarre as to be almost impossible, and so they already put us in mind of an attitude quite out of the ordinary. To bring Sandeep's, Alisha's, and Amir's delusions into line, let us stipulate for the moment that these attitudes are *false*, and not supported by anything that an observer would take to be evidence. Sandeep cites as evidence for Taylor Swift's love that she sends her coded messages on the number plates of purple cars in her local area. Alisha supports her claim of being followed by MI6 by pointing out that she sees the same red car on her way to work every day, except when she leaves early and 'tricks the agent'. (The driver of the car is someone who lives nearby who drives to work at the same time each day.) Amir's case – insofar as it is a denial of impairment – might look slightly different. He may not produce positive evidence in favour of his delusion (which before his stroke was an unremarkable truth), he simply fails to be moved by evidence of his new impairment.

With these examples on the table, let us do what is commonly done, and turn to characterisations of delusion within the two most recent editions of the *Diagnostic and Statistical Manual of Mental Disorders* (DSM-IV and DSM-5). In the glossaries of each, the definition of delusions is given as

> a false belief based on incorrect inference about external reality that is firmly sustained despite what almost everyone else believes and despite what constitutes incontrovertible and obvious proof or evidence to the contrary. The belief is not one ordinarily accepted by other members of the person's culture or subculture (e.g., it is not an

article of religious faith). When a false belief involves a value judgment, it is regarded as a delusion only when the judgment is so extreme as to defy credibility.

*(DSM-IV 2000: 765, DSM-5 2013: 819)*

The *DSM-5* also characterises delusions when they appear in a list of key features of psychotic disorders. There they are described as

> fixed beliefs that are not amenable to change in light of conflicting evidence. Their content may include a variety of themes (e.g. persecutory, referential, somatic, religious, grandiose) [...] Delusions are deemed bizarre if they are clearly implausible and not understandable to same-culture peers and do not derive from ordinary life experiences [...] The distinction between a delusion and a strongly held idea is sometimes difficult to make and depends in part on the degree of conviction with which the belief is held despite clear or reasonable contradictory evidence regarding its veracity.

*(DSM-5 2013: 87)*

Concerns have been raised with almost all components of these characterisations. Let us air four of those now. First: *falsity*. It is of course obvious that not all false beliefs are delusions – yesterday I believed that *my car would start*, it didn't, but I was not deluded about the functionality of my car. It might be less obvious that there could be delusions which are true, or at least, that we ought to allow for the possibility of delusions with true contents, something ruled out by the glossary definitions in both the *DSM-IV* and *DSM-5*. To the first point, there are cases which might be interpreted as true delusions. Lisa Bortolotti discusses the case of Martha Mitchell, who was married to Richard Nixon's attorney general John Mitchell. Martha claimed that she had been kidnapped and sedated, claims which were interpreted as delusional but which turned out to be true. At the time of her claims, Martha was experiencing mental health issues and was under the care of a psychiatrist. Bortolotti points out that this case might be one of *fake delusion* rather than *true delusion*, that is, Martha didn't have a delusion that turned out to be true (*true delusion*), she had a true belief that turned out not to be a delusion (*fake delusion*) (Bortolotti 2023: 46). The *fake delusion* interpretation gave rise to the term *the Martha Mitchell Effect*, coined by Brendan Maher to pick out the misinterpretation of a person's true report as a delusion. Maher notes that cases of this kind are familiar to psychopathologists and involve subjects who 'seemed to be deluded' turning out not to be so (Maher 1988: 19).

Whether all apparent cases of true delusion turn out to be fake delusion will depend on the features of the context. Nevertheless, even if Martha's case and others like it are thought to be *fake* rather than *true*, we should probably not rule out the bare possibility of true delusions, lest we leave our understanding of these attitudes hostage to the operations of philosophical thought experiments. It is certainly coherent to suppose that we could have a case exactly like Alisha's delusion, which nevertheless happened to be true. Recall that Alisha believes that *MI6 are following her*. She claims to be innocent of any crime, but she wonders whether the agency's interest in her is based on her psychic abilities. This should sound fairly implausible to a neutral observer who might wonder whether Alisha has any evidence for her delusion. She certainly claims to. That *same red car*, every weekday, at 08:00. What else could explain why it's always there? As she waits for her bus to work each day, she spots that *same red car*. It must be an agent who knows which bus she takes,

3

ensuring that they drive by each day to monitor her activities. But now suppose that in a case of mistaken identity, MI6 really are tracking Alisha. An agent in various vehicles does indeed follow her each day, although she's never spotted them. Alisha's belief that *MI6 are following her* turns out to be true. Would we thus withdraw the status of delusionality? Probably not. As Martin Davies and colleagues point out:

> if a true belief is sustained in just the same way as a delusion is sustained, despite its implausibility and in the face of all the available evidence, then it seems that, for the purposes of a psychological theory, it should be grouped together with delusions.
>
> *(Davies et al. 2001: 133)*

If cases like these are possible (even if not very likely), it cannot be necessary to delusions that they are false.

Let us turn to the second controversial component of the *DSM* definitions: the relationship between delusion and evidence. In the glossaries of *DSM-IV* and *DSM-5* delusions are characterised as being 'firmly sustained despite what almost everyone else believes and despite what constitutes incontrovertible and obvious proof or evidence to the contrary', and in *DSM-5*, they are described as 'not amenable to change in light of conflicting evidence'. Once again, a poor relationship to evidence should not be taken to amount to a sufficiency condition on delusion, all sorts of everyday beliefs are based on poor evidence or resistant to counterevidence, without them being delusions. For example, religious beliefs have been argued to display an 'astonishing' lack of evidential responsiveness (Van Leeuwen 2017: 55, see also Ichino 2024: 84–86), and almost any characterisation of self-deceptive beliefs will build in the condition that such beliefs are held in the face of evidence available to the subject which would justify what they ought to believe, rather than what they self-deceptively believe (Van Leeuwen 2007: 422).

It might be thought that a sufficiency condition could be grounded on a difference in degree – perhaps everyday evidence-resistant beliefs are not held in the face of *incontrovertible* counterevidence, and it is this more precise relationship to evidence which is sufficient for delusion. However, even if we take evidence resistance to a strong degree to be the relevant condition, challenges abound from some quarters even with respect to this. For example, Brian F. Schaffner and Samantha Luks showed their experimental participants two photographs: one depicting Donald Trump's presidential inauguration and one depicting Barack Obama's. They took their question of which photograph contained more people to have an answer which is 'so clear and obvious to the respondents that nobody providing an honest response should answer incorrectly' (Schaffner and Luks 2018: 135). And yet, they found that 15% of Trump voters maintained that the photograph of his inauguration contained more people than the photograph of Obama's (Schaffner and Luks 2018: 139). One interpretation of this result is that Trump voters were not moved by incontrovertible counterevidence from their belief that Trump's inauguration attracted a larger crowd than Obama's.

An alternative explanation is that the Trump voters weren't expressing a genuine belief, but were rather engaging in *expressive responding*. Indeed, Schaffner and Luks take their findings to support the view that 'at least some of the misinformation reported in surveys is the result of partisan cheerleading rather than genuinely held misperceptions' (2018: 135). If that's right, this is not a case that can be appealed to as one of incontrovertible evidence-resistant belief. However, others, in reflecting on this finding, take expressive responding to be consistent with belief. Bortolotti suggests that 'it is plausible that some of our sincere reports have this expressing role', and that the experimental findings are 'surprising if the role of the belief were merely to represent reality accurately, but unsurprising if the role of the belief were also to express approval' (Bortolotti 2023: 81, see also Williams 2021).

Other kinds of belief might also put pressure on distinguishing delusions as especially evidence-irresponsive. Indeed, in their contribution, Ian Gold and Joel Gold, in reflecting on the *DSM-5*'s characterisation of delusions as 'fixed beliefs that are not amenable to change in light of conflicting evidence' note that this 'is no less true of a wide range of other beliefs [...] conspiracy theories provide a conspicuous example' (Chapter 36: 534), and Bortolotti has it that 'conspiracy beliefs are *as resistant* to counterevidence as clinical delusion' (2023: 64, my emphasis).

Can we at least safely take it that evidence-insensitivity is a necessary feature of delusions? One problem with this is that it might not capture all delusions, as Max Coltheart and colleagues have pointed out, 'incontrovertible proof against delusions is often not available' because some delusions are, at least in practice, unfalsifiable (2011: 274). They suggest delusions of control as a candidate for this. Recall Freya, who has the delusion that *her arm is being controlled by alien forces*. What 'incontrovertible and obvious proof or evidence to the contrary' can be brought to bear against this belief? What is the 'conflicting evidence' in light of which the delusion is not amenable? It is hard to say.

A final point about the relationship between delusion and evidence is this: it might be that people with delusions have the capacity to rationally respond to counterevidence to their delusion, but fail to put that capacity into practice due to features of the delusional context (we might think in terms of *masks* on that capacity). This idea has recently been developed by Carolina Flores, who argues that the 'puzzling responses' that subjects with delusions have to evidence supports the claim that they have the capacity to respond to it (Flores 2021: 6307). For example, subjects *incorporate* the evidence, rather than *dismiss* it. Recall Mira, who believes that *she has ceased existing* but recognises that her abilities to walk and talk are rare for those who don't exist. However, since she has these abilities, she reasons that some non-existing people simply must retain them (Mira's case is modelled on the case of J.K., reported in Young and Leafhead 1996: 158). As Flores points out, the subject engages with the evidence, and the pattern of reasoning that results is 'recognisable':

> If you observed, or were told about, something that looks like a violation of the laws of nature but were *certain* of what you saw or heard, you might find yourself reasoning in an analogous way. You know what you saw (or that someone else saw it), so the laws of nature must have been violated in that instance.
>
> *(Flores 2021: 6308)*

Flores further argues that subjects with delusions understand how evidence bears on their delusions, and indeed, which possible responses are epistemically permissible (Flores 2021: 6308), and they also display evidence-avoidance akin to what we find in other cases (e.g. confirmation bias) (Flores 2021: 6308–6309). Overall then, the claim that delusions are 'not amenable to change in light of conflicting evidence', however understood, faces significant challenges.

Third, in the glossary definitions, delusional beliefs are described as not 'ordinarily accepted by other members of the person's culture or subculture (e.g., it is not an article of religious faith)'. This clause has been criticised as atheoretical – it is not clear why we should exclude a belief from the category of delusion just on the basis that is shared, and indeed, this exemption excludes, by fiat, the possibility of group delusion (Hamilton 2006 220, Ross and McKay 2017: 317, Gipps and Clarke *forthcoming*). On the other hand, it has been argued that something in the vicinity of this clause is important because we should recognise the role of culture in normal belief formation:

> Our expectations about normal belief formation include expectations about the kinds of beliefs people are likely to acquire in the course of normal human development. [...] we think that it is normal for people to pick up beliefs that we find weird from the culture around them, and not normal for them to arrive at equivalently weird beliefs all by themselves in cultures that provide no support for such beliefs.
>
> *(Murphy 2013: 119)*

The ubiquity of religion plus cultural learning gives way to an explanation of why people might have religious beliefs, and perhaps legitimises the culture clause in the diagnostic criteria.

Finally, the *DSM* definitions capture delusions as *beliefs*. This is contentious because some characterisations of belief look to rule out delusions as part of that category. Beliefs are typically thought of as responsive to evidence at least to some degree, and efficacious with respect to behaviour. On the other hand, delusions are described as being irresponsive to evidence, and are not always efficacious in the way we would expect if they were beliefs. Broadly speaking, there are two strategies to pursue in light of these observations. One could remain committed to *doxasticism* about delusions, that is, to the view that delusions are beliefs, and think of delusions as a test case for accounts of the nature of belief. It might just turn out that our accounts of belief need adjusting in order to properly recognise delusions as a member of the set. Doxasticists have done this by loosening the strict ties between, for example, belief and rationality, allowing delusions to be seen as one kind of imperfect belief among others (Bortolotti 2009). Alternatively, one could embrace *non-doxasticism* about delusion, and have it that they are better understood not as beliefs but as something else (Currie 2000, Gallagher 2009, Dub 2017), or as somewhere in between two kinds of state (Egan 2008, cf. Kind 2024).

We have seen that characterisations of delusion in the last two iterations of the *DSM* are hugely imperfect, either in failing to properly characterise all and only delusions or in failing to properly capture key parts of their nature. Some of these issues occur as part of discussion in the chapters herein, giving the reader an up-to-date overview of the relevant debates. I turn now to the six parts of the Handbook and give some context for the chapters within them.

## 2. Overview of Parts

### 2.1  *Part I: Nature of delusion*

The opening part of the Handbook is focused on how we should think about delusion in the broader context of well-functioning human cognition. Many recent discussions of the topic begin by asserting the pathological status of delusion as a datum, and then proceed to give accounts of what makes it so (see e.g. Miyazono 2015: 561, Sakakibara 2016: 147,

Petrolini 2017: 502, Bortolotti 2018, cf. Bortolotti 2022). In the Handbook's opening contribution (Chapter 1), Valentina Petrolini identifies a tension between taking delusions to be continuous with other beliefs and taking them to be instances of pathology. After all, if delusions are continuous with other beliefs, on what grounds might we mark them out as pathological? Petrolini spells out this challenge and suggests that the question of pathology should be answered more broadly, by considering delusions in the wider context of a person and their environment.

The idea that delusions are instances of pathology is widely endorsed, but if that seems too bold or challenging to make good on, at the very least, delusions are often characterised negatively, that is, they are poor epistemically, they disrupt functioning or wellbeing, and so on. Bortolotti has recently suggested that a richer understanding of the nature of delusional beliefs can be had from paying attention to the *benefits* of delusion. One idea is that delusions are cases of *epistemically innocent* cognitions. A cognition that is epistemically innocent is one that is epistemically irrational, but nevertheless delivers some epistemic benefit to a subject, where the adoption of an epistemically better cognition is unavailable to the subject or would not deliver the same benefit (Bortolotti 2020: 13). This idea has been explored in the context of delusion, where it has been argued that some delusions are epistemically innocent (Bortolotti 2015a, 2015b, 2020: Chapters 4 and 5) and that this claim is available to various ways of thinking about delusion formation (Sullivan-Bissett 2018).

Another avenue for identifying benefits of delusions is to consider *meaning*. Psychologists have investigated the *Sense of Coherence* (SOC) in subjects with delusions which picks out a

> global orientation that expresses the extent to which one has a pervasive, enduring though dynamic, feeling of confidence that (1) the stimuli deriving from one's internal and external environments are structured, predictable, and explicable; (2) the resources are available to one to meet the demands posed by these stimuli; and (3) these demands are challenges, worth of investment and engagement.
>
> *(Antonovsky 1987: 19)*

Moshe Bergstein and colleagues found that subjects at the acute stage of experiencing delusions had an average SOC score similar to that of the non-delusional population. More illuminating perhaps was their finding that six months later those subjects in remission from their delusions had *lower* SOC scores than those subjects who retained their delusion. In reflecting on work suggesting that depression is associated with remission from delusional states, they note that this is unsurprising 'if remission from delusional states is accompanied by a reduction in the level of meaning and purpose … with a resultant decrease in psychological well-being' (2008: 289).

More recently, researchers have identified a couple of ways in which we might properly characterise delusions as *meaningful* (discussed in Ritunnano and Littlemore, Chapter 2). The first concerns the meaning experienced by the person with a delusion. Rosa Ritunnano and colleagues (2022) draw on a case study (Harry) to argue that delusions can enhance a person's sense of *meaningfulness*, understanding meaning as 'the extent to which one's life is subjectively experienced as making sense, and as being motivated and directed by valued goals' (Ritunnano et al. 2022: 110). The authors draw on several other recent sources of evidence suggestive of a relationship between delusions and enhanced sense of meaningfulness (2022: 113–114). The idea that delusions can confer meaningfulness on the person experiencing them has been argued to support a phenomenological approach in the clinical context, understood, at the very least, as one which pays careful attention to the experience of the subject, or *what the world feels like* to them (Ritunnano et al. 2022: 114). But of course, there's no reason why this call for attention to the experiential perspective of subjects with delusions could not be open to anyone who took seriously the idea that experience – often of an anomalous kind – is key to the formation and maintenance of delusions (see Chapters 26, 28, and 29). A less obvious way of relating delusions and meaning is from the perspective of the interpreter, whose capacity for constructing explanations and predictions of the subject's behaviour may be enhanced by engaging with delusional reports (Ritunnano and Bortolotti 2022: 950, see also Palafox-Harris, Chapter 17 for brief remarks on the relationship between subjective meaning and testimonial injustice).

The discussion concerning meaning in delusion has implications for how we think about the nature of delusion in the context of normal functioning or wellbeing. In reflecting on their case study of Harry, Ritunnano and colleagues note that they 'could agree on the fact that Harry's social and occupational function is impaired', but on the other hand, 'Harry is telling us that he is the happiest man in the world. He reports finding a highly significant meaning for leading his life, something that gives him coherence and purpose' (2022: 114).

Let us turn to the proper functioning of belief in the context of evolution. One question we can ask is whether delusional beliefs are adaptations or malfunctions of belief. Some researchers have suggested that delusions (or a subset of them) might be biological adaptations, where the mechanisms responsible for their formation were selected for their role in deceiving others into social alliances (Hagen 2008, cf. Gold and Gold 2014: 98–100). Another kind of adaptive approach can be located in the prediction error framework (see Chapter 30). According to such an approach, delusions are adaptive insofar as they maintain behavioural interactions in the face of abnormal prediction-error signalling (Mishara and Corlett 2009, Fineberg and Corlett 2016, cf. Lancellotta 2022). In their contribution (Chapter 3), Bortolotti and Martino Belvederi Murri investigate the potential adaptiveness of delusions as part of the explanation of the insight paradox (where insight into one's condition provides both costs and benefits). They suggest that delusions can sometimes support psychological and epistemic functionality, in the manner of helping the person respond to a crisis. This might be via its content (a rosier version of reality might help manage negative emotions) or via its offering an explanation of puzzling events or experiences. In some cases, a person's gaining insight into the delusionality of their belief can be harmful insofar as these emergency-oriented benefits are lost.

On the other hand, when thinking about delusion and proper functioning, the idea that delusions are instances of malfunction carries with it significant prima facie plausibility. Delusions are characterised across various literatures as extreme cases of *belief gone wrong*. They are proposed as cases of the most extreme forms of irrationality, and as we have already noted, it is often taken for granted in many discussions that delusions are the paradigmatic case of *pathological belief*. If one is attracted to integrating delusion into a broader programme of biologising human cognition, before we even get to the details, the idea that they are malfunctioning beliefs may strike one as appealing. Kengo Miyazono is a key proponent of the malfunction approach, in particular, the view that delusions are malfunctioning beliefs (2015, 2018). The account developed by Miyazono identifies three possible sites of malfunction: in mechanisms responsible for anomalous experiences, attention mechanisms (against a background of prediction error accounts), and second factors. In his contribution (Chapter 4), Miyazono identifies two questions about delusions: what mental state they are (the *nature question*), and what makes them pathological (*the pathology question*). He outlines his view which provides answers to both questions: delusions are *malfunctioning beliefs*.

Another question that might be asked concerning the nature of delusion is whether they constitute a natural kind (Samuels, Chapter 5), something that 'has been roundly rejected by many theorists' (Samuels 2009: 50). In the strongest terms, we might take natural kindhood to designate 'genuine scientifically interesting divisions in nature, worthy of investigation', and we might even think that 'identifying natural kinds and disregarding categories that are not natural kinds is a key source of progress in science as a whole' (Taylor 2020: 2074). Even if that's a little strong for some tastes, we might at least think that if delusions did not constitute a natural kind then there's a sense in which they are 'inappropriate for the purposes of scientific enquiry' (Samuels 2009: 49). Discussion on this question has tended to take Richard Boyd's (1991) homeostatic property cluster account as the relevant backdrop. The idea of delusions as a natural kind so understood has met with many objections, which primarily focus on elements of the nature of delusion which rule them out as a candidate for kindhood (e.g. their being continuous with non-delusional phenomena, their being heterogeneous, and more besides) (see Samuels 2009 for the most robust defence of the natural kind claim for delusions).

The chapters in this opening part explore the role of delusion in the context of normal functioning or wellbeing, and how we should understand them against a broadly naturalistic framework. We have seen that delusions are standardly taken to be instances of pathology, and this idea finds a natural home in accounts of them as malfunctioning beliefs. On the other hand, at least some delusions have also been hypothesised to imbue a subject's life or experience with meaning, to deliver epistemic benefits not otherwise available, and to operate as emergency responses which keep the subject functioning in unusual or difficult circumstances. Some of these more positive features might be harnessed into a view which casts delusions as evolutionarily adaptive, or, even if they do not change what we want to say about the functional status of delusions, at the very least they suggest a more nuanced picture of the effect of delusions on a subject's overall wellbeing. It might be thought that getting closer to a unified account of the nature of delusion would, at the same time, resolve questions regarding pathology, adaptation, and malfunction. However, even if we take delusions to represent a unified kind – a natural kind even – the case for this nevertheless leaves room for substantial disagreement about how best to understand them in the context of proper functioning and overall wellbeing.

## 2.2  *Part II: Delusions in disorders*

Part of the richness of the topic of delusion is the role of the wider contexts in which they appear. One key contextual feature of any given case is whether the delusion occurs as part of a wider mental disorder, manifesting as one symptom among others. It might seem surprising that sometimes they do not, but so-called *monothematic* delusions are those concerning a single theme which arise in otherwise healthy individuals (Coltheart et al. 2007: 642). This second part is devoted to delusions as they occur across a range of mental disorders, including, most obviously, delusional disorders (Grassi and Folesani, Chapter 6), as well as psychosis (Broeker and Broome, Chapter 7), anorexia nervosa (Gadsby, Chapter 8), obsessive compulsive disorder (OCD) (Szalai, Chapter 9), depression (Bortolan, Chapter 10), and disorders of old age (Hughes, Chapter 11). Contextualising delusions in this way can help us better understand their nature, how they interact with the conditions of which they are a part or a consequence, and indeed, the nature of the conditions themselves.

A subject with delusional disorder is someone whose condition is characterised by the presence of at least one delusional belief, indeed, other than the influence of the delusion on the subject's broader mental state and behaviour, they are otherwise functionally normal. Types of delusional disorders are distinguished based on the content or theme of the delusions present, for example, *persecutory, somatic, misidentification,* and so on. The heterogeneity of content or theme is underpinned by a range of hypothesised causes: biopsychological, neurobiological, and psychological (explored by Grassi and Folesani, Chapter 6).

Turning now to broader conditions in which delusions can sometimes or often be a symptom. Let us begin with psychosis, something difficult to define, but most narrowly can be understood as picking out 'the presence of delusions, hallucinations without insight, or both' (Arciniegas 2015: 717). *Psychosis* is an umbrella term which includes, most obviously, schizophrenia, or schizophrenia spectrum disorders. Just like with delusional disorders, delusions in psychosis take a variety of forms (with respect to content) and have been hypothesised to arise from a range of causes (discussed by Broeker and Broome, Chapter 7). A recent review and qualitative evidence synthesis focusing on first person accounts of lived experience of delusions in psychosis concluded:

> Delusions in psychosis are best understood as strongly individualised and inherently complex phenomena emerging from a dynamic interplay between interdependent subpersonal, personal, interpersonal, and sociocultural processes.
>
> *(Ritunnano et al. 2022: 472)*

Several of these processes as related to delusion more broadly are discussed later in the Handbook (see Parts V and VI).

For other conditions explored in this part, with respect to the beliefs involved, which are often harmful, it is sometimes contested whether they are properly characterised as delusions. Let us turn to the distinction between *overvalued ideas* and *delusions*. In the *DSM-5*'s glossary, an *overvalued idea* is understood as

> an unreasonable and sustained belief that is maintained with less than delusional intensity (i.e., the person is able to acknowledge the possibility that the belief may not be true). The belief is not one that is ordinarily accepted by other members of the person's culture or subculture.
>
> *(DSM-5 2013: 826)*

The difference between these two kinds of beliefs comes down to the former 'leav[ing] room for some element of doubt when challenged by contradictory evidence' (Barton et al. 2022: 2), whilst, as we have seen, delusions are typically understood as held with significant conviction in the face of overwhelming counterevidence.[3] This distinction appears in the literature on anorexia nervosa (see Gadsby, Chapter 8 for a critique of its usefulness), and has been suggested as a distinction that might map onto severity of symptomology. That is, where beliefs reach the level of delusional intensity (something found in at least some subjects with anorexia nervosa), some researchers have suggested that it would be fruitful to discover whether such cases represent an increased risk (Barton et al. 2022: 8).

The notion of an *overvalued idea* has also appeared in discussions of the nature of OCD, although in this context, it appears alongside delusion rather than in contrast to it. Whereas it was once commonly thought that subjects with OCD were able to rationally assess their obsessive concerns, in a significant minority of cases, it has been found that this is not the case (Kozak and Foa 1994, O'Dwyer and Marks 2000). The nature of such concerns in these cases then has been thought better captured as overvalued ideas or delusions, and this has implications, not least for the clinical context. For example, Edna Foa found that behavioural treatment was less effective in those subjects with OCD who manifested *overvalued ideation* (Foa 1979, see also Salkovskis and Warwick 1985). Even if this is not so, and OCD involving overvalued ideas or delusions does respond to traditional treatments (as suggested by some case studies presented in O'Dwyer and Marks 2000), the character of the cognitive components of the condition is surely key to our understanding of its nature (as explored in Szalai, Chapter 9).

Delusions as they occur alongside depression represent a different kind of taxonomical challenge. Whereas with anorexia nervosa and OCD delusions (or overvalued ideas, or something weaker still) are considered part of these conditions (with associated implications for clinical management), things aren't so clear for delusions as they occur alongside depression. Some researchers understand this in a way akin to anorexia nervosa and OCD, that is, some severe forms of unipolar depression involve usually mood-congruent delusions (i.e. involving themes of persecution, inadequacy, or disease), whilst others have it that unipolar depression (even severe) is a different condition from delusional depression. That is, depressive delusions ought not be conceptualised as a symptom of (severe) unipolar depression, rather, their presence indicates the appropriateness of a different or additional diagnosis. As well as discussing this issue in her contribution (Chapter 10), Anna Bortolan also defends the idea that we can better understand delusions in depression by attending to the bodily and affective experiences that may ground some of the delusional thoughts associated with the condition, with delusions of worthlessness being a key example.

Let us turn finally to delusions as they occur in disorders specifically old age. Perhaps it will be wondered why this is a marked out as an independent topic of interest. A tempting thought might be that the nature of delusions, notwithstanding their heterogeneity elsewhere, is not usefully discovered or understood by looking in particular at those which are *late-onset*. In fact, though, this is up for grabs, and there has been significant debate over the term *paraphrenia,* used by Emil Kraepelin (1920) to pick out 'a condition characterised by a strong delusional component with preservation of thought and personality' (Casanova 2010: 196[4]). It has been proposed that paraphrenia is associated with late onset (people over 60), but this has been contested on the grounds of insufficient data to support it (see e.g. Casanova 2010: 196, Ravindran et al. 1998: 134). The term was excluded from the previous two editions of the *DSM*, which, according to some researchers, 'only serves to worsen the overinclusiveness of the schizophrenia category and to discourage original research on paraphrenia' (Ravindran et al. 1998: 133, see also Howard and Rabins 1997). If we do not have a diagnostic label for the phenomenon Kraepelin took to be of interest, we risk losing out on a proper understanding of at least some cases of delusions in old age which are ill-suited to our taxonomy (for discussion see Hughes, Chapter 11).

We have, in this part of the Handbook then, discussions of delusions as they occur in various wider disorders. We have seen that the questions that arise in these discussions are as heterogeneous as the disorders themselves. Sometimes the presence of delusions is the primary or significant feature of a condition (as in delusional disorders or psychosis), and a key point of interest here is how such delusions arise, concerning which a range of causes have been hypothesised. For other conditions which involve strange and often harmful beliefs, capturing such beliefs as *delusions* might help map the severity of symptoms (as in anorexia nervosa), or might be a way of better capturing and understanding the cognitive component of a condition (as in OCD). Sometimes it is contested whether a given disorder might involve delusions or whether the presence of delusions in fact indicates the presence of an additional disorder (as in severe depression), and there has also been significant debate over whether delusions which appear later in life should be of particular theoretical interest. We see then that discussing delusions in the broader context of disorders in which they might appear does not provide a homogeneous bunch of theoretical fruit in each such context. Rather, these discussions allow for a range of further questions and research programmes directed at better understanding delusions themselves, as well as the conditions of which they might be a part.

## 2.3   Part III: Epistemology of delusion

We turn now to epistemological questions concerning delusion. As we have already noted, the question of whether delusions are best understood as beliefs has been one of the major concerns in philosophical work on delusion. The epistemology of delusions is of course relevant to this question, with some epistemic features of delusions thought to put pressure on their doxastic status. We saw earlier (Section 1) that delusions are often defined in terms of their poor relationship to evidence, and indeed, the difference between an *overvalued idea* and a *delusion* according to the *DSM-5* hinges on the relationship to counterevidence. Notwithstanding limitations of this already noted, this feature of delusion has played a major role in discussions regarding delusion's doxastic status (Noordhof, Chapters 19 and 20), what we can say about its rationality (Gibson and Bradley, Chapter 14), and how many factors must be posited to explain their formation and maintenance (Sullivan-Bissett, Chapter 28, Davies and Coltheart, Chapter 29).

As noted earlier section, Flores (2021) has recently argued that delusions are in fact evidence-responsive, a claim she supports by drawing on the epistemic behaviour of subjects with delusions. First, these subjects often engage with such evidence. That engagement might not be rational or epistemically ideal, but it is engagement nonetheless: 'Patients may state that they are an exception to generalizations, bite the bullet on implausible conclusions, or contrive stories that explain away the evidence' (Flores 2021: 6307). We see these patterns in our earlier cases of Mira (who takes herself to be an exception to a generalisation about the capacities of non-existence people), and Amir (who explains away evidence of his apparent incapacities). Flores also canvasses evidence that subjects with delusions understand the way in which a piece of evidence bears on their delusion, and that these subjects engage in evidence-avoidant behaviours (Flores 2021: 6308–6309).

For those who want to resist the idea delusions are evidence-resistant to any remarkable or inexplicable extent, some have reflected on the fact that they are often accompanied by highly anomalous experiences, which might be a source of (apparent) evidence for their content (Flores 2021: 6315, Noordhof and Sullivan-Bissett 2021: 10280). Our grounds for saying this may depend in part on the conception of evidence in play (i.e. internalist or externalist, something explored by Flores, Chapter 12). And of course, it's one thing to identify a source of evidence for delusional belief; it might be quite another for a belief to seem utterly incalcitrant to a range of other sources of evidence, like that presented in one's background beliefs or testimony (Coltheart and Davies 2021: 222).

Another epistemic feature that has put pressure on doxasticism about delusion is *double bookkeeping*, a term used to capture what might be going on in a subject with a delusion who appears to demonstrate internal incoherence (Sass 1994: 21). We are to imagine two mental *books* kept by the subject, one concerning most of her ordinary beliefs, appropriately linked up with action and so on, whilst the second book is one where 'intersubjective standards of confirmation are suspended, as are the usual connections to the patient's other mental states, action, and emotion' (Porcher 2019: 113). The phenomenon of double bookkeeping has played a role in the debate about the doxastic status of delusion, particularly with respect to behaviour and phenomenology (these issues, as well as the possibility of phenomenologically centred approaches to delusion which might evade them, are explored in Porcher, Chapter 13).

Let us turn now to irrationality. Maher, father of the one-factor approach (see Chapter 28), is often cited as claiming that forming a delusional belief on the basis of an anomalous experience is a *rational* response to that experience (see e.g. Davies and Coltheart 2000: 8, Bentall et al. 2001: 1149, Bortolotti 2009: 47). Maher makes a claim of this kind in one place (Maher 1974: 104), but taking his body of work as a whole (including the 1974 paper), this does not appear to be his considered view. Rather, Maher is interested in *normality*, and he defends the claim that the cognitive activity of people with delusions is 'essentially indistinguishable' from that employed by people without delusions. He also talks of delusions being developed 'through the operation of *normal cognitive processes*' (Maher 1974: 103, my emphasis), which, of course, is home to a whole suite of irrationalities. It is fairly uncontroversial that delusions are irrational beliefs (although see Noordhof and Sullivan-Bissett 2021, Section 5.1 for a speculative challenge to this), and the above-mentioned features of their relationship to evidence and the phenomenon of double bookkeeping have been explored as part of an assessment of delusion's rationality (in e.g. Sakakibara 2016). But of course there's room for disagreement even here, in particular, with respect to whether the irrationality displayed by subjects with delusions is anything beyond the ordinary. It is answering this question in the negative which best captures Maher's position.

In their contribution (Chapter 14), Quinn Hiroshi Gibson and Adam Bradley consider how best to understand the irrationality of delusion. They begin with the claim that delusions are beliefs, and thus appropriate targets for rational evaluation. They consider the ways in which delusions fall short of epistemic and structural rationality, before turning to whether the irrationality of delusion is abnormal. Finally, they overview an account of delusion they have defended elsewhere, according to which delusional beliefs arise 'through the non-rational processes involved in figurative or metaphorical thought and language' (Bradley and Gibson 2023: 824) and 'serve an expressive function' (Bradley and Gibson 2023: 824, fn. 13). Gibson and Bradley argue that their view is apt to explain (better than endorsement and explanationist accounts, see Bongiorno and Parrott, Chapter 26) how it is that subjects with delusions fall short of rationality. Although they label their view an *expressivist* one (to capture how delusions *function* as figurative expressions of experience (Bradley and Gibson 2023: 825)), the target of their arguments is the nature of delusion itself (and the processes responsible for it), rather than a claim regarding what it is that we're up to when we talk about or ascribe delusion. In this sense then, their overall project is perfectly descriptivist.

In contrast to descriptivist projects, expressivist views about a given domain have it that 'although it looks like the domain is in the business of describing facts, it is actually doing something else' (Wilkinson 2020: 67). Expressivism in this sense has also been explored with respect to delusion. Sam Wilkinson has argued that when we look to at least some of the considerations appealed to in the service of moral expressivism (regarding parsimony, motivation, and disagreement), we find that they also apply to delusion ascription (Wilkinson 2020: 70–72). In his contribution (Chapter 15), Wilkinson explores what we're up to when we describe something as a delusion, beginning with the more orthodox descriptivist approach, according to which a delusion is something in the world that satisfies certain criteria, which successful ascription accurately detects. He moves on to discuss an alternative expressivist picture, according to which delusion attribution functions not to describe what the world is like, but rather to give expression to an evaluation.

Turning now to epistemological challenges raised by *introspection,* where we might think that beliefs based on it stand on firmer (perhaps the firmest) epistemic grounds than beliefs based on, for example, perception. As Chiara Caporuscio notes, there is a 'long philosophical tradition [which] attributes to introspection at least some epistemic privileges, including infallibility, omniscience, incorrigibility, indubitability, truth-sufficiency or self-warrant', and yet, on the other side, 'empiricists and philosophers alike have pointed out how we often cannot trust our judgments about the contents of our minds' (Caporuscio 2023: 166–167). Caporuscio argues for an account on which beliefs formed via introspection are susceptible to failure conditions similar to beliefs formed in other ways. If this is right, mistaken beliefs concerning one's internal life (e.g. Anton-Babinski which involves denial of vision loss) could arise from the same doxastic failures as mistaken beliefs about the external world (Caporuscio 2023: 181). Just then as we have delusions about the external world, (e.g. Capgras), so too could we have *introspective delusions* (a possibility explored in Caporuscio, Chapter 16).

We turn finally to an epistemological concept which is only recently gaining traction in debates around delusion: *epistemic injustice,* a term introduced by Miranda Fricker (2007) to pick out a particular kind of injustice related to how one is treated qua an epistemic agent. On Fricker's account, within this umbrella term are two types of epistemic injustice: *testimonial* (where someone is unjustly viewed as less epistemically credible than they are) (Fricker 2007: 28) and *hermeneutical* (where someone's understanding of their experience is inhibited due to structural issues leading to gaps in hermeneutical resources)(Fricker 2007: 155). The *injustice* of *epistemic injustice,* most obviously in the testimonial case, lies at least in part on the subject having their epistemic credibility underestimated. When we're thinking about epistemic injustice in the context of delusion, a natural thought is that in such cases, there is no injustice after all (people with delusions are *correctly* treated as poor epistemic agents). On the other hand, perhaps particular stereotypes that might be applied to people with delusions encourage unjust assessments of epistemic credibility (Sanati and Kyratsous 2015, and explored by Palafox-Harris, Chapter 17).

In this part of the Handbook, the chapters explore epistemological questions about the nature of delusion, how the exercise of certain epistemic abilities might give rise to delusion, and more broadly what we're up to when we ascribe delusions, and the possibility of epistemic injustice. We have seen that epistemological diagnoses of delusions regarding their relationship to evidence and the strength of their irrationality are not settled by appeal to observable epistemic behaviour. That is, one person's evidence engagement might be another person's evidence evasion (concerning phenomena like taking oneself to be an exception to a generalisation). One person's normal range irrationality might be another person's justification for positing abnormal irrationality or even non-rational processes at the root of delusion. The ways in which certain epistemic behaviours are likely interpreted may also play into our practices of delusion attribution, as well as contribute to a distinctive kind of injustice to which people with delusions may be especially vulnerable.

## 2.4  *Part IV: Delusion's place in the mind*

This part of the Handbook is devoted to how delusion fits into a general folk psychological theory of mind. As noted already, there is a live debate concerning the doxastic status of delusions, a topic which occurs in many of the chapters herein. One of the features of delusion that has played a role in this debate is its relationship to action (explored by Tumulty, Chapter 18). Now, it might be thought that the debate can only turn on the nature of belief, given agreement on the first-order facts regarding delusions' influence on behaviour. However, things are more complicated, since often the first-order facts here do not have the status of broad agreement. For example, whilst some folk will point to the motivational impotence of delusions as evidence against doxasticism (e.g. Hamilton 2006, Tumulty 2011: 612–613), others have described the idea that delusions are motivationally inert as 'a philosophical myth rather than a fact needing explanation' (Bortolotti 2009: 171), noting that plenty of work demonstrates clear correlations between delusional belief and behaviour, often violent (Bortolotti 2009: 164–167). With respect to erotomanic delusions for example, the *DSM-5* notes that 'efforts to contact the object of delusion are common' (DSM-5 2013: 91), and Flores has argued that understanding the delusion to be a belief can help explain particular behaviours (Flores 2021: 6302). Of course, not all delusions are so correlated, but all clinical delusions are at least *minimally* manifested in behaviour insofar as they are 'reported and diagnosed *as delusions* partially for the negative consequences that follow from the subject's conviction that the content of the delusion is true' (Bortolotti 2009: 163).

Furthermore, even when the first-order facts are agreed upon – perhaps we can agree that some delusions do not appear to be hooked up to action in the manner of belief – it is possible to nevertheless salvage doxasticism by appealing to defeaters or excusing conditions (see e.g. Bayne and Pacherie 2005: 184). The latter are understood as non-standard features of a situation. When an attitude fails to play an action-guiding role, we can ask whether that might be explained by appeal to non-standard features of the situation. In the case of delusion, subjects may recognise that if they were to act on their attitudes in the usual way, they could end up institutionalised (Bayne and Pacherie 2005: 185), or in any case, negatively judged by their peers. Maura Tumulty, working in a dispositionalist framework, has objected to this way of capturing delusions as beliefs. She argues that when it comes to *manifestation-failure* (i.e., a subject failing to manifest a disposition constitutive of her believing that *p*), we should distinguish between an *excuse* and an *explanation*. Knowing that one is likely to be involuntarily institutionalised if one acts on one's delusional belief is an example of an *excuse* – the belief may still be ascribed, but its dispositional profile is inhibited due to features of the context. However, other cases involve an *explanation* which understands the subject not as inhibiting a disposition, but as not having it in the first place. According to Tumulty, some of the other non-standard features of the delusional context to which Tim Bayne and Elisabeth Pacherie appeal (e.g. anomalous experiences) look better understood as *explanations* rather than *excuses*. In which case it is not by appeal to these non-standard features that we can explain why a subject with a delusion fails to manifest the dispositions relevant to that delusion, understood as a belief (Tumulty 2011: 602ff).

Let us turn now to various folk psychological states of mind to which the chapters in this part are devoted. The most obvious question we can ask in this context is which of the states of mind is the correct one for modelling delusion? Insofar as there is an orthodoxy regarding the attitudinal nature of delusion, we have seen that it has it that they are *beliefs* (this is represented in diagnostic definitions of delusions, as well as most discussions of delusions in philosophy and psychology). In philosophy, non-doxasticism, although the less popular approach, has its defenders, and comes in many varieties, for example, it has been argued that delusions are best understood as *imaginings* (Currie 2000, Gallagher 2009), *bimaginings* (Egan 2008), and *cognitive feelings* (Dub 2017). In his dual contribution, Paul Noordhof considers delusions as doxastic (Chapter 19), and non-doxastic (Chapter 20) (it is recommended to read these chapters as a pair). Across these chapters, Noordhof considers the case for each position in general (rather than with respect to particular types of delusion). He notes that successful resolution of the question requires a proper characterisation of the nature of belief, a task he discharges by considering several approaches (phenomenological, representationalist, normative, and functional), before bringing doxastic and non-doxastic arguments to bear against this careful background. In both chapters, Noordhof considers three arguments which have been used against doxasticism and in favour of non-doxasticism. These appeal to delusions having an inappropriate epistemic basis, delusions being poorly integrated, and delusions not playing the motivational role of belief. In his first chapter, drawing on earlier material on the nature of belief, as well as empirical evidence, Noordhof argues that the case against doxasticism from such quarters is weak. In the second chapter, he strengthens part of the case for non-doxasticism by considering recent doxasticist responses to the argument from inappropriate epistemic basis (Spinozan doxasticism and Flores (2021) on delusions as evidence-responsive). He then turns to critically evaluate several non-doxastic accounts grouped as those which include meta-cognitive states (i.e. delusion as an imagining mistaken as belief), those with hybrid first-orders states (i.e. bimagining, in-between believing), and those appealing to two levels of cognition (i.e. delusion as acceptance). He concludes with some recommendations for how a successful non-doxasticist position could be developed.

One non-doxastic alternative discussed in further detail in the Handbook is the view that delusions are imaginings. The nature of imagination is a bit more flexible than that of belief, and we can see this by comparing the two with respect to a couple of features. For example, belief is taken to hold a strong connection to truth or evidence, whilst imagination is not, either as a matter of psychological capacities (I *can* imagine something I know to be false) or as a matter of normative evaluation (all else equal, *I am not criticisable* for imagining false propositions, or for not revising an imagining in the light of evidence that that which is imagined is false). Imagination is also not connected to action in the manner of belief.[5] Imagination might strike one as an especially plausible non-doxastic attitude for modelling delusion since some of the features of delusion which suggest they are not beliefs are features which edge them into the scope of the imagination instead. In her contribution (Chapter 21), like Noordhof in the chapters before, Amy Kind takes a proper assessment of an account which models delusion on cognitive state $x$, to require as its starting point a proper consideration of the nature of $x$. Kind provides a characterisation of imagination against which she discusses the imagination model, clarifying its core commitments and considering versions offered by Gregory Currie (2000) and Shaun Gallagher (2009).

Aside from what cognitive states delusions *are*, another question that might be asked in this context is how delusions relate to other folk psychological mental states. For example, many authors have drawn comparisons between delusion and self-deception (not least Tim Bayne and Jordi Fernández in their 2009 edited volume *Delusion and Self-Deception*). Why the comparison? At the broadest level, beliefs arising from self-deception and delusion are both cases of 'belief that has gone wrong in some way' (Bayne and Fernández 2009: 2). Might we be more specific? At the very least, and before we do much theorising, we might think both kinds of belief are epistemically irrational,[6] insofar as they exhibit a poor relationship to evidence. This is, as we have discussed, definitional of delusion, but so too of self-deception. Although difficult to define in uncontroversial terms – one key feature of self-deceptive beliefs is that they are formed in the presence of information which would justify a different belief (Van Leeuwen 2007: 422). Another key feature helps us explain this – it is definitional of self-deception that it results in beliefs influenced by motivation or desire, most straightforwardly, the desire *that p is true* influences the formation of the belief that *p* (either as a result of intention, or as a result of cognitive biases which influence how the subject interacts with evidence). The etiology of delusion has also been claimed to involve motivation, at least in some cases. Such cases may include Reverse Othello Delusion (the belief that *one's partner is faithful*, see a famous case in Butler 2000), anosognosia, and perhaps others which contribute to increased self-esteem, e.g. erotomania and delusions of grandeur (Bortolotti and Mameli 2012: 208–209). Such cases might be considered ones of *extreme self-deception*. Of course, the influence of motivation on the formation of a delusional belief isn't sufficient for that belief to be an instance of self-deception. Davies has argued that for a delusional belief to count as self-deception, not only must there be motivational influences on its formation but must also involve a motivationally biased handling of evidence (Davies 2009: 84).

Many delusions might not look to involve anything obviously motivational in their formation, and so even those sympathetic to the idea that some delusions are cases of extreme self-deception, or at least, involve similar processes, will nonetheless recognise that more broadly, there are distinct phenomena here. And indeed, even in cases where delusions have motivational provenance, and strike us as similar to self-deception, there are nevertheless important differences that one should keep in sight relating to etiology, impact, normativity, and psychopathology (as discussed by Fernández, Chapter 22).

Let us turn to another folk psychological mental state: memory. Research on delusion and memory has primarily focused on confabulation. *Confabulations* or *confabulatory explanations* are explanations offered by subjects which are *ill-grounded*,[7] *provoked* (which is to say, offered as a response to a question), and *motivated* (where the subject is motivated to give an answer *at all* to avoid dumbfounding or is motivated to give an answer with a particular content). They are also hypothesised to *fill a gap* (either to 'cover gaps in memory' (Hirstein 2005: 32), or more broadly to help produce 'complete, coherent representations of the world' (Hirstein 2005: 30)), and are offered with no intention to deceive (confabulators are not liars). Sometimes the *filling a gap* component of confabulation is best understood as filling a gap *in memory*, and when memory *pathology* is in play, the confabulation may count as *delusional* (see Langdon and Bayne 2010 for discussion).

A less explored area of research in which delusion and memory intersect is the role of memory in delusion formation. We said earlier that some delusions are accompanied by anomalous experiences which may provide a source of evidence for the belief. What about *memories of* such experiences? Might they have a similar epistemic import? Fabrice Berna and colleagues investigated the phenomenological characteristics (specifically: vividness and emotions brought about from retrieval) of such memories. They found that in people with high delusional proneness and people diagnosed with schizophrenia with delusion, memories of delusion-like experiences were 'more vivid, more emotionally intense and considered more central to the self' than other memories (Berna et al. 2017: 38). This is important when we're thinking about delusional maintenance since these memories may contribute to a delusion being maintained by continuing to provide evidence speaking in favour of it (Berna et al. 2017: 40).

A more specific case of the role of memory and delusion formation is in duplication syndromes (e.g. Capgras), where such delusions have been explained by appeal to a deficit in memory updating. Such an idea can be traced back to R. Dennis Staton, Roger A. Brumback, and Helen Wilson (1982), whose case study patient had reduplicative paramnesia and Capgras symptoms. They suggested that in reduplicative paramnesia, the underlying functional impairment is a disconnection between past memory stories and new memory registration (Staton et al. 1982: 31). Although this view has had relatively little uptake in the contemporary literature, Sarah Robins and Si-Won Song argue that it is worthy of consideration, and explore and elaborate on the approach in their contribution (Chapter 23).

Turning now to delusions and dreaming, where perhaps the connection is less obvious. One way of seeing the relevance of one to the other is to consider *reality testing,* an ability that some have suggested is absent during episodes of dreaming. For example, Edward F. Pace-Schott has argued that in dreaming (and confabulation), the 'innate human tendency' that we have to create stories which organise reality (past, present, and future) is released from executive constraint, due to altered function of the pre-frontal cortex (Pace Schott 2013: 2). Impaired doxastic reality testing, that is, our ability to test beliefs formed on the basis of experience against background beliefs, has also been appealed to in the explanation of delusions (see Gerrans 2014 for discussion). We can also think about features of anomalous experiences involved in delusion, which look to have dream correlates. For example, Philip Gerrans (2012) has argued that feature binding anomalies in facial recognition occur in both the anomalous experience associated with delusions of misidentification (e.g. Capgras) and dreaming. There may also be neurological similarities, in particular, a neural substrate of dreaming has been identified in the default mode network (DMN) (Pace-Schott 2013) and the DMN has also been identified as playing a role in delusion formation (Gerrans 2014). We may then have found a neurological basis for both delusions and dreams (a view explored in Gerrans, Chapter 24).

The chapters in this part discuss delusion's place in the mind with reference to a range of mental states which find a home in *folk psychology.* This is the term given to 'denote our everyday way of understanding, or rationalising, intentional actions in mentalistic terms' (Hutto and Ravenscroft 2021). With respect to mental disorder more broadly, Pascal Boyer has argued that folk detection of mental disorder proceeds on the basis of intuitive principles which guide our understanding of the behaviour of others. He argues that folk intuition of mental disorder or dysfunction 'is triggered by observed (repeated, otherwise inexplicable) violations of tacit psychological expectations' (Boyer 2011: 113). In his contribution (Chapter 25) Murphy overviews the philosophical debate regarding the usefulness and accuracy of folk psychology, before turning to its relevance for delusion, exploring the application of Boyer's broader picture in this context. He suggests that such a picture does not accommodate our recognition of various ways ordinary belief formation is vulnerable to non-justifying causes (e.g. bias, loyalty). In expanding the remit of folk psychology beyond *rational* states, we can make sense of our willingness to accept such ways of forming beliefs. Delusions though are attributed when we have run out of road to explain why somebody believes what they profess to believe with the tools of folk psychology (see also Murphy 2012: 22).

When thinking about delusion's place in the mind, in particular, its place in the folk psychological landscape, there are broadly two questions one might ask. The first, and certainly the one which has captured the attention of philosophers, is which of these folk psychological attitudes is best placed to include delusion as one of its token instances? The scope of possible answers to this question has been relatively narrow, they are taken as either beliefs, or, less commonly, imaginings, among a small handful of other non-doxastic options. Our first question in this context doesn't require an exploration of the *breadth* of folk psychological options, although, as we have seen, it has called for significant theoretical *depth* with respect to a narrow range of those options. Another broad question we might ask in this context is how do delusions *relate to* various posits of folk psychology? Here we cast the net wider and consider whether the mechanisms underlying other folk psychological posits might also find a home in explaining delusion (dreams), or indeed, might suggest that delusions sometimes naturally fall under the remit of something else (self-deception). Dysfunction in other parts of the mind might also be appealed to in an explanation of particular kinds of delusion (memory). Taking a step back, we see that folk psychology is not married to a rational picture of the mind, it is a familiar fact that we fail to believe what we should believe, that we misremember, that we act against our better judgement, and we've conjured explanations for these failings which maintain interpretability (by appeal to bias, motivation, fatigue, inattention, and so on). Folk psychological explanations then are flexible, but whether they are sufficiently flexible to accommodate delusion, or whether delusion represents the limits of the interpretative system, is still up for grabs.

## 2.5  *Part V: Delusion formation*

In the penultimate part of the Handbook, we turn to the way in which delusions are formed and maintained. Theories of delusion formation have been primarily constructed in the context of *monothematic* delusion, and so the focus in this part mostly falls on such delusions. Empiricism has it that delusions are grounded in abnormal experiences.[8] In their contribution (Chapter 26), Federico Bongiorno and Matthew Parrott suggest that empiricism unites positions through a shared idea that sensory experiences are causally involved in the generation of delusion, but it is otherwise a natural home for a heterogeneous collection of positions. Given this, Bongiorno and Parrott identify three ways of understanding the role of sensory experience in the empiricist framework: as a source of justification, as a part of a causal mechanism, or as a source of meaning. In addition, they consider the rationalising role experience might be taken to play in delusion, such that the experience provides *reasons for the delusion*, or that the delusion *represents a rational response* to experience.

An alternative to empiricism is rationalism, which has it that anomalous experiences are downstream of delusions and play no role in generating them. John Campbell (2001) is probably the most recognised proponent of this view, arguing that delusions result from top-down organic malfunction which can subsequently affect experience. Part of the motivation for Campbell's view is the idea that the ascription of attitudes (including belief) requires that we take the subject to be (at least broadly) rational (Campbell 2001: 89). More important still, he argues, is the relationship between belief and meaning, with the latter being ascribed in a way that the subject comes out as broadly rational. The problem for empiricism, says Campbell, is that we cannot identify the content of a delusional belief in a way that satisfies this constraint – that is, we cannot capture the meaning of a delusional belief in a way that retains at least broad rationality for the subject with the belief (Campbell 2001: 91). On a rationalist approach on the other hand, delusions behave like Wittgenstein's *framework propositions,* understood as propositions which function as background assumptions required before we can do any testing of other propositions (Campbell 2001: 96). A change in beliefs expressing framework propositions (as a top-down result of organic malfunction) may well 'bring with it a change in the meanings of the terms used' (Campbell 2001: 98, see Bayne and Pacherie 2004, and Ohlhorst, Chapter 27 for further discussion).

Returning now to empiricism, within which there is a further question for those who take the anomalous experience to play a causal role in the formation of a delusion. This is the question of how many *factors* are taken to be required for delusion. According to the one-factor approach, the only factor to which we need to appeal in explaining delusion is anomalous experience (such a view can be found in Maher 1974, 1988, 1999, and has recently been defended by Sullivan-Bissett 2020, Noordhof and Sullivan-Bissett 2021, 2023, Sullivan-Bissett and Noordhof 2024). Two-factor views argue that in addition to anomalous experience, we need to appeal to a bias, deficit, or performance error in the mechanisms of belief formation or evaluation. Within empiricism, the two-factor approach certainly represents the current orthodoxy, and its appeal can be seen by looking to two questions we might ask about monothematic delusion (as noted by Davies and Coltheart, Chapter 29). The first is what prompted the delusion (understood as a question about the delusion's *content*), and the second is why was the delusion taken up (and maintained) in belief (rather than being rejected)? It is argued that the empiricist approach – by giving a role to anomalous experience – helps us articulate an answer to the first question, and on this one- and two-factor theorists are in agreement. The anomalous experience prompts the delusional idea. The second question gives us a way of getting a handle on the basis of the disagreement between one- and two-factor theorists, in particular, is a second factor needed in order to satisfactorily answer it? The one-factor theorist will say no – the adoption and maintenance of the delusional idea in belief can be explained in much the same way as we might explain the adoption and maintenance of other strange or irrational beliefs, that is, without positing a factor at the level of belief (see Sullivan-Bissett, Chapter 28). The two-factor theorist will say yes – answering the second question requires us to posit a second factor of this kind (for reasons for this, and details of the nature of the second factor, see Davies and Coltheart, Chapter 29).

The positions on delusion formation overviewed to this point endorse (at least implicitly) a distinction between perception and belief. An alternative framework for thinking about delusion formation comes from prediction error theories. Such theories have it that perceptual processing involves generating predictions about sensory input based on hypotheses about the world. To minimise the error of these predictions on the basis of comparison between them and sensory input, hypotheses are updated. One way of being a prediction-error theorist in this context is to have it that delusions result from a malfunctioning of this process. In his contribution, Philip Corlett (Chapter 30) overviews how the prediction error model of delusion has developed, and looks at current challenges, as well as how work in this area might go forward.

Another approach draws on a feature of at least some delusions: an *overattribution of salience,* first proposed by Shitij Kapur (2003) in the context of delusions in psychosis (explored by McKenna, Chapter 31). He proposed that inappropriate salience is assigned to external and internal stimuli due to an exaggerated release of dopamine (Kapur 2003: 15).

This leads to a 'novel and perplexing state marked by exaggerated importance of certain percepts and ideas' (Kapur 2003: 15). Delusions are then taken to be explanations of these experiences, which help the subject make sense of them.

The role of salience in delusion has also been appealed to by Coltheart in his discussions of erotomania. This delusion looks different from many other monothematic delusions in two ways. The first is that it looks not to involve neuropsychological impairment. And the second is that it doesn't involve anomalous experiences, rather, it is hypothesised that perfectly ordinary experiences are interpreted in such a way as to support the delusional belief. For example, in Sandeep's case, licence plates of purple cars in her area might be taken as messages of love (this case is roughly modelled on one reported by Jordan et al. 2006: 788). Salience has played the theoretical role of retaining continuity for erotomania with monothematic delusions. With respect to neuropsychological origins, Coltheart, following Corlett and colleagues (2006: 619), notes that these can be understood as involving 'altered salience of environmental stimuli arising from disturbed firing in the mesolimbic dopamine system' (Coltheart 2010: 24). With respect to anomalous experience, Coltheart suggests that erotomania might arise from an erroneous attribution of salience to events in experience (Coltheart 2010: 24–25). If these suggestions are right, we get continuity with other monothematic delusions. Salience then can help us understand the origin of delusions, perhaps in particular those that look, on the surface, to manifest slightly differently.

The final two chapters in this part turn from the broader picture of delusion formation, to particular features of it (inference, Laukaityte and Colombo, Chapter 32), or to ways we might usefully model it (hypnosis, Connors, Chapter 33). To the first, we find in the *DSM* a relationship between delusion and inference, where delusions are characterised as beliefs 'based on incorrect inference about external reality' (DSM-IV 2000: 765, DSM-5 2013: 819), and so one way into the topic is to think about why the inference is incorrect, that is, what is going wrong when people draw inferences that terminate in a delusional belief. One way of plugging the gap here has been by appeal to various candidate second factors, for example, the idea that people with delusions *jump to conclusions* or privilege certain kinds of evidence (i.e. perceptual) over minimising adjustments to one's beliefs. An incorrect inference is made, helped along by these biases. It might be thought, however, that the appeal to *inference* here (incorrect or otherwise) over-intellectualises the processes which move someone to a delusion, since the notion of inference that is commonly used requires propositional content, conscious deliberation, and epistemic standards of appraisal. In their chapter, Urte Laukaityte and Matteo Colombo interrogate what we might usefully mean by *inference* in this context. Drawing from the basal cognition research paradigm, they suggest that by adopting a more minimalist conception of inference, we can make progress in thinking about delusions (and possibly other psychiatric conditions) across multiple scales of organisation – from non-human cognitive systems and indeed perhaps through to human collective agents.

Turning now to hypnosis. Insofar as it is understood as a way of producing 'compelling alterations in belief' (Connors 2015: 27), hypnosis has been thought able to provide insight into delusions. For example, some studies have produced beliefs via hypnosis (*hypnotic delusion*) which share some surface features of delusion (strong conviction and resistance to challenge) (for an overview see Connors 2015). In his chapter (Chapter 33), Michael Connors overviews hypnotic delusions and how they have been used to model the processes involved in the formation of clinical delusions.

One of the more immediate questions one might have when introduced to delusions is *why? Why* does Fred believe that *his wife is an imposter? Why* does Alisha believe that

*MI6 are following her?* Delusions may strike us as so bizarre, implausible, or even (as some folk have been tempted to say) *unintelligible* that finding out how it is that they came to be might naturally be thought the theoretical priority. In this part, we have seen various approaches to this question, which, although they might agree on the raw materials present in many cases of delusion, they disagree on the explanatory priority of those materials, or even whether they play an explanatory role at all. In some cases, the disagreement plausibly arises from differing characterisations of what it is that needs explaining. If you think the irrationality displayed by subjects with delusions is within the normal range, then your approach to explaining their formation will not go beyond the explanatory resources used in other cases of ordinarily irrational belief. If, on the other hand, you take delusions to be beliefs which are sufficiently epistemically poor to evade ordinary explanation, you'll want in your explanatory toolbox a more robust cognitive ingredient. We see then that approaches discussed in this part must be tuned into wider discussions about the nature of delusion more generally.

### 2.6  Part VI: Responsibility, culture, and society

In the final part, authors look more broadly to the role of delusions in the moral and social sphere, and indeed the role played in their genesis by social and cultural factors. Although there is some disagreement about the role delusions play in action, there are at least some cases where delusions play a decisive role in the subject's actions, which can sometimes be violent, with dreadful consequences. We might ask: What implications does holding delusional beliefs have for one's moral responsibility? One answer is that the presence of delusional beliefs which lead to problematic actions directly absolves the subject of responsibility for those actions. Such a view though might be thought too crude, particularly in light of the popular idea that, at least in some respects, delusions are continuous with non-delusional beliefs. The presence of a delusion might help explain some action, but depending on the case, such beliefs may or may not do work of *justifying* or *excusing* that behaviour (Sullivan-Bissett et al. 2017). Mere delusion then, doesn't yet get us to a judgement regarding whether moral responsibility is diminished or absent – more is needed before we can make a judgement of this kind. In his contribution (Chapter 34), Matthé Scholten focuses on this issue, and discusses in which additional criteria must be fulfilled for someone to be absolved from responsibility when they act on their delusional beliefs.

The next two chapters of the Handbook can be seen, at least broadly, as contributing to what we might call a *social turn* in delusion research, which draws on social sources of evidence, cultural influences on delusion, and more generally resists approaches which zoom in on the individual. As Daniel Williams notes in his contribution (Chapter 35), although the social dimension of delusions has been taken key to their understanding before (he offers Freeman 2016 on paranoid delusions as an example) there is nevertheless a relatively recent research programme which aims to identify a role for the social in understanding delusion (a robust defence of such an approach forms the basis for Williams et al. *forthcoming*). Most broadly, those taking a social approach to delusion have it that such beliefs are better understood by appeal to disturbances in social cognition. This pivot to understanding delusions as, at least in part, a social phenomenon has been argued to provide an explanation for several features of them, including the fact that their contents are often socially themed (Gold and Gold 2014, Bell et al. 2021).

Taking their leave from research on the function of belief understood in social organisational terms (e.g. see Williams 2021), Vaughan Bell and colleagues argue that when modelling the causal roots of delusions, we should attend to the functioning of *coalitional cognition,* understood as the 'social cognitive processes involved in social influence, affiliation, interaction with groups, and the management of relationships' (Bell et al. 2021: 25). They give several examples of cases of 'mass delusion' where it is adaptive social processes that hold the key for an explanation of their formation, rather than impairments in an individual's rationality (Bell et al. 2021 26–27). Their positive view is that dysfunction in coalitional cognition can be appealed to in the explanation of delusion, both with respect to their resistance to social influence as well as with respect to their contents (Bell et al. 2021: 30). Williams explores precisely what is meant by claims like these, and identifies some possible issues. He also broadens what social theorists of delusion should take as their remit, arguing that the theories paying due attention to the social dimension of delusion need not limit their work to the positing of sociocognitive dysfunction.

One line of research which naturally falls into a framework of the above kind is work which looks to culture to understand why delusions have the contents that they do. Social themes have been identified as 'overwhelmingly the most common presentation' in delusion (Bell et al. 2021: 27). Most obviously this includes those delusions involving social actors (persecution, reference, erotomania), but as Bell and colleagues point out, some delusions which are not socially themed by definition, nevertheless have a social presentation. For example, a grandiose delusion might cast someone in a particular (elevated) position *relative to others,* and a delusion of alien control might posit control by *an external agent* (for more examples see Bell et al. 2021: 27–28). In their contribution (Chapter 36), Gold and Gold identify four features of delusion: the first is that they have social themes (as just noted). The remaining features are that they are sensitive to culture, they are often far-fetched, and they violate standards of belief. Gold and Gold elaborate on these features and suggest that a theory of delusion which pays due attention to them will need to be one which gives culture a central explanatory role.

Let us turn now to comparisons between delusions and other strange beliefs. We saw earlier (Section 2.4) that delusion had been compared to self-deception, and noted the shared features of irresponsiveness to evidence and motivational influence. The comparison here is to a class of beliefs with a particular genesis, but delusions have also been compared to beliefs with particular kinds of content. One comparison thought particularly instructive is conspiracy beliefs (e.g. Bortolotti et al. 2021, Pierre *forthcoming*). Both delusions and beliefs of this kind exhibit what can seem an extreme resistance to counterevidence. Indeed, conspiracy theorists' hasty dismissal of counterevidence has been described as 'arguably the most important feature of conspiracy theories' (McKenna 2017: 57) and, as already noted, it has been claimed that 'conspiracy beliefs are *as resistant* to counterevidence as clinical delusion' (Bortolotti 2023: 64, my emphasis). Persecutory delusions might be thought the most natural comparison point, with such beliefs and beliefs in conspiracies existing on what has been called a *spectrum of mistrust-related phenomena* (for discussion see Starcevic and Brakoulias 2021: 537–538). There are, of course, key differences, and even those who see the utility of the comparison are not in the business of denying those (for reviews see Bortolotti et al. 2021, Starcevic and Brakoulias 2021, Pierre *forthcoming*). Notwithstanding these differences, it is a useful project to look at delusions and conspiracy beliefs alongside one another, not least because such a project may illuminate the heterogeneity of these categories, where they intersect or overlap, and offer challenges to attempts to properly define them (see Pierre, Chapter 37).

We have already seen some concerns with existing definitions of delusions which appear in diagnostic criteria, and some comparisons to other kinds of belief (those arising from self-deception and conspiratorial ideation) which might suggest that features commonly attributed to delusion are shared and not ones on which we might delineate delusional belief. In the closing contribution of the Handbook, Richard Bentall (Chapter 38) suggests that in trying to identify what's unique about delusions, it is common for an *unrealistic comparator* to be called into service. Bentall sketches three features of belief which can help us better understand what is distinctive about delusions in particular: certainty, organisation, and transmissibility. It is especially the third feature with respect to which delusions stand out as different – they are almost always believed by a single person, do not arise from testimony, and do not get transmitted to others (the contrast with political and religious ideologies along this dimension is clear).

In the final part of the Handbook, we have seen the lens widen to place delusions into context, both with respect to society and culture and with respect to their implications for evaluating an agent's moral responsibility when acting on the basis of a delusional belief. Socially sanctioned strange beliefs are natural comparators to delusions – at least insofar as they have a wayward relationship to evidence and bizarre contents. But key differences remain (not least that such social sanctioning has implications for the rational status of such beliefs). The social world more generally might give us a better understanding of various dimensions of delusion, especially why they have the contents they do. But it can also help us understand the ways in which delusions are distinctive when compared with religious, political, or conspiracy beliefs.

## 3.   Concluding remarks

Although delusion is a topic in its own right within academic philosophy, a recent and welcome trend has been for interdisciplinary work in this area, with cross-discipline collaboration in publishing, as well as empirically informed philosophy, and philosophically rich work in psychology and cognitive science. My hope for this Handbook is that it properly represents this rich interdisciplinary landscape and that it serves as a useful compendium for researchers interested in such a wide-ranging and fascinating topic.

## Acknowledgements

I acknowledge the support of the Arts and Humanities Research Council (*Deluded by Experience,* grant no. AH/T013486/10). I am grateful to all the contributors for engaging with the introduction to ensure their accurate representation, and to Matteo Colombo, Jordi Fernández, Peter McKenna, Maura Tumulty, and Sam Wilkinson for their encouraging comments. Special thanks to Kengo Miyazono for several helpful comments on an earlier version.

## Notes

1 Omissions arise from various factors including space constraints and availability of authors to produce chapters on these topics. Here are some topics I would otherwise have liked to have included, with a recommendation for something interested readers might like to consult instead.

   *Delusion and emotion.* See Richard Dub's 'Delusions, Acceptances, and Cognitive Feelings' (2017).

*Delusion and pain.* See Jennifer Radden's 'Imagined and Delusional Pain' (2021), as well as accompanying four commentaries and Radden's replies.

*Delusion and Spinozan theories of belief.* See brief discussions in Chapters 26 and 29. A fuller treatment can be found in Federico Bongiorno's 'Spinozan Doxasticism about Delusions' (2022).

*Delusion and testimony.* See brief discussions in Chapters 32 and 35. For a more comprehensive treatment see Miyazono and Alessandro Salice (2021).

2 Capgras delusion is one of the most common examples discussed in the philosophical literature on delusion, but it is worth noting (in case its first place position in our list of examples suggests otherwise) that it is extremely rare, even in the psychiatric population (as noted by Hirstein and Ramachandran 1997: 437, see also Shah, Shailesh, and Wadhwa 2023 for recent discussion).

3 Of course, recent pressure exerted on this conception of delusion may also bring into question the utility of distinguishing delusion from overvalued ideas along these lines.

4 See here also for a history of the term before Kraepelin's (1920) use.

5 This is more controversial, with some philosophers arguing that imagination and belief share a motivational role, and so cannot be distinguished on such grounds (Velleman 2000, Ichino 2019). Of course, it might well be granted that imaginings can influence our action, but this power is restricted to certain contexts (Noordhof 2001: 253, 2024: 270–271, O'Brien 2005: 59, Glüer and Wikforss 2013: 143–145). Other will say that belief is the practical ground for imagining having an influence of this kind (Van Leeuwen 2009).

6 It has recently been argued that sometimes self-deception exhibits a greater irrationality than delusion (Noordhof and Sullivan-Bissett 2023).

7 And almost always false. However, it is safer to pick out the epistemic fault in a way that is less hostage to the target case being accidentally true. In the case of confabulation, subjects with Korsakoff's syndrome have given true confabulations (Hirstein 2005: 3), and we might also imagine a subject confabulating about his biographical information, happening to get it right (McKay and Kinsbourne 2010: 289).

8 Empiricism can be usefully seen as encompassing two kinds of view of the relationship between the anomalous experience and the content of the delusion. According to endorsement models, the content of the anomalous experience is *identical to* the content of the delusion (the delusion is an *endorsement of* the content of the experience). Explanationist models on the other hand have it that the content of the anomalous experience falls short of the delusion. Rather, the delusion *explains* the anomalous experience (Bayne and Pacherie 2004: 3).

# References


American Psychiatric Association 2000: *Diagnostic and Statistical Manual of Mental Disorders: DSM-IV-TR*. Washington, DC: American Psychiatric Association.

American Psychiatric Association 2013: *Diagnostic and Statistical Manual of Mental Disorders. DSM-5*. Washington, DC: American Psychiatric Association. Antonovsky, Aaron 1987: *Unravelling the Mystery of Health*. San Francisco: Jossey-Bass.

Arciniegas, David B. 2015: 'Psychosis'. *Continuum*. Vol. 21, no. 3, pp. 715–736.

Barton, Rachel, Aouad, Phillip, Hay, Phillipa, Buckett, Geoffrey, Russell, Janice, Sheridan, Margaret, Brakoulias, Vlasios, and Touyz, Stephen 2022: 'Distinguishing Delusional Beliefs from Overvalued Ideas in Anorexia Nervosa: An Exploratory Pilot Study'. *Journal of Eating Disorders*. Vol. 10, no. 85, pp. 1–10.

Bayne, Tim and Fernández, Jordi 2009 (eds.) *Delusion and Self-Deception*. Psychology Press.

Bayne, Tim and Pacherie, Elisabeth 2005: 'In Defence of the Doxastic Conception of Delusion'. *Mind & Language*. Vol. 20, no. 2, pp. 163–188.

Bayne, Tim and Pacherie, Elisabeth 2004: 'Bottom-Up or Top-Down: Campbell's Rationalist Account of Monothematic Delusions'. *Philosophy, Psychiatry, and Psychology*. Vol. 11, no. 1, pp. 1–11.

Bell, Vaughan, Raihani, Nichola, and Wilkinson, Sam 2021: 'Derationalizing Delusions'. *Clinical Psychological Science*. Vol. 9, no. 1, pp. 24–37.

Bentall, Richard P., Corcoran, Rhiannon, Howard, Robert, Blackwood, Nigel, and Kinderman, Peter 2001: 'Persecutory Delusions: A Review and Theoretical Integration'. *Clinical Psychology Review*. Vol. 21, no. 8, pp. 1143–1192.

Bergstein, Moshe, Weizman, Abraham, and Solomon, Zehava 2008: 'Sense of Coherence Among Delusional Patients: Prediction of Remission and Risk of Relapse'. *Comprehensive Psychiatry*. Vol. 49, pp. 288–296.

Berna, Fabrice, Evrard, Renaud, Coutelle, Romain, Kobayashi, Hiroshi, Laprévote, Vincent, and Danion, Jean-Marie 2017: 'Characteristics of Memories of Delusion-like Experiences within the Psychosis Continuum: Pilot Studies Providing New Insight on the Relationship between Self and Delusion'. *Journal of Behavior Theory and Experimental Psychiatry*. Vol. 56, pp. 33–41.

Bongiorno, Federico 2022: 'Spinozan Doxasticism about Delusions'. *Pacific Philosophical Quarterly*. Vol. 103, no. 4, pp. 720–752.

Bortolotti, Lisa 2009: *Delusions and Other Irrational Beliefs*. Oxford: Oxford University Press.

Bortolotti, Lisa 2015a: 'Epistemic Benefits of Elaborated and Systematized Delusions in Schizophrenia'. *British Journal for the Philosophy of Science*. Vol. 67, no. 3, pp. 879–900.

Bortolotti, Lisa 2015b: 'The Epistemic Innocence of Motivated Delusions'. *Consciousness and Cognition*. Vol. 33, pp. 490–499.

Bortolotti, Lisa 2018: 'Delusion'. *The Stanford Encyclopedia of Philosophy*. Zalta, Edward (ed.) https://plato.stanford.edu/archives/sum2022/entries/delusion/

Bortolotti, Lisa 2020: *The Epistemic Innocence of Irrational Beliefs*. Oxford: Oxford University Press.

Bortolotti, Lisa 2022: 'Are Delusions Pathological Beliefs'? *Asian Journal of Philosophy*. Vol. 1, article no. 31, pp. 1–10.

Bortolotti, Lisa 2023: *Why Delusions Matter*. London: Bloomsbury.

Bortolotti, Lisa, Ichino, Anna, and Mameli, Matteo 2021: 'Conspiracy Theories and Delusions'. *Italian Journal of Cognitive Science*. Vol. VIII, no. 2, pp. 183–200.

Bortolotti, Lisa and Mameli, Matteo 2012: 'Self-Deception, Delusion and the Boundaries of Folk Psychology'. *Humanamentre*. Vol. 20, pp. 203–221.

Boyd, Richard 1991: 'Realism, Anti-Foundationalism and the Enthusiasm for Natural Kinds'. *Philosophical Studies*. Vol. 61, pp. 127–148.

Boyer, Pascal 2011: 'Intuitive Expectations and the Detection of Mental Disorder: A Cognitive Background to Folk-Psychiatries'. *Philosophical Psychology*. Vol. 24, no. 1, pp. 85–118.

Bradley, Adam and Gibson, Quinn Hiroshi 2023: 'Monothematic Delusions and the Limits of Rationality'. *British Journal for the Philosophy of Science*. Vol. 74, no. 3, pp. 811–835.

Butler, P V. 2000: Reverse Othello Syndrome Subsequent to Traumatic Brain Injury'. *Psychiatry: Interpersonal and Biological Processes*. Vol. 63, no. 1, pp. 85–92.

Campbell, John 2001: 'Rationality, Meaning, and the Analysis of Delusion'. *Philosophy, Psychiatry & Psychology*. Vol. 8, pp. 89–100.

Caporuscio, Chiara 2023: 'Introspection and Belief: Failures of Introspective Belief Formation'. *Review of Philosophy and Psychology*. Vol. 14, pp. 165–184.

Casanova, Manuel F. 2010: 'The Pathology of Paraphrenia'. *Current Psychiatry Reports*. Vo. 12, pp. 196–201.

Coltheart, Max 2010: 'The Neuropsychology of Delusions'. *Annals of the New York Academy of Sciences*. Vol. 1191, pp. 16–26.

Coltheart, Max and Davies, Martin 2021: 'Failure of Hypothesis Evaluation as a Factor in Delusional Belief'. *Cognitive Neuropsychiatry*. Vol. 26, no. 4, pp. 213–260.

Coltheart, Max, Landon, Robyn, and McKay, Ryan 2007: 'Schizophrenia and Monothematic Delusions'. *Schizophrenia Bulletin*. Vol. 33, pp. 642–647.

Coltheart, Max, Langdon, Robyn, and McKay, Ryan 2011: 'Delusional Belief'. *Annual Review of Psychology*. Vol. 62, pp. 271–298.

Connors, Michael 2015: 'Hypnosis and Belief: A Review of Hypnotic Delusions'. *Consciousness and Cognition*. Vol. 36, pp. 27–43.

Corlett, Philip R., Honey, Garry D., Aitken, Michael R. F., Dickingson, Anthony, Shanks, David R., Absalon, Anthony R., Lee, Michael, Pomarol-Clotet, Edith, Murray, Graham K., McKenna, Peter J., Robbins, Trevor W., Bullmore, Edward T. and Fletcher, Paul C. 2006: 'Frontal Responses During Learning Predict Vulnerability to the Psychotogenic Effects of Ketamine: Linking Cognition, Brain Activity, and Psychosis'. *Archives of General Psychiatry*. Vol. 63, pp. 611–621.

Currie, Gregory 2000: 'Imagination, Hallucination and Delusion'. *Mind and Language*. Vol. 15, pp. 168–183.

Davies, Martin 2009: 'Delusion and Motivationally Biased Belief. Self-Deception in the Two-Factor Framework'. In Bayne, Tim and Fernández, Jordi (eds.) *Delusion and Self-Deception*. Psychology Press, pp. 71–86.

Davies, Martin and Coltheart, Max 2000: 'Introduction: Pathologies of Belief'. *Mind and Language*. Vol. 15, no. 1, pp. 1–46.

Davies, Martin, Coltheart, Max, Langdon, Robyn, and Breen, Nora 2001: 'Monothematic Delusions: Towards a Two-Factor Account'. *Philosophy, Psychiatry, &Psychology*. Vol. 8, no. 2/3, pp. 133–158.

Dub, Richard 2017: 'Delusions, Acceptances, and Cognitive Feelings'. *Philosophy and Phenomenological Research*. Vol. 94, no. 1, pp. 27–60.

Egan, Andy 2008: 'Imagination, Delusion, and Self-deception'. In Bayne, Tim and Fernández, Jordi (eds.) *Delusion and Self-deception: Affective and Motivational Influences on Belief Formation*. New York: Psychology Press, pp. 263–280.

Flores, Carolina 2021: 'Delusional Evidence-responsiveness'. *Synthese*. Vol. 199, no. 3–4, pp. 6299–330.

Foa, Edna B. 1979: 'Failure in Treating Obsessive-Compulsives'. *Behaviour Research and Therapy*. Vol. 17, no. 3, pp. 169–176.

Freeman, Daniel 2016: 'Persecutory Delusions: A Cognitive Perspective on Understanding and Treatment'. *The Lancet Psychiatry*. Vol. 3, no. 7, pp. 685–692.

Fricker, Miranda 2007: *Epistemic Injustice: Power and the Ethics of Knowing*. Oxford: Oxford University Press.

Gallagher, Shaun 2009: 'Delusional Realities'. In Bortolotti, Lisa and Broome, Matthew (eds.) *Psychiatry and Cognitive Neuroscience*. Oxford: Oxford University Press, pp. 245–266.

Gerrans, Philip 2012: 'Dream Experience and a Revisionist Account of Delusions'. *Consciousness and Cognition*. Vol. 21, pp. 217–227.

Gerrans, Philip 2014: 'Pathologies of Hyperfamiliarity in Dreams, Delusions and Déjà Vu'. *Frontiers in Psychology*. Vol. 5, article 97, pp. 1–10.

Gipps, Richard and Clarke, Simon *forthcoming*: 'Religious Delusion or Religious Belief?' *Philosophical Psychology*. doi. 10.1080/09515089.2024.2302519

Glüer, Kathrin and Wikforss, Åsa 2013: 'Aiming at Truth: On the Role of Belief'. *Teorema*. Vol. 42, no. 3, pp. 137–162.

Gold, Joel and Gold, Ian 2014: *Suspicious Minds: How Culture Shapes Madness*. New York: Free Press.

Hamilton, Andy 2006: 'Against the Belief Model of Delusion'. In Chung, Man Cheung, Fulford, Bill, and Graham, George (eds.) *Reconceiving Schizophrenia*. Oxford: Oxford University Press, pp. 217–234.

Hirstein, William 2005: *Brain Fiction: Self-deception and the Riddle of Confabulation*. MIT Press.

Hirstein, William and Ramachandran, V. S. 1997: 'Capgras Syndrome: A Novel Probe for Understanding the Neural Representation of the Identity and Familiarity of Persons'. *Proceedings: Biological Sciences*. Vol. 264, no. 1380, pp. 437–444.

Howard, Robert and Rabins, Peter 1997: 'Late Paraphrenia Revisited'. *The British Journal of Psychiatry*. Vol. 171, no. 5, pp. 406–408.

Hutto, Daniel and Ravenscroft, Ian 2021: 'Folk Psychology as a Theory'. In Zalta, Edward N. (ed.) *The Stanford Encyclopedia of Philosophy*. (Fall 2021 Edition) https://plato.stanford.edu/archives/fall2021/entries/folkpsych-theory/

Ichino, Anna 2019: 'Imagination and Belief in Action'. *Philosophia*. Vol. 47, no. 5, pp. 1517–1534.

Ichino, Anna 2024: 'Religious Imaginings'. In Sullivan-Bissett, Ema (ed.) *Belief, Imagination, and Delusion*. Oxford: Oxford University Press, pp. 81–106.

Jordan, Harold W., Lockert, Edna W., Johnson-Warren, Marjorie, Cabell, Courtney, Cooke, Tiffany, Greer, William, and Howe, Gary 2006: 'Erotomania Revisited: Thirty-Four Years Later'. *Journal of the National Medical Association*. Vol. 98, no. 5, pp. 787–793.

Kapur, Shitij 2003: 'Psychosis as a State of Aberrant Salience: A Framework for Linking Biology, Phenomenology, and Pharmacology in Schizophrenia'. *American Journal of Psychiatry*. Vol. 160, no. 1, pp. 13–23.

Kind, Amy 2024: 'Contrast or Continuum? The Case of Belief and Imagination'. In Sullivan-Bissett, Ema (ed.) *Belief, Imagination, and Delusion*. Oxford: Oxford University Press, pp. 42–59.

Kozak, Michael J and Foa, Edna B 1994: 'Obsessions, Overvalued Ideas, and Delusions in Obsessive-Compulsive Disorder'. *Behaviour Research and Therapy*. Vol. 32, no. 3, pp. 343–353.

Kraepelin, Emil 1920: 'Die Erscheinungsformen des Irreseins'. *Zeitschrift für Gesammte Neurologie und Psychiatrie*. Vol. 62, pp. 1–29.

Lancellotta, Eugenia 2022: 'Is the Biological Adaptiveness of Delusions Doomed?' *Review of Philosophy and Psychology*. Vol. 13, no. 1, pp. 47–63.

Langdon, Robyn and Bayne, Tim 2010: 'Delusion and Confabulation: Mistakes of Perceiving, Remembering and Believing'. *Cognitive Neuropsychiatry*. Vol. 15, no. 1–3, pp. 319–345.

Maher, Brendan 1974: 'Delusional Thinking and Perceptual Disorder'. *Journal of Individual Psychology*. Vol. 30, no. 1, pp. 98–113.

Maher, Brendan 1988: 'Anomalous Experience and Delusional Thinking: The Logic of Explanations.' In Oltmanns, T. and Maher, B. (eds.) *Delusional Beliefs*. John Wiley and Sons.

Maher, Brendan 1999: 'Anomalous Experience in Everyday Life: Its Significance for Psychopathology'. *The Monist*. Vol. 82, no. 4, pp. 547–570.

McKay, Ryan and Kinsbourne, Marcel 2010: 'Confabulation, Delusion, and Anosognosia: Motivational Factors and False Claims'. *Cognitive Neuropsychiatry*. Vol. 50, nos. 1–3, pp. 288–318.

McKenna, Peter 2017: *Delusions: Understanding the Un-understandable*. Cambridge: Cambridge University Press.

Miyazono, Kengo 2015: 'Delusions as Harmful Malfunctioning Beliefs'. *Consciousness and Cognition*. Vol. 33, pp. 561–573.

Miyazono, Kengo 2019: *Delusions and Beliefs*. Oxon: Routledge.

Miyazono, Kengo and Salice, Alessandro 2021: 'Social Epistemological Conception of Delusion'. *Synthese*. Vol. 199, pp. 1831–1851.

Murphy, Dominic 2012: 'The Folk Epistemology of Delusions'. *Neuroethics*. Vol. 5, pp. 19–22.

Murphy, Dominic 2013: 'Delusions, Modernist Epistemology and Irrational Belief'. *Mind & Language*. Vol. 28, no. 1, pp. 113–124.

Noordhof, Paul 2001: 'Believe What You Want'. *Proceedings of the Aristotelian Society*, Vol. 101, no. 1, pp. 247–265.

Noordhof, Paul 2024: 'Irrationality and the Failures of Consciousness'. In Sullivan-Bissett, Ema (ed.) *Belief, Imagination, and Delusion*. Oxford: Oxford University Press, pp. 266–304.

Noordhof, Paul and Sullivan-Bissett, Ema 2021: 'The Clinical Significance of Anomalous Experience in the Explanation of Monothematic Delusion'. *Synthese*. Vol. 199, pp. 10277–10309.

Noordhof, Paul and Sullivan-Bissett, Ema 2023: 'The Everyday Irrationality of Monothematic Delusion'. In Henne, Paul and Murray, Sam (eds.) Advances in Experimental Philosophy of Action. London: Bloomsbury, pp. 87–111.

O'Brien, Lucy 2005: 'Imagination and the Motivational View of Belief'. *Analysis*. Vol. 65, no. 1, pp. 55–62.

O'Dwyer, Anne-Marie and Marks, Isaac 2000: 'Obsessive-compulsive Disorder and Delusions Revisited'. *British Journal of Psychiatry*. Vol. 176, no. 3, pp. 281–284.

Pace-Schott, Edward F. 2013: 'Dreaming as a Story-telling Instinct'. *Frontiers in Psychology*. Vol. 4, article 159, pp. 1–4.

Petrolini, Valentina 2017: 'What Makes Delusions Pathological?' *Philosophical Psychology*. Voll. 30, no. 4, pp. 1–22.

Pierre, Joseph *forthcoming*: 'Conspiracy Theory Belief: A Sane Response to an Insane World?'. *The Review of Philosophy and Psychology*. doi: 10.1007/s13164-023-00716-7

Porcher, José Eduardo 2019: 'Double Bookkeeping and Doxasticism about Delusion'. *Philosophy, Psychiatry, and Psychology*. Vol. 26, no. 2, pp. 111–119.

Radden, Jennifer 2021: 'Imagined and Delusional Pain'. *Revista Internazionale di Filosofia e Psicologia*. Vol. 12, no. 2, pp. 151–166.

Ravindran, Arun V., Yatham, Lakshmi, N. and Munro, Alistair 1998: 'Paraphrenia Redefined'. *The Canadian Journal of Psychiatry*. Vol. 44, no. 2, pp. 131–192.

Ritunnano, Rosa and Bortolotti, Lisa 2022: 'Do Delusions Have and Give Meaning?' *Phenomenology and the Cognitive Sciences*. Vol. 21, pp. 949–68.

Ritunnano, Rosa, Humpston, Clara, and Broome, Matthew R. 2022: 'Finding Order Within the Disorder: A Case Study Exploring the Meaningfulness of Delusions'. *BJPsych Bulletin*. Vol. 46, pp. 109–115.

Ritunnano, Rosa, Kleinman, Joshua, Oshadi, Daniella Whyte, Michail, Maria, Nelson, Barnaby, Humpston, Clara S. and Broome, Matthew R. 2022: 'Subjective Experience and Meaning of Delusions in Psychosis: A Systematic Review and Qualitative Evidence Synthesis'. *The Lancet Psychiatry*. Vol. 9, no. 6, pp. 458–476.

Ross, Robert M. and McKay, Ryan 2017: 'Why is Belief in God not a Delusion?' *Religion, Brain & Behavior*. Vol. 7, no. 4, pp. 316–319.

Sakakibara, Eisuke 2016: 'Irrationality and Pathology of Beliefs'. *Neuroethics*. Vol. 9, no. 2, pp. 147–157.

Salkovskis, Paul M. and Warwick, Hilary M. C. 1985: 'Cognitive Therapy of Obsessive-compulsive Disorder: Treating Treatment Failures'. *Behavioural Psychotherapy*. Vol. 13, pp. 243–255.

Samuels, Richard 2009: 'Delusions as a Natural Kind'. In Broome, Matthew and Bortolotti, Lisa (eds.) *Psychiatry as Cognitive Neuroscience: Philosophical Perspectives*. Oxford: Oxford University Press.

Sanati, Abdi and Kyratsous, Michalis 2015: 'Epistemic Injustice in Assessment of Delusions'. *Journal of Evaluation in Clinical Practice*. Vol. 21, no. 3, pp. 479–485.

Sass, Louis 1994: *The Paradoxes of Delusion: Wittgenstein, Schreber, and the Schizophrenic Mind*. New York: Cornell University Press.

Schaffner, Brian F. and Luks, Samantha 2018: 'Misinformation or Expressive Responding? What an Inauguration Crowd Can Tell Us About the Source of Political Misinformation in Surveys'. *Public Opinion Quarterly*. Vol. 82, no. 1, pp. 135–147.

Shah, Kaushal, Shailesh, B., and Wadhwa, Roopma [updated 29th May 2023]: 'Capgras Syndome'. *StatPearls*. Available from: https://www.ncbi.nlm.nih.gov/books/NBK570557/

Starcevic, Vladan and Brakoulias, Vlasios 2021: '"Things are Not What They Seem to Be": A Proposal for the Spectrum Approach to Conspiracy Beliefs'. *Australasian Psychiatry*. Vol. 29, pp. 535–539.

Staton, R. Dennis, Brumack, Roger A. and Wilson, Helen 1982: 'Reduplicative Paramnesia: A Disconnection Syndrome of Memory'. *Cortex*. Vol. 18, pp. 23–36.

Sullivan-Bissett, Ema 2018: 'Monothematic Delusion: A Case of Innocence from Experience'. *Philosophical Psychology*. Vol. 31, no. 6, pp. 920–947.

Sullivan-Bissett, Ema 2020: 'Unimpaired Abduction to Alien Abduction: Lessons on Delusion Formation'. *Philosophical Psychology*. Vol. 33, no. 5, pp. 679–704.

Sullivan-Bissett, Ema, Bortolotti, Lisa, Broome, Matthew, and Mameli, Matteo 2017: 'Moral and Legal Implications of the Continuity between Delusional and Non-delusional Beliefs'. In Keil, Geert, Keuck, Lara, and Hauswald, Rico (eds.) *Vagueness in Psychiatry*. Oxford: Oxford University Press, pp. 191–210.

Sullivan-Bissett, Ema and Noordhof, Paul 2024: 'Revisiting Maher's One-Factor Theory of Delusion, Again'. *Neuroethics*. Vol. 17, article no. 1, pp. 1–8.

Taylor, Henry 2020: 'Emotions, Concepts and the Indeterminacy of Natural Kinds'. *Synthese*. Vol. 197, pp. 2073–2093.

Tumulty, Maura 2011: 'Delusions and Dispositionalism About Belief'. *Mind & Language*. Vol. 26, no. 5, pp. 596–628.

Van Leeuwen, Neil 2007: 'The Product of Self-Deception'. *Erkenntnis*. Vol. 67, pp. 419–437.

Van Leeuwen, Neil 2009: 'The Motivational Role of Belief'. *Philosophical Papers*. Vol. 38, no. 2, pp. 219–246.

Van Leeuwen, Neil 2017: 'Do Religious Beliefs Respond to Evidence?' *Philosophical Explorations*. Vol. 20, pp. 52–72.

Velleman, J. David *The Possibility of Practical Reason*. Oxford: Oxford University Press.

Wilkinson, Sam 2020: 'Expressivism about Delusion Attribution'. *European Journal of Analytic Philosophy*. Vol. 16, no. 1, pp. 59–78.

Williams, Daniel 2021: 'Socially Adaptive Belief'. *Mind & Language*. Vol. 36, pp. 333–354.

Williams, Daniel, Wilkinson, Sam, and Miyazono, Kengo *forthcoming*: *The Social Roots of Delusions*. Oxford: Oxford University Press.

Young, Andrew W. and Leafhead, Kate M. 1996: 'Betwixt Life and Death: Case Studies of the Cotard Delusion'. In Halligan, Peter and Marshall, John C. (eds.) *Methods in madness: Case Studies in Cognitive Neuropsychiatry*. Hove: Psychology Press, pp. 147–171.

# PART 1

# The nature of delusion

# 1
# DELUSION AND PATHOLOGY

*Valentina Petrolini*

The burgeoning debate about delusions in philosophy and psychiatry has mostly revolved around three questions, summarized by Kengo Miyazono (2018) as follows. The *nature* question inquires about the kind of mental states we should take delusions to be – e.g., beliefs, imaginings, or something else entirely. The *etiology* question explores how delusions come about and the processes that underlie their formation, such as abnormal experiences or cognitive biases. Finally, the *pathology* question asks whether delusions are pathological states and how we can successfully distinguish them from healthy – or otherwise 'normal' – ones. As Miyazono emphasizes, these three questions have been discussed independently for quite some time. While epistemologists and philosophers of mind seemed mostly interested in the nature question – and specifically in establishing whether delusions *really* are beliefs – the etiology and the pathology questions were usually under the purview of philosophy of psychiatry, cognitive science, neuroscience, and clinical psychiatry. However, these three questions are conceptually linked in important ways. For instance, in order to determine what delusions are, it might be relevant to understand how they develop. Moreover, both the nature and the etiology of a mental state are likely to affect our understanding of whether that state should be understood as pathological.

In this chapter, I focus on one specific connection between *nature* and *pathology*, one that underscores a potential tension in the philosophical debate about delusions. Here's how the tension arises. One popular – and in my view convincing – answer to the nature question consists in regarding delusions as beliefs (doxasticism). Some versions of doxasticism – most notably the strand originally defended by Lisa Bortolotti (2010, 2012a) – also subscribe to the *Continuity Thesis*, that is, to the idea that delusions are importantly continuous with other irrational beliefs. Yet, most defenders of doxasticism also take delusions to be *pathological* beliefs (cf. Bortolotti 2022). A standard way to make good on the idea that delusions are pathological beliefs, as I illustrate in Section 1, is to appeal to their failing to live up to norms of rationality. I overview these ideas before arguing that the joint commitment to doxasticism and continuity makes it difficult to answer the pathology question satisfactorily. In a nutshell: if delusions are continuous with other beliefs, what makes them distinctively pathological? (Petrolini 2017; Miyazono 2018).

   DOI: 10.4324/9781003296386-3

Before moving forward, however, one clarification is in order. Although I assume so in this chapter, I do not take it for granted that the pathology question needs to be answered in the affirmative. In fact, one may very well deny that there is something distinctively pathological about delusions. In other words, a firm commitment to continuity may lead one to reconsider the very idea that delusions should be regarded as pathological. Recent developments of Bortolotti's work (Bortolotti 2022), as well as several other contributions, seem to go in this direction. Some researchers have defended the idea that delusions should be understood as epistemically innocent (Bortolotti 2015, 2016), as psychologically adaptive or meaningful (Lancellotta & Bortolotti 2019, 2020; Ritunnano & Bortolotti 2022, see Ritunnano & Littlemore, Chapter 2 for more on delusion and meaning, and Bortolotti & Murri, Chapter 3 for more on delusion and adaptiveness), and even as biologically adaptive at least in some circumstances (see Lancellotta 2022 for discussion). Although these lines of research are undoubtedly promising, in this chapter I flesh out an alternative. What I ultimately want to show is that we need not call into question the pathological import of delusions, even if we embrace some version of doxasticism and continuity.

My argument unfolds as follows. I start by rehearsing Bortolotti's early answer to the nature question (2010, 2012a): the upshot is a doxastic picture where delusions are in many important ways continuous with other beliefs. I then show that committing to a doxastic view *and* to some version of continuity creates the tension mentioned above, or at least makes it particularly difficult to offer a satisfactory answer to the pathology question. As a consequence, Bortolotti's later work (Bortolotti 2015, 2016; Lancellotta & Bortolotti 2019, 2020), as well as other contributions (McKay & Dennett 2009; Mishara & Corlett 2009; Fineberg & Corlett 2016), have moved towards exploring the epistemically innocent or adaptive nature of delusional beliefs. Yet, I argue that the joint commitment to doxasticism and continuity does not imply a rejection of the pathological nature of delusions. Rather, I outline a position that takes delusions to be beliefs *and* takes delusions to be pathological, without committing to them being *pathological beliefs*. On this view, the pathological import of delusions does not lie in their nature, but rather in their *functioning* – i.e., in how they work within a person's mental economy and how they interact with a person's global situation. This explains why we encounter beliefs whose features may be indistinguishable from delusional ones, which still fail to qualify as pathological in a clinical sense.

One key aspect of the account I propose is the following: no belief can qualify as pathological *in itself*, neither in virtue of its content nor in virtue of its quantitative features (e.g., intensity, frequency, duration). To further corroborate this position, I draw on some insights from psychoanalysis and pragmatism, and more specifically on Sigmund Freud's (Freud & Breuer 1895) and John Dewey's (1894, 1895) reflections on the pathology of emotions. These contributions substantiate the idea that mental states cannot qualify as pathological when taken in isolation. What makes a belief or an emotion pathological is rather the way in which they are embedded in a situation or context, or more precisely the way in which a whole person relates to a situation. These insights nicely complement recent contributions in the delusions debate (Bortolotti et al. 2016; Bortolotti 2022), which underscore the importance of beliefs being assessed in a context as well as the difficulty of determining the pathological import of beliefs in a vacuum. The account I offer yields some important consequences for these debates as well as for the classic questions on the nature and pathology of delusions.

In the next section, I first reconstruct Bortolotti's original argument in favor of a doxastic view of delusions, and then I show that the conclusions of her argument leave defenders of doxasticism in a difficult spot with respect to the pathology question.

## 1.  Delusions and other irrational beliefs

In *Delusions and Other Irrational Beliefs* (2010), Bortolotti convincingly argues that we cannot distinguish delusions from other irrational beliefs in virtue of their epistemic features. The argument hinges on two core claims. First, she offers reasons to reject the rationality constraint thesis (RCT) – initially formulated by Donald Davidson (2004) – that unduly ties together the criteria for belief ascription and the criteria for rationality. Second, she shows that delusions share their distinctive epistemic features – including their failure to live up to rational norms – with other paradigmatically irrational beliefs such as superstitions, religious beliefs, biases, and so on. This brings about the *Continuity Thesis* (CT), according to which all beliefs lie on a continuum of rationality, with delusions at the most irrational end of the spectrum.

Bortolotti rejects RCT by showing that belief ascription should not be constrained by whether a given belief is rational. To the contrary, a plethora of beliefs that we encounter in our everyday lives blatantly violate the canonical norms of rationality. For instance, people routinely hold sets of beliefs that are incompatible with one another, like the superstitious doctor who believes that a night of a full moon causes more accidents (Bortolotti 2010: 85). This is a common violation of the *procedural* rationality norm, which requires a certain degree of coherence or integration among beliefs. People are also often unresponsive – or at least insufficiently responsive – to contrary evidence. For instance, both racial prejudice and religious beliefs tend to be remarkably resistant to evidence pointing towards their falsehood (Bortolotti 2010: 149–153). These are violations of the *epistemic* rationality norm, which requires that beliefs are minimally responsive to supporting as well as disconfirmatory events. Finally, individuals often fail to appropriately connect their beliefs with their actions: politicians do not act according to their own policies, people fail to follow-up on their diet or workout plans, and do not wear masks or condoms although they believe it would prevent contagion. These are all violations of the *agential* rationality norm, according to which beliefs should be action-guiding – i.e., endorsing a belief should also imply displaying behaviors in accordance with such a belief. All these examples – along with many others – cannot but convince us that the violations of canonical norms of rationality 'are not the exception to the rule, but widespread and systematic' (Bortolotti 2010: 78). As a consequence, RCT seems to set too high of a bar, and subscribing to it would imply denying the status of belief to way too many convictions that people hold in their everyday life.

Where does this leave us with respect to delusions? Most clinical descriptions of delusions, including the *DSM-5-TR* (APA [American Psychiatric Association] 2022) characterization, appeal exactly to the sort of violations described above. Although delusions are usually described in terms of epistemic irrationality – e.g., as 'fixed beliefs that are not amenable to change in light of conflicting evidence' (APA 2022) – they also break procedural and agential norms. For instance, some delusional individuals hold mutually incoherent sets of beliefs – e.g., 'I am in Paris and Berlin at the same time'; 'I am dead although I can walk and talk'. Some also fail to perform actions that would naturally follow from endorsing their delusion, as when individuals claim that their spouse has been replaced by an impostor without taking any appropriate action such as calling the police or looking for the missing person (see Tumulty, Chapter 18 for more on delusion and action).

These examples show that delusions and ordinary beliefs share crucial epistemic features and often fail to meet the standards of canonical norms of rationality. An important step follows from this analysis: once we take a closer look, delusions and ordinary beliefs appear to be more similar than we previously thought. As a consequence, we might end up supporting some version of the CT: given that the line between delusions and (some) ordinary beliefs does not appear to be clear-cut, we should regard the difference between them as one of degree. As Bortolotti concludes: 'delusions appear typically irrational *to a greater extent* or irrational *across more dimensions* than non-delusional beliefs, but they are irrational *roughly in the same way*' (Bortolotti 2012b: 39, my emphasis, see Bradley and Gibson, Chapter 14 for more on delusion and rationality).

The upshot of Bortolotti's arguments may thus be summarized as follows:

a  Delusions are beliefs (rejection of RCT and endorsement of doxasticism);
b  Delusions resemble other irrational beliefs because they violate canonical norms of rationality in a similar way (endorsement of CT).

Although both arguments are ultimately successful, their combination ends up creating a tension between the questions on the nature and pathology of delusions.[1] If delusions cannot be distinguished from other irrational beliefs by their failure to live up to rational norms, what makes them pathological? This tension has been underscored in different ways in the literature (Petrolini 2017; Miyazono 2018), but a core insight remains. A specific answer to the nature question – i.e., delusions are beliefs – combined with an endorsement of CT, makes it particularly challenging to determine what makes delusions distinctively pathological. Bortolotti herself grants that the answer to the pathology question is far from straightforward. However, she feels confident about one thing. The pathological import of delusional beliefs surely does not lie in their *irrationality*, as they clearly share such a feature with everyday beliefs (Bortolotti 2010: 259). In the next section, I show that things are even more complicated for the doxasticist. If appealing to rationality is not going to help us distinguish between delusions and other beliefs, the appeal to other features pertaining to beliefs – e.g., their content, frequency, intensity – proves equally bound to failure. As a consequence, I conclude that no belief may qualify as pathological when considered in isolation.

## 2.  Doubling down on continuity: other features of beliefs

As discussed above, the joint commitment to doxasticism and continuity makes it difficult to pry apart delusions and other irrational beliefs. As Bortolotti argues, the appeal to *irrationality* is not going to yield a satisfactory answer, as both delusions and ordinary beliefs constantly violate the norms of procedural, evidential, and agential rationality. Yet, other features of delusions may help us to draw such a distinction. For instance, Bortolotti (2012a, 2012b) suggests we distinguish delusions from other beliefs as follows: 'Clinical delusions are typically irrational *to a greater extent* or irrational *across more dimensions* than non-delusional beliefs' (2012a: 39).

Yet, within a continuity view, what would it take for a belief to be irrational 'to a greater extent' and 'across more dimensions' with respect to another? One obvious candidate would be to look at the *content* of beliefs to assess where they stand along the mundane-bizarre dimension. Yet, as Bortolotti and others readily acknowledge (Bortolotti 2018; Gunn & Bortolotti 2018), delusions are often *less* puzzling in terms of content than other irrational beliefs. Believing that my partner is cheating on me (Othello syndrome) seems far more plausible than believing that a full moon is responsible for more accidents, or that my job interview went well because I wore my grandmother's necklace. Another option would be to formulate a *functional* criterion, according to which delusions are more detrimental to a person's overall functioning and wellbeing.

However, the past ten years of debates on delusions have contributed to amassing evidence against such a claim. Recent work has shown that delusions may be understood as being adaptive or beneficial in some sense (Fineberg & Corlett 2016; Lancellotta & Bortolotti 2019; Garson 2022; Ritunnano & Bortolotti 2022). At times, delusions may be seen as epistemically and psychologically beneficial because they perform a defensive function by preventing the person from adopting a more harmful set of beliefs (Bortolotti 2015, 2016; Bortolotti & Lancellotta 2020). The main example usually marshaled in support of this view is the case of an individual who develops reverse Othello syndrome – i.e., the belief that one's partner is faithful when they are not. In some cases, the endorsement of the delusional belief 'my partner still loves me' can be described as an adaptive response that helps the person cope with an unbearable situation – such as being abandoned by one's partner following a serious car accident – without falling prey to depression and anxiety (Bortolotti 2015: 4). This and other examples show that delusions are not always harmful and distressing (Bortolotti et al. 2016). Even paradigmatically distressing cases such as the Capgras delusion – i.e., coming to believe that your partner has been replaced by an impostor – are amenable to an adaptive explanation. Some psychodynamic accounts offer defensive explanations of Capgras (Capgras & Carette 1924; Bell 2003), and it is plausible to suppose that such a belief might arise as a response to challenging emotional circumstances. For instance, in a particularly difficult marital relationship, believing that the person in front of you is *not* your spouse may help to preserve a positive image of the actual spouse.

On the flip side, recent historical events have shown that non-clinical beliefs can be detrimental both to individuals and to society at large. In previous work, I speculated that some forms of superstition, as well as the endorsement of extreme forms of racism and sexism, may affect wellbeing to a significant degree and cause various degrees of social isolation (Petrolini 2017: 4). After a few years, the point ceased to be speculative, given the overwhelming evidence about the individual and social harm caused by the adherence to conspiracy theories (Cassam 2019), and the degree of self-isolation provided by epistemic bubbles (Nguyen 2020). It is now apparent that a range of beliefs that have been traditionally considered non-delusional – and that, in most cases, do not arise in the context of a psychiatric diagnosis – can cause significant harm at the individual, social, and political levels. A purely functional criterion, based on the degree of harm caused by a given belief, therefore fails to address the pathology question satisfactorily. Some delusional beliefs can be beneficial to the person – at least in some sense and temporarily – while some non-delusional beliefs can be harmful.

In her reply to critics (2012b), Bortolotti offers yet another suggestion to reconcile the commitment to continuity with a positive answer to the pathology question. She does so by attempting to pinpoint more precisely what it would mean for a delusional belief to be at the most irrational end of the spectrum: 'the degree of rationality tracks both *how much they deviate* from norms of rationality for beliefs and *how many norms* of rationality they deviate from' (2012b: 4, my emphasis). However, even this more specific answer fails to draw a meaningful boundary between pathological and non-pathological beliefs. In fact, several beliefs that are not ordinarily classified as pathological are nonetheless irrational to the greatest possible degree or across many dimensions. Religious beliefs are a paradigmatic example: maintaining that someone has resurrected from death, or that their body is *literally* present in a piece of bread (transubstantiation) seems at the same time practically impossible (procedural), unsupported by evidence (epistemic), and problematic to endorse in practice (agential). Religious beliefs are an interesting example also because they are difficult to distinguish from delusions by appealing to merely *quantitative* factors: both experiences tend to be intense, somewhat long lasting, and play a relevant role in a person's life (for more on delusion and religious belief, see Bentall, Chapter 38).[2]

Taking stock: Bortolotti's early suggestions about tackling the pathology question by appealing to other features of individual beliefs have miscarried. As I stress above, a true, mundane, and motivated belief may be delusional, whereas a false, bizarre, and potentially harmful belief may be non-delusional. Later work by Bortolotti and others (Bortolotti et al. 2016; Bortolotti 2022) seemingly agrees with such a conclusion, and advises caution when it comes to demarcating delusions from other irrational beliefs. In many cases, however, such caution translates into a doubling down with respect to continuity: 'there is more continuity than is commonly thought between experiences and beliefs that are classified as clinically significant, and those that characterize the non-clinical population' (Bortolotti et al. 2016: 48).

In what follows, I argue that we should resist a radical embracement of continuity, especially one that risks erasing the pathological nature of delusions. After all, many delusions *do* arise in the context of a psychiatric disorder, negatively affect a person's life, and are – at least generally speaking – harmful. In the next section, I take some preliminary steps towards developing an account that does justice to these facts. My starting point grants the conclusions reached by Bortolotti and colleagues with respect to the continuity between delusions and other irrational beliefs, as well as about the doxastic nature of delusions. Delusional beliefs may be continuous with non-delusional ones in terms of content, epistemic features (e.g., truth value, degree of irrationality), and quantitative features such as intensity or frequency. Yet, many delusions are also *pathological*, although they are not pathological *qua* beliefs. In the next section, I unpack this seemingly puzzling claim by exploring a more general question on what makes a mental state pathological. I do so primarily by drawing on insights from psychoanalysis and pragmatism about pathological emotions.

## 3.   What makes a *mental state* pathological?

Both Freud and Dewey – interestingly around the same time (Dewey 1894, 1895; Freud & Breuer 1895) – have struggled with a version of the pathology question surrounding emotions, and have reflected on the conditions under which an affective experience may qualify as pathological. Their answer may be generalized as follows: mental states cannot qualify as pathological *in themselves*, but rather become pathological in virtue of specific relations that unfold between an individual and their environment over time.[3]

Before delving deeper into their view, it is important to keep in mind that both Freud and Dewey subscribe to a Darwinian picture of emotions, according to which these experiences have an evolutionary purpose (Darwin 1872). In some cases, such a purpose may be immediately transparent (e.g., fear = flight), whereas in others it might be more difficult to discern (e.g., happiness = laughter). On their view, emotions are thus 'habits which, upon the whole, were evolved as useful' (Dewey 1894: 563) or 'actions which originally had a meaning and served a purpose' (Freud & Breuer 1895: 181). More specifically, Freud describes affective life as being characterized by the ebbs and flows of a particular sort of energy – 'a quota of affect' (Freud & Breuer 1895: 166) or 'sum of excitation' (Freud & Breuer 1895: 86) – that psychologists would nowadays discuss in terms of arousal or activation (Russell & Barrett 1999; Russell 2003). What matters for our current purposes is that this affective dimension interacts with an individual's environment in complex ways. As a result, some increases in energy – i.e., higher arousal states – are functional, whereas others are dysfunctional: this fine line separates an engaging conversation with a friend from a verbal dispute that ends in a fight (see Freud & Breuer 1895: 199 for a similar example involving coffee and alcohol). In functional cases, affective energy seems to 'rise uniformly' and at the service of a common goal, while in dysfunctional cases stimulation gives way to 'agitation' and affective energy ends up inhibiting one's relevant goals and actions. Dewey similarly discusses the example of a crowd watching a game: by observing the people and their movements, we can form a quite accurate picture of who is winning and losing. The winners' movements are characterized by 'frictionless lines of action, harmonized activity [...] postures are erect, lungs frequently expanded, movements quick, abrupt, and determined' (Dewey 1894: 557). By contrast, the losers' movements appear more disjointed and follow 'opposed lines of activity'; everyone's energy and attention are directed inwards, and people sit by themselves while they rethink the game, make hypothetical changes, recall blunders, and so on. To sum up: in the former group, activity appears to be unified towards a common goal, while in the latter the observer perceives a tension between the goal and its achievement.

These examples allow us to understand something crucial about emotions *qua* psychological states. First, emotions – and affective states more generally – are better described in terms of interactions between an individual and their environment. They are actions or movements that arise in response to stimuli and that interact with such stimuli in complex ways. Some responses are intrinsically teleological (e.g., throwing up after having ingested something toxic) while others may be only figuratively so – e.g., storming out of a room even if no immediate threat is present. Once we grant this point, it becomes easier to see how an affective state may qualify as disruptive – and in some cases, as pathological. In Dewey's view, an emotion becomes pathological when we witness a 'breakdown of teleological coordination' (1894: 560). In some cases, the actions connected to our increase (or decrease) of affective energy become not only useless – e.g., we storm out of a room although we are not in danger – but also harmful and counterproductive. The example developed by Dewey concerns a panic attack. A set of movements are elicited (e.g., breath accelerates, muscles become tense), but they are not working harmonically towards a goal (e.g., flight) and actually end up being inefficient or counterproductive to that very purpose: we end up being paralyzed by fear in a way that makes it impossible for us to accomplish the relevant goals at hand.[4] Obviously, in all these cases, there is nothing about the emotions or set of actions *in themselves* that allows us to determine their degree of harm or appropriateness. After all, we can definitely imagine a situation in which being paralyzed by fear turns out to be an adaptive response – e.g., if we are hiding from a predator. This is why the assessment of the *situation* becomes central.

Dewey offers yet another suggestion as to how affective states can become pathological. In his essays devoted to emotions (1894, 1895), he distinguishes three dimensions of emotion that usually coexist with one another: a *bodily* aspect (the Jamesian 'feeling' – e.g., breath, muscle activation), a *practical* aspect (a disposition or readiness to act in a certain way – e.g., to attack one's opponent when angry), and an *objective* aspect (an intentional, but also broadly situational character – i.e., an emotion is always "about" or "toward" something). According to some readings, these dimensions of emotion typically coexist in a relation of productive tension with one another, but a pathological situation ensues when one of them ends up 'colonizing' the others (Santarelli & Serrano Zamora 2020: 255). To illustrate the point, let us consider the panic attack described above. In this case, the bodily aspect of an emotion – arguably fear – colonizes the other two: fear becomes purely bodily, disconnected from action and deprived of a proper object. In cases of obsessions or phobias, the objective aspect prevails over the others, so that the object of the obsession becomes the gravitational center of one's intentional life, thereby corroding the appropriate connections with bodily and practical aspects. In cases of manipulation or antisocial behavior, we may witness a domination of the practical over the bodily and the objective: what matters is the course of action – i.e., what the relevant emotion can make us (or others) *do* – as opposed to its balance with bodily and objective components.

Let us now circle back to delusional beliefs to assess whether Freud's and Dewey's suggestions on emotions can be applied to the pathology question. One general take-home message concerns the very nature of emotions and beliefs: rather than mental states to be analyzed and understood in isolation, we should conceive of them as *relations between individuals and their environment*. As I propose elsewhere (Petrolini 2017), beliefs are intimately tied with the notion of relevance detection or salience. The way in which we experience something in our environment as relevant is bound to have a profound effect on the beliefs we form, as well as on their appropriateness in a given context. As several first-person accounts of delusions suggest (Reina 2009; Freeman et al., 2019), delusion formation is usually preceded by a more or less extended stretch of time where the person experiences subtle – albeit gradually more invasive – changes in relevance detection (Kapur 2003; Mishara 2010). In this phase of heightened awareness – at times described in terms of hypervigilance (Freeman et al., 2000; Ibanez-Casas et al., 2013) or perplexity (Humpston & Broome 2016) – specific experiences or ideas acquire more importance. People's faces may appear more threatening, seemingly unrelated objects and events may be seen as more meaningful, and other people's actions or words may be experienced as directed to oneself (see McKenna, Chapter 31 for more on delusion and salience). Similarly to emotions, beliefs are therefore better understood as complex relations between individuals and their environment.

This suggestion helps us bring the pathology question into sharper focus: what qualifies as pathological is hardly ever a belief taken in isolation, but rather the way in which such belief is embedded in a situation or context. For example, the belief: "I am being followed by the FBI" may – and perhaps should – qualify as delusional in many contexts, but Malcolm X and James Baldwin (among many others) were justified in believing that that was the case. Similarly, a religious belief such as: "This piece of bread is the body of Christ" may not qualify as pathological when it is embedded in an intersubjectively shared situation where it acquires a specific meaning – e.g., Catholic mass. However, the same belief showing up in a different context, such as a dinner with friends, may be rightfully regarded as more problematic. When it comes to tackling the pathology question, our perspective should move away from individual beliefs and turn to the whole person along with the situation in which they are embedded. As I already mentioned above, Bortolotti has recently reached a similar conclusion: "beliefs are not the right kind of thing to attract judgments about dysfunction and harmfulness out of context" (Bortolotti 2022: 31). She then advocates for a model of pathology that encompasses the person as a whole, and their capacity for agency in particular (Bolton & Gillett 2019). The discussion above allows us to expand such an approach and move towards a more complex picture that involves multiple dimensions of interaction between individual and environment besides agency.

More specific aspects of Freud's and Dewey's contributions may also be applied to the pathology question concerning delusions. For instance, the idea of "breakdown of teleological coordination" (Dewey 1894, but also Freud & Breuer 1895) helps us see that one hallmark of pathological beliefs would be their weakened or otherwise disrupted relation to their original purpose (Miyazono 2015, 2019, see also Miyazono, Chapter 4 for more on delusion and malfunction). If emotions arise as actions that are functional insofar as they contribute to accomplishing our goals, beliefs are similarly formed to track our relationship with evidence, reality, and ultimately other people. A "breakdown of teleological coordination", in the case of beliefs, may thus occur when a given belief ceases to play one or more of these roles. As in the case of the panic attack, the belief machinery is set in motion but fails to be working towards the goal of tracking the environment in a way that is sufficiently reliable and harmonious. In many cases – as it happens with pathological emotions – this generates individual harm or suffering and also makes it difficult for the delusional person to carry out their everyday activities as well as to relate to other people. Delusional beliefs become sealed off from other sources of evidence and are paradigmatically unresponsive to them. Following Santarelli and Serrano Zamora's suggestion, these difficulties may be additionally interpreted as a consequence of a "colonization" process of one belief – or a group of beliefs – over others. Some violations of the rational norms discussed above may be described precisely along these lines. For instance, delusional beliefs may fail to cohere with other beliefs because they acquire – be it gradually or suddenly – an exaggerated importance for the person, to the point that they act as "hinges" around which all the other beliefs revolve (Wittgenstein 1953; Rhodes & Gipps 2008, see Ohlhurst, Chapter 27 for more on delusions as hinge beliefs). Similarly, epistemic violations – i.e., the paradigmatic lack of responsiveness to evidence – may be seen as a consequence of the delusional beliefs developing a "colonizer" status, where all the pieces of evidence that would potentially contradict it get automatically discredited and discarded (but see Flores 2021 and Chapter 12 for a critical perspective).

These insights from pragmatism and psychoanalysis help us chart a more promising response to the pathology question. We can happily grant – following the doxasticist – that delusions are beliefs that may be more or less irrational, like many others. Yet, their pathological nature lies elsewhere, namely in their interaction with the person's specific situation and with other aspects of the person's psychological makeup, i.e., their other beliefs, affective experiences, goals, and so on. I conclude the chapter by illustrating some broader implications of this view for the debate on delusions.

## 4. Conclusion and implications

In this chapter, I focused on a specific tension between the nature and pathology of delusions. If we subscribe to doxasticism *and* to some version of continuity, we naturally come to see delusions as more or less continuous with other irrational beliefs. As a consequence, we may be tempted to discount or minimize their pathological status and to treat them on a par with beliefs that we regard as non-clinical – e.g., religious beliefs and conspiracy theories. I argue that we should resist such a temptation. In fact, the joint commitment to doxasticism and continuity need not imply an eliminativist answer to the pathology question. We may avoid such an answer by giving up on the idea that delusions are individual beliefs whose pathological status may be determined in isolation. By contrast, drawing on the pragmatist and psychoanalytic traditions, I suggest we see delusions as *beliefs embedded in a situation.* This shift allows us to tackle the pathology question more successfully, by taking the relationship between a person and their environment into account when assessing whether pathological elements are present. Notably, such an approach also more accurately reflects clinical practice, where diagnostic processes take place over time and draw on a variety of sources such as in-depth interviews, behavioral observation, batteries of tests, and so on.

This proposal has some important consequences for the broader debate on delusions. First, it suggests that some irrational beliefs that are typically *not* regarded as delusional have the potential of crossing the threshold to pathology. This possibility is granted by the fact that a belief does not qualify as pathological in virtue of its epistemic or quantitative features (Section 2), but rather due to its relationship with a specific situation (Section 3). Consider the members of the Manson Family, who committed a series of murders in the late 1960s because they believed that an apocalyptic race war (known as Helter Skelter, from the Beatles song released in 1968) was upon them. Or consider the subset of participants in the Jan. 6 Capitol insurrection (2021) who subscribed to the QAnon conspiracy theory, according to which a global child sex trafficking ring had conspired against Donald Trump's re-election. These beliefs may not have arisen in the context of a psychiatric condition (at least not in all cases) but they should probably be characterized as delusional due to their interaction with the psychology and the environment of the people who subscribed to them. In both cases, a dramatic breakdown seems to have occurred at the level of relevance detection, so that these beliefs have become entrenched and sealed off from all sources of disconfirmatory evidence. They have also acquired a "colonizer status" with respect to other beliefs, as they have gradually become the gravitational center of cognition and action, to the point that people were willing to sacrifice their life – and other people's – in their name. It is exactly in virtue of these complex interactions with other beliefs and the overall situation that beliefs may qualify as pathological. By contrast, the features of beliefs themselves – their strangeness, intensity, and so on – do not have such power. With a bit of effort, we can imagine a scenario where the members of the Manson Family voiced their concerns about race within an open participatory dialogue, and where QAnon subscribers filed a petition to make sure that no irregularities took place during the 2020 Presidential Election.

Second, in virtue of the same reasoning, some beliefs that qualify as delusional in the context of a psychiatric diagnosis may not rise to pathological status. Consider the very examples discussed by the literature on the adaptiveness of delusions (Bortolotti 2015, 2016; Ritunnano & Bortolotti 2022), where delusional beliefs arise for defensive reasons and provide the person with epistemic and existential tools to navigate a difficult psychological condition. Once again, the assessment of pathology would hinge on the way in which the relevant belief interacts with other beliefs as well as with the person's overall context. In many cases, the endorsement of a delusional belief engenders some kind of trade-off: it provides the person with a short-term psychological benefit while proving detrimental in the long run. This might be the case of the person with reverse Othello syndrome who – thanks to the delusional belief – holds on to the idea of being loved and part of a meaningful relationship. In other cases, such as the ones recently discussed by Garson (2022), we should be open to the idea of delusions playing a more fundamental, meaning-making role that has the potential to support individuals while they attempt to cope with traumatic life circumstances.

To conclude, neither the pathological nor the adaptive nature of delusions can be established in a vacuum. More so than to the epistemic and quantitative features of beliefs, we should pay attention to the overall situation in which they are embedded as well as to the complex dynamics between them and other aspects of the person's psychological functioning. By doing so, we will probably find not only that many delusions are pathological for a reason but also that many exceptions exist. While some pathological beliefs may hide in plain sight, some delusions may turn out to be truly adaptive and beneficial.

## Notes

1  The rejection of either (a) or (b) would make it easier to argue that delusions are pathological. By rejecting (a), for instance, one might argue that delusions are pathological because they are illusions (Hohwy & Rajan 2012), imaginings (Currie 2000), or disturbances of lower-level processes (Gerrans 2014). By rejecting (b), one might rather endorse a categorical view that understands delusions as being qualitatively different from other beliefs. I won't discuss these possibilities any further in this chapter, as I am primarily interested in exploring the pathology question in the context of the endorsement of *both* (a) and (b).

2  According to some interpretations, the endorsement of religious beliefs is reinforced by the fact that a broader community of people also subscribes to them and keeps them alive through rituals and ceremonies to be performed according to specific rules and schedules (Freud 1907). Yet, the very fact that religious beliefs are intersubjectively shared sets them apart from delusions in an important sense. For instance, according to Dominic Murphy: 'Numbers matter with delusions. If only a tiny minority of humans were religious we might be more tempted to call them delusional [...] The fewer people believe in something, the less natural it seems' (Murphy 2006: 182). This idea also shows up in the *DSM-5* (APA 2013), which allows for exclusion clauses in case the allegedly delusional belief can be understood as part of the person's cultural repertoire.

3  In previous work, I argued that we should take a step forward from Bortolotti's argument on norms of rationality to offer an etiological account of what makes delusions pathological (Petrolini 2017). On that occasion, I proposed to turn to *emotions* to see delusions as arising from an affective dysfunction. If one subscribes to that view, it becomes even more apparent why Freud's and Dewey's insights on emotions can be successfully applied to beliefs – and hence to delusions. However, one need not be convinced by that argument to draw some interesting parallels between Freud and Dewey's work on emotions and the debate surrounding the pathological nature of delusional beliefs.

4  Freud and Breuer (1895) similarly distinguish between active (*sthenic*) and passive (*asthenic*) forms of affect. The former can be leveled out by actions directed towards *discharge*– e.g., shouting, jumping, and crying – while the latter cannot be directly discharged – e.g., anxiety and phobias. Although the notion of discharge latches onto an outdated view of psychological functioning – the so-called hydraulic model (Kitcher 1995) – it still tells us something important about emotions *qua* mental states. Some emotions simply 'run their course' and can be successfully directed towards one's goals and endeavors (e.g., we vent with a friend and move on with our life), while others tend to fester in the mind and body until they acquire a different form – e.g., they resurface as psychiatric symptoms.

## References

American Psychiatric Association [APA] (2013). Diagnostic and statistical manual of mental disorders: DSM-5. 5th ed. Washington, DC: American Psychiatric Association.

American Psychiatric Association [APA] (2022). *Diagnostic and Statistical Manual of Mental Disorders*: DSM-5-TR. 5th ed. revised, Washington, DC: American Psychiatric Association.

Bell, D. (2003). *Paranoia*. Cambridge: Icon.

Bolton, D., & Gillett, G. (2019). *The Biopsychosocial Model of Health and Disease: New Philosophical and Scientific Developments*. Cham: Springer Nature.

Bortolotti, L. (2022). "Are delusions pathological beliefs?". *Asian Journal of Philosophy* 1: 1–31.

Bortolotti, L. (2018). "Delusions and three myths of irrational belief". In L. Bortolotti (ed.) *Delusions in Context*. Cham: Palgrave MacMillan, pp. 97–116.

Bortolotti, L. (2016). "Epistemic benefits of elaborated and systematized delusions in schizophrenia". *The British Journal for the Philosophy of Science* 67(3): 879–900.

Bortolotti, L. (2015). "The epistemic innocence of motivated delusions". *Consciousness and Cognition* 33: 490–499.

Bortolotti, L. (2012b). "Reply to critics". *Neuroethics* 5(1): 39–53.

Bortolotti, L. (2012a). "Précis of delusions and other irrational beliefs". *Neuroethics* 5(1): 1–4.

Bortolotti, L. (2010). *Delusions and Other Irrational Beliefs*. Oxford: Oxford University Press.

Bortolotti, L., Gunn, R., & Sullivan-Bissett, E. (2016). "What makes a belief delusional?". In I. McCarthy, K. Sellevold & O. Smith (eds.) *Cognitive Confusions*. Cambridge: Cambridge University Press, pp. 37–51.

Capgras, J., & Carette, P. (1924). "Illusion de sosie et complexe d'Oedipe". *Annales Medico-Psychologiques* 82: 48–68.

Cassam, Q. (2019). *Conspiracy Theories*. Cambridge: Polity Press.

Currie, G. (2000). "Imagination, delusion and hallucinations". *Mind & Language* 15(1): 168–183.

Darwin, C. (1872). *The Expression of Emotions in Man and Animals*. London: John Murray.

Davidson, D. (2004). *Problems of Irrationality*. Oxford: Oxford University Press.

Dewey, J. (1895). "The theory of emotion". *Psychological Review* 2(1): 169–188.

Dewey, J. (1894). "The theory of emotion: I: emotional attitudes". *Psychological Review* 1(6): 553–569.

Fineberg, S. K., & Corlett, P. R. (2016). "The doxastic shear pin: delusions as errors of learning and memory". *Cognitive Neuropsychiatry* 21(1): 73–89.

Flores, C. (2021). "Delusional evidence-responsiveness". *Synthese* 199(3): 6299–6330.

Freeman, D., Garety, P., & Phillips, M. (2000). "An examination of hypervigilance for external threat in individuals with generalized anxiety disorder and individuals with persecutory delusions using visual scan paths". *The Quarterly Journal of Experimental Psychology Section A* 53(2): 549–567.

Freeman, D., Morrison, A., Bird, J. C., Chadwick, E., Bold, E., Taylor, K. M.,…, & Waite, F. (2019). "The weeks before 100 persecutory delusions: the presence of many potential contributory causal factors". *British Journal of Psychiatry Open* 5(5): 1–7.

Freud, S. (1907). "Obsessive actions and religious practices". In J. Strachey (ed. & trans.) *The Standard Edition of the Complete Psychological Works of Sigmund Freud*, Vol. 9: pp. 47–56 London: Hogarth.

Freud, S., & Breuer, J. (1895). "Studies on hysteria". In J. Strachey (ed. & trans.) *The Standard Edition of the Complete Psychological Works of Sigmund Freud*, Vol. 2: pp. 1–335. London: Hogarth.

Garson, J. (2022). *The Helpful Delusion*. Melbourne: AEON Psyche.

Gerrans, P. (2014). *The Measure of Madness. Philosophy of Mind, Cognitive Neuroscience and Delusional Thought*. Cambridge: MIT Press.

Gunn, R., & Bortolotti, L. (2018). "Can delusions play a protective role?". *Phenomenology and the Cognitive Sciences* 17(4): 813–833.

Hohwy, J., & Rajan, V. (2012). "Delusions as forensically disturbing perceptual inferences". *Neuroethics* 5: 5–11.

Humpston, C. S., & Broome, M. R. (2016). "Perplexity". In G. Stanghellini and M. Aragona (eds.) *An Experiential Approach to Psychopathology*. Cham: Springer, pp. 245–264.

Ibanez-Casas, I., De Portugal, E., Gonzalez, N., McKenney, K. A., Haro, J. M., Usall, J.,…, & Cervilla, J. A. (2013). "Deficits in executive and memory processes in delusional disorder: a case-control study". *PLoS One* 8(7): 1–8.

Kapur, S. (2003). "Psychosis as a state of aberrant salience: a framework for linking biology, phenomenology and pharmacology in schizophrenia". *American Journal of Psychiatry* 160(1): 13–23.

Kitcher, P. (1995). *Freud's Dream: A Complete Interdisciplinary Science of Mind*. Cambridge: MIT Press.

Lancellotta, E. (2022). "Is the biological adaptiveness of delusions doomed?". *Review of Philosophy and Psychology* 13(1): 47–63.

Lancellotta, E., & Bortolotti, L. (2020). "Delusions in the two-factor theory: pathological or adaptive?". *European Journal of Analytic Philosophy* 16(2): 37–57.

Lancellotta, E., & Bortolotti, L. (2019). "Are clinical delusions adaptive?" *Wiley Interdisciplinary Reviews: Cognitive Science* 10(5): 1–15.

McKay, R. T., & Dennett, D. C. (2009). "The evolution of misbelieve". *Behavioral and Brain Sciences* 32(6): 493–510.

Mishara, A. L. (2010). "Klaus Conrad (1905–1961): delusional mood, psychosis, and beginning schizophrenia". *Schizophrenia Bulletin* 36(1): 9–13.

Mishara, A. L., & Corlett, P. (2009). "Are delusions biologically adaptive? Salvaging the doxastic shear pin". *Behavioral and Brain Sciences* 32(6): 530–531.

Miyazono, K., & Mckay, R. (2019). Explaining delusional beliefs: A hybrid model. *Cognitive Neuropsychiatry*, 24(5): 335–346.

Miyazono, K. (2018). *Delusions and Beliefs: A Philosophical Inquiry*. London: Routledge.

Miyazono, K. (2015). "Delusions as harmful malfunctioning beliefs". *Consciousness and Cognition* 33: 561–573.

Murphy, D. (2006). *Psychiatry in the Scientific Image*. Cambridge: MIT Press.

Nguyen, C. T. (2020). "Echo chambers and epistemic bubbles". *Episteme* 17(2): 141–161.

Petrolini, V. (2017). "What makes delusions pathological?". *Philosophical Psychology* 30(4): 502–523.

Rhodes, J., & Gipps, R. G. (2008). "Delusions, certainty, and the background". *Philosophy, Psychiatry, & Psychology* 15(4): 295–310.

Ritunnano, R., & Bortolotti, L. (2022). "Do delusions have and give meaning?". *Phenomenology and the Cognitive Sciences* 21(4): 949–968.

Russell, J. A. (2003). "Core affect and the psychological construction of emotion". *Psychological Review* 110(1): 145–7172.

Russell, J. A., & Barrett, L. F. (1999). "Core affect, prototypical emotional episodes, and other things called emotion: dissecting the elephant". *Journal of Personality and Social Psychology* 76(5): 805–819.

Santarelli, M., & Serrano Zamora, J. (2020). "The affective side of political identities: pragmatism, populism, and European social theory". In M. Festl (ed.) *Pragmatism and Social Philosophy*. London: Routledge, pp. 248–264.

Wittgenstein, L. (1953). *On Certainty*. Oxford: Blackwell.

# 2
# DELUSION AND MEANING

*Rosa Ritunnano and Jeannette Littlemore*

What is it to speak of 'meaning' in relation to delusions? The study of meaning does not fall neatly within the boundaries of any single scholarly field. Across philosophy, psychology, linguistics, and psychiatry, we may use 'meaning' and 'meaningfulness' in a variety of senses, and for different purposes. Depending on the target of the enquiry—be it, for instance, life as a whole, a state of affairs, a mental state or linguistic expression—these different senses of 'meaning' give rise to different philosophical questions. With regard to life, we may ask: What is the meaning of life? Or, what makes life meaningful? With regard to a particular occurrence such as a traumatic life event, we may wonder: What significance does this have for me? Why me? Conversely, if we are referring to a linguistic expression, we may be concerned with a further sense of the word 'meaning' and we may ask what someone 'actually means', where 'they are coming from', what meaning they intended to articulate when they expressed something in that particular way (e.g., using a certain word, gesture, metaphor), and how the context of use shaped that meaning.

In the case of delusions, and partly due to their contested and multidimensional nature, all the above questions apply and more could be asked. We may be interested in knowing more about what makes a delusion meaningful in the context of someone's life but may also wonder where meaning comes from in a delusion. In addition, we may ask whether someone uttering a delusional expression means it literally or metaphorically. In this chapter, we briefly review some of the recent empirical and philosophical literature addressing the first question, concerned with the psychological *meaningfulness* of delusions. We then turn to phenomenological accounts of delusion formation, for a more in-depth exploration of felt experiencing as a *source of meaning* in delusions. Finally, the third and last section explores the contested issue of *metaphorical meanings* in delusional thinking and expression.

## 1.   What is it for a delusion to be 'meaningful'?

The idea that delusions are more than just 'false beliefs', that they have a meaning, or a function for the individual who holds them, is not new. A tradition that dates from the 1800s involves thinking about delusions as coping, or strategic mechanisms, and plausibly is found in Shakespeare (cf., Garson 2022: 127–144). Variations on the same idea are

DOI: 10.4324/9781003296386-4

found aplenty among psychoanalysts, beginning with Sigmund Freud, and including Frieda Fromm-Reichmann, Harry Stuck Sullivan, and Jacques Lacan among others. Within this tradition, the conception of madness as a strategic retreat from unconscious conflicts, or painful experiences, is most evident in the analysis of delusional phenomena—here viewed less as 'symptoms' of mental illness than efforts to repair.

However, the dominant conception of delusion in contemporary psychiatry is one that is best captured by the so-called *madness-as-dysfunction* paradigm—as formulated by Justin Garson (2022). This view, which has been present all along but has become predominant since psychiatry's operational revolution in the 1970s, carries a fundamental assumption: When someone has a symptom of mental illness, such as a delusion, there is a 'deficit' or a 'dysfunction' in that person's mind or brain which is responsible for delusional pathology (for more on delusion and pathology see Petrolini, Chapter 1, for more on delusion and malfunction see Miyazono, Chapter 4). Thus, much psychiatric research, at least in the past 50 years, has been engaged in the search for this putative cognitive dysfunction, with the idea that, once the dysfunction is corrected (via psychological or pharmacological means), then the delusion will be 'cured'. In parallel, much work in the area of philosophy of psychology and psychopathology has been devoted to clarifying the nature of those malfunctioning cognitive mechanisms, or factors, that can account for the pathological character of delusions (Corlett 2018; Langdon 2011; Miyazono 2015; Petrolini 2017; see also, Sullivan-Bissett, Chapter 28, and Davies & Coltheart, Chapter 29).

If we work strictly under the assumptions of *madness-as-dysfunction*, then speaking of 'meaning' in delusions may only conjure up the psychopathological expressions of delusion as a 'symptom' of severe mental illnesses such as schizophrenia and other psychoses. In this case, we would be left with a narrow and deficit-oriented conception of meaning as either something missing altogether from delusional phenomena (as in Berrios' 'empty speech acts' 1991) or as something broadly overlapping with the 'cause' of delusions, as in the mechanisms that are thought to explain their onset and maintenance (see chapters in Part 5 for further reading on delusion formation and maintenance).

When considering psychotic disorders, it is undeniable that clinical delusions are often associated with emotional distress, depression, and harm (Upthegrove 2018). But it is also true that, at certain times and within certain autobiographical and socio-cultural contexts, they can serve to enhance a person's sense of coherence, meaning and significance. A rapidly expanding body of literature, and supporting empirical evidence, can now be cited in support of this claim (Bergstein, Weizman, & Solomon 2008; Gunn & Bortolotti 2018; Gunn & Larkin 2020; Isham et al. 2022; Lancellotta & Bortolotti 2019; Ritunnano & Bortolotti 2022; Ritunnano et al. 2022; Roberts 1991).

Rachel Gunn and Lisa Bortolotti (2018) argue that even seemingly implausible beliefs can be made sense of in the context of the person's life and can play a protective role, albeit temporarily. Drawing on the findings of in-depth phenomenological interviews with people experiencing delusions in psychosis, they conclude that a psychological adaptive role can be ascribed to these phenomena: in times of upheaval, they protect the person from unbearable feelings of despair and powerlessness, which may otherwise potentially lead to depression and suicide. Similarly, the idea that delusions have and give meaning has been defended by Rosa Ritunnano and Bortolotti (2022). Integrating evidence from cognitive psychology and phenomenology, they argue that delusions are not only meaningful—in spite of the fact that they represent significant failures of rationality—but they can also enhance the sense that one's life is meaningful, supporting agency and creativity in some circumstances.

This echoes Glenn Roberts's view that delusion formation can be seen, at least initially, as an 'adaptive process of attributing meaning to experience through which order and security are gained, [...] and the occult potential of its mystery is defused' (Roberts 1992). In his own clinical study on the relationship between the delusional beliefs system and the need for meaning in life, Roberts used self-administered psychometric scales such as the Purpose in Life Test (Crumbaugh 1968), the Life Regard Index (Battista & Almond 1973), and the Beck Depression Inventory, Shortened Form (Beck & Beck 1972) to measure respectively perceived meaning and purpose in life, positive life regard, and level of depression in a group of individuals with chronic delusions who met the criteria for a diagnosis within the schizophrenia spectrum. Measures were compared with a group of previously deluded patients in remission, and two non-clinical control groups: psychiatric rehabilitation nurses and Anglican Ordinands. Findings showed that patients in remission (no longer holding the delusions) were both more depressed and found their lives less meaningful than individuals who were currently deluded. There also was a higher degree of verbalised suicidal ideation in the former group. Meaning in life scores were not significantly different across the clinical group with chronic delusions, the ordinands, and the nursing group. The author suggested that the benefits associated with the chronic delusional systems may have contributed to their maintenance, thus deterring recovery. When looking at the descriptive (qualitative) answers obtained from the questionnaire items, patients with chronic delusions often reported a new sense of identity, a clearer sense of duty and allegiance to a higher purpose, and an affective change from feeling bored, frightened, and depressed, towards feeling lively and enthusiastic (Roberts 1991: 27–28). When asked 'what would your life be like without these beliefs / if one day you discovered they were not true / were false' (Roberts 1991: 27), many stated they would have nothing to live for:

If I am not Jesus I have nothing to live for...if it is not true I would be a nobody.

*(Roberts 1991: 27)*

I should be shattered—I've devoted so much time and effort to it [...] I'd have nothing to keep me going...if it's proved wrong what am I going to do? I'd be left with nothing.

*(Roberts 1991: 27, abridged)*

I'd miss the excitement of life, life has no drama in it or reality. Life would not be worth living.

*(Roberts 1991: 27)*

A more recent study by Louise Isham and colleagues (2022) focused more specifically on 'grandiose' delusions—a group of delusions linked together by the common theme of having special abilities, wealth, power, or a unique mission. Using newly developed measures to investigate both the experience of meaning and the sources of meaning, they found that grandiose delusions provided three types of meaning: a sense that life makes sense (coherence), a sense of directedness in life (purpose), and a sense that life matters and is worthwhile (significance). Sources of meaning overlapped with those commonly sought by anyone (with or without delusions): doing things for the greater good, supporting loved ones, overcoming adversity, gaining self-confidence when among others, having a positive social perception, and gaining spirituality. They concluded that, while meaning seems to be a significant maintenance factor for grandiose delusions, attempts to medically address the delusions without supporting the person's search for alternative sources of meaning could be both difficult and harmful.

A tension seems to arise here. On the one hand, delusions seem to foster a sense of meaningfulness in the face of adversity, at least for some people, at the time of adoption, if not in the long term (as in the study by Roberts 1991). But there are also many ways in which delusions are harmful or can lead to harm. For instance, a person believing that they can fly might attempt to 'walk' off a cliff or into traffic, with catastrophic consequences. Or, believing the entire world is conspiring against them, they may experience increased anxiety and distress, and may gradually withdraw from others, avoid working or leaving their house, which in turn might intensify feelings isolation, disconnectedness, and depression.

This tension can be resolved if we think that delusions are neither static entities, nor that they happen in a vacuum; rather, they are complex, dynamic, and situated phenomena arising through multiple layers of meaning-making across embodied, psychological, linguistic, and social levels of analysis. This dynamic perspective, embraced by the Emergence Model of Delusions (Ritunnano et al. 2022), is apt because it immediately solves the tension between strategy and dysfunction, between meaningfulness and harmfulness: what is dysfunctional at one level, may show adaptive properties at another level, and vice versa. In this model, delusions are understood as strongly individualised and inherently complex phenomena emerging from a dynamic interplay between interdependent subpersonal, personal, interpersonal, and sociocultural processes. On this view, meaning emerges through

> interdependent layers or strata of increasing organisational complexity—each depending in part on the properties of the lower levels, but irreducible to it or them. The boundaries between layers are porous to indicate interdependence and reciprocal interactions. Each layer is autonomous, in the sense of being governed by its irreducible set of laws and mechanisms, which can be studied by different disciplines using different concepts.
>
> *(Ritunnano et al. 2022: 473)*

A dynamic perspective sees how these multiple, nested meaning-making processes continuously unfold and interact in non-linear ways. In this sense, the recovery of meaning in delusion not only requires an effort towards understanding the content of a delusion or its reason for the individual person, but also recognises that meaning is the result of a constant exchange between the person and their environment as they reciprocally condition one another. In the Emergence Model of Delusions, 'Delusional phenomena are emergent in the sense that their meanings are rooted in and emergent from the person's phenomenal consciousness, through an engagement with others and the sociocultural context that is mediated by language and affect' (Ritunnano et al. 2022: 472).

The above reference to the person's 'phenomenal consciousness' should not be interpreted as a suggestion that meanings reside in the person's head (Kusters 2022), but rather that they are *lived through* and *enacted* in the relationship between self and world, as well as expressed through language and performed in the 'liminal' spaces between action, thought, belief, and perception. The person's phenomenal consciousness should be understood here as only one among many possible points of *entry into* meaning; one that begins with an effort to understand how intentional states may shape experiential contents and acts through interaction with others, and through participation in the symbolic systems of the culture (Bruner 1990). Meaning cannot be constituted independently, through individual and un-shareable intentional acts; it is relationally constituted through bodily, affective, and communicative practices.

To further explore this bodily, affective, and non-propositional dimension of meaning, we must take a step back from the kind of moral-epistemic considerations implicit in discussions of meaningfulness and harmfulness. Here, we take—as our unit of investigation— the person with delusions and their *lived world*. Following phenomenology's commitment to interrogate even the most familiar features of our everyday experience as 'perpetual beginners', we try and set aside those preconceptions often placed on the meaning of delusions in advance, to let the phenomenon show itself for what it is.

## 2.  Where does meaning come from in delusions?

To begin with, let us consider a quote extracted from a memoir of a young woman, Renee, with schizophrenia:

> Objects are stage trappings, placed here and there, geometric cubes *without meaning*. People turn weirdly about, they make gestures, movements without sense; they are phantoms whirling on an infinite plain, crushed by the pitiless electric light. And I - I am lost in it, isolated, cold, stripped purposeless under the light. A wall of brass separates me from everybody and everything. [...] Madness was finding oneself permanently in an all embracing Unreality.
>
> *(Sechehaye 1970: 33; our emphasis)*

Now consider another excerpt, this time written by Erin Hawkes, neuroscientist and patient with schizophrenia:

> Ah, another clue! I bent down reverently and picked up the piece of blue plastic that was lying innocently on the sidewalk. It was the shape and size of a bullet, signifying by the Deep Meaning that I was going to be sniper shot soon. Alarmed, I walked on, faster, and then—another one. This one was a piece of wood; a minute later, another plastic bullet shape. I was in grave danger.
>
> *(Hawkes 2012: 1109)*

She explains:

> Insight into the Deep Meaning had been with me for a while, around the time I had stopped taking the 1400 mg of daily Seroquel I was supposed to take for my paranoid schizophrenia. I was being messaged by various things I found on the sidewalk: a red elastic band, intact, meant that I would not have to open my wrist and bleed out again; a yellow strip of plastic prophesied that my body would become a crime scene with that 'Do not enter' warning. I collect them, keep them in a little drawstring bag.
>
> *(Hawkes 2012: 1109)*

These accounts may appear, at first, to differ in significant ways to the point that we may consider them to be the expression of a different phenomenon altogether. From a phenomenological psychopathology perspective, they may, indeed, indicate different phases in the course of the development of delusions (though not always chronologically linked): the first one suggestive of 'delusional mood' or 'delusional atmosphere', often described by individuals in the early stages of psychosis, and the second one describing a fully-formed delusion of reference as well as a delusional perception (Fuchs 2005). But there is also a way in which these two accounts can be seen as two sides of the same coin, or alterations along the same experiential continuum. Both involve a transformed sense of *felt significance, vitality* or *relevance* of the surrounding objects and world more generally, in the context of a dynamic sense of engagement between self and world (Sass & Ratcliffe 2017). What is at stake here then is an all-encompassing, *ontological* change in the experience of reality as either devoid of meaning (hypo-real), or imbued with a sense of uncanny particularity and felt meaningfulness (hyper-real) (Van Duppen 2016).

In an attempt to closely investigate these transformations of reality-experience and their subjective apprehension, Jasper Feyaerts and colleagues (2021) interviewed patients with lived experience of delusions who had attracted a diagnosis of schizophrenia. Following the methods of Interpretative Phenomenological Analysis (Smith et al. 2021), they found that, in most cases, the participants' descriptions did not point to a particular cognitive or perceptual content. Rather, they often stressed the mood-like (or atmospheric) character of the experiential changes, as opening up a whole new world or reality—dominated in some cases by a sense of mystical unity and love:

> My psychosis was a total experience. It was not merely my beliefs or thoughts that changed, but also my behaviour, my feeling, [...] it was a complete and total form of experiencing.
>
> *(Feyaerts et al. 2021: 4)*

> In one single instance, everything was totally different. I found myself in an entirely different world.
>
> *(Feyaerts et al. 2021: 4)*

In the context of this all-enveloping, atmospheric transformation—often dominated by a sense of unreality and perplexity—Rob Sips and colleagues describe similar experiences of 'insight' or 'aha-experiences':

> So there is no one there at that moment, but normally it is a busy street. And I thought... *It felt so weird...* And suddenly I think: *'It's happened. I have died'.* (...) It is as if... As if you thought this was not possible, and then you are startled and frightened by the thought that it might be possible.
>
> *(Sips et al. 2021: 5; our emphasis)*

Here, within what appears like an overall, elusive, and perplexing transformation of the lived world ('it felt so weird'), the participant has a sudden insight experience ('It's happened. I have died') that manifest as an immediate certainty of reality involving the *seeing of meaning*. This experience is famously described by Jasper, in his discussion of 'primary delusions' or 'delusions proper' characteristic of schizophrenia (in contrast with the with the more mundane 'delusion-like ideas') (Jaspers 1963: 96–99):

> Now, the *experiences of primary delusion are analogous to this seeing of meaning*, but the awareness of meaning undergoes a radical transformation. There is an

immediate, intrusive knowledge of the meaning and it is this which is itself the delusional experience.

*(Jaspers 1963: 99; emphasis in original)*

There remain open questions as to the nature of this experience of felt meaning or seeing of meaning. Kasper Møller Nielsen, Julie Nordgaard, and Mads Gram Henriksen (2022) have recently revisited classical psychopathological accounts of delusional perception, as the prototypical example of primary delusions, and asked whether it is essentially a normal perception which triggers an abnormal interpretation or whether the delusional meaning is rather contained within a changed perception. Although different accounts exist, most seem to converge with the idea that these insight experiences emerge within an unfamiliar experiential framework where the ordinary meaning structures that link subject and objects are changed or destabilised.

This implicit, meaningful relationship between self and world, as the experiential foundation for meaning-making, is central to phenomenological philosophy and has been variously articulated by Husserl, Heidegger, Merleau-Ponty, and Sartre among others. Central to the work of Merleau-Ponty (1945/2013) in particular is the idea that this form of tacit knowledge, guiding our behaviour, is fundamentally *embodied*: it is through the 'knowing-body', and not through a disembodied intelligence, that I grasp the meaning of a given object or scene. Using Merleau-Ponty's words, felt meaning can thus be conceived as a bodily 'grip' or 'hold' (*prise*) on a given perceptual scene or the world of perception more generally. Perceptual knowledge then unfolds through intentional interlocking of body and world as two sides of a single act, which cannot be reduced to the conceptual processing of a sensory experience given through a detached act of judgment.

Inextricable from and complementary to the role of bodily intentionality is an emphasis—found predominantly in the work of Heidegger—on the role of *moods*[1] or 'existential feelings'[2] (Ratcliffe 2008). In this view, moods are an essential ingredient of what allows the world to *matter* in a certain way for us; that is, filled with meaning and structured by a sense of our future possibilities. For Matthew Ratcliffe, existential feelings are both 'bodily states', in that they are experienced as *feelings* through bodily engagement with the world, and 'ways of finding oneself in the world' as background orientations through which our experience of the world is structured. Alterations of existential feelings have been proposed as a fruitful explanatory framework for many psychopathological experiences frequently interpreted (in propositional terms) as pathologies of belief (Ratcliffe 2009).

As we move from sources of dysfunction to sources of meaning, it is our contention that felt experiencing can be regarded as a generative locus of meaning in delusions in multiple ways. Certain feelings and emotions may not only carry with them a sense of reality (so that the meaning perceived in this direct, felt way, has the character of reality) and shape the very structure of delusional realities—thus affecting the thematic content of the delusions. They may also affect the ways in which delusions are articulated through communicative acts, as we will see in the next section. In those cases where delusions may appear 'implausible' or resistant to empathic understanding, the recognition that they may have developed from changes in the form of experience (i.e., alterations of felt experiencing) rather than aberrant reasoning, may improve our ability to engage with others' testimonies with openness, care, and respect. In these cases, it may be helpful to think about delusional utterances not (always or necessarily) as *assertions* of truth,[3] as their orthodox definition would seem to suggest, but rather as expressive attempts at articulating felt meaning and understanding,

52

which may involve metaphorical and metonymic thinking (see Littlemore 2015). Here, we are particularly interested in the meaning-generative and meaning-shaping relationship between metaphorical thinking and the formation of the delusion itself.

## 3.   The articulation of meaning in delusion: literal, metaphorical, or both?

Several philosophers and psychopathologists have appreciated the challenges inherent in using language to express the kinds of ineffable transformations of experience just described (for a review, see Pienkos, Škodlar, & Sass 2022). Figurative language, in these cases, may aid the articulation and communication of novel and highly unusual bodily experiences, and thus have a *meaning-generative* effect that allows the interlocutor to gain a glimpse of the *what-it-is-likeness* of occurrent (delusional) experiential states (Nordgaard, Sass, & Parnas 2013). In addition, it has been suggested that metaphorical thinking accounts for the nature of some delusions found in psychosis, and that it plays a role in the inner speech patterns of people with psychosis that link real-world experiences to the creation of delusions (Deamer & Wilkinson 2021). Felicity Deamer and Sam Wilkinson suggest that under certain conditions, non-literal inner speech may come to be understood literally, and that these literally understood inner utterances lead the individual to believe in the truth of their delusion. They point to the large body of literature showing that figurative thinking is a natural response to emotional distress.

Indeed, there is a large body of literature showing that people often reach for metaphors when attempting to describe or make sense of the qualitative aspects of their emotional experiences (Gibbs & Franks 2002; Littlemore & Turner 2019). It can be very difficult, and in some cases impossible, to describe the exact nature of an emotional experience (e.g. what it feels like to be sad) using only literal language (Stanley et al. 2021)—which is why people often use metaphors (e.g. 'I felt empty'). Metaphors provide information about the rich detail and complexity of human emotional experience in a way that literal language does not (Colston & Gibbs 2021). They allow us to describe ineffable experiences in concrete, tangible, and often physical terms. For this reason, people have been found to use more metaphors when talking about personal emotional experiences than when talking about other types of experience (Gibbs & Franks 2002; Williams-Whitney, Mio, & Whitney 1992), with intense emotions leading to more metaphors than mild emotions (Fainsilber & Ortony 1987).

When considering the role played by metaphors in delusions, a question that is of central interest is whether metaphorical thinking plays a role in the inception of the delusional idea, and if so, whether this original 'metaphoricity' is preserved (to a degree) in the delusional expression here and now. Following on from this, it is important to consider whether the meaning of the delusional expression is 'metaphorical or literal', and whether the answer to this question can really be taken at face value in the assessment of 'delusionality'. For example, someone may describe an anomalous sensation in their spine 'as if there are electric vibrations'. In this case, an external observer may take the 'as if' designation to be indicative of metaphoricity, thus pointing to a preserved clinical 'insight' or 'grip' on the sense of reality. In contrast, the same interlocutor, listening to the claim 'I *know* that there are electric vibrations in my spine', may take that as unequivocally expressive of literal meaning and therefore suggestive of the delusionality of their experience (Nordgaard, Sass, & Parnas 2013: 360). The line, however, between metaphorical and literal meanings, may not be so easily drawn by an external observer solely on the basis of a decontextualised linguistic expression, detached from its phenomenological context—that is, from the individual's subjective experience of the lived world, including their experience of language. Rather, metaphoricity may be best thought of as being on a cline (Goatly 1997; Hanks 2006), where the same expression may be *lived through* more or less literally by the speaker and subject of experience. Variations along the cline may depend upon different factors, such as whether the subject is indeed in the midst of a delusional reality (not uncommonly experienced in parallel with and simultaneous to the shared 'ordinary' reality) at the time of the speech event, whether they have long theorised about it perhaps developing a systematised narrative, or whether the subject has taken some emotional and experiential 'distance' from the perceptual or quasi-perceptual event that initially gave rise to the delusion and is now recollecting a memory of it for a specific communicative purpose.[4] Indeed, as happens with novel metaphors entering a language for the first time (consistent with the 'career of the metaphor hypothesis' advanced by Dedre Gentner et al. 2001), it is tempting to speculate on potential differences in cognitive processing (from comparison to categorisation) occurring at different stages of the life of a metaphor adopted within the more localised system of meanings for an individual experiencing a delusion. According to this view, it is possible that expressions such as 'I have insects crawling under my skin' may initially be adopted as a metaphorical understanding of a delusional bodily experience, only to become a literal expression at a later stage in the life of the metaphor (and, concurrently, of the delusion), when metaphor processing shifts 'from online active interpretation to retrieval of stored meaning' (Gentner et al. 2001: 216) and the metaphorical roots of the delusional thought disappear (see Gibbs & Santa Cruz, 2012).

There is now increasing recognition of the fact that a good number of metaphors draw on physical experiences (e.g., in English, 'understanding' is often talked about in terms of 'seeing', 'time' is often talked about in terms of 'space' and 'advancement' is often talked about in terms of upward movement) (Lakoff & Johnson 1980/2003). Metaphors such as these are part of our conceptual system, and without them, we would find it virtually impossible to reason and communicate about abstract concepts. These metaphors are not just part of our language but they have the potential to be 'experienced' at a subconscious level. In other words, when we encounter them under certain conditions (see Littlemore 2019), subconscious sensory-motor responses are triggered that are similar to those that would be triggered if we actually observed or experienced these actions and senses in the real world (Gibbs, Lima, & Francozo 2004). These metaphors therefore have the potential to be experienced on a physical level, rather than being purely an external, objective phenomenon. Raymond W. Gibbs (2006) suggests that part of our ability to make sense of metaphors such as these 'resides in the automatic construction of a simulation whereby we imagine performing the bodily actions referred to in these excerpts' (Gibbs 2006: 435). He goes on to argue that 'people's intuitive, felt, phenomenological experiences of their own bodies shape large portions of metaphoric thought and language use' (Gibbs 2006: 436). For this reason, metaphors such as these are often described as 'embodied'. The degree of embodiment can range from full-on sensory-motor activation through to the use of bodily knowledge in shaping our metaphorical thought processes (see Littlemore 2019).

Sarah Turner and Jeannette Littlemore (2023) argue that at times, people's use of metaphor goes beyond *talking about* something as if it were something else, and they actually *experience* it as if it were something else, or even *believe* that it actually *is* something else. The fact that metaphors can be experienced in this way is not a trivial observation for, as we have just seen, physical human experiences form the basis of a very large number of metaphors. Most, if not all, abstract phenomena are understood through metaphors, many of which are based on bodily experiences. If, as the above authors suggest, we live and embody metaphor, then when we speak in metaphors we also have the potential to experience them as real, which means that the divide between the 'literal' and the 'metaphorical' may not be as clear-cut as we think.

The blurring of the boundaries between the literal and the metaphorical is particularly common in situations where people are attempting to come to terms with emotional trauma, such as in the case of bereavement and grief (see Turner & Littlemore 2023). This blurring also appears to be present in delusions. In all these cases (bereavement, grief and delusions), the world may appear profoundly different and unfamiliar as a result of the 'loss of a system of possibilities' (Ratcliffe 2019). While an experience of grief is focused upon the loss of a particular person, both the case of grief and delusion appear to involve (at least at some stage) markedly similar, profound, and all-encompassing changes in the way one experiences and relates to the world as affording practical meanings. Sometimes described as lost 'assumptions' in the context of grief (Parkes & Prigerson 2013), it has been variously characterised as lost 'background' (Rhodes & Gipps 2008), 'common sense', or 'disembodiment' in the case of schizophrenic delusions (Stanghellini 2008). A central phenomenological theme, across these emotional kinds of trauma, is the dissolution of practical meanings so that things are no longer seen as *mattering* to us in the light of our concerns (i.e., as *pragmata*) but simply as bare 'things' with no practical relevance. The world, as a result, takes on an unfamiliar and *unhomelike* character that resists propositional understanding and literal articulation. It invites, instead, a narrative and metaphorical articulation of *felt* meaning as a form of tacit, embodied and affective understanding (as discussed in Section 2). Through this process of metaphorical thinking and articulation, new meanings are created that can ultimately shape experience as it is *lived through*. For instance, in their investigation into the use of metaphorical language, thought, and behaviour by parents coming to terms with the death of their child, Littlemore and Turner (2019) report cases where people imbued literal actions with metaphorical meaning, experienced metaphors as if they were literally true, or experienced phenomena as both literal and metaphorical at the same time. As suggested by the authors, this again speaks to the 'fuzzy nature of the boundaries between the literal and the metaphorical in situations where what was "real" has become "unreal" and what was "unreal" has become "real"' (Littlemore & Turner 2019: 407).

In psychiatry, we often find an implicit assumption associated with metaphors and psychopathological expressions of anomalous experiences, especially if these defy the limits of imagination (Jeppsson 2022). We may think that if someone is using (what looks like) a metaphorical expression, then this means that it does not reflect their experiential reality, rather they are abstracting from it. In other words, they cannot mean what they have said literally. For instance, in the case of psychosis, it is often assumed that talking metaphorically would not lead to 'acting' on the delusion (e.g., in a delusion of persecution, that is, a person would not respond behaviourally to a threatening stimulus). Or that when someone indicates, with bodily gestures or with an assertion, that they are experiencing something as 'real' or 'true', then it must bear literal meaning and should be fully concordant (and non-contradictory) with their actions, beliefs, and behaviours. However, as we have just seen, the line between the 'literal' and the 'metaphorical' can sometimes become blurred; metaphorical expressions can lose their metaphorical roots and can acquire literal meanings. Pointedly, in their empirical work on the linguistic markers used by adolescents at risk of psychosis, Lise Baklund, Jan Ivar Røssberg, and Paul Møller (2023: 7) noted 'a fuzzy border between the symbolic and literal meaning of metaphors'.

This has important implications for the phenomenological concept of 'double-bookkeeping', where the delusional individual appears to accept that both the delusion and an inconsistent reality are true, and seems unconcerned by the apparent inconsistency (Deamer & Wilkinson 2021; see also Porcher, Chapter 13); when literal and metaphorical meanings converge, the inconsistency disappears. In psychosis, the blurring of the boundaries between literal and metaphorical language, thought and behaviour, must be understood in the context of the complex relationship between the radical and all-encompassing changes in one's reality-experience and the person's simultaneous exposure to the shared-social world and the linguistic rules thereof. As Gert Jensen suggests (2022), drawing on his own experience of schizophrenic delusions, what may look to an outsider like a flaw in reasoning (and concurrently, something unconceivable or ontologically impossible as discussed by Humpston 2022), 'If anything [...] is an expression of a compromise of one's changed set of preferences, following changes in one's subjective lifeworld due to alterations in one's exposure to both worlds' (Jensen 2022: 3).

In addition to blurring the boundaries between the literal and the metaphorical, another characteristic of metaphorical thinking in delusions is that it is often highly unconventional. This is perhaps unsurprising; when we share relatively common states and feelings, conventional metaphors are largely sufficient (e.g., 'I felt my blood boil'), but when sharing our more nuanced and deeper personal experiences, which are not universal, we often need to use more novel metaphors (Semino 2011). For example, someone might say 'it felt like organ rejection' (Littlemore, Turner, & Tuck 2023) to individuate their personal experience from the general experience of exclusion. Novel metaphors allow us to employ a finite set of linguistic resources to express an infinite range of experiences (see Colston & Gibbs 2021). Using metaphors in novel ways is therefore key in making sense of the nature of unshared experience and in creating rapport (Reisfield & Wilson 2004). Indeed, it has been shown that people generate more novel metaphors when writing about their own emotional experiences than when writing about the feelings of others (Williams-Whitney, Mio, & Whitney 1992). The experiences that give rise to psychosis are often highly individualised, and it is therefore unsurprising that they give rise to novels forms of metaphorical thinking.

Several factors are likely to affect the extent to which, and the ways in which people use metaphors in novel ways when sharing or making sense of their emotional experiences. These include: emotional valence (Jovanovic et al. 2016), mood state (Russ 2013), medium of expression (Deignan, Littlemore, & Semino 2013), and level of interaction (Cameron & Deignan 2006). All of these factors are relevant to the case of delusions and the contexts in which delusional content is discussed. But what forms do these novel metaphors tend to take? It has been noted that novel uses of metaphor rarely involve a completely new mapping from one domain to another (Littlemore, Turner, and Tuck 2023). Rather, they involve extensions and alternative uses of existing metaphorical mappings. In their work on the novel 'uses' that people made of metaphor when describing and evaluating emotionally charged workplace experiences, Littlemore, Turner, and Tuck (2023) found that they could involve: introducing more detail into a conventional metaphorical mapping; combining metaphor with hyperbole; appropriating a well-known idiom, using a conventional metaphor to talk about something that it is not usually used to talk about; employing a metaphor that interacts with metonymy in a novel way; combining two or more metaphors; making use of strong or unexpected personification; employing metaphors that work on both a metaphorical and a literal level at once; and making use of creative contrast.

We can see evidence of some of these novel ways of using metaphor in John Rhodes and Simon Jakes's (2004) study of the role played by metaphor and metonymy in the formation of delusions. For example, one of their participants, who had experienced high levels of family violence, poverty, and insecurity as a child, reported that he watched numerous superhero cartoons and that these were his only source of comfort. His subsequent delusion involved him seeing himself as a superhero (which is a metaphor for how he would like to see himself in an ideal world) and that his body was based on 'hydrogen', which is a metonym for his super-powerful body. This delusion, in which the source and target domain merge in the face of emotional pain, involves a novel combination of metaphor and metonymy. Another participant, who felt guilty for having abandoned multiple romantic partners, began to see himself as the Devil. He found himself pacing up and down and swallowing (in this case an expression of anxiety), and immediately interpreted this action within the metaphorical framework that he had established, and thought that he was 'swallowing God's medicine'. He then reported 'seeing' horns on his head and concluded that he was the Devil, condemned to Hell. These metaphorical thinking patterns appear to involve the addition of entailments to an existing metaphor ('God's medicine' and the 'Devil horns'), as well as a hyperbolic extension of a conventional metaphor (I am the Devil), which he experiences both literally and metaphorically. Another participant reported that in her a delusion, an unspecified 'man' was using a rope to pull her into a coffin. This man was thought to be a Christian who did not like God. The 'man' in her delusion appears to be a strong, unexpected personification of some of her fears, and perhaps of her previous negative experiences with respect to organised religion. All these narratives provide interesting insights into the complex processes of literal, metaphorical and metonymic articulation of the felt and intersubjective experience of meaning in delusions.

## 4. Conclusion

In this chapter, we have explored different senses of the word 'meaning' in relation to delusions, which give rise to different philosophical questions, such as those concerning the psychological meaningfulness of delusions, their felt sources of meaning, and the articulation of these meanings through figurative language. We have reviewed a growing body of philosophical and empirical literature, supporting the idea that delusions can be both harmful *and* meaningful for the person experiencing them, and argued that this can be explained by the dynamic constitution of meaning across interdependent subpersonal, personal, interpersonal, and sociocultural layers. Taking the person's phenomenal consciousness as a point of entry to explore the intersubjective constitution of meaning, we then turned to phenomenology to examine meaning in its *felt*, non-propositional dimension. Here, phenomenological accounts are helpful inasmuch as they contribute to our understanding of the atmospheric alterations of the sense of reality within which sudden insight experiences are often dialectically embedded, in the context of psychosis. Finally, we have shown how the expression and articulation of this felt dimension of meaning is performed in the 'liminal' spaces between action, thought, belief, and perception. In these spaces, the boundaries between the literal and the metaphorical become easily blurred, and people may resort to novel uses of metaphor to aid understanding and communication of such complex and intense emotional experiences. Guided by these insights, we become better placed to engage with delusional thought and discourse as expressive attempts at articulating felt meaning and understanding, rather than unshakeable assertions of truth. Future delusion research may benefit from embracing their complex, dynamic, and situated nature through direct engagement with lived expertise and cross-disciplinary knowledge expansion.

## Acknowledgements

We are grateful to Pablo Hubacher Haerle and Sofia Jeppsson for helpful conversations and feedback on an earlier version of the manuscript.

## Notes

1 For Heidegger, 'mood' is not a specifically directed intentional state but is rather a 'disposition' that is presupposed by all such intentional states, and allows us to encounter things as mattering in a certain way. As Ratcliffe (2008) puts it, mood is 'what opens up a world in the first place; it is through mood that we find ourselves in a world' (Ratcliffe 2008: 48).
2 See Ratcliffe's *Feelings of Being* (2008) for an account of the nature and role of 'existential feelings' as a phenomenological category drawing on Heidegger's notion of mood.
3 For a novel and thoroughgoing examination of the linguistic meaning of delusional utterances, as performing different illocutionary acts beyond that of mere assertives, see Hofmann, Hubacher Haerle, and Maatz (2023).
4 We are indebted to Sofia Jeppsson (personal communication) for emphasising the need to distinguish between the initial cause or process leading up to the formation and adoption of a delusion, and the experience as it is lived and uttered in the 'here and now'. For instance, someone looking at their reflection in the mirror may say: 'I don't recognise myself' in a metaphorical sense because they weren't feeling themselves on that day, or because they behaved in an unusual or unexpected manner that does not reflect their 'normal' self. Although we cannot be entirely sure, this may also have happened at some point at the origin of a delusion (e.g., during childhood or at the onset of psychosis). However, here and now, the same person may be looking at the mirror and saying: 'It doesn't look like my face', meaning it literally as in: 'It looks like another face which is very similar to mine, but it's not perfectly similar (even though I can't say exactly where it differs)'.

## References

Baklund, L., Røssberg, J. I. and Møller, P. 2023. Linguistic markers and basic self-disturbances among adolescents at risk of psychosis. A qualitative study. *EClinicalMedicine* 55: 101733.

Battista, J. and Almond, R. 1973. The development of meaning in life. *Psychiatry* 36(4): 409–427.

Beck, A. T. and Beck, R. W. 1972. Screening depressed patients in family practice: A rapid technic. *Postgraduate Medicine* 52(6): 81–85.

Bergstein, M., Weizman, A. and Solomon, Z. 2008. Sense of coherence among delusional patients: Prediction of remission and risk of relapse. *Comprehensive Psychiatry* 49(3): 288–296.

Berrios, G. E. 1991. Delusions as "wrong beliefs": A conceptual history. *The British Journal of Psychiatry* 159(S14): 6–13.

Bruner, J. 1990. *Acts of Meaning*. Cambridge, MA: Harvard University Press.

Cameron, L. and Deignan, A. 2006. The emergence of metaphor in discourse. *Applied Linguistics* 27(4): 671–690.

Colston, H. L. and Gibbs, R. W. 2021. Figurative language communicates directly because it precisely demonstrates what we mean. *Canadian Journal of Experimental Psychology/Revue canadienne de psychologie expérimentale* 75(2): 228.

Corlett, P. 2018. Delusions and prediction error. In L. Bortolotti, ed., *Delusions in Context*. Cham: Springer International Publishing, pp. 35–66.

Crumbaugh, J. C. 1968. Cross-validation of purpose-in-life test based on Frankl's concepts. *Journal of Individual Psychology* 24(1): 74.

Deamer, F. and Wilkinson, S. 2021. Metaphorical thinking and delusions in psychosis. In M. Amblard, M. Musiol and M. Rebuschi, eds. *(In)coherence of Discourse: Formal and Conceptual Issues of Language*. Cham: Springer International Publishing, pp. 119–130.

Deignan, A., Littlemore, J. and Semino, E. 2013. *Figurative Language, Genre and Register*. Cambridge: Cambridge University Press.

Fainsilber, L. and Ortony, A. 1987. Metaphorical uses of language in the expression of emotions. *Metaphor and Symbol* 2(4): 239–250.

Feyaerts, J., Kusters, W., Van Duppen, Z., Vanheule, S., Myin-Germeys, I. and Sass, L. 2021. Uncovering the realities of delusional experience in schizophrenia: A qualitative phenomenological study in Belgium. *The Lancet Psychiatry* 8(9): 784–796.

Fuchs, T. 2005. Delusional mood and delusional perception – A phenomenological analysis. *Psychopathology* 38(3): 133–139.

Garson, J. 2022. *Madness: A Philosophical Exploration*. Oxford: Oxford University Press.

Gentner, D., Bowdle, B., Wolff, P. and Boronat C. 2001. Metaphor is like analogy. In D. Gentner, K.J. Holyoak and B.N. Kokinov, eds., *The Analogical Mind: Perspectives from Cognitive Science*. Cambridge: MIT Press, pp. 199–254.

Gibbs Jr, R. W. 2006. Metaphor interpretation as embodied simulation. *Mind and Language* 21(3): 434–458.

Gibbs Jr, R. W. and Franks, H. 2002. Embodied metaphor in women's narratives about their experiences with cancer. *Health Communication* 14(2): 139–165.

Gibbs Jr, R. W. and Santa Cruz, M. J. 2012. Temporal unfolding of conceptual metaphoric experience. *Metaphor and Symbol* 27(4): 299–311.

Gibbs Jr, R.W., Lima, P.L.C. and Francozo, E. 2004. Metaphor is grounded in embodied experience. *Journal of Pragmatics* 36(7): 1189–1210.

Goatly, A. 1997. *The Language of Metaphors*. London: Routledge.

Gunn, R. and Bortolotti, L. 2018. Can delusions play a protective role? *Phenomenology and the Cognitive Sciences* 17(4): 813–833.

Gunn, R. and Larkin, M. 2020. Delusion formation as an inevitable consequence of a radical alteration in lived experience. *Psychosis* 12(2): 151–161.

Hanks, P. 2006. Metaphoricity is gradable. In A. Stefanowitsch and S. Gries, eds., *Corpora in Cognitive Linguistics. Vol. 1: Metaphor and Metonymy*. Berlin and New York: Mouton de Gruyter, pp 17–35.

Hawkes, E. 2012. Making meaning. *Schizophrenia Bulletin* 38(6): 1109–1110.

Hofmann, J., Hubacher Haerle, P. and Maatz, A. 2023. What's the linguistic meaning of delusional utterances? Speech act theory as a tool for understanding delusions. *Philosophical Psychology*. DOI: 10.1080/09515089.2023.2174424.

Humpston, C. S. 2022. Isolated by oneself: Ontologically impossible experiences in schizophrenia. *Philosophy, Psychiatry, & Psychology* 29(1): 5–15.

Isham, L., Loe, B. S., Hicks, A., Wilson, N., Bird, J. C., Bentall, R. P. and Freeman, D. 2022. The meaning in grandiose delusions: Measure development and cohort studies in clinical psychosis and non-clinical general population groups in the UK and Ireland. *The Lancet Psychiatry* 9(10): 792–803.

Jaspers, K. 1963. *General Psychopathology*, J. Hoenig, and M.W. Hamilton, trans. Manchester: Manchester University Press.

Jensen, G. 2022. Delusion and reason: An argument for a phenomenological model for understanding schizophrenic delusion. *Schizophrenia Bulletin*: sbac185.

Jeppsson, S. 2022 (unpublished). Presented at the conference "Philosophy, Disability and Social Change 3" on December 8, 2022. https://www.bsg.ox.ac.uk/events/philosophy-disability-and-social-change-3

Jovanovic, T., Meinel, M., Schrödel, S. and Voigt, K. I. 2016. The influence of affects on creativity: What do we know by now? *Journal of Creativity and Business Innovation* 2: 46–64.

Kusters, W. 2022. On understanding madness: A paradoxical view. *Philosophical Psychology*. DOI: 10.1080/09515089.2022.2146491

Lakoff, G. and Johnson, M. 1980/2003. *Metaphors We Live By*. Chicago, IL: University of Chicago Press.

Lancellotta, E. and Bortolotti, L. 2019. Are clinical delusions adaptive? *Wiley Interdisciplinary Reviews: Cognitive Science* 10(5): e1502.

Langdon, R. 2011. The cognitive neuropsychiatry of delusional belief. *Wiley Interdisciplinary Reviews-Cognitive Science* 2(5): 449–460.

Littlemore, J. 2015. *Metonymy: Hidden Shortcuts in Language, Thought and Communication*. Cambridge: Cambridge University Press.

Littlemore, J. 2019. *Metaphors in the Mind: Sources of Variation in Embodied Metaphor*. Cambridge: Cambridge University Press.

Littlemore, J. and Turner, S. 2019. Metaphors in communication about pregnancy loss. *Metaphor and the Social World* 10(1): 45–75.

Littlemore, J., Turner, S. and Tuck, P. 2023. *Creative Metaphor, Emotion and Evaluation in Conversations about Work*. London: Routledge.

Merleau-Ponty, M. 1945/2013. *Phenomenology of Perception*, D.A. Landes, trans. London: Routledge.

Miyazono, K. 2015. Delusions as harmful malfunctioning beliefs. *Consciousness and Cognition* 33: 561–573.

Nielsen, K. M., Nordgaard, J. and Henriksen, M. G. 2022. Delusional perception revisited. *Psychopathology* 55(6): 325–334.

Nordgaard, J., Sass, L. A. and Parnas, J. 2013. The psychiatric interview: Validity, structure, and subjectivity. *European Archives of Psychiatry and Clinical Neuroscience* 263: 353–364.

Parkes, C. M. and Prigerson H. G. 2013. *Bereavement: Studies of Grief in Adult Life*. London: Routledge.

Petrolini, V. 2017. What makes delusions pathological? *Philosophical Psychology* 30(4): 502–523.

Pienkos, E., Škodlar, B. and Sass, L. 2022. Expressing experience: The promise and perils of the phenomenological interview. *Phenomenology and the Cognitive Sciences* 21(1): 53–71.

Ratcliffe, M. 2008. *Feelings of Being: Phenomenology, Psychiatry and the Sense of Reality*. Oxford: Oxford University Press.

Ratcliffe, M. 2009. Existential feeling and psychopathology. *Philosophy, Psychiatry, & Psychology* 16(2): 179–194.

Ratcliffe, M. J. 2019. The phenomenological clarification of grief and its relevance for psychiatry. In G. Stanghellini, M. Broome, A. Raballo, A.V. Fernandez, P. Fusar-Poli and R. Rosfort, R., eds., *Oxford Handbook of Phenomenological Psychopathology*. Oxford: Oxford University Press, pp. 538–551.

Reisfield, G. M. and Wilson, G. R. 2004. Use of metaphor in the discourse on cancer. *Journal of Clinical Oncology* 22(19): 4024–4027.

Rhodes, J. and Gipps R. G. T. 2008. Delusions, certainty, and the background. *Philosophy, Psychiatry, & Psychology* 15(4): 295–310.

Rhodes, J. E. and Jakes, S. 2004. The contribution of metaphor and metonymy to delusions. *Psychology and Psychotherapy: Theory, Research and Practice* 77(1): 1–17.

Ritunnano, R. and Bortolotti, L. 2022. Do delusions have and give meaning? *Phenomenology and the Cognitive Sciences* 21(4): 949–968.

Ritunnano, R., Kleinman, J., Oshodi, D. W., Michail, M., Nelson, B., Humpston, C. S. and Broome, M. R. 2022. Subjective experience and meaning of delusions in psychosis: A systematic review and qualitative evidence synthesis. *The Lancet Psychiatry* 9(6): 458–476.

Roberts, G. 1991. Delusional belief systems and meaning in life: A preferred reality? *British Journal of Psychiatry* 159(S14): 19–28.

Roberts, G. 1992. The origins of delusion. *British Journal of Psychiatry* 161(3): 298–308.

Russ, S. W. 2013. *Affect and Creativity: The Role of Affect and Play in the Creative Process*. Hillsdale, NJ: Routledge.

Sass, L. and Ratcliffe, M. 2017. Atmosphere: On the phenomenology of "atmospheric" alterations in Schizophrenia-Overall sense of reality, familiarity, vitality, meaning, or relevance (Ancillary Article to EAWE Domain 5). *Psychopathology* 50(1): 90–97.

Sechehaye, M. 1970. *Autobiography of a Schizophrenic Girl*. New York: New American Library.

Semino, E. 2011. Metaphor, creativity, and the experience of pain across genres. In J. Swann, R. Pope and R. Carter, eds., *Creativity in Language & Literature: The State of the Art*. London: Palgrave Macmillan, pp. 83–102.

Sips, R., Van Duppen, Z., Kasanova, Z., De Thurah, L., Teixeira, A., Feyaerts, J. and Myin-Germeys, I. 2021. Psychosis as a dialectic of aha-and anti-aha-experiences: A qualitative study. *Psychosis* 13(1): 47–57.

Smith, J. A., Larkin, M. and Flowers, P. 2021. *Interpretative Phenomenological Analysis: Theory, Method and Research*. London: SAGE Publications Ltd.

Stanghellini, G. 2008. Schizophrenic delusions, embodiment, and the background. *Philosophy, Psychiatry, & Psychology* 15(4): 311–314.

Stanley, B. L., Zanin, A. C., Avalos, B. L., Tracy, S. J. and Town, S. 2021. Collective emotion during collective trauma: A metaphor analysis of the COVID-19 pandemic. *Qualitative Health Research* 31(10): 1890–1903.

Turner, S. and Littlemore, J. 2023. Literal or metaphorical? Conventional or creative? Contested metaphoricity in intense emotional experiences. *Metaphor and the Social World* 13(1): 37–58.

Upthegrove, R. 2018. Delusional beliefs in the clinical context. In L. Bortolotti, ed., *Delusions in Context*. Cham: Springer International Publishing, pp. 1–34.

Van Duppen, Z. 2016. The phenomenology of hypo- and hyperreality in psychopathology. *Phenomenology and the Cognitive Sciences* 15(3): 423–441.

Williams-Whitney, D., Mio, J. S. and Whitney, P. 1992. Metaphor production in creative writing. *Journal of of Psycholinguistic Research* 21(6): 497–509.

# 3

# DELUSION AND ADAPTIVENESS

*Lisa Bortolotti and Martino Belvederi Murri*

## 1.  Introduction

In this chapter, we discuss the potential adaptiveness of delusions as a relevant factor in the explanation of the insight paradox. When people first take distance from their psychotic symptoms and start acknowledging that they have mental health problems, they gain insight. Gaining insight is supposed to be a good outcome as insight facilitates help-seeking and access to treatment. However, with insight, depression and demoralisation ensue and the person may experience low mood, poor self-esteem, and a sense of hopelessness. Understanding why this happens can help us support people who gain insight and prevent them from experiencing the adverse effects of severe depression.

One reason why people become vulnerable to depression and demoralisation is that they realise that they are or have been mentally unwell and this negatively affects their conception of themselves. Another reason may lie in the potential adaptiveness of delusions. If beliefs that are considered as symptoms of mental disorders play an important psychological and epistemic role at a critical time, when they start being recognised as delusions by the person and gradually subside, they leave a gap which the person needs to fill by other means. Acknowledging the potential adaptiveness of delusions brings home the importance of providing support to people gaining insight and informs decisions about what clinical interventions are most effective.

In Section 2, we will describe the phenomenon of the insight paradox in more detail, with a special focus on delusions. In Section 3, we will consider two views of the relationship between accurate representations of reality and wellbeing. According to the traditional view, our wellbeing depends on the accuracy of our representations of reality. This would explain why insight is conducive to good clinical outcomes but does not explain why insight brings depression and demoralisation. According to the trade-off view, some distortions of reality are necessary to our wellbeing. This would explain why insight causes depression and demoralisation but does not explain the positive effects of insight on clinical outcomes. In Section 4, we explore a third approach, based on the recognition of the complex role of delusional beliefs in temporarily and imperfectly supporting the person's functionality at a critical time. Finally, in Section 5, we ask how a better

DOI: 10.4324/9781003296386-5

understanding of the insight paradox based on the adaptiveness of delusions can help justify clinical interventions aimed at supporting people who gain insight after experiencing psychosis. A careful consideration of the insight paradox supports the view that delusions can be adaptive.

## 2.   The insight paradox

*J., a 19-year-old student of Engineering, is a regular cannabis smoker with erratic sleep/ wake rhythms. He has an uncle who supposedly suffered from 'depression' in his youth, and who died by suicide. He lives away from his family of origin and has few close friends. When the first difficult exams approach, J. starts noticing mysterious coincidences, begins feeling observed by neighbours, and gradually develops persecutory delusions about being controlled through his phone. His mental conditions further deteriorate in a matter of days, until he is admitted to the inpatient psychiatric unit, being chased by the police for exhibiting clamorous behaviour in the streets. J. receives antipsychotic treatment and his delusions resolve within a couple of weeks. In those days, he mulls over and re-elaborates his ideas, realising their unrealistic, delusional nature. One day he suddenly falls into despair and verbalises that he is 'a useless, mad chap who will not accomplish any of his goals', that he 'won't ever find a girlfriend and probably will die by suicide'. For several days he stops eating and is unable to sleep. J. is thus diagnosed with post-psychotic depression and starts psychotherapy. Eventually, J. recovers a sense of worth, improves his social life and learns to cope with the idea that he has suffered from a psychotic episode. A year later, J. claims that he should have not defined himself by that episode, which steered his life course and made him even stronger in perspective.*

J.'s story is not unusual. How can we best understand what happens to J.?

Insight is a key element of the psychiatric evaluation, especially among people who experience psychotic symptoms. The expression 'lack of insight' usually indicates that the person being evaluated is *unaware* of having a mental disorder, at least to some extent. Since psychotic disorders entail some degree of *loss of contact with reality* or distorted inferences (Benrimoh and Friston 2020), people who experience delusions or hallucinations are at greater risk of presenting lack of insight.

In clinical practice, lack of insight may become evident during a consultation as a reduced propensity or ability to elaborate on the topic of one's own mental health. Generally, but not necessarily, people lacking insight into their psychiatric condition also refuse psychiatric treatment, including admission to hospital, drug treatment, psychotherapy, or other forms of clinical management. Treatment refusal may take the form of gracious declinations or outright, sometimes violent, protests.

Good insight is generally a sign of a more favourable illness course (Latalova 2012; Lincoln et al. 2007; Manoli et al. 2021). Empirical research examining the clinical outcomes of people with severe mental illnesses finds that awareness of illness facilitates help-seeking, thus reducing delays of access to pharmacological or non-pharmacological treatment (Albert and Weibell 2019; Ferrara et al. 2021; Freeman et al. 2013; Kaminga et al. 2019). In addition to the assumed benefits of treatment, having good insight may be a sign of possessing better cognitive abilities (Amador and David 2013; David 2020). More recently, it was suggested that good insight is an epiphenomenon of being more generally keen to introspect and being more cognitively flexible. This is indicated with the term of *cognitive insight*, one facet of so-called meta-cognitive skills that also predict better recovery from psychosis (Moritz et al. 2019; Nair et al. 2014).

Better insight, however, might also be accompanied by negative features, namely depression or demoralisation. This phenomenon is known as the 'insight paradox': patients who display better levels of awareness 'paradoxically' present another problem, such as feelings of shame, sadness, and hopelessness (Belvederi Murri and Amore 2018; Belvederi Murri et al. 2015). This should not be considered paradoxical, however, since the realisation of suffering from a mental illness, or just appreciating the psychotic nature of one's beliefs, understandably leads to questioning one's sanity and can lower morale too.

Low mood might take the form of 'post-psychotic depression', a state of angst, hopelessness, and existential crisis that might appear when delusions subside. Post-psychotic depression is a highly debilitating condition, associated with a severe suicide risk, especially among young patients experiencing their first episode of psychosis (Upthegrove et al. 2014). The awareness of suffering from psychotic symptoms may slowly and inexorably dampen self-esteem, paving the way to demoralisation. Demoralisation is linked with disability, loss of purpose, and frustration, and haunts people suffering from all kinds of diseases; mental disorders are no exception (Belvederi Murri et al. 2020; Birchwood et al. 1993; Clarke et al. 2005).

Several authors investigated the reasons why insight can be a double-edged sword: unsurprisingly, detrimental effects on wellbeing seem more frequent among people who tend to stigmatise mental illness, are less optimistic about the effects of treatment, or tend to disengage from mental healthcare providers (Belvederi Murri et al. 2016; Cavelti et al. 2012; Lysaker et al. 2007). This might indicate an overall tendency to *be aware of*, but not to *accept*, mental illness.

Another important interpretation of the link between insight and depression lies in so-called defence theories. From psychodynamic theories onwards, the field of psychology has formalised the notion that knowledge about the world or about oneself can sometimes be too harsh to accept, and would necessarily entail a state of low mood. Denial and other primitive distortions of how we perceive reality would instead serve to maintain euthymia ('normal mood') in the face of adversities. Hence, psychosis could also play a protective role for the self in some situations (Hingley 1997). This view is in line with the effect of depressive realism, when people who are depressed are less biased in the appraisal of some self-related information (Moore and Fresco 2012). Clearly, this effect does not exclude that people with depression may have other cognitive biases that manifest in excessive pessimism (Bortolotti and Antrobus 2015). Having good insight means having a more realistic view of oneself ('these ideas are delusional, after all') at the expense of one's self-esteem ('I am ill', or worse 'I am mad') (Amore et al. 2020). Due to the difficulty of examining unconscious beliefs, few empirical studies have tested these hypotheses empirically, with mixed results (Kruck et al. 2009; Moore et al. 1999). A similar formulation has been proposed where low insight represents a different way of coping (Mcglashan et al. 1975).

To sum up, having good insight is generally good for treatment adherence but might bring depression and demoralisation. This suggests that acquiring insight should be conceived as a delicate process with costs and benefits. Gaining insight is not the end of the story for people who experience or have experienced psychosis: they may need further support to avoid the effects of low mood.

## 3. Accuracy and wellbeing in the traditional and the trade-off view

Traditionally, the capacity to accurately represent and predict reality has been seen as a necessary condition for mental health. The view that people cannot thrive unless they have a good understanding of the world around them has implications for the goals of medicine. For many, an accurate representation of reality is to be pursued as a means to effective functioning (e.g. Jourard and Landsman 1980). An example of the application of the traditional view is the account of depression according to which low mood and a sense of helplessness are due to negative biases in processing information or to false beliefs about lack of control—as seen in the classic work of Aaron Beck (1967) and Martin Seligman (1974). The message is that distortions of reality contribute to poor mental health and, if people could correct those distortions, their mental health would also improve. So good mental health outcomes come from accurate and well-grounded beliefs.

The trade-off view offers an alternative to the traditional view, arguing that the capacity to see the world accurately is not always conducive to better mental health. The claim is that, in some circumstances, reality distortions contribute to mental health. A very widely discussed application of the trade-off view is the discussion of the overall biological and psychological adaptiveness of the optimism bias—as seen in the influential work of Tali Sharot (2011). People who are unrealistically optimistic have all the marks of good mental health and successful agency, whereas those who are more realistic are prone to anxiety and depression. The trade-off view also has implications for the goals of medicine. Mental health is enhanced when the right kind of distortion is introduced or reinstated. For instance, according to Shelley Taylor (1989), people are psychologically healthy when they see things as they would like them to be and their motivation to pursue and achieve their goals is supported by 'positive illusions'. Positive illusions include overly optimistic beliefs about their skills and talents, an inflated sense of control, and a rosier picture of their future than is warranted by the evidence. Such positive illusions are supposed to protect against anxiety and depression. So good mental health outcomes can come from biased and ill-grounded beliefs.

Both the traditional view and the trade-off view seem to have only limited applications in their simplified versions (Bortolotti 2020; Bortolotti et al. 2019). The traditional view is uncomfortable with emerging evidence that neurodivergent ways of thinking and processing information are associated with more accurate representations of reality in some contexts. Examples include the depressive realism effect and the recognition that people with diagnoses of autism and schizophrenia are less vulnerable than controls to certain reasoning biases and framing effects (Brown et al. 2013; Shah et al. 2016).

The trade-off view cannot account for a more nuanced evaluation of the effects of unrealistic optimism on people's mental health. It may be true that accurate evaluations of oneself and reliable predictions of one's future come at the cost of accepting a reality that is somehow sub-optimal and causes low mood in the short run. However, the literature on unrealistic optimism also tells us that some forms of optimism, such as the denial of an existing threat, may invite risk-taking behaviour and have psychological costs in the long run, making people less prepared to face challenges and cope effectively with adversity (Bortolotti and Antrobus 2015; Sweeny et al. 2006).

More to the point, neither the traditional view nor the trade-off view satisfactorily explains the insight paradox. Take J. who is slowly realising that his beliefs about people persecuting him are in fact delusional. The traditional view can capture the value of insight: insight helps J. align his representation of reality with reality itself. But J. experiences depression and demoralisation. The traditional view finds it harder to explain how J.'s coming to grips with reality leads him to despair. The trade-off view can explain why being newly acquainted with the delusional nature of his beliefs makes J. vulnerable to depression and demoralisation but has less to say about the value of insight as an integral part of J.'s recovery. Ultimately, what seems to be problematic in the traditional and trade-off approaches is the overly simplified account of the effects of accurate representations of reality on mental health. For the traditional view, representing reality accurately is a precondition for mental health. For the trade-off view, representing reality accurately is in some contexts an obstacle to mental health. But the phenomenon of the insight paradox tells us that for people with delusions coming to a more accurate representation of reality at the same time contributes to and hinders mental health.

Recent work on the potential biological, psychological, and epistemic benefits of delusions can shed some light on the complexities of the relationship between a good grasp of reality and mental health.

## 4.    The adaptiveness of delusions

Some beliefs involving distortions of reality may be either poorly supported by evidence or incorrigible, or both, and yet have significant benefits for a person that at the time could not be easily attained by other means. Such benefits could be interpreted in terms of biological, psychological, or epistemic adaptiveness (Lancellotta and Bortolotti 2019, 2020).

Recognising the positive role of a person's belief may mean that we don't challenge the belief head-on for the time that we feel it is playing its positive role or that we challenge the belief in gradual and sensitive ways, making sure that the person is supported in the transition from a distorted to a more accurate model of reality. But in the case of delusions, which are widely recognised as pathological beliefs (see Petrolini, Chapter 1), what could be the positive role of the belief? What emergency can a delusion contribute to averting?

Some authors have argued that the delusion has the potential to be biologically adaptive. In some evolutionary accounts, non-bizarre delusions emerged as deceptions serving an important function, namely, responding to the threat of 'severe social failure' (Hagen 2008). An example of social failure is being ostracised by the group and the risk is to lose a mate and have fewer opportunities for reproduction. When this happens, people form beliefs that increase their 'social value': in paranoia, they fathom an external threat to gain people's support and cooperation; in erotomania they make themselves appear more desirable to potential mates. Another explanation that focuses on the relationship between the person and the surrounding environment is that at least some delusions emerge as an attempt to protect the person from the malicious intentions of others and from the costs of life adversities. For instance, being suspicious is beneficial in an environment where our competitors aim to mislead us to access our share of resources, may this be food or mating partners (Gold and Gold 2014).

Another argument for the potential biological adaptiveness of delusions comes from the predictive coding approach. Sarah Fineberg and Philip Corlett (2016) argue that, due to problems with prediction-error signalling, in the prodromal phase of psychosis, the person experiences salient events that are confusing and do not have an explanation. This compromises automated learning and drains attention. The delusional belief is adopted as a default explanation for the unsettling experiences (see Corlett, Chapter 30 for more on prediction error models of delusion). Thus, it enables automated learning to resume and attention to be directed elsewhere. For the authors, this means that delusions serve the function of restoring an interaction with the world that was disrupted by the signalling of prediction errors. Whether the claim that delusions have a role in reinstating automated learning is sufficient to identify a biologically adaptive role for them is debated (see e.g. Lancellotta 2021).

Ryan McKay and Daniel Dennett (2009) deny the potential for the biological adaptiveness of delusions on the basis of the tension that a radical distortion of reality creates in a person's life. Their view is that the delusion may appear as a designed response to overwhelming negative emotions, but its representation of reality is so inaccurate that it cannot support the reproductive and survival interests of the individual. However, a weaker claim that is gaining some traction in some contexts is that delusional beliefs can support a person's psychological and epistemic functionality. That is, delusions enable the person to interact with the surrounding environment in a way that is conducive to overcoming negative emotions and preserving the motivation to pursue their goals by maintaining a sufficiently positive view of the self (Bortolotti 2020).

It is not inconceivable that something that is judged overall as a bad thing also has some redeeming features. Consider as an analogy the legal notion of *innocence defence*. In the UK and US legal contexts, a person may not be deemed as liable for an act that appears to be wrongful if the act prevents serious harm. The act may have been an effective response to an emergency, as in cases of self-defence. If the only way available to us to stop a terrorist from detonating a bomb is to push them to the floor, our physical assault may be condoned in the circumstances. If we apply the notion of innocence-defence to our representations of the world, then we can say that there are circumstances when a belief that distorts reality and is either poorly supported by evidence or incorrigible confers some benefit that cannot be easily gained by adopting a less distorted, a better supported, or a more evidence-responsive belief. A distorted representation of reality, just like physical assault, remains a non-ideal way of dealing with a crisis. But in some junctures, it may be the response that is most readily available to the agent. The belief remains problematic given its failure to represent reality, ill-groundedness, and incorrigibility. Nonetheless, appreciating the belief's positive role helps us understand the disruption that ensues when the belief subsides. This idea has been captured by the claim that delusions, along with some other irrational beliefs, can be *epistemically innocent* (see e.g. Bortolotti 2016; Sullivan-Bissett 2018).

An example that helps us understand the potential for psychological and epistemic adaptiveness is the often-cited Reverse Othello syndrome (Butler 2000; McKay et al. 2005). The Reverse Othello syndrome is described as a *motivated delusion*—a delusion that acts as a defence mechanism, protecting the person from an unpleasant reality—and consists in a person believing that their ex-life partner is still romantically involved with them and faithful to them. A talented musician (B.X.) became severely disabled due to an accident. He formed the delusion that his girlfriend at the time of the accident, who had left him soon after, was still romantically involved with him and had recently become his wife. His clinical team argued that the delusion was playing a protective role, enabling B.X. to come to terms with his new disability by creating the illusion that his romantic life had not be shattered together with his professional life. The team claimed that the delusion helped B.X. cope with negative emotions and cooperate in rehabilitation. Just before B.X. was able to leave hospital, his delusion faded spontaneously. The delusion that the woman he loved was still in a relationship with him enabled B.X. to fend off suicidal thoughts and overcome a very critical moment in his life. Crucially, it provided not only psychological benefits such as relieving anxiety and low mood, but also epistemic ones, enabling the level of engagement with the surrounding environment that was necessary for cooperation with the clinical team and successful rehabilitation.

Does the acknowledgement that some delusional beliefs have a potentially positive role to play help us understand the insight paradox? Take J. coming to believe that the neighbours are spying on him and that he is controlled through his phone. Although these are distressing thoughts to have, for J. they may serve as an explanation of the mysterious coincidences he had recently experienced and serve as a way to impose some meaning on a world that was turning increasingly bleak and confusing to him. In addition, he might feel less alone, or have the sensation of being important to other human beings, although imaginary. Once J. appreciates the delusional nature of his beliefs, he is left to tackle his life difficulties, the exams, and the loneliness, with a new image of himself as someone who is 'mad' and does not have a good grasp on reality.

We could see the insight paradox as a dynamic case of depressive realism. Gaining a more realistic and less distorted belief about the self or the world ('She is no longer my girlfriend and will never be my wife', 'My neighbours are not spying on me') enhances a person's grasp on reality, but compromises the person's self-esteem, especially if the reality to be acquainted with is difficult for the person to accept ('I can no longer make music and I am alone', 'I cannot cope with my exams, and nobody can help me'). But different from the trade-off reading of the depressive realism effect, the reading from the perspective of the adaptiveness of delusions concedes that costs and benefits cannot be straight-forwardly traded and that they are strictly dependent on the context in which the person finds themselves. The delusion ('She is my wife') does not merely have psychological effects: for a time (during rehabilitation), it also contributes to epistemic functionality by enabling the person to respond to a crisis and continue to interact with the world in a meaningful way. And the accurate, realistic interpretation of reality ('She is no longer my girlfriend') does not merely have epistemic benefits, but once the crisis is averted (after rehabilitation) it also contributes to the mind frame that is necessary for the person to live an authentic and flourishing life.

In a typical insight-paradox situation, where a person who recognises the delusional nature of their beliefs becomes depressed and demoralised, what might be happening is that insight wipes out an emergency response to a crisis before the person is ready to cope with the crisis itself. That is, the delusion is left behind, but there is nothing else in its place that can play a positive function by supporting the person's psychological and epistemic functionality. In Butler's Reverse Othello syndrome case, one might argue that B.X. did not experience depression and demoralisation at the time of relinquishing the delusion, because he had already accepted his disability, had regained self-esteem by successfully engaging in rehabilitation, and had something to look forward to, that is, leaving the hospital and attaining self-sufficiency.

In the case of J., the realisation that his persecutory beliefs were not an accurate representation of reality comes at a point where he is not ready to go back to his life challenges because he has no confidence in himself being able to face them. The solution is not to reinstate the delusion but to support J. to develop better coping mechanisms so he can rely on a more positive sense of himself.


## 5.  Implications for clinical practice and conclusions

In this chapter, we considered the claim that clinical delusions can be adaptive through the lens of the insight paradox. Delusions are undeniably distressing for those who experience them and are regarded in popular culture as the most extreme and inexplicable form of irrationality. However, a more nuanced assessment of their role in a person's life can help us understand better what support people with delusions need at different stages of their illness.

Delusions are an important test case for the idea that madness is not (merely) a dysfunction but (also) a strategy. Justin Garson (2022) reconstructs the fascinating history of madness pointing out how in some authors and traditions of thought mental illness is characterised mechanistically as the failure of a process to work as it should. However, in the work of other authors and traditions of thought, mental illness is explained teleologically as a response to a crisis. Sigmund Freud (1911), for instance, stated that 'delusional formation, which we take to be the pathological product, is in reality an attempt at recovery, a process of reconstruction'. What would it mean to take the approach of 'madness-as-strategy' seriously?

When people start appreciating the delusional nature of their beliefs and gain insight into their mental illness, they can be affected by severe depression and demoralisation. If delusional beliefs were merely the harmful output of a dysfunctional process, realising their delusional nature and giving them up should be a positive development, ensuring better treatment adherence and long-term clinical outcomes. However, the risk of severe depression and demoralisation which increases when the delusion subsides suggests that the delusion may be adaptive in some sense. We saw that the prospects for delusion to be biologically adaptive are uncertain, but delusions may play some local and temporary role in supporting psychological and epistemic functionality, enabling the person to respond to a crisis. The delusion may help overcome negative emotions by constructing a more desirable version of reality or may help make sense of puzzling events by providing an all-things considered implausible but fitting explanation of what the person experiences.

The explanation we have proposed for the insight paradox can inform some responses to it, and in particular clinical efforts to support people who are gaining insight into their beliefs being delusional. If a belief that is subsiding has a positive psychological and epistemic function to play, then something else needs to be in its place to support the person to interact successfully with the surrounding environment.

Clinically, in Freudian terms, insight starts the process of 'mourning'—a re-elaboration that is necessary for the patient to come to terms with their new reality and to find new sources of hope as much as possible. Thomas H. Mcglashan et al. (1975) have provided the paradigm of 'recovery styles' for a comprehensive description of how patients cope with the occurrence of psychosis. In particular, the style of 'integration', unlike 'sealing over', indicates those cases where the person can coherently elaborate the changes of the self that are derived from acknowledging their illness, bearing the weight of painful realisations that accompany this delicate process. Recovery styles, however, may not just reflect the individual condition but may also be particularly sensitive to the surrounding context. Not surprisingly, people with good insight seem at higher risk of depression if they have lower socioeconomic status, more severe illness, and worse service engagement (Belvederi Murri et al. 2016).

The clinical implications people have drawn from the insight paradox are compatible with viewing the fading delusions as an (imperfect) emergency response to a crisis. Gaining insight is a process during which the person needs to receive support, for instance in the form of psychotherapy or psychoeducation. Such interventions should be carefully timed, delivered in the context of a good therapeutic relationship, and centred on the person's values and culture. Narrative psychotherapeutic approaches seem particularly fit to promote re-elaboration on the meaning of psychosis within the framework of the individual life trajectory, thus ensuring that insight dampens the person's self-esteem as little as possible. In some cases, psychotherapy may even prevent the acquisition of insight from turning into an existential crisis without hope (Lopez-Morinigo et al. 2020; Pijnenborg et al. 2013).

# References


Albert, N. and Weibell, M.A. (2019). The outcome of early intervention in first episode psychosis. *International Review of Psychiatry* 31 (5–6): 413–424.

Amador, X.F. and David A.S. (2013). *Insight and Psychosis*. Oxford: Oxford University Press.

Amore, M., Belvederi Murri, M., Calcagno, P., et al. (2020). The association between insight and depressive symptoms in schizophrenia: Undirected and Bayesian network analyses. *European Psychiatry* 63 (1): E46.

Beck, A.T. (1967). *Depression: Causes and Treatment*. Philadelphia: University of Pennsylvania Press.

Belvederi Murri, M. and Amore, M. (2018). The multiple dimensions of insight in schizophrenia-spectrum disorders. *Schizophrenia Bulletin* 45 (2): 277–283.

Belvederi Murri, M., Amore, M., Calcagno, P., et al. (2016). The "insight paradox" in schizophrenia: Magnitude, moderators and mediators of the association between insight and depression. *Schizophrenia Bulletin* 42 (5): 1225–1233.

Belvederi Murri, M., Caruso, R., Ounalli, H., et al. (2020). The relationship between demoralization and depressive symptoms among patients from the general hospital: Network and exploratory graph analysis: Demoralization and depression symptom network. *Journal of Affective Disorders* 276: 137–146.

Belvederi Murri, M., Respino, M., Innamorati, M., et al. (2015). Is good insight associated with depression among patients with schizophrenia? Systematic review and meta-analysis. *Schizophrenia Research* 162: 234–247.

Benrimoh, D.A. and Friston, K.J. (2020). All grown up: Computational theories of psychosis, complexity, and progress. *Journal of Abnormal Psychology* 129 (6): 624–628.

Birchwood, M., Mason, R., MacMillan, F., et al. (1993). Depression, demoralization and control over psychotic illness: A comparison of depressed and non-depressed patients with a chronic psychosis. *Psychological Medicine* 23: 387–395.

Bortolotti, L. (2016). Epistemic benefits of elaborated and systematised delusions in schizophrenia. *British Journal for the Philosophy of Science* 67 (3): 879–900.

Bortolotti, L. (2020). *The Epistemic Innocence of Irrational Beliefs*. Oxford: Oxford University Press.

Bortolotti, L. and Antrobus, M. (2015). Costs and benefits of realism and optimism. *Current Opinion in Psychiatry* 28 (2): 194–198.

Bortolotti, L., Sullivan-Bissett, E. and Antrobus, M. (2019). The epistemic innocence of optimistically biased beliefs. In M. Balcerak Jackson and B. Balcerak Jackson (eds.) *Reasoning: Essays on Theoretical and Practical Thinking* (Chapter 12). Oxford: Oxford University Press, pages 232–247.

Brown, J.K., Waltz, J.A., Strauss, G.P., McMahon, R.P., Frank, M.J. and Gold, J.M. (2013). Hypothetical decision making in schizophrenia: The role of expected value computation and "irrational" biases. *Psychiatry Research* 209 (2): 142–149.

Butler, P.V. (2000). Reverse othello syndrome subsequent to traumatic brain injury. *Psychiatry* 63 (1): 85–92.

Cavelti, M., Kvrgic, S., Beck, E.-M., et al. (2012). Self-stigma and its relationship with insight, demoralization, and clinical outcome among people with schizophrenia spectrum disorders. *Comprehensive Psychiatry* 53 (5): 468–479.

Clarke, D.M., Kissane, D.W., Trauer, T., et al. (2005). Demoralization, anhedonia and grief in patients with severe physical illness. *World Psychiatry* 4: 96–105.

David, A.S. (2020). Insight and psychosis: The next 30 years. *British Journal of Psychiatry* 217: 521–523.

Ferrara, M., Guloksuz, S., Mathis, W.S., et al. (2021). First help-seeking attempt before and after psychosis onset: Measures of delay and aversive pathways to care. *Social Psychiatry and Psychiatric Epidemiology* 56 (8): 1359–1369.

Fineberg, S.K. and Corlett, P.R. (2016). The doxastic shear pin: Delusions as errors of learning and memory. *Cognitive Neuropsychiatry* 21 (1): 73–89.

Freeman, D., Dunn, G., Garety, P., et al. (2013). Patients' beliefs about the causes, persistence and control of psychotic experiences predict take-up of effective cognitive behaviour therapy for psychosis. *Psychological Medicine* 43: 269–277.

Freud, S. (1911). Psychoanalytic notes on an autobiographical account of a case of paranoia (Dementia Paranoides). In Translated from the German by J. Strachey in collaboration with A Freud. Vol. XII. *The Standard Edition of the Complete Psychological Works of Sigmund Freud*. London: Vintage, 1999.

Garson, J. (2022). *Madness: A Philosophical Exploration*. New York: Oxford University Press.

Gold, J. and Gold, I. (2014). *Suspicious Minds*. New York: Free Press.

Hagen, E.H. (2008). Non-bizarre delusions as strategic deceptions. In S. Elton and P. O'Higgins (eds.) *Medicine and Evolution: Current Applications, Future Prospects*. London Routledge: CRC Press, Chapter 9, pages 181–216.

Hingley, S.M. (1997). Psychodynamic perspectives on psychosis and psychotherapy I: Theory. *British Journal of Medical Psychology* 70: 301–312.

Jourard, S.M. and Landsman, T. (1980). *Healthy Personality: An Approach from the Viewpoint of Humanistic Psychology*. New York: Macmillan.

Kaminga, A.C., Dai, W., Liu, A., et al. (2019). Effects of socio-demographic characteristics, premorbid functioning, and insight on duration of untreated psychosis in first-episode schizophrenia or schizophreniform disorder in Northern Malawi. *Early Intervention in Psychiatry* 13 (6): 1455–1464.

Kruck, C.L., Flashman, L.A., Roth, R.M., et al. (2009). Lack of relationship between psychological denial and unawareness of illness in schizophrenia-spectrum disorders. *Psychiatry Research* 169: 33–38.

Lancellotta, E. (2021). Is the biological adaptiveness of delusions doomed? *Review of Philosophy and Psychology*. https://doi.org/10.1007/s13164-021-00545-6

Lancellotta, E. and Bortolotti, L. (2019). Are delusions adaptive? *WIREs in the Cognitive Sciences* 10 (5): e1502.

Lancellotta, E. and Bortolotti, L. (2020). Delusions in the two-factor theory: Pathological or adaptive? *European Journal of Analytic Philosophy* 16 (2): 37–57.

Latalova, K. (2012). Insight in bipolar disorder. *The Psychiatric Quarterly* 83 (3): 293–310.

Lincoln, T.M., Lullmann, E. and Rief, W. (2007). Correlates and long-term consequences of poor insight in patients with schizophrenia. A systematic review. *Schizophrenia Bulletin* 33 (6): 1324–1342.

Lopez-Morinigo, J.D., Ajnakina, O., Martínez, A.S., et al. (2020). Can metacognitive interventions improve insight in schizophrenia spectrum disorders? A systematic review and meta-analysis. *Psychological Medicine* 50 (14): 2289–2301.

Lysaker, P.H., Roe, D. and Yanos, P.T. (2007). Toward understanding the insight paradox: Internalized stigma moderates the association between insight and social functioning, hope, and self-esteem among people with schizophrenia spectrum disorders. *Schizophrenia Bulletin* 33: 192–199.

Manoli, R., Cervello, S. and Franck, N. (2021). Impact of insight and metacognition on vocational rehabilitation of individuals with severe mental illness: A systematic review. *Psychiatric Rehabilitation Journal* 44 (4): 337–353.

Mcglashan, T.H., Levy, S.T. and Carpenter, W.T. (1975). Integration and sealing over: Clinically distinct recovery styles from schizophrenia. *Archives of General Psychiatry* 32: 1269–1272.

McKay, R.T. and Dennett, D.C. (2009). The evolution of misbelief. *Behavioral and Brain Sciences* 32 (6): 493–510.

McKay, R., Langdon, R. and Coltheart, M. (2005). "Sleights of mind": Delusions, defences and self-deception. *Cognitive Neuropsychiatry* 10 (4): 305–326.

Moore, M.T. and Fresco, D.M. (2012). Depressive realism: A meta-analytic review. *Clinical Psychology Review* 32: 496–509.

Moore, O., Cassidy, E., Carr, A., et al. (1999). Unawareness of illness and its relationship with depression and self-deception in schizophrenia. *European Psychiatry* 14: 264–269.

Moritz, S., Klein, J., Lysaker, P.H., et al. (2019). Metacognitive and cognitive-behavioral interventions for psychosis: New developments. *Dialogues in Clinical Neuroscience* 21: 309–317.

Nair, A., Palmer, E.C., Aleman, A., et al. (2014). Relationship between cognition, clinical and cognitive insight in psychotic disorders: A review and meta-analysis. *Schizophrenia Research* 152: 191–200.

Pijnenborg, G.H., van Donkersgoed, R.J., David, A.S., et al. (2013). Changes in insight during treatment for psychotic disorders: A meta-analysis. *Schizophrenia Research* 144 (1–3): 109–117.

Seligman, M.E. (1974). *Depression and Learned Helplessness*. Oxford: John Wiley & Sons.

Shah, P., Catmur, C. and Bird, G. (2016). Emotional decision-making in autism spectrum disorder: The roles of interoception and alexithymia. *Molecular Autism* 7: 43.

Sharot, T. (2011). The optimism bias. *Current Biology* 21 (23): R941–R945.

Sullivan-Bissett, E. (2018). Monothematic delusions. A case of innocence from experience. *Philosophical Psychology* 31 (6): 920–947.

Sweeny, K., Carroll, P.J. and Shepperd, J.A. (2006). Is optimism always best? Future outlooks and preparedness. *Current Directions in Psychological Science* 15 (6): 302–306.

Taylor, S.E. (1989). *Positive Illusions: Creative Self-Deception and the Healthy Mind*. New York: Basic Books.

Upthegrove, R., Ross, K., Brunet, K., et al. (2014). Depression in first episode psychosis: The role of subordination and shame. *Psychiatry Research* 217: 177–184.

# 4

# DELUSION AND MALFUNCTION

*Kengo Miyazono*

## 1. Introduction

This chapter discusses the idea of delusions as malfunctioning beliefs. This idea, which is called 'malfunction doxasticism' in this chapter, consists of two claims; that delusions are beliefs (e.g. Bayne & Pacherie 2005; Bortolotti 2009, 2012) and that delusions are malfunctioning (e.g. McKay & Dennett 2009; Miyazono 2015). As we will see below, both claims are philosophically and empirically controversial, and addressing these controversies is part of the aim of this chapter.

Malfunction doxasticism is based on an analogy between a delusion and a diseased internal organ such as a diseased kidney. On the one hand, a diseased kidney is a kidney, or it belongs to the category of kidney; it has the functions in terms of which the category of kidney is individuated (e.g. the function of filtering metabolic wastes from blood). On the other hand, the diseased kidney is malfunctioning; it fails to perform some of its functions (e.g. fails to filter metabolic wastes from blood). Analogously, on the one hand, a delusion is a belief, or it belongs to the category of belief; it has the functions in terms of which the category of belief is individuated (e.g. the function of representing states of affairs). On the other hand, the delusion is malfunctioning; it fails to perform some of its functions (e.g. fails to represent states of affairs).

My discussion will proceed as follows. In Section 2, I introduce two questions about delusions; the Nature Question (which is about what kind of mental state a delusion is) and the Pathology Question (which is about what makes a delusion a pathological mental state). Answers to the Nature Question can be divided into two groups; doxasticism (which regards delusions as beliefs) and non-doxasticism (which regards delusions as some non-doxastic mental states). As we will see, both doxastcism and non-doxasticism face prima facie difficulties in answering the Pathology Question. In Section 3, I present malfunction doxasticism and show how it answers the Nature Question and the Pathology Question. With regard to the Nature Question (Section 4), malfunction doxasticism implies that delusions are beliefs. Malfunction doxasticism is committed to teleo-functionalism (e.g. Sober 1985; Lycan, 1987; Sterelny, 1990) about belief, which supports the doxastic idea that delusions are beliefs because they have the right kind of functions. With regard

73        DOI: 10.4324/9781003296386-6

to the Pathology Question (Section 5), malfunction doxasticism implies that delusions are malfunctioning, which explains the pathological nature of delusions. Malfunction doxasticism is committed to the harmful-dysfunction analysis of disorders (e.g. Wakefield 1992a, 1992b), which supports the idea that delusions are pathological because they involve (harmful) dysfunctions or malfunctions. ('Dysfunction' and 'malfunction' are interchangeable in this chapter.)

## 2. Nature and pathology

*The Nature Question*: What kind of mental state is a delusion? Answers to this question can be classified into two groups; doxasticism (e.g. Bayne & Pacherie 2005; Bortolotti 2009, 2012; Clutton 2018; Miyazono 2018; Flores 2021; Bongiorno 2022) and non-doxasticism (e.g. Berrios 1991; Currie 2000; Currie & Jureidini 2001; Currie & Ravenscroft 2002; Egan 2009; Tumulty 2011; Hohwy & Rajan 2012; Schwitzgebel 2012; Dub 2017). According to the former, delusions are beliefs; i.e. a person with the delusion with the content P *believes* that P. According to the latter, delusions are some non-doxastic mental states; i.e. a person with the delusion that P is *in a non-doxastic mental state* (e.g. the state of imagining, the state of accepting) with the content P. Doxasticism is the default position in psychiatry. The definitions of delusion in psychiatry, in diagnostic manuals, textbooks, and research papers, presuppose doxasticism.[1] However, delusions have a number of peculiar features that are not belief-like, including the insensitivity to evidence (i.e. compared to non-delusional beliefs, delusions are remarkably insensitive to evidence) (see Flores, Chapter 12 for more on delusion and evidence) or the incoherence with non-verbal behaviour (i.e. unlike a person with the belief that P, a person with the delusion that P sometimes fail to behave as if P is the case) (see Tumulty, Chapter 18 for more on delusion and action). Non-doxasticism is motivated by the observation of these peculiar features.

*The Pathology Question*: What makes a delusion a pathological mental state?[2] What distinguishes pathological delusions (such as the grandiose delusion that God gives you the special ability to predict future events) from mundane irrational beliefs (such as the mundane irrational optimism that you are better than average drivers)?[3] A possible answer would be that the delusions are more irrational than mundane irrational beliefs. The mundane optimism about driving skills are irrational, but the grandiose delusion about predicting future events is significantly more irrational, which makes it pathological. Another possible view would be that delusions are more harmful than mundane irrational beliefs. The mundane optimism about driving skills can enhance self-esteem, while the grandiose delusion about predicting future events, despite its grandiose content, can bring worries, anxieties, preoccupations, etc., which makes it pathological (see Petrolini, Chapter 1 for more on delusion and pathology).

The Nature Question and the Pathology Question jointly constitute a challenge, which can be summarised as follows. With regard to the Nature Question, we adopt either doxasticism or anti-doxasticism. Either way, we face a prima facie difficulty in answering the Pathology Question.

Doxasticists regard delusions (such as the grandiose delusion about predicting future events) and mundane irrational beliefs (such as the mundane optimism about driving skills) as continuous such that they belong to the same mental category (i.e. the category of belief). In her defence of doxasticism, Lisa Bortolotti writes: 'there is continuity between everyday beliefs and clinical delusions. Clinical delusions are typically irrational to a greater extent or irrational across more dimensions than non-delusional beliefs, but they are irrational in roughly the same way' (Bortolotti 2012: 39). This raises a question with regard to the Pathology Question: Why are delusions pathological if they are continuous with mundane irrational beliefs? What distinguishes pathological delusions from mundane irrational beliefs? (Petrolini 2017, Petrolini, Chapter 1).[4] The explanatory task for doxasticists seems to be challenging. On the one hand, they need to identify the continuity between delusions and mundane irrational beliefs in virtue of which they belong to the same mental category and, on the other hand, explain why, unlike mundane irrational beliefs, delusions are pathological despite the continuity between the former and the latter.

Bortolotti (2009) is aware of this explanatory challenge. She tentatively suggests that delusions are pathological because they have significant negative impact on wellbeing:

> One possibility is that delusions are pathological in that they negatively affect the well-being and the health of the subjects who report them (as many have already argued). Irrational beliefs that are not delusions seem less distressing, and don't seem to exhaust the cognitive resources of the subjects in the same way delusions do.
>
> *(Bortolotti 2009: 260)*

In more recent work, Bortolotti (2020b, 2022) explores a different response to the explanatory challenge; she rejects the project of giving a coherent account of what makes delusions pathological, and insists that delusions can be a proper target of medical attention and medical care regardless of whether they are pathological.

Non-doxasticists, in contrast, regard delusions and mundane irrational beliefs as discontinuous such that they belong to different mental categories (e.g. the latter belong to the category of belief, while the former belong to the category of imagining). In his defence of non-doxasticism, Andy Egan (2009) writes: 'Categorizing delusions as straightforward cases of belief faces some pretty serious obstacles. The role that delusions play in their subjects' cognitive economies differs pretty dramatically from the role that we'd expect beliefs to play' (Egan 2009: 266). This raises a question with regard to the Pathology Question: Why are delusions pathological if they are discontinuous from non-delusional beliefs such that they are excluded from the category of belief? Delusions are (regarded as) pathological partly because they are (regarded as) beliefs. For instance, the grandiose delusion about predicting future events is (regarded as) pathological partly because the grandiose delusion is (regarded as) a belief. We regard it as pathological because, we assume, there is something pathological in seriously *believing* that God gives you the special ability to predict future events. (In contrast, probably there is nothing pathological in *imagining* or *hoping* that God gives you the special ability to predict future events.) The explanatory task for non-doxasticists seems to be challenging too, but for a different reason. On the one hand, they need to identify the discontinuity between delusions and non-delusional beliefs in virtue of which delusions are excluded from the category of belief and, on the other hand, explain why delusions are pathological despite that they are excluded from the category of belief.

Gregory Currie and colleagues (Currie 2000; Currie & Jureidini 2001; Currie & Ravenscroft 2002), who argue that delusions are imaginings, face the challenge of explaining why, for instance, the grandiose delusion about predicting future events is pathological; on the face of it, there is nothing pathological in *imagining* that God gives you the special ability to predict future events. I can easily imagine, without compromising my mental health, that

God gives me the special ability to predict future events.[5] Egan (2009), who argues that delusions are bimaginings (i.e. the intermediate states with some belief-like features and some imagining-like features), faces a similar challenge of explaining why, for instance, the grandiose delusion about predicting future events is pathological; it is unclear whether there is something pathological in *bimagining* that God gives you the special ability to predict future events. Tim Bayne and Jordi Fernández express a similar worry about Egan's proposal:

> Theorizing about delusion (and, to a lesser extent, self-deception) typically begins with the thought that these states are pathological beliefs – they violate certain norms of belief-formation. It is unclear how Egan's account might accommodate this thought, for nothing can be a pathological belief unless it is also a belief.
>
> *(Bayne & Fernández 2009: 17)*

## 3.  Malfunction doxasticism

### *3.1  Basic ideas*

As I noted in Section 2, the explanatory challenge for doxasticists is this: with regard to the Nature Question, they need to identify the continuity between delusions and mundane irrational beliefs in virtue of which, just like the latter, the former are regarded as beliefs and, with respect to the Pathology Question, identify the discontinuity between delusions and mundane irrational beliefs in virtue of which, unlike the latter, the former are pathological. Malfunction doxasticism provides us with an attractive response to this challenge.

To see how malfunction doxasticism works, let us first think about diseased kidneys. On the one hand, diseased kidneys are kidneys; and thus there has to be some continuity between diseased kidneys and healthy kidneys in virtue of which, just like the latter, the former are regarded as kidneys. On the other hand, diseased kidneys are pathological; and thus there has to be some discontinuity between diseased kidneys and healthy kidneys in virtue of which, unlike the latter, the former are pathological. What exactly are the 'continuity between diseased kidneys and healthy kidneys in virtue of which, just like the latter, the former are regarded as kidneys' and the 'discontinuity between diseased kidneys and healthy kidneys in virtue of which, unlike the latter, the former are pathological'?

Here is a possible answer to these questions. Diseased kidneys are malfunctioning kidneys; i.e. they *have* some functions that they *fail to perform* (see Section 3.2 for more about functions). On the one hand, diseased kidneys are kidneys because they *have* the right kind of functions (e.g. the function of filtering metabolic wastes from blood). In other words, having the right kind of functions is the 'continuity between diseased kidneys and healthy kidneys in virtue of which, just like the latter, the former are regarded as kidneys'. On the other hand, diseased kidneys are pathological (partly) because they *fail to perform* some of their functions (e.g. fail to filter metabolic wastes from blood). In other words, failing to perform some of their functions is (part of) the 'discontinuity between diseased kidneys and healthy kidneys in virtue of which, unlike the latter, the former are pathological'.

Let us now think about delusions. On the one hand, delusions are beliefs (at least according to doxasticism); and thus there has to be some continuity between delusions and mundane irrational beliefs in virtue of which, just like the latter, the former are regarded as beliefs. On the other hand, delusions are pathological; and thus there has to be some discontinuity between delusions and mundane irrational beliefs in virtue of which, unlike the latter, the former are pathological. What exactly are the 'continuity between delusions and mundane irrational beliefs in virtue of which, just like the latter, the former are regarded as beliefs' and the 'discontinuity between delusions and mundane irrational beliefs in virtue of which, unlike the latter, the former are pathological'?

According to malfunction doxasticism, delusions are malfunctioning beliefs; i.e. they *have* some functions that they *fail to perform*. On the one hand, delusions are beliefs because they *have* the right kind of functions. In other words, having the right kind of functions is the 'continuity between delusions and mundane irrational beliefs in virtue of which, just like the latter, the former are regarded as beliefs'. This is the answer to the Nature Question by malfunction doxasticism (see Section 4 for more details). On the other hand, delusions are pathological (partly) because they *fail to perform* some of their functions. In other words, failing to perform some of their functions is (part of) the 'discontinuity between delusions and mundane irrational beliefs in virtue of which, unlike the latter, the former are pathological'. This is the answer to the Pathology Question by malfunction doxasticism (see Section 5 for more details).

## 3.2 *Function and malfunction*

Some clarifications on 'function' and 'malfunction' are necessary.

In this chapter, the term 'function' is used in an etiological sense (Millikan 1984, 1989a; Neander 1991a, 1991b); i.e. the functions of X (or the functions X has) are the effects, consequences, or performances for which X has been selected in evolutionary history. Having a particular function, etiologically defined, is a historical property. Having the function of filtering metabolic wastes from blood, for instance, is a historical property; i.e. the property of having some ancestors that were selected in evolutionary history for filtering metabolic wastes from blood. Malfunction can be understood as a case in which something *has* a particular function (where 'having a function' is understood as having the right kind of history) and *fails to perform* the function (where 'performing a function' is understood as behaving in the right kind of way).[6] For instance, a malfunctioning kidney *has* the function of filtering metabolic wastes from blood (because it has the right kind of history) and *fails to perform* the function (because it does not behave in the right kind of way).

The etiological account of function, thus, can easily make sense of malfunction,[7] which is often taken to be an advantage of the etiological account (especially in the context of accounting for misrepresentation: Millikan 1984, 1989b; Neander 1995). In this chapter, we do not go into the 'function debate' between the etiological and other accounts of functions, including the systemic account (Cummins 1975, 1983) and the modal account (Nanay 2010, 2014). The function debate often focuses on the analysis of the concept 'function' that is actually used in the field of biology (e.g. Neander 1991b). We can be neutral on this issue for our purpose. We can simply adopt an etiological notion of 'function', not necessarily because the concept 'function' in the field of biology is an etiological one, but rather because the etiological notion is useful for our theoretical purpose; i.e. the purpose of understanding delusions. We can follow Ruth Millikan's (1989a) pragmatism according to which we adopt an etiological notion of function 'mainly to gather together certain phenomena under a heading or category that can be used productively in the construction of various explanatory theories', and 'the ultimate defense of such a definition can only be a series of illustration of its usefulness' (Millikan 1989a: 289).

## 4.  Delusions as beliefs

Delusions are beliefs, according to malfunction doxasticism, because they *have* the right kind of functions. This claim presupposes a teleo-functionalist idea that the category of belief is individuated by functions.

Following Peter Godfrey-Smith (1998), we can distinguish two forms of functionalism: dry-functionalism and teleo-functionalism. According to the former, mental states are individuated by the causal roles that they play (or are disposed to play), where 'causal roles' of a mental state are the roles the state plays in its causal interaction with (sensory) inputs, (behavioural) outputs, and other mental states. According to the latter, mental states are individuated by the functions they have, where 'functions' of a mental state are the effects, consequences, or performances for which the state has been selected in evolutionary history.[8]

Dry-functionalism and teleo-functionalism have different implications for the Nature Question. Indeed, many non-doxasticists adopt some form of dry-functionalism (e.g. Currie & Jureidini 2001; Egan 2009; Tumulty 2011; Schwitzgebel 2012). According to dry-functionalism, the category of belief is individuated by causal roles; to be a belief is to play belief-like causal roles. Delusions, however, do not seem to play belief-like causal roles. As we noted above, delusions have a number of peculiar features that are not belief-like, including the remarkable insensitivity to evidence or the incoherence with non-verbal behaviour. This seems to suggest that dry-functionalism supports non-doxasticism (the 'functional role argument' against doxasticism; Bayne 2011).

Teleo-functionalism, in contrast, opens up a different perspective on the Nature Question. According to teleo-functionalism, the category of belief is individuated by functions; to be a belief is to have the right kind of functions (or, to have the right kind of history). As we will see below, it can be argued that delusions have the right kind of functions (or, have the right kind of history) and thus belong to the category of belief.

Here is the crucial question for malfunction doxasticists: How do we know that delusions have the right kind of functions? This question can be divided into two sub-questions: (1) What are the 'right kind of functions', exactly? (2) How do we know that delusions have those functions?

Let us begin with the first question, which is about what 'the right kind of functions' are. A reasonable starting point would be F. P. Ramsey's (1931) famous statement that a belief is 'a map of neighbouring space by which we steer'. Ramsey's analogy between beliefs and maps suggests that beliefs, just like maps, are supposed to represent something accurately. And his statement that we steer by beliefs suggests that beliefs, just like maps, are supposed to guide our actions. A proposal, then, is that the functions of beliefs include the function representing accurately and the function of guiding actions.

However, the idea of beliefs having the function of representing accurately is controversial. As Stephen Stich notes, 'natural selection does not care about truth; it cares only about reproductive success' (Stich 1990: 62). The idea of beliefs having the function of representing accurately is relatively plausible when it comes to some factual beliefs, including the beliefs about whether predators are nearby or not, or beliefs about whether a mushroom is edible or not, where accurate representing is conducive to reproductive success. However, it is less plausible when it comes to other beliefs where accurate representing is not tied to reproductive success very closely. For instance, it is not very likely that the function of religious beliefs or moral judgments is to represent religious entities or mind-independent moral truths accurately. Their function is more likely to be related to coordinating people and regulating their behaviour. Again, accurate representation might not be the function of self-appraisals. Ryan McKay and Daniel Dennett (2009) maintain that positive illusions (i.e. unrealistically positive self-appraisals) are 'adaptive misbeliefs'; in other words, they are false beliefs that are adaptive in themselves.

For our purpose, we can set aside these controversies about the functions of belief. It turns out that identifying the functions of belief is not necessary for answering the second question. It is possible to show that delusions have the right kind of functions (the second question) without identifying exactly what the 'right kind of functions' are (the first question).

We need two assumptions here. The first assumption is that non-delusional beliefs, the ones that are uncontroversially classified in the category of belief, have the right kind of functions, whatever they are. Otherwise, teleo-functionalism would be radically revisionary; i.e. it has the implausible implication that non-delusional beliefs that are uncontroversially classified as beliefs are excluded from the category of belief. The second assumption is that the functions of mental states (such as the functions of belief) are derived from the functions of underlying mechanisms (Millikan 1984). For instance, a mental state's function of representing accurately is derived from an underlying mechanism's function of producing accurate representations.

With the first assumption, we can show that delusions have the right kind of functions by revealing that delusions and non-delusional beliefs share the same functions, whatever they are. And with the second assumption, we can show that delusions and non-delusional beliefs share the same functions by showing that delusions and non-delusional beliefs share the same underlying mechanisms; i.e. both delusions and non-delusional beliefs are produced and consumed by the same set of cognitive mechanisms.

Thus, we can show that delusions have the right kind of functions, without specifying what they are, by showing that delusions and non-delusional beliefs share the same underlying mechanisms. Now, the empirical research of delusion formation strongly supports the idea that delusions and non-delusional beliefs are produced by the same underlying mechanisms. The empirical research supports the idea, called 'empiricism' (Bayne & Pacherie 2004, see Bongiorno & Parrott, Chapter 26 for more on empiricism), that delusions are formed, in response to some abnormal experience, processed in (roughly) the same way that normal experience is processed in the case of non-delusional belief formation. There are different versions of empiricism. For example, the one-factor theory (e.g. Maher, 1974; Sakakibara 2019; Sullivan-Bissett 2020; Noordhof & Sullivan-Bissett 2021, 2023, Sullivan-Bissett, Chapter 28) is consistent with the idea that the producer mechanism is functioning properly both in producing non-delusional beliefs and in producing delusions. In contrast, the two-factor theory (e.g. Davies et al., 2001; Coltheart, 2007; Coltheart et al. 2010; Coltheart et al., 2011; Davies & Coltheart, Chapter 29) is consistent with the idea that the producer mechanism is functioning properly in producing non-delusional beliefs but malfunctioning in producing delusions (but see Bortolotti 2020b, 2022; Lancellotta & Bortolotti 2020). Either way, empiricism supports the idea that delusions and non-delusional beliefs are produced by the same underlying (functioning or malfunctioning) mechanisms.

## 5.  Delusions as malfunctions

### *5.1  Harmfulness thesis*

Delusions are malfunctioning, according to malfunction doxasticism, which explains the fact that delusions are pathological. More precisely, delusions are pathological because they involve harmful malfunctions. This claim depends on Jerome Wakefield's harmful dysfunction analysis (HDA; Wakefield 1992a, 1992b), according to which disorders are harmful dysfunctions or malfunctions.

HDA regards disorders as harmful dysfunctions. They are harmful in the sense that they have a negative impact on well-being, and they are dysfunctions in the sense that they involve a failure of performing functions. A kidney disease, for instance, is harmful in the sense that it has a negative impact on wellbeing, and it is a dysfunction in the sense that it involves a failure of performing the function of filtering metabolic wastes from blood. Analogously, according to malfunction doxasticism, a delusion is harmful in the sense that it has a negative impact on wellbeing (let us call this the 'harmfulness thesis'), and it is a dysfunction in the sense that it involves a failure of performing relevant functions (let us call this the 'malfunction thesis') (Miyazono 2015, 2018).[9]

According to the harmfulness thesis, a delusion is harmful in the sense that it has a negative impact on well-being. Delusions negatively influence the well-being of people with delusions in many ways; e.g. a person might be stressed and anxious because of her delusion of reference that strangers in a bus are always talking about her; a person might lose his dream job because of his persecutory delusion that his co-workers are harassing him, etc.

One might think, however, that some delusions, such as the grandiose delusion, are not harmful at all; e.g. a person with the grandiose delusion is perfectly happy with the thought that God gave him a special ability to predict future events. I have two responses to this. First, a delusion might cause harm to others rather than to the person with the delusion. Even if the person himself is not harmed by his grandiose delusion, people around him, such as family members, friends, colleagues, or neighbours, can be harmed by it. Second, the harmful aspect of delusions might not be captured in terms of hedonistic factors such as pains or pleasures. For instance, the life with the grandiose delusion can be pleasurable, at least for a while, from a hedonistic point of view (which is analogous to the fact that the life in Nozick's experience machine is pleasurable from a hedonistic point of view); still his delusion can be described as being harmful.

Bortolotti, whose recent work focuses on the psychological and epistemic benefits of delusional and irrational beliefs (Bortolotti 2015, 2016, 2020a), is sceptical about the harmfulness thesis (Bortolotti 2022; see also Lancellotta & Bortolotti 2020). She argues that 'for a belief to count as pathological, the belief itself should be the cause of the harm' (Bortolotti 2022: 7), but that delusional beliefs themselves are not the cause of the harm; rather they can be conceived as a psychologically adaptive response to some prior harmful events. She also argues that one's state of having some delusions is not more harmful than one's counterfactual state of having no delusions (in some close possible worlds);

> for some people at least, life without the delusion may be difficult in a different way, not always less difficult, than life with the delusion. The delusion may have enabled them to keep at bay some negative feelings that are ready to reemerge when the delusion fades if adequate support is not offered.
>
> *(Bortolotti 2022: 8)*

I do not think, however, that Bortolotti's claims undermine the harmfulness thesis (see Miyazono 2022 for a more detailed discussion). First, it is one thing to say that delusions are harmful (which is endorsed by the harmfulness thesis), and it is another to say that delusions are the causal source of the harm (which is not endorsed by the harmfulness thesis). The former can still be true even if the latter is false; e.g. the state of having delusional beliefs can still be harmful even if delusions are not the causal source of the harm. Bortolotti denies the latter, not the former.

Second, it is one thing to say that delusions are harmful (which is endorsed by the harmfulness thesis), and it is another to say that the one's state of having some delusions is more harmful than one's counterfactual state of having no delusions (which is not endorsed by the harmfulness thesis). The former can still be true even if the latter is false; e.g. delusions can still be harmful even if having delusions is less harmful than having no delusions. Bortolotti denies the latter, not the former.

Third, delusions might be adaptive only for a short period of time, and their adaptiveness can easily be overridden by the subsequent negative impact on well-being. Lancellotta and Bortolotti write; 'many delusions are in the long run psychologically harmful and biologically maladaptive, but that their adoption can be understood in context as offering some short-term benefits, as a response to an emergency situation' (Lancellotta & Bortolotti 2019: 12, see also Bortolotti & Murri, Chapter 3 for more on delusion and adaptiveness). But, then, the harmfulness thesis is true after all, as a claim about delusions' overall impact on well-being.

## 5.2 *Malfunction thesis*

According to the malfunction thesis, delusions are malfunctioning in the sense that they involve a failure of performing functions. In McKay and Dennett's terminology, delusions are 'doxastic dysfunctions': '[Delusional] misbeliefs result from breakdowns in the machinery of belief formation [...] these misbeliefs arise from dysfunction in the system – doxastic dysfunction. Such misbeliefs are the faulty output of a disordered, defective, abnormal cognitive system' (McKay & Dennett 2009: 496).

There are open empirical issues that are directly or indirectly relevant to the malfunction thesis. One of these issues is whether it is the one-factor theory or the two-factor theory that gives the correct account of delusion formation. One might think that the one-factor theory does not support the malfunction thesis. If, for example, delusions 'are derived by cognitive activity that is essentially indistinguishable from that employed by non-patients, by scientists, and by people generally' (Maher 1974: 103), then there is no malfunction in belief forming processes; rather malfunctions are only in perceptual processes. Strictly speaking, then, delusional beliefs are not malfunctioning. With my own terminology (Miyazono 2018), they are only misfunctioning (i.e. failing to perform a function due to some external or contextual misfortune) rather than malfunctioning (i.e. failing to perform a function due to some intrinsic damage). The two-factor theory, in contrast, is more consistent with the malfunction thesis. The theory seems to support the view that in addition to the malfunctions in perceptual processes (which give rise to the first factor), there are also some malfunctions in belief forming processes (which give rise to the second factor).

The debate between the one-factor theory and the two-factor theory is beyond the scope of this chapter.[10] Here I set aside the one-factor theory, and discuss whether the two-factor theory really supports the malfunction thesis. Take, for example, the version of the two-factor theory according to which the second factor is the 'bias towards observational adequacy' (Stone & Young 1997; McKay 2012), which is a bias of inappropriately prioritising the demand of incorporating observational inputs into the belief system (observational adequacy) against the demand of maintaining prior beliefs as long as possible (doxastic conservatism). Bortolotti (2020b, 2022; see also Lancellotta & Bortolotti 2020) argues that this version of the two-factor theory does not support the malfunction thesis because the bias towards observational adequacy is just a 'bias', not a 'malfunction'.

I have two responses to Bortolotti's challenge (see Miyazono 2022 for a more detailed discussion). First, Bortolotti assumes that 'bias' does not involve 'malfunction'. This is certainly reasonable when the term 'bias' is used in a particular way, referring to a deviation from *relevant logical or mathematical standards*. For instance, 'biases' in the heuristic and biases research such as the base-rate neglect or the conjunction fallacy (Tversky & Kahneman 1974) are biases in this sense. However, the term 'bias' is typically not used in that sense in the study of delusions. Rather the term typically refers to a deviation from *a statistically or biologically normal performance*. For instance, the 'jumping-to-conclusion bias' (Huq et al. 1988; Garety & Hemsley 1997) refers to a statistical difference between the amount of evidence that people in the delusional group need for reaching a conclusion and the amount of evidence that people in control groups need for reaching it. Note that the jumping-to-conclusion bias might not be a 'bias' in the first sense; i.e. it might not deviate from relevant logical or mathematical standards. In fact, as S. F. Huq et al. (1988) point out, the performance of people in the delusional group appears to be rational from a Bayesian point of view.

It is certainly reasonable to think that the 'biases' in the former sense, such as the base-rate neglect or the conjunction fallacy, do not involve any malfunction; after all they are widely shared in the non-clinical population. But the same thing does not apply to 'biases' in the latter sense, which is relevant to the study of delusions. For instance, there might be some underlying malfunctions in reasoning processes that explain the jumping-to-conclusion bias. In short, Bortolotti conflates two different senses of 'bias'; and her claim (i.e. 'bias' does not imply 'malfunction') applies to one sense of 'bias', not to the other, which is relevant to the study of delusions.

Second, even if Bortolotti is correct that there are no apparent malfunctions, there can be some malfunctions in a deeper level in the cognitive architecture. One might think, for example, that viral infection and appendicitis are counterexamples to Wakefield's HDA; on the face of it, viral infection does not involve any malfunction of organs (Tengland 2001), and appendicitis does not involve any malfunction because the appendix, a vestigial organ, has no function in the first place (Murphy & Woolfolk 2000). In response, Wakefield argues that in these conditions relevant malfunctions are not in a superficial (organ) level but rather in a deeper level; viral infection involves malfunctions at the cellular level, and appendicitis involves malfunctions at the tissue level.

A similar response to Bortolotti seems to be possible. Even if Bortolotti is correct that the bias towards observational adequacy is not malfunctional at a superficial (psychological) level, the bias can still be due to some underlying malfunctions at a deep (neurophysiological) level. Elsewhere (Miyazono 2018: Chapter 4; Miyazono & McKay 2019), I presented a hybrid theory of delusion formation which combines the two-factor theory and the prediction error theory (Fletcher & Frith 2009; Corlett et al. 2010; Sterzer et al. 2018). This theory has it that the first factor and the second factor in the two-factor framework correspond to the prediction error and its estimated precision in the prediction-error framework respectively. In particular, the bias towards observational adequacy, which is the second factor at the psychological level of description, is grounded in the overestimation of the precision of prediction-errors, which is an abnormality at a neurophysiological level of description, which might involve some malfunctions in that level.

## 6. Conclusion

According to malfunction doxasticism, delusions are malfunctioning beliefs. On the one hand, delusions are beliefs because they have the right kind of functions. On the other hand, delusions are malfunctioning, which is part of the reason why delusions are pathological.

## Notes

1 DSM-5 defines delusions as 'a false belief based on incorrect inference about external reality that is firmly held despite what almost everyone else believes and despite what constitutes incontrovertible and obvious proof or evidence to the contrary' (American Psychiatric Association 2013: 819).
2 Obviously, this question presupposes that delusions are pathological states. A strong interpretation of this is that *all* delusions are pathological, while a weak interpretation is that *many or most* delusions are pathological (which allows for the possibility of healthy delusions in non-clinical populations). See Bortolotti (2020b, 2022) for a scepticism about the very idea of pathological states of mind.
3 Strictly speaking, this question is for doxasticists. Non-doxasticists face different versions of the Pathology Question depending on their commitments. For instance, a question for non-doxasticists who regard delusions as imaginings (Currie 2000; Currie & Jureidini 2001; Currie & Ravenscroft 2002) would be: What distinguishes pathological delusions, such as the grandiose delusion about the special ability to predict future events, from the mundane fantastic imaginings, such as the one that Pixie Dust makes you fly?
4 In her contribution to this Handbook, Valentina Petrolini argues in response to this challenge that we can retain the combination of doxasticism and the continuity of delusional and non-delusional beliefs by appealing not to the nature of delusions, but the way in which they function within a person's broader mental economy and situation.
5 In response, Currie and colleagues might argue that the pathology of delusions is due to a pathological metacognitive failure where delusions, which are imaginings, are misidentified as beliefs (Currie 2000; Currie & Ravenscroft 2002). Currie and colleagues' metacognitive account of delusions, however, has been controversial (Bayne & Pacherie 2005). For delusions and metacognition, see Miyazono (2024).
6 Stricky speaking, a failure of performing a function due to some external or contextual factors does not constitute malfunction. For instance, a coffee machine is not regarded as malfunctional when it fails to peform its function (of producing coffee) simply because nobody has put water in it. See Section 5.2 for a related issue.
7 For an argument to the contrary, see Davies (2000, 2001). See also Sullivan-Bissett (2017) for a response to Davies.
8 Teleo-functionalism can take different forms, including homuncular teleo-functionalism (e.g., Lycan 1987; Sterelny 1990) and teleosemantics (e.g. Millikan 1984, 1989b; Neander 1995; Dretske 1997). The aim account of belief (e.g. Velleman 2000), according to which beliefs have a distinctive aim, is also a form of teleo-functionalism when the 'aim' is defined in terms of functions.
9 For HDA and delusions, see also Sakakibara (2016) and Clutton and Gadsby (2018).
10 I defended the two-factor theory elsewhere (Miyazono 2018, Chap. 4). See also Miyazono (2022), Sakakibara (2022) and Sullivan-Bissett (2022).

## References

American Psychiatric Association (2013). *Diagnostic and Statistical Manual of Mental Disorders*, 5th Edition. Washington, DC: American Psychiatric Publishing.
Bayne, T. (2011). Delusions as doxastic states: Contexts, compartments, and commitments. *Philosophy, Psychiatry, & Psychology*, 17(4), 329–336.

Bayne, T., & Fernández, J. (2009). Delusion and self-deception: Mapping the terrain. In T. Bayne & J. Fernández (eds.), *Delusions and Self-Deception: Motivational and Affective Influences on Belief Formation*. Hove: Psychology Press, 1–21.

Bayne, T., & Pacherie, E. (2004). Bottom-up or top-down: Campbell's rationalist account of monothematic delusions. *Philosophy, Psychiatry, & Psychology*, 11(1), 1–11.

Bayne, T., & Pacherie, E. (2005). In defence of the doxastic conception of delusions. *Mind & Language*, 20(2), 163–188.

Berrios, G. E. (1991). Delusions as "wrong beliefs": A conceptual history. *The British Journal of Psychiatry*, 159(S14), 6–13.

Bongiorno, F. (2022). Spinozan doxasticism about delusions. *Pacific Philosophical Quarterly*, 103(4), 720–752.

Bortolotti, L. (2009). *Delusions and Other Irrational Beliefs*. Oxford: Oxford University Press.

Bortolotti, L. (2012). In defence of modest doxasticism about delusions. *Neuroethics*, 5(1), 39–53.

Bortolotti, L. (2015). The epistemic innocence of motivated delusions. *Consciousness and Cognition*, 33, 490–499.

Bortolotti, L. (2016). Epistemic benefits of elaborated and systematized delusions in schizophrenia. *The British Journal for the Philosophy of Science*, 67(3), 879–900.

Bortolotti, L. (2020a). *The Epistemic Innocence of Irrational Beliefs*. Oxford: Oxford University Press.

Bortolotti, L. (2020b). Doctors without 'disorders'. *Aristotelian Society Supplementary Volume*, 94(1), 163–184.

Bortolotti, L. (2022). Are delusions pathological beliefs? *Asian Journal of Philosophy*. https://doi.org/10.1007/s44204-022-00033-3

Clutton, P. (2018). A new defence of doxasticism about delusions: The cognitive phenomenological defence. *Mind & Language*, 33(2), 198–217.

Clutton, P., & Gadsby, S. (2018). Delusions, harmful dysfunctions, and treatable conditions. *Neuroethics*, 11(2), 167–181.

Coltheart, M. (2007). Cognitive neuropsychiatry and delusional belief. *Quarterly Journal of Experimental Psychology*, 60(8), 1041–1062.

Coltheart, M., Menzies, P., & Sutton, J. (2010). Abductive inference and delusional belief. *Cognitive Neuropsychiatry*, 15(1–3), 261–287.

Coltheart, M., Langdon, R., & McKay, R. (2011). Delusional belief. *Annual Review of Psychology*, 62(1), 271–298.

Corlett, P. R., Taylor, J. R., Wang, X. J., Fletcher, P. C., & Krystal, J. H. (2010). Toward a neurobiology of delusions. *Progress in Neurobiology*, 92(3), 345–369.

Cummins, R. (1975). Functional analysis. *The Journal of Philosophy*, 72, 741–764.

Cummins, R. (1983). *The Nature of Psychological Explanation*. Cambridge MA: MIT Press.

Currie, G. (2000). Imagination, delusion and hallucinations. *Mind & Language*, 15(1), 168–183.

Currie, G., & Jureidini, J. (2001). Delusion, rationality, empathy: Commentary on Martin Davies et al. *Philosophy, Psychiatry, & Psychology*, 8(2), 159–162.

Currie, G., & Ravenscroft, I. (2002). *Recreative Minds: Imagination in Philosophy and Psychology*. Oxford: Oxford University Press.

Davies, P. S. (2000). Malfunctions. *Biology and Philosophy*, 15(1), 19–38.

Davies, P. S. (2001). *Norms of Nature: Naturalism and the Nature of Functions*. Cambridge, MA: MIT Press.

Davies, M., Coltheart, M., Langdon, R., & Breen, N. (2001). Monothematic delusions: Towards a two-factor account. *Philosophy, Psychiatry, & Psychology*, 8(2), 133–158.

Dretske, F. (1997). *Naturalizing the Mind*. Cambridge, MA: MIT Press.

Dub, R. (2017). Delusions, acceptances, and cognitive feelings. *Philosophy and Phenomenological Research*, 94(1), 27–60.

Egan, A. (2009). Imagination, delusion, and self-deception. In T. Bayne & J. Fernández (eds.), *Delusions and Self-Deception: Motivational and Affective Influences on Belief Formation*. Hove: Psychology Press, 263–280.

Fletcher, P. C., & Frith, C. D. (2009). Perceiving is believing: A bayesian approach to explaining the positive symptoms of schizophrenia. *Nature Reviews Neuroscience*, 10(1), 48–58.

Flores, C. (2021). Delusional evidence-responsiveness. *Synthese*, 199(3), 6299–6330.

Garety, P. A., & Hemsley, D. R. (1997). *Delusions: Investigations into the Psychology of Delusional Reasoning*. Hove: Psychology Press.

Godfrey-Smith, P. (1998). *Complexity and the Function of Mind in Nature*. Cambridge: Cambridge University Press.

Hohwy, J., & Rajan, V. (2012). Delusions as forensically disturbing perceptual inferences. *Neuroethics*, 5(1), 5–11.

Huq, S. F., Garety, P. A., & Hemsley, D. R. (1988). Probabilistic judgements in deluded and non-deluded subjects. *The Quarterly Journal of Experimental Psychology Section A*, 40(4), 801–812.

Lancellotta, E., & Bortolotti, L. (2019). Are clinical delusions adaptive? *Wiley Interdisciplinary Reviews: Cognitive Science*, 10(5), e1502.

Lancellotta, E., & Bortolotti, L. (2020). Delusions in the two-factor theory: Pathological or adaptive? *European Journal of Analytic Philosophy*, 16(2), 37–57.

Lycan, W. G. (1987). *Consciousness*. Cambridge, MA: MIT Press.

Maher, B. A. (1974). Delusional thinking and perceptual disorder. *Journal of Individual Psychology*, 30(1), 98–113.

McKay, R. (2012). Delusional inference. *Mind & Language*, 27(3), 330–355.

McKay, R. T., & Dennett, D. C. (2009). The evolution of misbelief. *Behavioral and Brain Sciences*, 32(6), 493–510.

Millikan, R. G. (1984). *Language, Thought, and Other Biological Categories: New Foundations for Realism*. Cambridge MA: MIT Press.

Millikan, R. G. (1989a). In defense of proper functions. *Philosophy of Science*, 56(2), 288–302.

Millikan, R. G. (1989b). Biosemantics. *The Journal of Philosophy*, 86(6), 281–297.

Miyazono, K. (2015). Delusions as harmful malfunctioning beliefs. *Consciousness and Cognition*, 33, 561–573.

Miyazono, K. (2018). *Delusions and Beliefs: A Philosophical Inquiry*. Abingdon: Routledge.

Miyazono, K. (2022). Replies to critics. *Asian Journal of Philosophy*. https://doi.org/10.1007/s44204-022-00048-w

Miyazono, K. (2024). Delusion and self-knowledge. In E. Sullivan-Bissett (ed.), *Belief, Imagination, and Delusion*. Oxford: Oxford University Press, 21–41.

Miyazono, K., & McKay, R. (2019). Explaining delusional beliefs: A hybrid model. *Cognitive Neuropsychiatry*, 24(5), 335–346.

Murphy, D., & Woolfolk, R. L. (2000). The harmful dysfunction analysis of mental disorder. *Philosophy, Psychiatry, & Psychology*, 7(4), 241–252.

Nanay, B. (2010). A modal theory of function. *The Journal of Philosophy*, 107(8), 412–431.

Nanay, B. (2014). Teleosemantics without etiology. *Philosophy of Science*, 81(5), 798–810.

Neander, K. (1991a). The teleological notion of 'function'. *Australasian Journal of Philosophy*, 69(4), 454–468.

Neander, K. (1991b). Functions as selected effects: The conceptual analyst's defense. *Philosophy of Science*, 58(2), 168–184.

Neander, K. (1995). Misrepresenting & malfunctioning. *Philosophical Studies*, 79(2), 109–141.

Noordhof, P., & Sullivan-Bissett, E. (2021). The clinical significance of anomalous experience in the explanation of monothematic delusions. *Synthese*, 199(3), 10277–10309.

Noordhof, P., & Sullivan-Bissett, E. (2023). The everyday irrationality of monothematic delusion. In P. Henne & S. Murray (eds.), *Advances in Experimental Philosophy of Action*. London: Bloomsbury, 87–111.

Petrolini, V. (2017). What makes delusions pathological? *Philosophical Psychology*, 30(4), 502–523.

Ramsey, F. P. (1931). *The Foundations of Mathematics and Other Logical Essays*. Abingdon: Routledge

Sakakibara, E. (2016). Irrationality and pathology of beliefs. *Neuroethics*, 9(2), 147–157.

Sakakibara, E. (2019). Intensity of experience: Maher's theory of schizophrenic delusion revisited. *Neuroethics*, 12(2), 171–182.

Sakakibara, E. (2022). On the nature, pathology, and etiology of delusions: Comments on Miyazono's Delusions and Beliefs. *Asian Journal of Philosophy*. https://doi.org/10.1007/s44204-022-00034-2

Schwitzgebel, E. (2012). Mad belief? *Neuroethics*, 5(1), 13–17.

Sober, E. (1985). Panglossian functionalism and the philosophy of mind. *Synthese*, 64(2), 165–193.

Sterelny, K. (1990). *The Representational Theory of Mind: An Introduction*. Oxford: Basil Blackwell.

Sterzer, P., Adams, R. A., Fletcher, P., Frith, C., Lawrie, S. M., Muckli, L.,…, & Corlett, P. R. (2018). The predictive coding account of psychosis. *Biological Psychiatry*, 84(9), 634–643.

Stich, S. P. (1990). *The Fragmentation of Reason: Preface to a Pragmatic Theory of Cognitive Evaluation*. Cambridge, MA: MIT Press.

Stone, T., & Young, A. W. (1997). Delusions and brain injury: The philosophy and psychology of belief. *Mind & Language*, 12(3&4), 327–364.

Sullivan-Bissett, E. (2017). Malfunction defended. *Synthese*, 194(7), 2501–2522.

Sullivan-Bissett, E. (2020). Unimpaired abduction to alien abduction: Lessons on delusion formation. *Philosophical Psychology*, 33(5), 679–704.

Sullivan-Bissett, E. (2022). Against a second factor. *Asian Journal of Philosophy*. https://doi.org/10.1007/s44204-022-00036-0

Tengland, P. A. (2001). *Mental Health: A Philosophical Analysis*. Dordrecht: Kluwer Academic.

Tumulty, M. (2011). Delusions and dispositionalism about belief. *Mind & Language*, 26(5), 596–628.

Tversky, A., & Kahneman, D. (1974). Judgment under uncertainty: Heuristics and biases. *Science*, 185(4157), 1124–1131.

Velleman, J. D. (2000). *The Possibility of Practical Reason*. Oxford: Oxford University Press.

Wakefield, J. C. (1992a). The concept of mental disorder: On the boundary between biological facts and social values. *American Psychologist*, 47(3), 373–388.

Wakefield, J. C. (1992b). Disorder as harmful dysfunction: A conceptual critique of DSM-III-R's definition of mental disorder. *Psychological Review*, 99(2), 232–247.

*5*

# DELUSION AND NATURAL KINDS

*Richard Samuels*

The status of psychiatric kinds has long been a focus of dispute (Szasz 1960). Debates regarding the status of *diagnostic* categories, such as schizophrenia and borderline personality disorder, are testimony to such concerns (Pickard 2009). But so too are discussions of categories of *symptoms* – especially, first-rank symptoms, such as delusion. To a first, very rough approximation, what lies at the heart of such disputes is whether the kinds of psychiatry are, in an appropriate sense, real divisions or groupings in the world, or whether they are arbitrary or merely conventional groupings. Though such issues may be framed in quite different ways, one familiar approach frames the issue in terms of whether the salient psychiatric kind is a *natural kind*.

In this chapter, I consider an instance of this sort of issue – whether *delusion* is a natural kind. In doing so, I make a pair of assumptions. First, I assume there are at least some natural kinds. That is, for present purposes, I disregard eliminativism about natural kinds (Hacking 2007; Ludwig 2018). Unless we do so, it makes little sense to assess the specific claim that delusion is a natural kind. Indeed, and for similar reasons, I assume for present purposes that the paradigm candidates of natural kinds – chemical elements, atomic particles, and biological species, for example – are, in fact, natural kinds. For if we reject such relatively uncontentious candidates, it makes little sense to assess whether a highly contentious candidate, like delusion, is a natural kind.

Second, I assume that it is commonplace for natural kinds to exhibit some form of taxonomic organization. This is apparent in the case of paradigmatic candidates of natural kinds, such as those of chemistry, particle physics, and biological systematics (Ellis 2001).[1] Consider the periodic table. Magnesium is plausibly a natural kind. But metal is also a natural kind – a relatively superordinate kind that has magnesium, iron, aluminium, etc. as subordinate kinds. Moreover, *chemical element* is also a plausible candidate for natural kindhood, albeit one that has magnesium and metal as nested subordinate kinds.

Kinds of delusion also appear to exhibit nesting relations. Notoriously, the clinical literature is replete with many sorts of delusions – persecutory delusions, erotomanic delusions, Othello syndrome, Capgras delusion, and delusions of passivity, to name but a few – which may themselves be organized into relatively superordinate categories – e.g. monothematic and polythematic; bizarre and mundane. Now, we may ask of the above kinds whether they

87

DOI: 10.4324/9781003296386-7

are natural kinds. But in the present chapter, my primary focus will be on delusion *as such*. That is, I will be concerned with what I call the *NK thesis*: Delusion *as such* is a natural kind.

Clarifying and assessing this thesis involves the coordination of two quite different sorts of issue. First, we must consider an array of broadly empirical issues regarding delusions. Second, we must consider the general matter of what natural kinds are. As we will see, there are several extant accounts, which impose quite different requirements on being a natural kind. In view of this, I propose to index discussion of the NK thesis to specific conceptions of natural kinds and consider the matter of whether the thesis is plausible on *that* construal of natural kinds. More specifically, I consider the thesis in the light of three views about natural kinds: *natural kind essentialism*; Richard Boyd's *homeostatic property cluster* account of natural kinds; and what Muhammad Ali Khalidi calls *the simple casual account*.

Here's how I proceed. In Section1, I consider the plausibility of the NK thesis on the assumption that natural kind essentialism is true. I argue that on this assumption, the thesis is *very implausible*. But in Section 2, I argue that the fault lies with natural kind essentialism, which should be rejected in favour of some alternative account of natural kinds. In Section 3, I consider the merits of the suggestion that delusion is a natural kind in the sense articulated by the *Homeostatic Property Cluster* (HPC) account. Finally, in Section 4, I consider the plausibility of the NK thesis, on the assumption that the simple causal account is correct.

## 1.  Natural kind essentialism and delusion

According to one influential view, natural kinds are to be characterized in terms of *the possession of common essences* (Barnes 1984; Kripke 1972; Putnam 1973). Though *Natural Kind Essentialism* (NKE) may be formulated in different ways, one typical rendering maintains the following:

*NKE:* A kind K is a natural kind if and only if (and because):
- *Individuation:* All and only the members of K share a common essence E.
- *Necessity:* E is a property, or collection of properties, that all and only K members *must* have.
- *Intrinsicality:* E properties are intrinsic as opposed to extrinsic or relational.
- *Causal Centrality:* E properties cause the instantiation of other properties associated with members of K.[2]

Some philosophers maintain that NKE applies well to the kinds of some sciences. For example, Brian Ellis (2001) maintains that the chemical elements have essences and, hence, are natural kinds in this sense.[3] However, it is implausible to maintain that delusions have essences of the sort articulated by NKE (Ghaemi 2004).

### 1.1  *Delusions and the individuation condition*

One reason to doubt that delusions possess an essence is that there's little reason to suppose they satisfy Individuation. Reflection upon the dismal track record of efforts to define delusion is relevant here.[4] Despite extensive efforts, it's highly doubtful that any extant proposal provides satisfactory necessary and sufficient conditions for delusion; and certainly, no such proposal garners consensus from the relevant scientific communities.[5]

To illustrate the problem, consider what is arguably the closest thing we have to a consensus definition of delusion – what I call the *Standard Account* – because it's found in many texts, including *DSM-IV*, the glossary of *DSM-5*, and ICD-11. On this view, delusion is a species of *belief*, whose instances possess the following characteristics:

1 *Falsity:* A delusion is a *false* belief.
2 *Conviction:* Delusions are *firmly held* by the patient.
3 *Doxastic Isolation:* A patient's delusion is not accepted by other members of the person's culture or subculture.
4 *Resistance to Rational Persuasion:* Delusions cannot be dispelled by argument – including *good* argument – to the contrary.
5 *Resistance to Incompatible Information:* Delusions are maintained in the face of available, incompatible information.

Satisfying Individuation would require that the Standard Account provide necessary and sufficient conditions for delusion. Yet it does not plausibly do so. First, as many have noted, most – perhaps even all – of 1–5 are unnecessary for delusion:

- Not all delusions are false. For example, there are reported cases of hypochondriacal delusions ('I am ill') and Othello Syndrome ('My partner is unfaithful'), where the belief is true but nevertheless delusional (Gipps and Fulford 2004).
- Not all delusions are doxastically isolated. Sometimes – as in the case of folie à deux – the very same delusion is held by multiple individuals.
- There's ample evidence that the conviction with which delusions are held can vary, and at times fail to be strong (Garety and Freeman 1999).
- Though delusions are often resistant to argument, the efficacy of cognitive therapy casts doubt on the claim that they *always* are. As Richard Gipps and Bill Fulford (2004: 227) note 'in some ways people with delusions can be brought to reflect on their delusional beliefs and, with patience and support, be brought to question them'.

Second, it is far from clear that the Standard Account provides a sufficient condition for delusion. To illustrate, consider the following case:

*Stubborn Philosopher:* Prof. Smith is deeply invested both personally and professionally in a 'pet theory' (PT) that they alone defend. Unbeknownst to Smith, PT is false, and was arrived at by faulty reasoning. Moreover, despite strong argument and evidence to the contrary, Smith has remained ardent in his commitment to PT. Indeed, he has become quite well-known within his subfield for defending this view.[6]

Philosophy, I suspect, is replete with Smith-like figures; and yet no psychiatrist would return a diagnosis of psychosis for Smith merely because they exhibit the profile sketched above. Mere bullish commitment to a pet theory – even when false, implausible, and singularly held – need not be delusional.

### *1.2  Delusion and the intrinsicality condition*

A second reason to doubt that delusion satisfies NKE is that even if clinicians were to identify a set of properties that satisfy Individuation, there's little reason to suppose that these properties would be *intrinsic*. This is because psychiatric kinds quite generally – delusion, in particular – are almost invariably characterized *relationally*. Again, reflection on the Standard Account is useful here, since the sorts of properties it cites are quite typical of extant approaches to delusion:

- *Doxastic Isolation* requires that a patient's delusion is not accepted by other members of the person's culture or subculture. Yet this quite explicitly articulates a requirement concerning the *relation* between the delusion and the patient's cultural context.
- *Resistance to Rational Persuasion* and *Resistance to Incompatible Information* are also relational. Specifically, they involve relations to accessible arguments and available information.
- *Falsity* is plausibly a relational property. Specifically, on almost every philosophical theory of truth, falsity is characterized in terms of the *absence* of a relation. According to correspondence theories, for example, the falsity of a belief consists in its failure to correspond to the facts; and according to coherence theories, the falsity of a belief consists in its failure to cohere with other beliefs.
- *Belief*: Perhaps less obviously, on almost every account of what beliefs are, being a belief is a relational property. For example, according to functionalism – arguably the dominant approach over the past half century – being a belief is a functional property specified in terms of how beliefs tend to relate to environmental stimuli, behavioural responses, and other mental states. In which case, delusions as a species of belief will of course inherit this relationality.
- *Intentional Content*: Perhaps even less obviously, for delusions to be the sorts of states that could have truth values, they will need to have *intentional contents*: they would need to represent or be *about* something. Yet on almost everyone's view, intentionality is itself relational.

Of course, none of the above precludes the bare possibility of a future psychiatry that characterizes delusion non-relationally. But if extant practice is any guide, this outcome would be quite remarkable.

## 2.  Natural kinds without traditional essentialism

The upshot of Section 1 is that delusion is not plausibly a natural kind by the lights of NKE. Yet reflection on scientific kinds quite broadly has led philosophers of science to view NKE as highly problematic, and to reject it in favour of less demanding accounts of natural kinds. In view of this, the possibility remains that the NK thesis is correct, albeit relative to some more credible account of natural kinds. In this section, I first say more about the dominant assumptions that underwrite most extant views of natural kinds, and then rehearse some of the main reasons for rejecting NKE.

### *2.1  Some dominant assumptions about natural kinds*

Though the notion of a natural kind has had a chequered intellectual history, it regained some semblance of respectability among philosophers of science, largely due to its utility in understanding core aspects of scientific practice (Boyd 1991; Quine 1969). Such philosophers very typically adopt the following three assumptions.[7] First, they assume that the division of phenomena into kinds – i.e. classification and taxonomy – is a central aspect of scientific practice: one that's important in its own right, but also a prerequisite for other core aspects of science, including the production of generalizations, theories, models, and explanations. Second, they commonly assume a form of *methodological naturalism*. Methodological naturalists typically suppose that science is our best – albeit defeasible – guide to empirical reality. For present purposes, the crucial and widely shared assumption is that scientific classification is our best guide to what *kinds* of things there are in the Universe. Finally, following John Venn (1866), contemporary philosophers of science typically construe natural kinds as the denotations of scientific classificatory terms.[8] Thus chemical elements, biological species, and subatomic particles (e.g. leptons, neutrons, and electrons) are paradigmatic natural kinds, since they are among the kinds acknowledged by the classificatory schemes of apparently successful science.

Given the above assumptions, a good first step in developing a philosophical account of natural kinds is to identify common features of the (putative) kinds that scientific terms denote. In doing this, philosophers of science have proposed several candidate features, with the following related ones being perhaps the most widely endorsed:

*Inductive potential*: Natural kinds are denoted by terms that can enter into successful inductive inference. As such, natural kind *terms* are *projectible*
*(Goodman 1955; Magnus 2012)*

*Fecundity*: Natural kinds are, at least pragmatically, the subject of many scientifically relevant, empirical generalizations
*(Machery 2005; Mill 1843/1882; Quine 1969)*

*'Stickiness'*: Natural kinds are 'sticky' in the sense that they are associated with clusters of properties (and relations) that, while logically unrelated, reliably covary (Khalidi 2023). As a result, instances of each specific natural kind – e.g. specific samples of gold, or individual electrons – tend to have lots of properties (and relations) in common
*(Boyd 1991; Khalidi 2023; Mill 1843/1882)*

Though we need not address the precise relationship between these three features, they will each be relevant to later discussion.[9]

## 2.2   *Reasons to reject NKE*

In view of the above comments, the principal reason to reject NKE is easily stated. If scientific classification is our best guide to what natural kinds there are, then the conception of natural kinds afforded by NKE is manifestly *too restrictive*. For while it might hold of (say) the elements of the periodic table, it clearly does not apply more broadly to the kinds denoted in scientific classifications. One reason is that many such kinds are not plausibly characterizable in terms of their intrinsic properties. This is true of biological kinds, such as species, but also true of the kinds of psychology, materials science, and arguably physics (Boyd 1991; Griffiths 1997; Khalidi 2023; Magnus 2012; Samuels 2009). A second reason is that even if we reject intrinsicality and allow essences to contain relational properties, the modified view is still overly restrictive. Specifically, it's doubtful that natural kind membership is always definable in terms of the causally central characteristics of kind members. This is plausibly true, for example, of the kinds cell and neuron. Finally, as Boyd (1991) and others have observed, there is not the slightest reason to suppose that all the (presumed) natural kinds denoted by scientific terms can be defined by sets of individually necessary and jointly sufficient conditions – i.e. that Individuation is true. Boyd's parade case is biological species; but the point is almost certainly true of many other plausible candidates for natural kindhood, including the kinds of psychology, anatomy, and ecology.

The above has clear implications for the present discussion of delusion. First, if NKE is unacceptable as an account of natural kinds, then the considerations rehearsed in Section 1 provide no grounds for rejecting the NK thesis. But second, if NKE is unacceptable, then we would do well to consider the plausibility of the NK thesis in the light of other, more plausible accounts of natural kinds. In the remainder of this chapter, I do just this. Specifically, I focus on a pair of views about natural kinds that are often regarded as more plausible characterizations of special science kinds, especially those that figure in the brain and behavioural sciences. In Section 3, I consider the plausibility of the NK thesis in light of Boyd's well-known *homeostatic property cluster* (HPC) view; and in Section 4 I consider it in the light of what's sometimes called the *simple causal theory* (SCT) of natural kinds (Craver 2009; Khalidi 2013, 2023).

## 3.    Delusion as a homeostatic property cluster

The HPC view of natural kinds is often adopted by philosophers interested in assessing the naturalness of psychological and psychiatric kinds (Beebee and Sabbarton-Leary 2010; Griffiths 1997; Machery 2005; Samuels 2009). In what follows I briefly sketch the view and consider the NK thesis in the light of this view.

### 3.1    *The HPC account of natural kinds*

According to the HPC account,[10] K is a natural kind if:

H1. K is associated with a property cluster P: a contingently co-varying collection of properties that tend to be co-instantiated by instances of the kind, but need not be necessary conditions for kind membership.

H2. There is *homeostatic mechanism*[11] – an empirically discoverable causal mechanism(s) that explain why members of K reliably exemplify the property cluster P.

H3. To the extent that there is any real definition of what it is for something to be a member of K, it is not the property cluster, as such, but the presence of the underlying homeostatic mechanism that defines membership of K.[12]

Consider an illness such as influenza. Influenza plausibly meets conditions H1–3: (a) it is associated with a range of characteristic symptoms – coughing, elevated body temperature, etc.; (b) there's a causal mechanism – roughly, the influenza virus – which explains the occurrence of such symptoms; and (c) to the extent that the kind, influenza, has a definition, it's not symptoms as such, but the virus that characterizes the kind.

As P. D. Magnus observes, the HPC view isn't plausible as a *definition* of natural kind – that 'natural kind = HPC' (Magnus 2012: 147). This is because some paradigmatic natural kinds appear not to be HPC kinds. Most obviously, the account won't apply to the kinds of fundamental physics – e.g. electron and quark. Although these are among the paradigm examples of natural kinds, it's hard to see how H2 could be true of such kinds since, *qua fundamental* entities, the covariation of their associated properties could not be explained by some causal mechanism, process, or structure. Nonetheless, as noted earlier, many have supposed the Boyd's proposal offers a plausible characterization of special science kinds – especially the kinds of biology and the behavioural sciences. In view of this, it makes sense to ask how plausible the NK thesis is, on the assumption that delusion must be an HPC kind.

### 3.2   *Prima facie grounds for optimism about the NK thesis*

Assuming the HPC account of natural kinds, the best evidence for the NK thesis would be an empirically attested account of the causal mechanism responsible for the co-variation of properties associated with delusion. Evidently, we have no such account. Nevertheless, in previous work, I suggest prima facie reasons to take seriously the view that delusion is an HPC kind, including the following (Samuels 2009):

*Consideration 1: Delusion is associated with a contingently covarying property cluster.* Earlier, when discussing the Standard Account of delusion, I noted that none of the five conditions it imposes are necessary for delusion and that collectively these conditions are insufficient. Nevertheless, it is very often the case that delusions instantiate *all* five properties. But this is precisely what we would expect if delusion is an HPC kind. In short, the suggestion is that, as per HPC, delusion has an associated covarying property cluster, and that the Standard Account specifies at least some of the properties which constitute it.

*Consideration 2: Empirical Regularities.* If the NK thesis is true, then we should expect appropriate methods of enquiry to yield a body of empirical generalizations concerning delusion. Though it is too early to tell with any certainty, there are grounds for optimism on this score. Over the past few decades, a wide array of results has emerged regarding delusions. For example, there is considerable evidence of cognitive abnormalities in the reasoning, attention, metacognition, and attributional tendencies of delusional patients (Bell et al. 2006; Garety & Freeman 20013). To illustrate, first consider the manifestation of a reasoning bias, known as *the jumping to conclusions (JTC) bias.* This bias consists in gather very limited information – far less than typical subjects – when making judgments and decisions. Moreover, it is strongly statically associated with the manifestation of delusions (Dudley et al. 2016). For a second, very different sort of illustration, consider the convergent neuroscientific evidence regarding the role of the dopamine system in the formation and maintenance of delusions (Weinberger 2022).

Evidently, such considerations do not provide strong grounds for accepting the NK thesis. Nevertheless, they may provide some prima facie reason to take the claim seriously.

### 3.3   *Some challenges for the view that delusion is a HPC kind*

There are also several potential challenges to the view that delusion is an HPC kind. Here are two.[13]

### 3.3.1 Continuity objections

For delusion to be a HPC kind, it needs to be a *kind*. However, some have challenged the categoricity of delusion, instead viewing delusion as *continuous* with non-delusions (Lincoln 2007; van Os 2003). It's important to see that the complaint is not merely that delusions comprise a kind with *vague* boundaries. After all, there's no obvious problem with kinds having borderline cases; and as Andrea Scarantino and Paul Griffiths (2011) note, Boyd's proposal is, in part, designed to accommodate the borderline cases of special science kinds. Rather, the claim is that delusion should be construed as a range on a continuum for which there exists no well-motivated boundaries – vague or otherwise – between delusion and other sorts of state. For example, it has been suggested that psychotic delusion is continuous with the sorts of 'delusional ideation' that occurs in ordinary experiences of the general population (Linscott and van Os 2013; Verdoux et al. 1998). In one review, for example, it was revealed that more than 8 per cent of the general population report psychotic experiences (van Os et al. 2009).

Whether such considerations pose a significant challenge to the NK thesis is unclear. This is because the observation that members of nonpathological populations have delusion-like experiences is wholly consistent with the NK thesis. First, the NK thesis in no way implies that delusions are always pathological. By widespread consensus, having a psychopathology presupposes that some *evaluative* condition is met – such as being *harmful* (Wakefield 1992). In which case, for all we have said so far, the delusion-like experiences of nonpathological subjects many be *bona fide* delusions – albeit nonpathological, because they fail to meet the relevant evaluative condition (for more on delusion and pathology, see Petrolini, Chapter 1). Second, the sort of continuity that the available evidence supports is a continuity of *symptoms*. Roughly put, non-pathological subjects have mental states whose properties are very similar to, or overlap with, those associated with psychotic delusion (Verdoux and van Os 2002). But such *symptomatic* continuity is wholly consistent with the NK thesis. After all, it's not symptoms, as such, but the instantiation of the salient homeostatic mechanism that determines category inclusion. And this, of course, permits many phenomena that are superficially similar to delusion and yet not genuine delusions. (Compare: influenza is symptomatically like many other illnesses, e.g., the common cold. But that does not mean that a continuum theory of influenza should be adopted.)

### 3.3.2 The unity problem

Perhaps the most serious challenge to the claim that delusion is a HPC kind is what I elsewhere call the *Unity Problem* (Samuels 2009). According to the HPC view, natural kinds are individuated by their associated homeostatic mechanisms (H3). But if this is so, then the absence of a shared homeostatic mechanism would be reason to deny that delusion is an HPC kind. The problem is that we currently have no well-developed account of what common mechanism(s) might be responsible for the formation and maintenance of delusion. Rather, the issue remains an ongoing and substantially unresolved empirical matter.

In view of this predicament, what might be said about the mechanisms responsible for the formation and maintenance of delusion? For the moment, I restrict myself to a single observation:[14]

*Determinable Type Unity:* We should expect the Unity Problem to be resolved by identifying a determinable, mechanism type, as opposed to some highly determinate mechanism.

Sometimes Unity Problems in the sciences are resolved by identifying some very specific sort of mechanism or process that produces instances of the kind. Consider, for example, the mechanism responsible for a typical form of colour-blindness, deuteranopia. This form of red-green colourblindness is explained by a relatively specific mechanism – the presence of functional retinal L-cones and S-cones, accompanied by an absence of functional M-cones ('green' cones). The relative specificity of this mechanism contrasts with the case of retinal colourblindness more broadly. Here, the type of primary mechanism consists in the reduction of function for *some* subset of retinal cone types. But crucially, the specific types of cones that are affected, and the degree to which they are impaired varies, thereby producing different forms of colour blindness (Bartolomeo 2021). In the case of retinal colourblindness, then, there is a kind of unity at the level of mechanism. But it takes the form of a *determinable* mechanism type, of which there are different *determinates* for different sorts of colour blindness.

What does any of this have to do with delusion? The suggestion is that, in view of the vast array of different sorts of delusion, a solution to the Unity Problem will likely be analogous to the case of retinal colourblindness. That is, the Unity Problem, if it is to be solved, will likely involve the specification of a determinable mechanism type.

One extant proposal that fits well with the above suggestion come from the Bayesian Brain research program (Adams et al. 2015). According to this influential approach, a central function of the brain is *predictive processing*. That is, a central function of the brain is to minimize *prediction error*: the disparity between the sensory signals the brain 'expects', based on its model of the world, and the sensory signals it actually receives (Bongiorno and Corlett 2024). Moreover, because of the brain's structural organization, especially in sensory cortex, proponents of the Bayesian Brain hypothesis often suggest that predictive coding is hierarchically organized into interacting layers where prior beliefs and hypotheses are conveyed via backward connections to predict inputs from the layer below.

Against these background commitments, several theorists defend what Sterzer and colleagues (2018) call the *canonical account* of delusion – that 'the relevant disturbance consists in an overweighting of sensory precision as compared to prior beliefs' with the result that 'prediction errors call for unneeded and sometimes profound revisions in an agent's model of the world' (Bongiorno and Corlett 2024). To illustrate, consider the case of Capgras delusion, where the patient believes that a loved one, such as a wife, has been replaced by an imposter. As Federico Bongiorno and Philip Corlett (2024) explain, according to the canonical account:

> In Capgras delusion, the connection between the face recognition system and the autonomic nervous system is damaged, so that seeing your wife's face does not elicit the appropriate level of autonomic response, as it does in healthy subjects (Ellis, Lewis, et al. 2000). The ensuing mismatch between the expected response and the actual lack of response gives rise to a prediction error indicating that your internal model is mistaken and needs to be updated. According to the canonical account, the misleading error signal would be afforded excessive precision and allotted undue influence on model revision. This would cause rejection of the hypothesis that is most compatible with their prior beliefs ('this person is my wife') in favour of one which is delusional but more observationally adequate ('this person is an imposter').

The point of the present illustration is not to argue that the canonical account is correct. Rather, my point is that the canonical account, construed as a general account of delusion, fits well with the suggestion that the Unity Problem could be resolved at the level of determinable mechanism types. In the case of Capgras, it is the connection between face recognition and the autonomic nervous system that is disrupted, and the salient predictive hierarchy will involve these systems. In other cases, e.g. passivity phenomena or delusions of grandeur, the contents of the delusions will be quite different, and the salient predictive hierarchies will likely be different as well. Nevertheless, the mechanism that results in delusion will still, according to the canonical account, involve an overweighting of sensory precision as compared to prior belief. That is: we have sameness of determinable mechanism type, with a difference of determinate mechanism.

## 4. Delusion and the simple causal theory of natural kinds

Though the HPC account has been highly influential in recent debates about the status of special science kinds, it is not the only option. In this section, I close by considering the NK thesis in the light of an alternative view, which, following Carl Craver (2009), Khalidi calls the *Simple Causal Theory* (SCT) (Khalidi 2013, 2023).

### 4.1 *The simple causal theory of natural kinds*

One way to construe the SCT is that it results from relaxing a requirement imposed by Boyd's HPC account. Specifically, we drop the requirement for a homeostatic mechanism that explains the covariation of the kind's associated property cluster while insisting that

> natural kinds are the kinds appearing in generalizations that correctly describe the causal structure of the world regardless of whether a mechanism explains the clustering of properties definitive of the kind.
>
> *(Craver 2009: 579)*

As Khalidi explains, the suggestion is not that the *mere* presence of a property cluster suffices for natural kindhood. It would not suffice, for example, if the associations were merely conventional.[15] Instead, what's required is that 'causation … glues these properties together' (20023: 27). In this regard, the SCT is like the HPC account, which also supposes that the covariation of properties associated with a natural kind is a result of causation. But in contrast to Boyd's view, the SCT does not insist that the salient causal relations obtain in virtue of a homeostatic mechanism. Instead, it suffices that K and its associated properties be 'nodes' in 'recurring causal networks'.[16] We thus end up with something like the following view: K is a natural kind if:

S1. K has an associated cluster of properties, $P_1...P_n$ that contingently co-vary, and tend to be co-instantiated by instances of K.

S2. The covariation relations between K and $P_1...P_n$ obtain in virtue of their causal relations to each other – the fact that they are all nodes in a 'recurring causal network'.

S3. To the extent that there is any real definition of what it is for something to be a member of the natural kind, K, it is to be an instance of, K, where this kind is itself individuated by the salient recurring causal network within which $P_1...P_n$ are nodes.

## 4.2 Assessing the NK thesis in light of SCT

Suppose we adopt the SCT of natural kinds. What are the implications for the NK thesis? Let's start with the grounds for optimism. First, assuming SCT, the prima facie grounds for optimism rehearsed in Section 3.2 carry over. That is: the fact that (a) delusion is associated with a contingently covarying property cluster, and (b) researchers have identified various empirical regularities regarding delusion, comports well with the proposal that delusion is, by the lights of SCT, a natural kind.

Second, if we reject the HPC view in favour of the SCT, then a primary challenge to the NK thesis – the Unity Problem – no longer seems pressing. Recall, on the HPC account, natural kinds are individuated by an underlying homeostatic mechanism. Thus, the failure to identify such a mechanism for delusion is prima facie grounds to doubt the NK thesis itself. In contrast, since the SCT relaxes the demand for a homeostatic mechanism, failure to identify such a mechanism for delusion is no longer grounds to doubt the NK thesis. Thus, the switch from the HPC account to the SCT of natural kinds is accompanied by a reduction in the demands on defending the NK thesis. Defending this thesis no longer seems to require the specification of a homeostatic mechanism for delusion.

Nevertheless, the adoption of the SCT is accompanied by another, albeit quite different, problem. Specifically, it appears to give rise to indeterminacy worries for the NK thesis. The problem may be formulated as a dilemma:

> Horn 1: As typically presented, SCT is implausibly profligate as an account of natural kinds. As such, on such presentations, delusion will count as a natural kind, but only because SCT is implausibly profligate.

> Horn 2: If SCT is not to be implausibly profligate, then certain restrictions must be imposed – of which more below. But now – and until some plausible restriction is identified – we have *no idea* whether delusion is a natural kind.

Either way, the transition to SCT appears not to aid us in determining whether the NK thesis is true.

To appreciate the first horn of the dilemma, consider Craver's original gloss on the SCT: 'natural kinds are the kinds appearing in generalizations that correctly describe the causal structure of the world' (2009: 579). Literally interpreted, this formulation generates an implausibly profligate conception of natural kinds. Almost any grouping will count as a natural kind. To illustrate, consider *constellation*. By broad consent, constellation – Orion, Leo, Aries, etc. – is not a natural kind. It is a kind (or category) that consists of arbitrary groupings of stars that we created, presumably because we can see gestalt patterns in arbitrary configurations of entities. Yet there are causal generalizations involving the kind constellation – e.g. that on looking at the night sky people with the requisite knowledge and intentions tend to make judgements regarding the presence of constellations. Since nothing prevents an arbitrary grouping of things from being a cause, the above characterization of SCT turns arbitrary groupings into natural kinds.

Of course, those sympathetic to SCT never thought that constellation counts as a natural kind. Among other things, they assume that bona fide natural kinds figure in *lots* of causal generalizations, not just a few. Or to put the point in terms of causal networks: They assume that natural kinds are 'highly connected vertices in directed causal graphs' – that they involve causal links to *many other* properties (Khalidi 2023). But now we confront the second horn of our dilemma. If the difference between natural kinds and other kinds is to be understood in terms of the *richness* of their causal connections, then we appear to need some principled way of specifying when the connections are rich *enough*. And this is something that proponents of SCT are yet to provide.

Now, proponents of SCT are fully aware of this sort of issue.[17] Moreover, the failure to specify such a principled distinction need not be a problem for many purposes. Suppose, for example, we are concerned with the kind *electron*. Here we might suppose that the richness of the causal connections is *so great* as to render it as clear-cut a case of a natural kind as anything is. But the situation is very different when we turn to delusion. As noted earlier, researchers have identified some causal regularities involving delusion. Yet extant formulations of the SCT provide no guidance regarding whether these regularities are rich *enough* to confer natural kind status on delusion. That is, without precisification of the SCT, the status of the NK thesis remains indeterminate.

## 5.   Conclusion

In the light of different conceptions of natural kinds, this chapter explored the issue of whether delusion is a natural kind – whether the NK thesis is true. I first argued that, on well-known essentialist accounts of natural kinds, the NK thesis is almost certainly false, but that this is due to the implausible stringency of natural kind essentialism. Next I argued that on Boyd's more plausible HPC account of natural kinds, there are *prima facie* reasons to take the NK thesis seriously. But I also noted that the thesis faces some significant explanatory challenges, most notably the Unity Problem. Finally, I argued that, on extant formulations of the recently popular SCT of natural kinds, the status of the NK thesis remains indeterminate. Combining the above, the status of the NK thesis remains unresolved. The issue of whether delusion is a natural kind will only be resolved in the light of further empirical study of delusion, but also – and crucially – sustained philosophical attention to the issue of what natural kinds are.

## Notes

1 Unlike Ellis (2001) I won't assume that organization into a taxonomic hierarchy is criterial for natural kinds.

2 For a formulation of this view see, for example, Khalidi (2023).

3 To illustration, if the kind *hydrogen atom* is a natural kind, then: (a) All and only members of the kind share a common property – e.g. having the atomic number one; (b) something *must* have this property to be a member of the kind; (c) this property will be intrinsic; and (d) having this atomic number, will cause the instantiation of other properties associated with hydrogen.

4 For a useful review, see Garety and Hemsley (1994). See also Radden (2011).

5 This is perhaps reflected in the most recent editions of the Diagnostic and Statistical Manual of Mental Disorders – DSM-5 and DSM-5-TR – in which little effort is made to provide a definition of delusion.

6 For discussion of a related phenomenon in science see Maher (1988: 20–22).

7 It should be noted that the sort of approach to natural kinds discussed here is not the only one. See Chapter 4 of Cooper (2007) for other approaches.

8 At any rate, the good ones. After all, not all the terms that figure in scientific classifications successfully denote. The terms 'caloric', 'phlogiston' and 'aether' readily come to mind.

9 One thought is that Stickiness explains Fecundity and Fecundity explains Inductive Potential. In more detail: It's because the instances of natural kinds reliably share a cluster of contingently related properties (and relations) that natural kinds tend to be subject of many true empirical generalizations. And it is because they are the subject of many such generalizations that one can reliably make inductive inferences about the instances of natural kinds.

10 For more extensive characterizations of the homeostatic cluster view see, for example, Boyd (1991, 1999).

11 Although Boyd often speaks of homeostatic mechanisms, it clear that he has an expansive conception of mechanisms that incorporates lots of things that are often called processes, states and structures.

12 In Boyd's words, '[t]he natural definition of …homeostatic property clusters kinds is determined by the members of a cluster of often co-occurring properties and by the ("homeostatic") mechanisms that bring about their co-occurrence' (Boyd 1999: 141).

13 For more extensive discussion see Samuels (2009).

14 In earlier work I further suggested that the salient mechanisms are likely cognitive mechanisms that are multiply realized by various neural processes (Samuels 2009).

15 To illustrate: *constellation* won't be a natural kind since our grouping of stars into constellations – Orion, Leo, Aries, etc. – is (merely) conventional.

16 Though I won't explore the issue here, the present view is clearly formulated in the light of recent developments in casual modelling. For details see, for example, Pearl (2000) and Woodward (2003).

17 Khalidi appears to view this sort of indeterminacy – or at any rate something very much like it – as more-or-less inevitable. See Khalidi (2023: 28).

# References

Adams, R. A., Brown, H. R. and Friston, K. J. (2015) "Bayesian Inference, Predictive Coding and Delusions", *Avant* 5: 51–88.

American Psychiatric Association (APA) (2000). *Diagnostic and statistical manual of mental disorders: DSM-IV-TR*. 4th ed. Washington, DC: American Psychiatric Association.

American Psychiatric Association (APA) (2013) *Diagnostic and Statistical Manual of Mental Disorders*: DSM-5. Washington, DC: American Psychiatric Association.

Barnes, J. (Ed.) (1984) *The Complete Works of Aristotle*. Aristotle, categories. Princeton, NJ: Princeton University Press.

Bartolomeo, P. (2021) "Color Vision Deficits", *Current Neurology and Neuroscience Reports* 21: 1–7.

Beebee, H. and Sabbarton-Leary, N. (2010) "Are Psychiatric Kinds Real?" *European Journal of Analytic Philosophy* 6(1): 11–27.

Bell, V., Halligan, P. W. and Ellis, H. D. (2006) "Explaining Delusions: A Cognitive Perspective", *Trends in Cognitive Sciences* 10(5): 219–226.

Bongiorno, F. and Corlett, P. R. (2024) "Delusions and the Predictive Mind", *Australasian Journal of Philosophy*, 1–16. https://doi-org.proxy.lib.ohio-state.edu/10.1080/00048402.2023.2293825

Boyd, R. (1991) "Realism, Anti-Foundationalism and the Enthusiasm for Natural Kinds", *Philosophical Studies* 61: 127–148.

Boyd, R. (1999) "Homeostasis, Species, and Higher Taxa", in R. Wilson (ed.), *Species: New Interdisciplinary Essays*. Cambridge: MIT Press, 141–186.

Cooper, R. (2007) *Psychiatry and Philosophy of Science*. Stockfield: Acumen.

Craver, C. F. (2009) "Mechanisms and Natural Kinds", *Philosophical Psychology* 22(5): 575–594.

Dudley, R., Taylor, P., Wickham, S. and Hutton, P. (2016 May) "Psychosis Delusions and the 'Jumping to Conclusions' Reasoning Bias: A Systematic Review and Metaanalysis", *Schizophrenia Bulletin* 42(3): 652–665.

Ellis, B. (2001) *Scientific Essentialism*. Cambridge: Cambridge University Press.

Ellis, H. D., Lewis, M. B., Moselhy, H. F. and Young, A. W. (2000) "Automatic without Autonomic Responses to Familiar Faces: Differential Components of Covert Face Recognition in a Case of Capgras Delusion", *Cognitive Neuropsychiatry* 5: 255–269.

Garety, P. and Freeman, D. (1999) "Cognitive Approaches to Delusions: A Critical Review of Theories and Evidence", *British Journal of Clinical Psychology* 38: 113–154.

Garety, P. A. and Freeman, D. (2013) "The Past and Future of Delusions Research: From the Inexplicable to the Treatable", *British Journal of Psychiatry* 203(5): 327–333.

Garety, P. A. and Hemsley, D. R. (1994) *Delusions: Investigations into the Psychology of Delusional Reasoning*. Oxford: Oxford University Press.

Ghaemi, S. Nassir (2004) "The Perils of Belief: Delusions Reexamined", *Philosophy, Psychiatry, and Psychology* 11(1): 49–54.

Gipps, R. G. and Fulford, K. W. M. (2004) "Understanding the Clinical Concept of Delusion: From an Estranged to an Engaged Epistemology", *International Review of Psychiatry* 16(3): 225–235.

Goodman, N. (1955/1983). *Fact, Fiction, and Forecast*. Cambridge, MA: Harvard University Press.

Griffiths, P. E. (1997) *What Emotions Really Are: The Problem of Psychological Categories*. Chicago: University of Chicago Press.

Hacking, I. (2007) "Natural Kinds: Rosy Dawn, Scholastic Twilight", *Royal Institute of Philosophy Supplement* 61: 203–239.

Khalidi, M. A. (2013) *Natural Categories and Human Kinds: Classification in the Natural and Social Sciences*. New York: Cambridge University Press.

Khalidi, M. A. (2023) *Natural Kinds*. Cambridge: Cambridge University Press.

Kripke, S. (1980) *Naming and Necessity* Cambridge, MA: Harvard University Press.

Lincoln, T. M. (2007) "Relevant Dimensions of Delusions: Continuing the Continuum Versus Category Debate", *Schizophrenia Research* 93(1–3): 211–220.

Linscott, R. J. and van Os, J. (2013) "An Updated and Conservative Systematic Review and Meta-Analysis of Epidemiological Evidence on Psychotic Experiences in Children and Adults: On the Pathway from Proneness to Persistence to Dimensional Expression across Mental Disorders", *Psychological Medicine* 43(6): 1133–1149.

Ludwig, D. (2018) "Letting Go of 'Natural Kind': Towards a Multidimensional Framework of Non-Arbitrary Classification", *Philosophy of Science* 85: 31–52.

Machery, E. (2005) "Concepts Are Not a Natural Kind", *Philosophy of Science* 72: 444–467.

Magnus, P. (2012) *Scientific Enquiry and Natural Kinds: From Planets to Mallards*. New York: Palgrave-Macmillan.

Maher, B. A. (1988) "Anomalous Experience and Delusional Thinking: The Logic of Explanations", in T. F. Oltmanns and B. A. Maher (eds.), *Delusional Beliefs*. New York: John Wiley & Sons, 15–33.

Mill, J. S. (1843/1882) *A System of Logic* (8th edition). New York: Harper & Brothers.

Pearl, J. (2000) *Causality*. Cambridge: Cambridge University Press.

Pickard, H. (2009) "Mental Illness Is Indeed a Myth", in M. Broome and L. Bortolotti (eds.), *Psychiatry as Cognitive Neuroscience: Philosophical Perspectives*. Oxford: Oxford University Press, 82–102.

Putnam, H. (1973), "Meaning and Reference", *Journal of Philosophy* 70, 699–711.

Quine, W. V. O. (1969) *Ontological Relativity and Other Essays*. New York: Columbia University Press.

Radden, J. (2011) *On Delusion*. New York: Routledge.

Samuels, R. (2009) "Delusions as a Natural Kind", in M. Broome and L. Bortolotti (eds.), *Psychiatry as Cognitive Neuroscience: Philosophical Perspectives*. Oxford: Oxford University Press, 49–79.

Scarantino, A. and Griffiths, P. (2011) "Don't Give Up on Basic Emotions", *Emotion Review* 3(4): 444–454.

Sterzer, P., Adams, R. A., Fletcher, P., Frith, C., Lawrie, S. M., Muckli, L., Petrovic, P., Uhlhaas, P., Voss, M. and Corlett, P. R. (2018) "The Predictive Coding Account of Psychosis", *Biological Psychiatry* 84(9): 634–643.

Szasz, T. S. (1960) "The Myth of Mental Illness", *American Psychologist* 15(2): 113–118.

van Os, J. (2003) "Is There a Continuum of Psychotic Experiences in the General Population?" *Epidemiologia e Psichiatria Sociale* 12: 242–252.

van Os, J., Linscott, R. J., Myin-Germeys, I., Delespaul, P. and Krabbendam, L. (2009 Feb) "A Systematic Review and Meta-Analysis of the Psychosis Continuum: Evidence for a Psychosis Proneness-Persistence-Impairment Model of Psychotic Disorder", *Psychological Medicine* 39(2): 179–195.

Venn, J. (1866/1888) *The Logic of Chance* (3rd edition). London: Macmillan.

Verdoux, H., Maurice-Tison, S., Gay, B., Van Os, J., Salamon, R. and Bourgeois, M. L. (1998) "A Survey of Delusional Ideation in Primary-Care Patients", *Psychological Medicine* 28(1): 127–134.

Verdoux, H. and van Os, J. (2002) "Psychotic Symptoms in Non-Clinical Populations and the Continuum of Psychosis", *Schizophrenia Research* 54(1–2): 59–65.

Wakefield, J. C. (1992) "Disorder as Harmful Dysfunction: A Conceptual Critique of DSM-III-R's Definition of Mental Disorder", *Psychological Review* 99(2): 232–247.

Weinberger, D. R. (2022) "It's Dopamine and Chizophrenia all Over again", *Biological Psychiatry* 92(10): 757–759.

Woodward, J. (2003) *Making Things Happen: A Theory of Causal Explanation*. Oxford: Oxford University Press.

# PART 2

# Delusion in disorders

# 6
# DELUSIONAL DISORDERS

*Luigi Grassi and Federica Folesani*

## 1.  Introduction

Delusional disorders have their roots in the concept of paranoia (from the Greek, παράνοια, from παρά, pará=beyond, beside, and νόος, nóos=mind) which denotes a general condition of being outside the normal (likewise the Latin *de-lirare:* de=besides; lira=furrow, from which Italian *delirio* comes). Paranoia, as a general descriptor of insanity, has been part of philosophical (e.g., Plato, Aristotle) and medical discussions (e.g., Hippocrates), and Greek tragedies (e.g., Aeschylus, Sophocles, Euripides), that represented human passions and psychological conditions including madness: psychotic episodes, confusional states, and delusions that affected the protagonists of the tragedies (e.g., Ajax, Orestes, Medea, the Bacchae) (Christopher Gill, 1996; Maieron, 2017; Padel, 1997; Theodorou, 1993).

Shakespeare magisterially presents a classic example of a delusion with morbid jealous characteristics in Othello. Convinced by Iago that his wife Desdemona is unfaithful and having an affair with Cassio, Othello grows increasingly jealous until, in the tragic conclusion, he strangles her (Oyebode, 2012).

Centuries later, paranoia and what are today called *delusional disorders* were more precisely studied and clinically characterized (Kendler, 2009), as discussed in this chapter where the development of delusional disorders in psychiatry, their clinical characteristics and current nosology, and the biopsychosocial co-causative factors will be described. We will conclude with the illustrative example of the tragic Jonestown mass suicide of November 18, 1978, caused by the delusional disorder of its leader.

## 2.  Development and conceptualization of paranoia (delusional disorders) in psychiatry

The clinical approach to paranoia and what are now defined as delusional disorders begins in the mid-19th century. In French, German, and Italian psychiatry, this disorder replaced the general concept of insanity (madness) and received the dignity of a defined mental

  DOI: 10.4324/9781003296386-9

illness that had different features in comparison with other psychotic disorders, especially schizophrenia (Castagnini, 2016; Dowbiggin, 2000; Schifferdecker & Peters, 1995).

Johann Christian Heinroth in 1818 (re)-introduced the term of *paranoia* in psychiatry, considering it 'partial insanity' or '*delire partial*', with preserved emotions and volition. These issues were part of what Etienne Esquirol (1838) observed and defined *monomanie intellectuelle*. According to Esquirol, this clinical condition differed from other forms of monomania he described (the *affective* and the *instinctive* ones) in that

> the patients start from a false principle, which they follow logically without devia-
> tion, and from which they derive legitimate consequences which modify their affects
> and acts of their volition; outside this partial delusion, they feel, reason and act as
> everybody else.

Likewise, Karl Kahlbaum in 1863 considered paranoia as an illness per se, with persistent delusions and a stable course (Opjordsmoen, 2014), while in 1860, Jules Baillarger described the fact that delusional beliefs could be shared by two or more people in a close relationship, coining the term '*folie communiquee*' (communicated psychosis). This condition was called '*folie à deux*' by Ernest Charlès Lasègue and Jules Falret (1877)) and '*Induziertes Irresein*' described in German psychiatry by Lehman in 1883.

The first more organized psychiatric nosology, Emil Kraepelin's *Psychiatrie*, edition 6 (1899), defined delusions as pathological erroneous beliefs that cannot be corrected by logical proof to the contrary, and suggested that beyond the core mental illnesses of dementia praecox, depression, and manic-depressive illness, paranoia also existed as a chronic condition. According to Kreapelin, the typical clinical symptoms of paranoia were: preserved thought process but with fixed and non-bizarre delusions; lack of deterioration over time; and relatively slight involvement of affect and volition. He also systematized the content of delusions, namely persecutory, erotomanic, grandiose, jealous, and hypochondriacal. In later editions, he considered in a sort of continuum, the existence of paranoia; paraphrenia, as an intermediate condition, with fantastic and bizarre delusions and hallucinations, but no personality deterioration; and the paranoid subtype of dementia praecox.

Karl Jaspers, in his essay on morbid (delusional) jealousy (*Eifersuchtswahn*, 1910) and subsequent psychopathology textbook (*Allgemeine Psychopathologie*, 1913), considered paranoia in a less specific fashion. For Jaspers' delusion, 'the basic characteristic of madness' had to meet three main criteria for diagnosis: (a) being held with strong subjective certainty, namely with unusual conviction; (b) being incorrigible despite logical demonstration of the impossibility of the conviction; and (c) having impossible or false content. However, Jaspers' differentiation of 'development' and 'process', 'understanding' and 'explaining', and 'content' and 'form' of psychopathologic symptoms complicated the isolation of paranoia from schizophrenia and other psychotic illnesses.

During the 20th century, the concept of paranoia in the schools of psychiatry in Europe and the United States diverged between some who maintained the Kraepelinian tradition and those who disagreed with it and subsumed the condition under schizophrenia. The first two, psychoanalytically oriented psychiatric classifications of the American Psychiatric Association (APA), the *Diagnostic and Statistical Manual of Mental Disorders* (*DSM*, first and second edition) considered paranoia a variant of schizophrenia (Kendler, 2017).

## 3.   Delusional disorders in the current psychiatric nosological systems

In the late 20th century, a series of papers indicated the need to re-examine and restore the concept of paranoia and delusional disorders (Kendler, 1988, 1980; Kendler & Tsuang, 1981; Lewis, 1970; Munro, 1982; Winokur, 1977).

In the United States, the reawakened interest in Kraepelin's work (neo-Kraepelinianism) in psychiatric classification constituted the main reason to propose a new *DSM* edition (*DSM-III*, 1980) with a categorical, atheoretical framework and a careful description of symptoms to create reliable criteria. The *DSM-III* made paranoia a possible exclusion diagnosis when delusions did not fit the criteria for schizophrenia, mood disorders, or other psychiatric conditions. *Folie a deux* was rescued and defined as shared paranoid disorder. Delusional disorders became a more specific separate chapter, with clear demarcation from schizophrenia, in the *DSM-III-Text Revised* edition (1987), *DSM-IV* (1994), and *DSM-IV-TR* (2000) (Fear et al., 1998). The World Health Organization International Classification of Disease (ICD) included both delusional disorders and shared psychotic disorders in its tenth edition (ICD-10, 1992) (Shimizu et al., 2007). Epidemiological studies using these criteria indicate that delusional disorders are a rare condition affecting about 0.2 per cent of the population, without differences between males and female, but a higher prevalence in late life (Kendler, 2017). Also, the mean age of presentation is in mid-to-late adult life (35–55 years old) with higher prevalence in women than men (female-to-male ratio about 1.5:1) (Kendler, 1982).

The *DSM-5* (2013) and the *DSM-5-Text Revised* (*DSM-5-TR*) (2023) now describe delusional disorders in a specific chapter as pathological conditions. Delusions, as false beliefs 'based on incorrect inference about external reality that is firmly sustained despite what almost everybody else believes and despite what constitutes incontrovertible and obvious proof or evidence to the contrary', are the main clinical characteristic. In these disorders, delusions have a powerful internal consistency, do not interfere with general logical reasoning or with behavioural disturbance (unless related to the delusional belief system), and are stable over time, making this a chronic disorder. Moreover: 'The belief is not one ordinarily accepted by other members of the person's culture or subculture (e.g., it is not an article of religious faith)' (*DSM-5TR*, pp. 421–423). Unlike the *DSM-III-TR* and the subsequent editions, the *DSM-5* and *DSM-5-TR* once again propose the possibility that the delusion can be bizarre and that sometimes perception disturbances (e.g., delusion-concordant, non-persistent hallucinations) are part of the syndrome.

Likewise, in the latest ICD-11 edition (2019), delusional disorders (par. 6A24) are confirmed as a specific disorder within the chapter on Schizophrenia and Other Primary Psychotic Disorders. The ICD-11 describes delusional disorders as characterized by

> the development of a delusion or set of related delusions, typically persisting for at least 3 months and often much longer [...]. The delusions are variable in content across individuals, but typically stable within individuals, although they may evolve over time.

The typical symptoms of depressive, manic, or mixed mood episode are absent, as well as those of schizophrenia (e.g., disorganized thinking, experiences of influence, passivity, or control, negative symptoms), although perceptual disturbances (e.g., hallucinations, illusions, misidentifications of persons) can be present especially if thematically related to the delusion. The *DSM-5-TR* and ICD-11 in part retain the subtypes that psychiatrists of 19th and 20th centuries described (Table 6.1), namely:

- Erotomania, characterized by a delusional belief is that one is the object of another person's love (de Clerambault's syndrome);
- Grandiosity, in which the delusion is represented by the conviction that one has some great but unrecognized talent or powers;
- Jealousy, a disorder where the main feature is an unshakeable, delusional conviction that one's partner is unfaithful (Othello syndrome);
- Persecution, defined by a delusion centred on the fact that one is spied, cheated, followed, poisoned maliciously maligned and so on;
- Bodily preoccupation, in which the theme of the delusion is that there is something happening in one's own body, such as severe bodily changes or organ functions, severe diseases, body modifications (Ekbom syndrome)

When no specific delusional theme predominates, the mixed type can be diagnosed, whereas if the dominant delusional belief is unclear (e.g., referential delusions without a prominent persecutory or grandiose component), the unspecified subtype applies. The *DSM* and ICD criteria do not consider a shared psychotic disorder (*folie à deux*) a discrete diagnosis but rather a rare possible manifestation of the disorder itself.

Regarding *severity*, the Clinician-Rated Dimensions of Psychosis Symptom Severity, an eight-item measure (each item rated on a 5-point scale, from 0 = none to 4 = present and severe) can be used. This allows rating the delusion as equivocal (severity or duration insufficient to be considered psychosis); present, but mild (little pressure to act upon delusional beliefs, not very bothered by beliefs); present and moderate (some pressure to act upon beliefs, or is somewhat bothered by beliefs); or present and severe (severe pressure to act upon beliefs, or is very bothered by beliefs).

With regard to *temporal* and *clinical* presentation, options include a first episode or multiple episodes, defined as acute episode; episode in partial remission; episode in full remission; or continuous (diagnostic criteria present for most of the illness course).

## 4. Biopsychosocial factors associated with delusional disorders

Studies of the origins of delusional disorders have indicated that many intervening factors influence the development and onset of delusions. Although the etiopathogenesis is still not clearly understood for some psychotic disorders and these factors differ across disorders (Kunert et al., 2007) (Figure 6.1), neurobiological, psychological, and interpersonal variables have been proposed.

### 4.1 Neurobiological basis of delusional disorder

Regarding neurobiological factors, delusional ideas may be rooted in *anomalous cerebral circuitries* and *neurotransmission*, especially those involving dopamine and serotonin. In delusional disorder, increased DA transmission could be related to dysfunction in the DA transporter that terminates synaptic DA activity (Guàrdia et al., 2021) and increased

*Table 6.1* Eponyms related to psychotic disorders (including delusional disorders)

| Name | Clinical features |
| --- | --- |
| Capgras syndrome (illusion des sosies) (described by Capgras and Reboul-Lachaux in 1923) | A delusional misidentification that a person closely related to the patient has been replaced by an impostor. |
| Fregoli syndrome (described by Courbon and Fail in 1927) | A delusional misidentification in which the patient identifies a familiar person in various other people he or she encounters. |
| Courbon syndrome or Intermetamorphosis (described by Courbon in 1932) | A delusional misidentification in which a patient believes he/she can see others change into someone else in both external appearance and internal personality. |
| Christodoulou syndrome (syndrome of subjective doubles) (described by Christodoulou in 1978) | A delusional misidentification in which a person believes to have a double (doppelgänger), a biologically unrelated look-alike, or a double of a living person with the same appearance, but usually with different character traits, that is leading a life of its own. |
| De Clérambault syndrome (erotomania, the phantom lover syndrome, psychose passionelle) (described by De Clerambault in 1885) | A delusion that an exalted yet inaccessible person is in love with the patient. These patients are convinced that the object of their affection is in love with them when the supposed lover is not, has indirect conversations with the patient, and behaves in a paradoxical and contradictory way. |
| Ekbom syndrome (delusional parasitosis) (originally described by Charcellay De Thours in 1843, then better described by Ekbom in 1938) | A delusion in which a patient believes to be infested by living or nonliving pathogens such as parasites, insects, or bugs. The delusion is characterized by sensation resembling insects crawling on or under the skin. |
| Cotard syndrome (délire de négation généralisée, nihilistic delusion) (described by Cotard in 1880) | A delusion, especially in psychotic depression with hypochondriasis, with bizarre and dramatic delusion that parts of their body are missing, or that they are dying, dead, or do not exist and nothing exists. |
| Lasegue and Falret syndrome or Folie impose (imposed psychosis) (described by Lasegue and Falret in 1877). | A delusion is transferred from an individual with psychosis to an individual without psychosis in an intimate relationship. The delusions in the induced individual soon disappear once the two are separated. |
| Lehmann syndrome or Folie induite (induced psychosis) (described by Lehmann in 1885) | A delusion is assumed by an individual with psychosis who is being influenced by another individual with psychosis |
| de Montyel syndrome or Folie communiquée (communicated psychosis) (described by de Montyel in 1881) | Similar to folie impose, with a delusion in the secondary partner occurs after a long period of resistance; the secondary partner will maintain the delusion even after separation from their partner. |
| Regis syndrome (Folie simultanee or simultaneous psychosis) (described by Regis in 1880) | Both partners share the psychosis simultaneously. They both have risk factors through long social interactions that predispose them to develop this condition. There are reports of sharing genetic risk factors among siblings. |

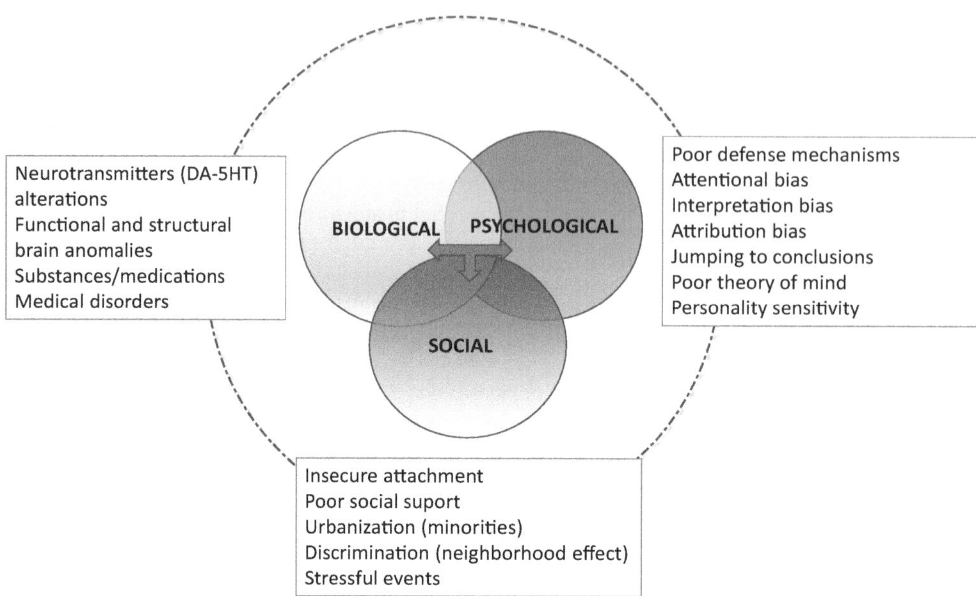


*Figure 6.1* Biopsychosocial factors associated with delusional disorders.

striatal dopaminergic synthesis (Cheng et al., 2020). Serotoninergic transmission also appears involved (Guàrdia et al., 2021). Although *several brain abnormalities* appear to be transdiagnostic across different psychiatric disorders, patients with delusional disorders display *structural and functional brain abnormalities*, such as reduced grey matter volume in the medial frontal/anterior cingulate cortex and the bilateral insula, and failure to de-activate medial frontal cortex during a working memory task (Vicens et al., 2016). For example, subjects with the delusion of infestation display increased right medial orbito-frontal gyrus cortical thickness associated with mistaken interpretation of somatic symptoms, and decreased temporoparietal surface area and cortical folding that could explain cognitive inflexibility and abnormal sensory perceptions (Hirjak et al., 2017). Also predictive coding and prediction errors have been described in delusion formation (see Corlett, Chapter 30).

Among biological mechanisms directly causing delusions, both the *DSM-5-TR* and the ICD-11 consider the existence of *delusional syndromes Due to Another Medical Condition or Substance/medication-induced delusions,* which should be ruled out in the diagnosis of primary delusional disorders we described.

### 4.2 *Psychological correlates of delusion*

Sigmund Freud considered delusions the result of a *psychological defense mechanism* against anxiety, namely projection. In his work on the psychosis of judge Daniel Paul Schreber, Freud (1911) suggested his paranoid delusion was traceable back to a profound conflict over unresolved homosexual impulses. The projection defence mechanism acted to protect the individual from the conflict-related anxiety. Different types of delusions could arise from the refusal of an unconscious homosexuality, contradicting the statement 'I (a man) love him (a man)'. Eventually, the unconscious feeling of loving another person of the same gender turns into hate justified by the persecution of the other. These theories appear nowadays as controversial at least, as well as not supported by research evidence (Chalus, 1977; Lester, 1975).

From a different perspective, models of delusion formation in delusional disorder focus on *cognitive styles*, neurocognitive *deficits*, and *perceptual deficits* (Abdel-Hamid & Brüne, 2008). Cognitive biases involved in the formation of persecutory delusions could relate to perceptual and inferential biases. The former include attentional biases characterized by the tendency to give greater weight to potentially threatening stimuli, whereas the latter include attributional biases, jumping to conclusions, and deficits in theory of mind (Blackwood et al., 2001) (see Davies and Coltheart, Chapter 29).

A further aspect regards *personality factors*, especially the *DSM*-defined cluster A (i.e., paranoid, schizoid, and schizotypal personality disorders) or C (i.e., obsessive-compulsive). Like Kretschmer's hypothesis that personality could confer greater vulnerability to delusional disorder, that is *sensitive delusion of reference,* cluster A disorders are characterized by bizarre thoughts and behaviours which may predispose to later development of a delusional disorder (de Portugal et al., 2009). However, it is not possible to clarify if prodromal characteristics of delusional disorder may be present from the early years of life or if specific affective dispositions (e.g., shame) can be part of delusional spectrum disorders (Pellegrini et al., 2022; Tonna et al., 2018).

As far as interpersonal and social factors issues, *attachment* is the paramount theory of psychiatrist and psychoanalyst John Bowlby (1982) who indicated the basic, intrinsic need for children to have a close bonding relationship with at least one primary caregiver to ensure normal development. Attachment has been investigated in practically all psychiatric disorders, including delusional disorders (Murphy et al., 2020). Although the direction of the relation is still unclear (i.e., what is the cause and what the consequence), several studies indicate that insecure attachment may favour paranoia via affective patterns (e.g. maladaptive emotion regulation) and cognitive factors (e.g., negative beliefs about self and others, poor self-esteem) (Lavin et al., 2020; Sood et al., 2022).

With regard to the *socio-demographic correlates*, compared to individuals with schizophrenia, those with delusional disorder differ significantly in the later illness onset, higher drug abuse rates before onset of the disorder, better daily functioning (Peralta & Cuesta, 2016), greater marital frequency, and higher premorbid IQ (Muñoz-Negro et al., 2018). Also, most people with delusional disorders are married immigrants of low socioeconomic and educational status (Kendler, 1982). The characteristics of the neighbourhood where people live are important in increasing or mitigating risk for psychotic symptoms (e.g. higher proportion of individuals of the same ethnicity could reduce individual risk for psychosis by reducing the negative effects of discrimination) (Brown, 2011). When examining a series of factors such as age, gender, disability, appearance, skin colour or ethnicity, and sexual orientation, the rate of delusions in the general population was 0.5 per cent, but higher in those who reported discrimination in one of the above-mentioned factors (0.9 per cent) or more than one factors (2.7 per cent) (Janssen et al., 2003). Social isolation constitutes a risk factor for development of delusional disorder, especially in the elderly (Nagendra & Snowdon, 2020). Sensory impairment is more common in individuals with delusional disorder and could further contribute to isolation and alteration in the interpretation of social situations, especially, but not only, in older individuals (Porras Segovia et al., 2016)

*Stressful life events* and traumatic experiences are associated with the risk for psychotic symptoms and disorders, even in the absence of post-traumatic stress disorder (Scott et al., 2007). Also, childhood traumas appear related to the severity of delusions in individuals with psychotic disorders (Bailey et al., 2018). Almost half of the individuals with delusional disorder report at least one stressful event before the onset of the disorder, and in one-third of cases the delusional content was related to the nature of the event (de Portugal et al., 2009; Pillmann et al., 2012), including highly traumatic events (Amsel et al., 2012). Individual characteristics, especially self-criticism and negative affectivity, may mediate the association between stressful life events and delusion formation and therefore could represent a treatment target (Kingston & Schuurmans-Stekhoven, 2016).

## 5.   Outcome and prognosis of delusional disorders

The *outcome* of delusional disorders largely depends upon early treatment (Fear, 2013). Although long considered a difficult-to-treat condition with a functional outcome intermediate between schizophrenia and affective disorders (Jørgensen, 1994; Opjordsmoen & Retterstöl, 1993), delusional disorders may respond to antipsychotic medications, with the somatic subtype showing a particularly favourable and marked response to pimozide among all antipsychotics (Manschreck & Khan, 2006; Muñoz-Negro & Cervilla, 2016). The main determinant of treatment response, however, is adherence, which appears to be critical in delusional disorders characterized by high levels of suspiciousness and fairly unimpaired real-world functioning (Fear, 2013; Manschreck & Khan, 2006). Regarding psychotherapy, Cognitive Behavioural Therapy (Mehl et al., 2015) and the combination of psychosocial and pharmacological approaches (Goodwin et al., 2020) hold promises for delusional disorders, although more evidence is needed (Skelton et al., 2015).

Delusional disorders, especially if untreated, have negative *consequences*, with outcome varying according by delusional disorder subtype, severity, and environmental factors (e.g., poor social support and occurrence of stressful life events). Although daily and social functioning can be maintained, especially in the so-called partial psychosis (with encapsulated, well-organized delusions), these disorders may worsen across time. For some forms (e.g., somatic type), depression is a possible consequence, often associated with social isolation and suicide risk (González-Rodríguez et al., 2014; Phillips et al., 2005). For others (e.g., jealous and persecutory types), legal consequences, violent acts and harm to others, including homicide, can be the end result (Darrell-Berry et al., 2016).

In some cases, paranoia and delusional disorders may produce tragedies because of the power of some leaders' delusional systems, as history teaches us. The Italian Jungian psychoanalyst Luigi Zoja (Zoja, 2011) analysed 'cases' of paranoia such as Hitler and Stalin, pointing out that, whereas most people with severe psychiatric disorders (e.g., schizophrenia, bipolar disorders) pass through history without leaving a trace, paranoia *can make history*, having the property of 'autotrophy' – an autonomous ability to multiply and infect.[1]

## 6.   Exemplifying delusional disorders: the tragedy and massacre
of Jonestown

The Jonestown massacre in Guyana, where 913 people of the agricultural commune Peoples Temple were found dead by mass suicide, is a striking example about delusional disorders and how the charisma of its paranoid leader, the Reverend Jim Jones, influenced others in the community through a sort of pandemic psychic contagion (Lasaga, 1980; Ulman & Abse, 1983).[2]

Five months before the tragedy, Deborah Layton Blakey, a former member and Financial Secretary of the Peoples Temple, made a series of declarations under penalty of perjury. From these declarations, the delusional features of Jim Jones clearly emerge [our emphases in bold].

6. The Rev. Jones saw himself as the **center of a conspiracy. The identity of the conspirators changed from day to day along with his erratic world vision.** [...] He convinced black Temple members that if they did not follow him to Guyana, they would be put into **concentration camps and killed.** White members **were instilled with the belief** that their names appeared on a **secret list of enemies** of the state that was kept by **the C.I.A.** and that they **would be tracked down, tortured, imprisoned, and subsequently killed** if they did not flee to Guyana.

7. Frequently, at Temple meetings, Rev. Jones **would talk non-stop for hours. At various times, he claimed that he was the reincarnation of either Lenin, Jesus Christ, or one of a variety of other religious or political figures.** He claimed that **he had divine powers** and **could heal the sick.** He stated that he had **extrasensory perception and could tell what everyone was thinking.** He said that he **had powerful connections the world over, including the Mafia, Idi Amin, and the Soviet government.**

8. [...] At other times, **he appeared to be deluded by a paranoid vision of the world.** He would not sleep for days at a time and **talk compulsively about the conspiracies against** him.

27. [...] **He was irate at the light in which he had been portrayed by the media. He felt that as a consequence of having been ridiculed and maligned, he would be denied a place in history.** His obsession with his place in history was maniacal.

31. At least once a week, Rev. Jones would declare a 'white night', or state of emergency. The entire population of Jonestown would be awakened by blaring sirens. Designated persons, approximately fifty in number, would arm themselves with rifles, move from cabin to cabin, and make certain that all members were responding. A mass meeting would ensue. Frequently during these crises, we would be told that the **jungle was swarming with mercenaries and that death could be expected at any minute.**

32. During one 'white night', we were informed that our situation had become hopeless and that the only course of action open to us was **a mass suicide for the glory of socialism.** We were told that we would **be tortured by mercenaries if we were taken alive.** Everyone, including the children, was told to line up. As we passed through the line, we were given a small glass of red liquid to drink. We were told that the liquid contained poison and that we would die within 45 minutes. We all did as we were told. When the time came when we should have dropped dead, Rev. Jones explained that the poison was not real and that we had just been through a **loyalty test.**

In the crisis after the assassination of Congressman Leo Ryan and other four people, on November 18, 1978, Reverend Jones convinced his people to commit mass suicide. His last 44-minute speech, recorded and kept, during the site inspection after the tragedy, by the FBI next to Jones' wooden throne chair on the stage of Jonestown's open-air pavilion, is instructive in depicting Jones' pathological condition (our emphasis in bold) (1993):

> Jones: We're in a compound situation, not only are there those who have left and **committed the betrayal of the century,** some have stolen children from others and then seek right now to kill them because they stole their children, and we are sitting here waiting on a powder keg [...] It **was said by the greatest of prophets, from time immemorial, 'No man takes my life from me, I lay my life down'.**
> Crowd: Yeah!
> [...]
> Jones: So, my opinion is that we be kind to children and be kind to seniors and **take the potion like they used to take in ancient Greece,** and step over quietly because we are not committing suicide. It's a revolutionary act. We can't go back. [...] Don't be afraid to die ... (unintelligible words) ... **if these people land out here, they'll torture some of our children here. They'll torture our people, they'll torture our seniors. We cannot have this.**
> Crowd: Right, right.
> [...]
> Jones: [...] (unintelligible words) ... take our life from us, we laid it down, we got tired. We didn't commit suicide. We committed an act of revolutionary suicide protesting the conditions of an inhumane world.

## 7.  Discussion and conclusions

In this chapter, we have presented the main issues related to delusional disorders as today classified and interpreted by psychiatry, including diagnostic features, possible biopsychosocial determinants and associated factors, and outcomes.

Some issues deserve discussion, considering that these complex mental disorders have still a series of questions to be answered. A first concerns the problem of the criteria used to diagnose delusion. As we said, the general conceptualization of delusion as a disturbance of the thinking process applies to delusional disorders: unusual persistence or force of the belief, even when evidence contradicts it; implausibility with respect to the individual's social, cultural, and religious background; the person's belief and behaviour is perceived as uncharacteristic and alien by people who know the patients; any attempt to contradict the idea or belief arouses an inappropriately strong emotional reaction and if the belief is acted upon can generate abnormal behaviours (even if sometimes understandable in light of the delusional belief), the undue influence of delusion on the person's life, often altering that way of life is to an inexplicable degree (Munro, 1988). However, the difference between healthy and pathological, normal and abnormal mental processes may prove difficult to demarcate in assessing subjective states (e.g., thought, perception, and feeling) in comparison with objective parameters (e.g., blood pressure and liver enzymes). Psychiatric diagnostic criteria are based on factors such as statistical frequency or infrequency (conformity to vs. deviance from norms), impact on 'normal' psychosocial functioning, adaptation/adjustment, the presence or absence of which is not neatly dichotomous (true/false; yes/no). When other factors are taken into consideration (e.g. cultural, ethical, and anthropological variables, social changes, and expectations about features like physical appearance, sexuality, and gender) the problem of categorization (normal/abnormal) is even bigger

(Bassett & Baker, 2015; Fabrega, 1989; Wakefield & First, 2013). The well-known experiment by Rosenhan (Rosenhan, 1973)[3] to provocatively show the unreliability of psychiatric diagnosis indicated that mentally healthy people miming psychiatric symptoms can receive the diagnosis of schizophrenia and treatment with antipsychotic medications. For these reasons, the clinical use of more reliable and precise categorical criteria, such as those proposed first by the Research Diagnostic Criteria group (Spitzer et al., 1978) and then by the *DSM-III*, was welcomed. In the last 20 years, however, *DSM* categorical criteria have themselves been criticized in favour of a more dimensional approach, which avoids the problem of a dichotomous approach (Kessler, 2002; Kraemer et al., 2004; Narrow & Kuhl, 2011). An example of this long ongoing and unsolved problem is the subjective psychiatrist's criterion proposed by Rümke (1941), the *praecox-gefühl* (praecox feeling), as a core symptom of schizophrenia. Emanating from the clinician, this indirect criterion describes a characteristic feeling of unease or bizarreness, an atmosphere of strangeness the clinician experiences in encountering and interviewing a person with schizophrenia. Rümke's conviction that the diagnosis of schizophrenia could often be reached through this passive and indescribable intuition was rejected by the *DSM* as a standard reflecting a-scientific psychiatry. However, there has been a recent upsurge of interest in *praecox-gefühl*, with authors supporting the reliability and value of this criterion, opening the question of the diagnostic process in psychiatry again (Gozé, 2022; Gozé et al., 2019; Pallagrosi & Fonzi, 2018).

A second related problem is that, as noted, delusional disorders secondary to medical diseases or medications/substances must be ruled out to diagnose primary (idiopathic) delusional disorders. Nevertheless, it remains germane that an objective condition (e.g., a Central Nervous System (CNS) lesion) may determine a phenomenological presentation similar or identical to a primary delusional condition. Does this indicate that we lack sufficiently sophisticated techniques to catch subtle neuronal network or cellular neurobiological alterations of primary delusions? Are primary and secondary delusional symptoms identical or similar epiphenomena of different processes? Can secondary delusional disorders enhance understanding of the pathophysiology of primary (idiopathic) delusional disorders (Joyce, 2018)? Again, using a dichotomous approach, in this case organic versus non-organic ('functional') or primary versus secondary, seems to compound the problem. Several recent attempts have been made to re-organize the nosology of psychiatric disorders, including delusional disorders, by using other approaches such as the Hierarchical Taxonomy of Psychopathology (HiTOP) or the network theory,[4] which contrast with the *DSM* and the ICD (Stein et al., 2022).

A third issue concerns the philosophical approach now emerging in the context of delusional beliefs (Bortolotti, 2018). It questions the concept of delusion and its descriptive characteristics. Specifically, regarding the *falsity* criterion, it is not at all obvious that all delusions are false. The separation of what is false or true in reality is more complex when a delusional experience relates to the external world and refers to 'object' (e.g., 'there are people spying and following me', more typical of persecutory delusions) than the inner world and the subjective experience about oneself (e.g., 'I am sure an occult cancer is growing in me', more typical of somatic delusions). Regarding *incorrigibility*, again, people not uncommonly have incorrigible beliefs without being delusional (e.g., Leeser & O'Donohue, 1999). The *content* criteria, including absurdity, implausibility, and absence of meaning of delusions can be also challenged: delusions may be not meaningless. Instead, they may relate to some painful experiences the person had prior to the delusion onset, with a precise personal meaning (Gunn & Bortolotti, 2018; Ritunnano & Bortolotti, 2022; Ritunnano et al., 2022, see also Ritunnano and Littlemore, Chapter 2). Regarding delusion's *rigidity* and *resistance to change,* data indicate that the opposite can be true, as shown by computational psychiatry (e.g., Ashinoff et al., 2022).

Last, there are delusional systems beyond the clinical context, the so-called 'everyday delusions' that share some features of delusional disorders but are not typically idiosyncratic to one person, and can be shared by groups of people in defined social groups whose views depart from those widely accepted in mainstream society (Grassi & Bortolotti, 2022). There are many examples in history that are usually triggered by societal crisis situations and events causing substantial uncertainty, fear, and a remarkable sense of personal vulnerability or threat (e.g., U.S. government to be complicit in 9/11 terrorist attack) (van Prooijen & Douglas, 2017; van Prooijen & van Vugt, 2018). The recent COVID-19 denialism and COVID-19 conspiracy beliefs have become part of a shared condition characterized by 'everyday delusions' associated with a rigid and firm conviction about the way in which the SARS-Co-V2 developed, the role of 5G technology, the deliberate threats to which people are exposed by receiving anti-COVID-19 vaccine (for more on delusion and conspiracy theories see Pierre, Chapter 37).

In summary, delusional disorders are a complex and heterogeneous group of mental disorders that can affect a single individual and sometimes more than one (shared psychotic disorder). Several forms have been described in terms of delusional content (e.g., persecutory and jealousy), severity, and clinical state (acute or persistent). They have significant consequences for personal functioning, although fewer than disorders such as schizophrenia. A series of shortcomings regarding this long-debated condition remain unsolved. Among these are the difficulty in clearly making the diagnosis by the psychiatric categorical approach; the evidence of a continuum of psychotic symptoms and disorders in the general population; and the problem of defining causes, given the overlapping and complex interaction between neurobiological, psychological, cognitive, social, and environmental factors, all deserving attention. More integrated approaches, including philosophical, phenomenological, neuroscientific, and precision and personalized models, should be implemented for clinical practice.

## Acknowledgements

The authors are deeply indebted to John C. Markowitz, M.D., Professor of Clinical Psychiatry at the Columbia University College of Physicians & Surgeons and Psychiatric Researcher at the New York State Psychiatric Institute, for his thoughtful comments on the chapter.

## Notes

1 As Luigi Zoja writes, 'Paranoia is infinitely more difficult to identify than other mental disorders because it is able to disguise itself, both within the personality of the paranoiac, who as a whole is far from mad, and among the individuals around him. What we see is the tip of an iceberg of unreason on which any ship of reason can founder. [...] Between mentally ill and sane people there is no leap, but continuity. But even in the madman's mind, thought usually slides from "normality" into delusion only by degrees, and this transition can be particularly imperceptible in the paranoiac' (2011: 11). 'paranoia is the only mental disorder that possesses *autotrophy* – an autonomous ability to multiply and infect. Only paranoia has a circular relationship with history. It is the cause and at the same time the consequence of mass events. It is the only illness capable

of making history. [...] The psychiatrist can stop the mad hand that grasps the knife, but not the hands of Hitler, Stalin and the masses who followed them; it cannot do so, precisely because the masses followed them. [...] paranoia outside the gates, mingled with everyday life, scattered in every part of society, has exterminated more human masses than the plague epidemics' (2011: 38).

2 James Warren Jones, known as Jim Jones, was an American cult leader who in 1955 established in Indianapolis a Pentacostal church, the Wings of Deliverance, later renamed the Peoples Temple. The church moved to different places in California, apparently from Jones' fears of nuclear war. He proclaimed himself 'the Prophet' and asserted he had psychic powers such as ability to foretell the future and heal the sick. After being accused of illegally diverting money from cult members, he and the People's Temple moved in 1977 to the Guyananese jungle to found an agricultural commune, Jonestown. Here people were manipulated, threatened, and blackmailed. Jones created an atmosphere of terror with nighttime rehearsals (so called 'white nights') for a ritual suicide as a sign of loyalty. After a few people left and made affidavits about the terrible conditions in Jonestown, Congressman Leo Ryan and a journalist flew to Jonestown on November 14, 1978 to investigate possible abuses perpetrated by Jones and his closest cult members there. After four days, Ryan and 14 cult members who wanted to flee the village prepared to fly back to the US. Jones then ordered their assassination by attacking them in the jungle en route to the airstrip. Ryan, three journalists and a fifth person were shot, while the others escaped. Fearing becoming a victim of prosecution by authorities, Jones convinced the Peoples Temple to commit suicide by dinking a potion with barbiturates and cyanide. Those who refused were killed by others. Jones also eventually died by gunshot, although authorities are still uncertain whether he took his own life.

3 The experiment was carried out in 12 US psychiatric hospitals. Mentally healthy people (8 individuals, including Rosenhan) pretended to be affected by mental disorders (reporting auditive hallucinations) and for that reason were admitted to a psychiatric unit. Although these pseudo-patients acted normally during their stay and said denied still having symptoms, they were given medication and had difficulty getting discharged, with lengths of stay ranging from 7 to 52 days, despite ongoing normal behaviour. Rosenhan concluded that diagnoses of psychiatric disorders were invalid and reliable, leaving room for significant mistakes and problems.

4 The HiTOP is a scientific effort to solve the problems of DSM and ICD in making psychiatric diagnoses (e.g. arbitrary boundaries between psychopathology and normality, frequent disorder co-occurrence, heterogeneity within disorders, and diagnostic instability), by combining individual signs and symptoms into homogeneous components or traits, assembling them into empirically-derived syndromes, and finally grouping them into psychopathology spectra. The Network theory conceptualizes psychiatric disorders as relatively stable networks of interacting symptoms, including non-symptom factors relevant, such as environmental factors (e.g. adverse life events, social relationships).

# References


Abdel-Hamid, M., & Brüne, M. (2008). Neuropsychological aspects of delusional disorder. *Current Psychiatry Reports*, 10(3), 229–234. https://doi.org/10.1007/s11920-008-0038-x

American Psychiatric Association (1980) *DSM-III. Diagnostic and Statistical Manual of Mental Disorders* (Third Edition). Washington, DC: American Psychiatric Publishing

Amsel, L. V., Hunter, N., Kim, S., Fodor, K. E., & Markowitz, J. C. (2012). Does a study focused on trauma encourage patients with psychotic symptoms to seek treatment? *Psychiatric Services (Washington, D.C.)*, 63(4), 386–389. https://doi.org/10.1176/appi.ps.201100251

Ashinoff, B. K., Singletary, N. M., Baker, S. C., & Horga, G. (2022). Rethinking delusions: A selective review of delusion research through a computational lens. *Schizophrenia Research*, 245, 23–41. https://doi.org/10.1016/j.schres.2021.01.023

Bailey, T., Alvarez-Jimenez, M., Garcia-Sanchez, A. M., Hulbert, C., Barlow, E., & Bendall, S. (2018). Childhood trauma is associated with severity of hallucinations and delusions in psychotic disorders: A systematic review and meta-analysis. *Schizophrenia Bulletin*, 44(5), 1111–1122. https://doi.org/10.1093/schbul/sbx161

Bassett, A. M., & Baker, C. (2015). Normal or abnormal? «Normative uncertainty» in psychiatric practice. *The Journal of Medical Humanities*, 36(2), 89–111. https://doi.org/10.1007/s10912-014-9324-2

Blackwood, N. J., Howard, R. J., Bentall, R. P., & Murray, R. M. (2001). Cognitive neuropsychiatric models of persecutory delusions. *American Journal of Psychiatry*, 158(4), 527–539. https://doi.org/10.1176/appi.ajp.158.4.527

Bortolotti, L. (2018). Delusions and three myths of irrational belief. In L. Bortolotti (A c. Di), *Delusions in Context* (pp. 97–116). Springer International Publishing. https://doi.org/10.1007/978-3-319-97202-2_4

Bowlby J (1982) Attachment and loss: retrospect and prospect *American Journal of Orthopsychiatry*, 52(4), 664–678. https://doi.org/ 10.1111/j.1939-0025.1982.tb01456.x.

Brown, A. S. (2011). The environment and susceptibility to schizophrenia. *Progress in Neurobiology*, 93(1), 23–58. https://doi.org/10.1016/j.pneurobio.2010.09.003

Castagnini, A. (2016). «Paranoia and its historical development (systematized delusion)», by Eugenio Tanzi (1884). *History of Psychiatry*, 27(2), 229–240. https://doi.org/10.1177/0957154X16630501

Chalus, G. A. (1977). An evaluation of the validity of the Freudian theory of paranoia. *Journal of Homosexuality*, 3(2), 171–188. https://doi.org/10.1300/j082v03n02_06

Cheng, P. W. C., Chang, W. C., Lo, G. G., Chan, K. W. S., Lee, H. M. E., Hui, L. M. C., Suen, Y. N., Leung, Y. L. E., Au Yeung, K. M. P., Chen, S., Mak, K. F. H., Sham, P. C., Santangelo, B., Veronese, M., Ho, C.-L., Chen, Y. H. E., & Howes, O. D. (2020). The role of dopamine dysregulation and evidence for the transdiagnostic nature of elevated dopamine synthesis in psychosis: A positron emission tomography (PET) study comparing schizophrenia, delusional disorder, and other psychotic disorders. *Neuropsychopharmacology*, 45(11), 1870–1876. https://doi.org/10.1038/s41386-020-0740-x

Darrell-Berry, H., Berry, K., & Bucci, S. (2016). The relationship between paranoia and aggression in psychosis: A systematic review. *Schizophrenia Research*, 172(1–3), 169–176. https://doi.org/10.1016/j.schres.2016.02.009

de Portugal, E., González, N., Vilaplana, M., Haro, J. M., Usall, J., & Cervilla, J. A. (2009). An empirical study of psychosocial and clinical correlates of delusional disorder: The DELIREMP study. *Revista de Psiquiatría y Salud Mental (English Edition)*, 2(2), 72–82. https://doi.org/10.1016/S2173-5050(09)70034-2

Dowbiggin, I. (2000). Delusional diagnosis? The history of paranoia as a disease concept in the modern era. *History of Psychiatry*, 11(41 Pt 1), 37–69. https://doi.org/10.1177/0957154X0001104103

Fabrega, H. (1989). Cultural relativism and psychiatric illness. *The Journal of Nervous and Mental Disease*, 177(7), 415–425; discussion 426–430. https://doi.org/10.1097/00005053-198907000-00005

Fear, C. F. (2013). Recent developments in the management of delusional disorders. *Advances in Psychiatric Treatment*, 19(3), 212–220. https://doi.org/10.1192/apt.bp.111.010082

Fear, C. F., McMonagle, T., & Healy, D. (1998). Delusional disorders: Boundaries of a concept. *European Psychiatry: The Journal of the Association of European Psychiatrists*, 13(4), 210–218. https://doi.org/10.1016/S0924-9338(98)80006-0

Freud, S (1911). *The Schreber Case*. Translated by Andrew Webber. New York: Penguin Classics Psychology, 2003. ISBN 0-14-243742-5.

Gill, C. (1996). Mind and madness in Greek tragedy. *Apeiron*, 29(3), 249–268. https://doi.org/10.1515/APEIRON.1996.29.3.249

González-Rodríguez, A., Molina-Andreu, O., Navarro Odriozola, V., Gastó Ferrer, C., Penadés, R., & Catalán, R. (2014). Suicidal ideation and suicidal behaviour in delusional disorder: A clinical overview. *Psychiatry Journal*, 2014, 834901. https://doi.org/10.1155/2014/834901

Goodwin, T.-A., Lowry, T. J., Meurk, C., & Neillie, D. (2020). Treating the untreatable? The biopsychosocial treatment of delusional disorder: A case study. *Australasian Psychiatry: Bulletin of Royal Australian and New Zealand College of Psychiatrists*, 28(4), 433–437. https://doi.org/10.1177/1039856220901463

Gozé, T. (2022). How to teach/learn praecox feeling? Through phenomenology to medical education. *Frontiers in Psychiatry*, 13. https://www.frontiersin.org/articles/10.3389/fpsyt.2022.819305

Gozé, T., Moskalewicz, M., Schwartz, M. A., Naudin, J., Micoulaud-Franchi, J.-A., & Cermolacce, M. (2019). Reassessing "praecox feeling" in diagnostic decision making in schizophrenia: A critical review. *Schizophrenia Bulletin*, 45(5), 966–970. https://doi.org/10.1093/schbul/sby172

Grassi, Luigi, & Bortolotti, Lisa (2024). Delusions across and beyond diagnoses. In Falcato A., GonçalvesJ (Eds) *The Philosophy and Psychology of Delusions. Historical and Contemporary Perspectives*. London: Routledge, pp. 1–13, London https://doi.org/10.4324/9781003288992.

Guàrdia, A., González-Rodríguez, A., Seeman, M. V., Álvarez, A., Estrada, F., Acebillo, S., Labad, J., & Monreal, J. A. (2021). Dopamine, serotonin, and structure/function brain defects as biological bases for treatment response in delusional disorder: A systematic review of cases and cohort studies. *Behavioral Sciences, 11*(10), 141. https://doi.org/10.3390/bs11100141

Gunn, R. L., & Bortolotti, L. (2018). Can delusions play a protective role? *Phenomenology and the Cognitive Sciences.* https://doi.org/10.1007/s11097-017-9555-6

Hirjak, D., Huber, M., Kirchler, E., Kubera, K. M., Karner, M., Sambataro, F., Freudenmann, R. W., & Wolf, R. C. (2017). Cortical features of distinct developmental trajectories in patients with delusional infestation. *Progress in Neuro-Psychopharmacology & Biological Psychiatry, 76,* 72–79. https://doi.org/10.1016/j.pnpbp.2017.02.018

Janssen, I., Hanssen, M., Bak, M., Bijl, R. V., De Graaf, R., Vollebergh, W., McKenzie, K., & Van Os, J. (2003). Discrimination and delusional ideation. *British Journal of Psychiatry, 182*(1), 71–76. https://doi.org/10.1192/bjp.182.1.71

Jaspers, K. (1913). *Allgemeine Psychopathologie Ein Leitfaden Fur Studierende, Arzte Und Psychologen.* Berlin: Springer Verlag

Jaspers, K (1910) Eifersuchtswahn. Ein Beitrag zur Frage: "Entwicklung einer PersiJnliehkeit" oder, "ProzeB"? *Zeitschrift für die gesamte Neurologie und Psychiatrie, 1,* 567–637 https://doi.org/10.1007/BF02895947.

Jones, J. (1993). *Jonestown Massacre: Transcript of Jim Jones' Last Speech, Guyana 1978.* Sussex: Temple Press

Jørgensen, P. (1994). Course and outcome in delusional disorders. *Psychopathology, 27*(1–2), 79–88. https://doi.org/10.1159/000284852

Joyce, E. M. (2018). Organic psychosis: The pathobiology and treatment of delusions. *CNS Neuroscience & Therapeutics, 24*(7), 598–603. https://doi.org/10.1111/cns.12973

Kendler, K. S. (1980). The nosologic validity of paranoia (simple delusional disorder). A review. *Archives of General Psychiatry, 37*(6), 699–706. https://doi.org/10.1001/archpsyc.1980.01780190097012

Kendler, K. S. (1982). Demography of paranoid psychosis (delusional disorder). *Archives of General Psychiatry, 39*(8), 890. https://doi.org/10.1001/archpsyc.1982.04290080012003

Kendler, K. S. (1988). Kraepelin and the diagnostic concept of paranoia. *Comprehensive Psychiatry, 29*(1). https://doi.org/10.1016/0010-440x(88)90031-4

Kendler, K. S. (2009). An historical framework for psychiatric nosology. *Psychological Medicine, 39*(12), 1935–1941. https://doi.org/10.1017/S0033291709005753

Kendler, K. S. (2017). The clinical features of paranoia in the 20th century and their representation in diagnostic criteria from DSM-III through DSM-5. *Schizophrenia Bulletin, 43*(2), 332–343. https://doi.org/10.1093/schbul/sbw161

Kendler, K. S., & Tsuang, M. T. (1981). Nosology of paranoid schizophrenia and other paranoid psychoses. *Schizophrenia Bulletin, 7*(4), 594–610. https://doi.org/10.1093/schbul/7.4.594

Kessler, R. C. (2002). The categorical versus dimensional assessment controversy in the sociology of mental illness. *Journal of Health and Social Behavior, 43*(2), 171–188.

Kingston, C., & Schuurmans-Stekhoven, J. (2016). Life hassles and delusional ideation: Scoping the potential role of cognitive and affective mediators. *Psychology and Psychotherapy: Theory, Research and Practice, 89*(4), 445–463. https://doi.org/10.1111/papt.12089

Kraepelin, E. (1899). *Psychiatrie: ein Lehrbuch für Studirende und AerzteJ.* Leipzig: Johann Ambrosius Barth, 1899.

Kraemer, H. C., Noda, A., & O'Hara, R. (2004). Categorical versus dimensional approaches to diagnosis: Methodological challenges. *Journal of Psychiatric Research, 38*(1), 17–25. https://doi.org/10.1016/s0022-3956(03)00097-9

Kunert, H. J., Norra, C., & Hoff, P. (2007). Theories of delusional disorders. An update and review. *Psychopathology, 40*(3), 191–202. https://doi.org/10.1159/000100367

Lasaga, J. I. (1980). Death in Jonestown: Techniques of political control by a paranoid leader. *Suicide & Life-Threatening Behavior, 10*(4), 210–213. https://doi.org/10.1111/j.1943-278x.1980.tb00701.x

Lasègue C, Falret J. (1877) La folie à deux. *Annales Médico-Psychologiques, 18,* 321–355

Lavin, R., Bucci, S., Varese, F., & Berry, K. (2020). The relationship between insecure attachment and paranoia in psychosis: A systematic literature review. *The British Journal of Clinical Psychology, 59*(1), 39–65. https://doi.org/10.1111/bjc.12231

Leeser, J., & O'Donohue, W. (1999). What is a delusion? Epistemological dimensions. *Journal of Abnormal Psychology, 108*, 687–694. https://doi.org/10.1037/0021-843X.108.4.687

Lehmann, G. (1883) Zur Kasuistik des induzierten Irreseins. *Archiv für die gesamte Psychologie, 14*, 145.

Lester, D. (1975). The relationship between paranoid delusions and homosexuality. *Archives of Sexual Behavior, 4*(3), 285–294. https://doi.org/10.1007/BF01541628

Lewis, A. (1970). Paranoia and paranoid: A historical perspective. *Psychological Medicine, 1*(1), 2–12. https://doi.org/10.1017/s0033291700039969

Maieron, M. A. (2017). The meaning of Madness in ancient Greek culture from Homer to Hippocrates and Plato. *Medicina Historica, 1*(2), Art. 2.

Manschreck, T. C., & Khan, N. L. (2006). Recent advances in the treatment of delusional disorder. *Canadian Journal of Psychiatry. Revue Canadienne De Psychiatrie, 51*(2), 114–119. https://doi.org/10.1177/070674370605100207

Mehl, S., Werner, D., & Lincoln, T. M. (2015). Does Cognitive Behavior Therapy for psychosis (CBTp) show a sustainable effect on delusions? A meta-analysis. *Frontiers in Psychology, 6*, 1450. https://doi.org/10.3389/fpsyg.2015.01450

Muñoz-Negro, J. E., & Cervilla, J. A. (2016). A systematic review on the pharmacological treatment of delusional disorder. *Journal of Clinical Psychopharmacology, 36*(6), 684–690. https://doi.org/10.1097/JCP.0000000000000595

Muñoz-Negro, J. E., Ibáñez-Casas, I., de Portugal, E., Lozano-Gutiérrez, V., Martínez-Leal, R., & Cervilla, J. A. (2018). A psychopathological comparison between delusional disorder and schizophrenia. *The Canadian Journal of Psychiatry, 63*(1), 12–19. https://doi.org/10.1177/0706743717706347

Munro, A. (1982). Paranoia revisited. *The British Journal of Psychiatry: The Journal of Mental Science, 141*, 344–349. https://doi.org/10.1192/bjp.141.4.344

Munro, A (1988) Delusional (paranoid) disorders. *Canadian Journal of Psychiatry, 33*(5), 399-404. doi: 10.1177/070674378803300516.

Murphy, R., Goodall, K., & Woodrow, A. (2020). The relationship between attachment insecurity and experiences on the paranoia continuum: A meta-analysis. *British Journal of Clinical Psychology, 59*(3), 290–318. https://doi.org/10.1111/bjc.12247

Nagendra, J., & Snowdon, J. (2020). An Australian study of delusional disorder in late life. *International Psychogeriatrics, 32*(4), 453–462. https://doi.org/10.1017/S1041610219000966

Narrow, W. E., & Kuhl, E. A. (2011). Dimensional approaches to psychiatric diagnosis in DSM-5. *The Journal of Mental Health Policy and Economics, 14*(4), 197–200.

Opjordsmoen, S. (2014). Delusional disorder as a partial psychosis. *Schizophrenia Bulletin, 40*(2), 244–247. https://doi.org/10.1093/schbul/sbt203

Opjordsmoen, S., & Retterstöl, N. (1993). Outcome in delusional disorder in different periods of time. Possible implications for treatment with neuroleptics. *Psychopathology, 26*(2), 90–94. https://doi.org/10.1159/000284805

Oyebode, Femi. (2012). Jealousy the green-eyed monster and madness in Shakespeare. In Femi Oyebode (Ed.), *Madness at the Theatre* (pp. 31–47). London: Cambridge University Press.

Padel, R. (1997). Whom gods destroy: Elements of Greek and tragic madness. *The Classical World.* https://www.academia.edu/78175573/Whom_Gods_Destroy_Elements_of_Greek_and_Tragic_Madness

Pallagrosi, M., & Fonzi, L. (2018). On the concept of praecox feeling. *Psychopathology, 51*(6), 353–361. https://doi.org/10.1159/000494088

Pellegrini, R., Negro, J. E. M., Ottoni, R., Cervilla, J. A., & Tonna, M. (2022). The affective core of delusional disorder. *Psychopathology, 55*(3–4), 244–250. https://doi.org/10.1159/000522344

Peralta, V., & Cuesta, M. J. (2016). Delusional disorder and schizophrenia: A comparative study across multiple domains. *Psychological Medicine, 46*(13), 2829–2839. https://doi.org/10.1017/S0033291716001501

Phillips, K. A., Coles, M. E., Menard, W., Yen, S., Fay, C., & Weisberg, R. B. (2005). Suicidal ideation and suicide attempts in body dysmorphic disorder. *The Journal of Clinical Psychiatry, 66*(6), 717–725. https://doi.org/10.4088/jcp.v66n0607

Pillmann, F., Wustmann, T., & Marneros, A. (2012). Clinical course and personality in reactive, compared with nonreactive, delusional disorder. *Canadian Journal of Psychiatry. Revue Canadienne De Psychiatrie, 57*(4), 216–222. https://doi.org/10.1177/070674371205700404

Porras Segovia, A., Guerrero Jimenez, M., Carrillo de Albornoz Calahorro, C., & Cervilla Ballesteros, J. (2016). Comorbidity between delusional disorder and sensory deficits. Results from the deliranda case register. *European Psychiatry, 33*, S144–S145. https://doi.org/10.1016/j.eurpsy.2016.01.249

Ritunnano, R., & Bortolotti, L. (2022). Do delusions have and give meaning? *Phenomenology and the Cognitive Sciences, 21*(4), 949–968. https://doi.org/10.1007/s11097-021-09764-9

Ritunnano, R., Kleinman, J., Whyte Oshodi, D., Michail, M., Nelson, B., Humpston, C. S., & Broome, M. R. (2022). Subjective experience and meaning of delusions in psychosis: A systematic review and qualitative evidence synthesis. *The Lancet Psychiatry, 9*(6), 458–476. https://doi.org/10.1016/S2215-0366(22)00104-3

Rosenhan, D. L. (1973). On being sane in insane places. *Science, 179*(4070), 250–258. https://doi.org/10.1126/science.179.4070.250

Rümke, H. C. (1941) Das Kernsymptom der Schizophrenie und das „Praecoxgefühl". *Nederlands Tijdschrift voor Geneeskunde*, 4516–4521

Schifferdecker, M., & Peters, U. H. (1995). The origin of the concept of paranoia. *The Psychiatric Clinics of North America, 18*(2), 231–249.

Scott, J., Chant, D., Andrews, G., Martin, G., & McGrath, J. (2007). Association between trauma exposure and delusional experiences in a large community-based sample. *British Journal of Psychiatry, 190*(4), 339–343. https://doi.org/10.1192/bjp.bp.106.026708

Shimizu, M., Kubota, Y., Toichi, M., & Baba, H. (2007). Folie à deux and shared psychotic disorder. *Current Psychiatry Reports, 9*(3), 200–205. https://doi.org/10.1007/s11920-007-0019-5

Skelton, M., Khokhar, W. A., & Thacker, S. P. (2015). Treatments for delusional disorder. *Schizophrenia Bulletin, 41*(5), 1010–1012. https://doi.org/10.1093/schbul/sbv080

Sood, M., Carnelley, K. B., & Newman-Taylor, K. (2022). How does insecure attachment lead to paranoia? A systematic critical review of cognitive, affective, and behavioural mechanisms. *The British Journal of Clinical Psychology, 61*(3), 781–815. https://doi.org/10.1111/bjc.12361

Spitzer, R. L., Endicott, J., & Robins, E. (1978). Research diagnostic criteria: Rationale and reliability. *Archives of General Psychiatry, 35*(6), 773–782. https://doi.org/10.1001/archpsyc.1978.01770300115013

Stein, D. J., Shoptaw, S. J., Vigo, D. V., Lund, C., Cuijpers, P., Bantjes, J., Sartorius, N., & Maj, M. (2022). Psychiatric diagnosis and treatment in the 21st century: Paradigm shifts versus incremental integration. *World Psychiatry: Official Journal of the World Psychiatric Association (WPA), 21*(3), 393–414. https://doi.org/10.1002/wps.20998

Theodorou, Z. (1993). Subject to emotion: Exploring madness in «Orestes». *Classical Quarterly, 43*(1), 32–46. https://doi.org/10.1017/s0009838800044153

Tonna, M., Paglia, F., Ottoni, R., Ossola, P., De Panfilis, C., & Marchesi, C. (2018). Delusional disorder: The role of personality and emotions on delusional ideation. *Comprehensive Psychiatry, 85*, 78–83. https://doi.org/10.1016/j.comppsych.2018.07.002

Ulman, R. B., & Abse, D. W. (1983). The group psychology of mass madness: Jonestown. *Political Psychology, 4*(4), 637. https://doi.org/10.2307/3791059

van Prooijen, J.-W., & Douglas, K. M. (2017). Conspiracy theories as part of history: The role of societal crisis situations. *Memory Studies, 10*(3), 323–333. https://doi.org/10.1177/1750698017701615

van Prooijen, J.-W., & van Vugt, M. (2018). Conspiracy theories: Evolved functions and psychological mechanisms. *Perspectives on Psychological Science: A Journal of the Association for Psychological Science, 13*(6), 770–788. https://doi.org/10.1177/1745691618774270

Vicens, V., Radua, J., Salvador, R., Anguera-Camós, M., Canales-Rodríguez, E. J., Sarró, S., Maristany, T., McKenna, P. J., & Pomarol-Clotet, E. (2016). Structural and functional brain changes in delusional disorder. *The British Journal of Psychiatry, 208*(2), 153–159. https://doi.org/10.1192/bjp.bp.114.159087

Wakefield, J. C., & First, M. B. (2013). Clarifying the boundary between normality and disorder: A fundamental conceptual challenge for psychiatry. *The Canadian Journal of Psychiatry, 58*(11), 603–605. https://doi.org/10.1177/070674371305801104

Winokur, G. (1977). Delusional disorder (paranoia). *Comprehensive Psychiatry, 18*(6), 511–521. https://doi.org/10.1016/S0010-440X(97)90001-8

Zoja, L. (2011). *Paranoia. La Follia che fa la storia*. Boringhieri, Milano (English Translation, 2017, Paranoia. the madness that makes history), Routledge, London.

# 7
# DELUSIONS IN PSYCHOSIS

*Marianne D. Broeker and Matthew Broome*

## 1. Introduction

It can be hard to find a clear definition of psychosis. The previous edition of the *DSM*, *DSM-IV* (American Psychiatric Association [APA], 1994), says cautiously that the term *psychotic* has had a number of definitions over time and goes on to say, 'The narrowest definition of *psychotic* is restricted to delusions or prominent hallucinations, with the hallucinations occurring in the absence of insight into their pathological nature' and a 'less restrictive definition would also include prominent hallucinations that the individual realizes are hallucinatory experiences. Broader still is a definition that includes other positive symptoms of schizophrenia (i.e., disorganized speech, grossly disorganized or catatonic behaviour)' (APA, 2000, DSM-4-TR, p. 827). Hence, psychosis is synonymous with delusions and/or hallucinations in the absence of insight, for the narrowest definition. This includes a range of particular diagnoses, and much of the work of the clinician is to determine the precise diagnosis and to rule out any other wider causes of psychosis. If we conceptualize psychosis as the presence of hallucinations and delusions then this is a state that any of us could be in: for example, with a head injury, when suffering a delirium from an infection, drug intoxication or withdrawal, or an endocrine disturbance. Once these and other problems have been excluded, then additional clinical features are important in determining the precise diagnosis, for example, clinical course over time, presence of affective disturbance, negative symptoms. The focus of our chapter is on psychosis as a disorder, and delusions in the context of 'functional' psychotic illnesses, and in particular, one of the commonest causes of psychotic illness, namely, schizophrenia. However, 'psychotic' can also be used to refer to the whole continuum of psychosis – from treatment-refractory chronic schizophrenia to fleeting unusual perceptions or thoughts in those who are not either distressed nor help-seeking. Hence, delusions are part of the diagnostic and conceptual features in schizophrenia and other psychotic disorders. They are very common, occurring in more than 90 per cent of psychotic cases (APA, 2013). The most prevalent type of delusion is persecutory (~70 per cent of first episode patients) but many different types have been observed in psychosis (APA, 2013).

DOI: 10.4324/9781003296386-10

In this chapter, we will first discuss how delusions in psychosis can be described and what characteristics have been assigned to them from various approaches ranging from doxastic, belief-based approaches, including cognitive error and prediction error approaches to delusions, that often highlight their dysfunctionality, to more phenomenological approaches, that also emphasize function, adaptiveness, and meaning of delusions in psychosis. Since most definitions make no reference to the mechanisms responsible for the formation of delusions, we will then turn to theories of causes of delusions in psychosis. Here, a plurality of different theories exists, whereas no ultimate conclusions have been settled on yet. As we will highlight multifactorial explanations, that also include socio-cultural factors, we will give some details about both biological as well as psychosocial explanatory accounts.

## 2. Experience of delusions in psychosis (lived experience, first-person account)

So people are like a family for me, it's like a safety blanket, they make me feel so comfortable now … If I found out that they are not watching me and reading my mind, I would feel alone and crazy like everyone else. To feel like I have everyone following me around, whether it's negative or positive, that alone is a force of power ….

These are the words of Harry, a 33-year-old man, whose case is described by Rosa Ritunnano and colleagues (2021b: 2). Harry believes that he possesses knowledge that nobody else has about the earth and things at large, which brings him into a powerful position. Besides that, people know who he is, they recognize him on the streets and follow him at times. Unimaginably to him, they choose to go about their days and remain blind to all the insights available to him. However, he discovered that he could influence their thoughts positively, making himself even more powerful.

### 2.1 How are delusions experienced?

As explained by Ritunnano and colleagues (2021b), delusions, besides often being linked to negative consequences, can enhance a person's sense of agency and belonging, with no distress necessarily reported in terms of the delusions themselves. In Harry's case, the delusion fundamentally changed how he sees himself, his relationship to the world and others, the delusion helped him to feel important and attended to. Communicating an experience of being the sole knower of some 'truth' that is elusive to others can convey a sense of unreality to others that surrounds the individual. Using metaphorical language, like Harry, individuals with delusions in psychosis may describe intrapsychic changes in words that reflect the world that surrounds them; thus, they may use materialistic sounding descriptions to depict inner psychological and experiential changes. They describe alterations in their subjective experience of the self, lived world, including dimensions of space, time, atmosphere, and other humans (Pienkos et al. 2017). Thus, a delusional meaning-making framework can be understood as establishing a new order within the 'disorder' (Ritunnano et al. 2021a, 2021b). Importantly, this can alleviate negative feelings and anxiety and can allow the person to reestablish a connection to the world. Crucially, the experienced alterations often arise as a secondary response to a person's personal, social, or structural system breaking down.

## 3. Characteristics of delusions in psychosis

Classification has long been thought of to reveal the nature of a disorder, as well as the structural features (Kendell and Jablensky 2003).

The characterization and description of delusions in psychosis has strongly been influenced by a separation into form and content, where the form focuses on the external criteria of delusions, and is thought to be culturally invariant, and the content refers to what the delusion is about and its personal significance. Of course, content can be highly varied between persons, and throughout history and cultures. In wider psychopathology, the same content may occur in a variety forms: for example, the content 'I have committed a terrible crime' could be not only a delusion but also an obsessive rumination or a depressive idea of guilt.

Whereas the *DSM* and empirical sciences have mainly focused on the form, philosophical, phenomenological, and first-person perspectives have highlighted the meaning and content of delusions in psychosis. More recently, this divide has incrementally been bridged, and the emphasis is shifting to first-person accounts, which is, however, still a process in its infancy. Such greater attention to the experience and meaning of delusions will also provide greater detail for subsequent empirical study, with findings more pertinent to those with lived experience and practitioners.

Having illustrated first-person accounts, we will now turn to scientific, psychiatric, and philosophical descriptions of the characteristics of delusions in psychosis and will thereby highlight that these do not necessarily and only partially overlap.

Psychiatric research typically searches for *core invariant features* (Broeker and Broome 2023), meaning characteristics of a phenomenon, such as particular symptoms and their underpinnings, which then typically become the criteria by which a disorder is defined and classified. In the case of delusions, this can be difficult due to the debate about the definition.

### *3.1 Delusions in psychosis in the DSM*

The *DSM*-based definition of delusions conceptualizes delusions as beliefs. This can also be called a 'doxastic account', and usually juxtaposes delusions to epistemically rational beliefs and thoughts (for more on delusion and doxasticism see Noordhof, Chapter 19). Generally, the *DSM* stays agnostic about causes and content of delusions and focuses mainly on the form. Central to the definition of delusions is that they are *beliefs*, which have been ascribed different attributions, from being *false* in DSM-IV (APA, 1994) to being *irrational*, to now being *rigid* and *certain*, hence, 'not amenable to change in light of conflicting evidence' (APA, 2013, DSM-5, p. 819) (for more on delusion and evidence see Flores, Chapter 12). These attributes typically gain their meaning in reference to objective, shared evidence and shared frameworks of meaning, that stipulate how to relate to that evidence, which can be called a *propositional framework* (see Ohlhurst, Chapter 27). In other words, we need a common understanding of how things are in the world, to deem certain beliefs, *false, irrational, rigid in the light of conflicting evidence*, based on shared and often normative assumptions of world and reality.

Due to the focus on the structural aspects of beliefs and thoughts, the *DSM* is based on a cognitive model of delusions. In sum, delusions in psychosis are conceptualized in terms of pathologically deviant beliefs that stand out in terms of their irrationality, stemming from cognitive errors (Bayne 2017). Alongside the emphasis on rigidity and certainty comes the focus on the form, the structural criteria, rather than content or meaning. However, content and meaning have also been proven important for delusions (Ritunnano et al. 2022, for more on delusion and meaning see Ritunnano and Littlemore, Chapter 2).

### 3.2  Delusions in psychosis and their appeal to rationality and computational approaches

Concepts such as *rigidity* and *certainty*, that do not seem to explicitly refer to (ir)rationality at first, can still appeal to the notion of rationality in a probabilistic sense. One form of probabilistic rationality is Bayesian rationality. The difference between logical rationality and probabilistic Bayesian rationality, as stated by Mike Oaksford and Nick Chater (2009) is that the former involves a monotonicity assumption, meaning that the inferential relations are held with certainty, are truth-preserving, and contingent facts cannot be accommodated. Whereas within the probabilistic Bayesian rationality approach, rationality is defined as the ability to reason about uncertainty, while accommodating contingent facts. This non-monotonicity seems to suit the everyday world better than an absolute certainty assumption. Within non-monotonicity, any conclusion can be overturned if more information is acquired, as inference itself is uncertain. Furthermore, probability itself refers to a degree of belief rather than to objective facts. In short, probability theory seems, as stated by Oaksford and Chater (2009), much more suitable to deal with the non-monotonic, uncertain character of everyday reasoning. However, although probability theory does not assume absolute certainty, it assumes certainty to a specific degree of precision. Thus, it assumes *truths* that are more or less likely and thereby builds on the same operational premises as logic, while taking away the absolute certainty of the assumptions made. Within non-monotonicity, statistical or probabilistic truth gets the pretence of absolute truth. This becomes apparent in the juxtaposition of deductive to abductive and inductive inference, whereas the former refers to premises as being true and conclusions being certain, the latter one refers to premises being possibly true and conclusions being probable. Computational approaches to delusions in psychosis rest on two main assumptions: next to a biological underpinning, cognitive errors are assumed to be the underlying causes of delusions, and these errors occur in a probabilistic fashion. Thus, computational approaches assume that domain-general rationality impairments underlie delusions in psychosis (Broeker and Broome 2023). In sum, within a computational approach to beliefs, the rationality of beliefs can either be logical or probabilistic, however, in the Bayesian Brain hypothesis, a common theoretical framework within computational psychiatry, rationality is thought of as being the latter.

In computational paradigms, such as the Bayesian brain hypothesis, the data collected in experimental tasks often isolate deliberate, hence active reasoning processes. The data is then looked at through a Bayesian, mathematical model that has two main parameters, one representing to what extent a decision relied on prior knowledge, the other one indicating to what extent the decision relied on momentarily given information. The model can also consider to what extent information gets integrated into a system of knowledge (priors). Since the model is a probabilistic, inferential model, it is hypothesized that the brain functions in a similar way, and aberrations in delusions in psychosis result from the probabilistic system functioning differently, hence, being dysfunctional. However, there is an inherent contradiction in computational psychiatry, which claims to look at underlying implicit, automatic inferential processes, as these were initially thought to be probabilistic (Helmholtz 1925), while experimentally isolating overt manifestations, hence explicit reasoning (Broeker and Broome 2023). In other words, domain-general reasoning impairments are the central part of computational paradigms. Computational psychiatry, though often trying to align itself closer with biological and neurological approaches, still entails a fundamental cognitive assumption about human psychology as rational agents and is thereby an extension to the cognitivist tradition in conjunction with the *DSM* definition it directly builds on. Thus, computational approaches can be located within approaches that look at cognitive 'deficit' or aberrations.

### 3.3 *Cognitive biases and rationality in delusions in psychosis*

Within doxastic and cognitive models of delusions, delusional beliefs are often thought of as taking place within domain-general deductive and/or probabilistic/inferential (reasoning) processes, as well as processes of interpreting sensory evidence, that are mostly deliberate and consciously accessible. When delusions in psychosis are conceptualized as in the *DSM-5*, underlying cognitive biases are often assumed as the cause on the functional level, next to a biological underpinning (Broome et al. 2007, 2012).

Common to all claims in terms of irrationality in delusions in psychosis is that causal factors are assumed to lay at the level of cognitive dysfunction, especially decision-making or higher-order cognition like decision-making that impacts processes like perception. Highlighting cognitive dysfunctions, hence, errors, represents a deficit-oriented approach to delusions in psychosis, which evolved from older assumptions of a two-stage impairment of perception and reasoning (Langdon and Coltheart 2000), to a hierarchical prediction error account, where one deficit (in inferential *reasoning/cognition*) impacts perception and reasoning at different hierarchical levels (Corlett et al. 2010, see Corlett, Chapter 30 for more on prediction error theories). The later prediction error account is also called a *computational approach* to delusions. Changes in deductive and/or probabilistic reasoning processes are then thought to behaviourally manifest through cognitive biases and errors: e.g. a cognitive bias that has gotten a lot of attention but recently has been strongly questioned (De Rossi and Georgiades 2022; Strube et al. 2021; Tripoli et al. 2021; Xenaki et al. 2022) is the jumping to conclusion (JTC) bias, representing a probabilistic reasoning bias, in delusions in psychosis (Huq et al. 1988). Recent meta-analyses (Dudley et al. 2015; So et al. 2015; Tripoli et al. 2021) have shown that the bias can be explained by general cognitive difficulties, not specific to delusions in psychosis, rather than concrete symptomology. Furthermore, although claiming that aberrations in inferential processes can occur at more implicit and automatical levels, most computational paradigms on delusions in psychosis still operationalize and isolate deliberate reasoning processes within their empirical paradigms and can therefore not make claims about changes in more automatic rather than deliberate cognitive processes (Broeker and Broome 2023). Another cognitive bias which is involved in delusions in psychosis is the lack of belief flexibility. Lack of belief flexibility indicates the difficulty to accept that one might be mistaken in accommodating alternative explanations (So et al. 2012). However, empirical results remain inconclusive.

More generally, a meta-analysis (McLean et al. 2017) that looked at various cognitive biases in delusions in schizophrenia, including JTC, bias against disconformity evidence, and others, showed only small effects in comparison to healthy controls, but did not control for general cognitive function. In sum, most people with delusions in psychosis do not seem to have a generalized problem with deductive or inferential reasoning. Neither do they seem to deviate from rationality in a more objective and socially shared sense. On the contrary, they seem to have aberrations in a very personal and circumscribed (ir)rationality, in which conclusions are ir/rational only in the context of the delusional belief system of an individual, rather than in a normative and socially shared way of making sense of world and self (Gold and Hohwy 2000). Recently, there have been some extensions of the cognitive approach to delusions that include social cognition: Vaughan Bell and colleagues (2020) argue within a cognitive model but for the emphasis on social and coalitional thinking as the cognitive domains where impairments occur, rather than within domain-general rationality. Their account can explain some of the missing gaps of other cognitive models, namely, that delusions are mainly socially themed and that delusions reduce sensitivity to social context, accounting for both content, and form.

Moving away from decision-making processes, the aberrant salience hypothesis and the role of Dopamine (Broome et al. 2005; Kapur 2003; Modinos et al. 2020; Ratcliffe and Broome 2022) have also been prominent in describing and categorizing cognitive processes in delusions. The initial aberrant salience hypothesis pertains to the tendency to attend to irrelevant internal and external stimuli and to the inability to correct one's interpretations of these perceptual stimuli accordingly. The aberrant salience hypothesis suggests that dopaminergic dysregulation (e.g. excessive dopamine signalling) in *psychosis* may disrupt the attribution of salience to otherwise normally inconspicuous events which then demand an explanation, consequently leading to delusions or delusional mood (for more on delusion and salience, see McKenna, Chapter 31).

### 3.4   Focus on content and meaning of delusions in psychosis

For the form of delusions, empirical science can design paradigms and test their hypotheses. However, when it comes to the content of delusions, we can mainly observe and gather clinical reports and first-person accounts. To include first-person accounts in the characterizing of delusions contributes to *epistemic justice* and *especially testimonial justice* (Fricker 2007; in delusions: Ritunnano 2022, see also Palafox-Harris, Chapter 17), which means that the voices of people experiencing delusions are actively included and they are valued as knowers. Furthermore, these accounts contribute to a more phenomenological model of delusions, which finds explanations through descriptions of experiences. In their systematic review and qualitative synthesis, Ritunnano and colleagues (2022), uncovered three main sub-themes of delusional content in schizophrenia: (a) A radical re-arrangement of the lived world that is bestride with intense emotions, which taps onto the experience of reality, uncertainty, and omnipresent mistrust. (b) Doubting, losing, and finding oneself again with delusional realities, which taps onto a state of self-doubt and fragmentation and changes in self-experience, self-interpretation, and identity construction. (c) Searches of meaning, belonging, and coherence beyond mere dysfunction. Here, meaning can also be co-constructed through testimonial exchange.

### 3.5   Delusional contents and themes

Different types of delusions in psychosis show different characteristics, especially in terms of the content: Delusions have a variety of different contents and themes. The commonest in clinical practice are those of persecution and reference, the latter referring to the experience where a neutral event is felt to have deep personal significance and relevance. This often takes the form where the person experiences their life being discussed in public media, for example, in the newspaper, TV, or radio. Other themes include grandiosity, hypochondriasisl, guilt, religious, nihilistic (Cotard's Syndrome), dysmorphophobic, infidelity (Othello Syndrome), erotomania (De Clerembeault's), and, of particular interest to philosophers, delusional misidentification (Capgras, Fregoli). Psychiatrists can also sometimes classify the 'passivity' experience of thought insertion, thought withdrawal, and thought broadcasting. The other ways of subclassifying delusions are as primary or secondary, or in Karl Jaspers's (1997) terminology, true delusions or delusion-like ideas, where secondary delusions arise from another abnormal mental state (e.g., a depressed mood or auditory hallucination) or arise as a primary phenomenon, *ex nihilo*, autochthonously. The subtypes of delusions tend to be more or less prevalent in different types of psychotic illness – delusions of reference and persecution, together with passivity experience, being most common in schizophrenia, whereas grandiose delusions can occur in a manic psychosis and delusions of guilt, or of illness, or Cotard's, in a severe depression with psychotic features. Historically, the other important way of classifying delusions was whether they were one of Schneider's First Rank Symptoms of Schizophrenia, a list of symptoms that had been thought historically to be most important, if not pathognomonic, for the diagnosis of schizophrenia. However, over the last several decades, it has been shown that these experiences occur in non-schizophrenia psychotic disorders as well, and hence their weighting in contemporary diagnostic systems has been reduced.

### 3.6   Can delusions be characterized in terms of being adaptive? Moving from the environment, reproduction, and the social realm to person-centered adaptiveness

Biological adaptiveness isn't easily established, however, Lancellotta and Bortolotti (2019) also looked at the psychological adaptiveness of delusions. This refers to their potential to give a sense of purpose, boost self-esteem (see, e.g., Peters et al. 1999;), and contribute to wellbeing (see Bortolotti and Murri, Chapter 3, for more on delusion and adaptiveness). Generally, delusions can have psychological and, indirectly, epistemic benefits (Bortolotti 2010, 2011), as delusions might enable people to keep pursing their epistemic goals. Eugenia Lancellotta and Lisa Bortolotti (2019) described four main functions under the umbrella of psychological adaptiveness, that exist mainly in the short-term. Two of which apply to delusions in psychosis, these are (a) the qualities of delusions of putting an end to uncertainty, e.g., in providing an explanation to the intense experiences a person undergoes, and (b) this explanation then has the potential to give some meaning to that person's life. In line with this, as pointed out by the others, it has been found that people in acute delusional state may have a greater "sense of coherence" than people with no psychiatric diagnosis (Bergstein et al. 2008). Other benefits are that delusions can help build a coherent self-image and identity, which includes the delusional beliefs (to some extent); delusions can further regulate emotions and guide behaviour; they can preserve a sense of one's rational agency, restoring intrapsychic coherence. However, generally, delusions often compromise functioning, at least in a very fundamental definition of the word, meaning in terms of living and being around others and in a shared reality. Importantly, the benefits of delusions highly depend on content and context, thus, they are quite circumscribed (Lancellotta and Bortolotti 2019). In sum, emphasizing content, meaning, and functionality of delusions contrasts with quite narrow models that characterize delusions mainly in terms of beliefs and irrationality, hence, cognitive and reasoning errors. Furthermore, looking at meaning and functionality of delusions in psychosis has the potential to move away from a deficit-oriented model to a more person-centred appreciation of the significance of delusions in psychosis.

## 4. Causes of delusions in psychosis (psychosocial and biological)

Delusions in psychosis do not have a single cause but arise from a complex interplay of sub-personal factors (such as a genetic predisposition), interpersonal and social factors as well as large scale societal factors (Broome et al. 2005). Thus, these various and quite diverse factors represent an explanatory pluralism.

### 4.1 Models favouring explanatory pluralism: bio-pheno-social model

Luis Sass and colleagues' (2018) Bio-Pheno-Social (BPS) model differentiates between primary and secondary factors that contribute to self-disorders, such as psychosis, in temporally different ways. Primary psychological factors are assumed to be more automatic, implicit, passively experienced, and potentially innate and more stable, hence, trait-like features or *neuro-vulnerabilities*, such as perceptual-(dis)integration. Secondary psychological factors are assumed to be more consequential, developing in short- and long-term responses to environmental factors (e.g., traumatic life events), or as an attempt to cope with more endogenous, innate, experiential disruptions of primary factors.

Next to the more passive and primary neuro-vulnerabilities, secondary factors thus entail a role of personhood in the pathogenetic model (Sass et al. 2018), e.g. a patient can adopt a change in attitude or orientation, for instance, involving active scrutiny of perceptual anomalies, this person-level attitude may have implications for the nature and course of the illness itself. The role of environmental factors (i.e. stressors as trauma or abuse) in the pathogenetic model of psychosis has also been backed up by a range of empirical evidence (Veling et al. 2016). According to Sass and colleagues (2018), manifestations of the self-disorder model, e.g., hyper-reflexivity and diminished self-affection, can occur in a primary or a secondary fashion. Thus, it could be concluded that primary factors constitute a neurological vulnerability in the self, which, triggered by external events (or endogenous causes), can lead to manifestations such as hyper-reflexivity, and other aspects of the self-disorder model.

We want to highlight that in Sass and colleagues' (2018) assumption, delusions arise from alterations in basic levels of awareness, hence, self/ipseity-related states (triggered by environmental events), rather than from objective and immediate, external perceptual or cognitive states. Sass and colleagues (2018) argue that symptoms unfolding in the immediate experience apply to specific delusions (i.e. paranoia); however, they cannot be extended to the entire ipseity-disorder model. Connectedly, the subjective ontological shift, instead of a shift in shared reality, remains almost always unaddressed in most cognitive approaches, leading to the conclusion that the immediate experience and shared external, epistemic, reality is the sphere in which aberrant saliences or other cognitive dysfunctions, e.g. prediction-error dysfunction and consecutively delusions evolve in.

Another model that emphasizes explanatory pluralism is the emergence model of delusions (Ritunnano et al. 2022), which includes multiple layers which all carry significance for the development of delusions in psychosis, these layers include: the sociocultural layer (norms, values, signifiers): interpersonal layer (testimonial interactions); personal layer (reflective, predicative, narrative); phenomenological layer (pre-reflective, pre-predicative); and sub personal layer (neural-embodied substrates).

## 4.2   *Individual factors contributing to delusions in psychosis*

When looking at individual factors that contribute to the development of delusions in psychosis, these can broadly be divided into psychosocial and biological factors. Psychosocial factors include social, systemic, and interpersonal factors, as well as developmental, whereas biological factors include neurological and genetic components (Broome et al. 2005). Both categories manifest in experiential, psychological, and cognitive symptomology and changed experiential and self-states.

### 4.2.1   *Socio-developmental factors*

A key advance in the understanding of the onset of schizophrenia and psychosis, and in the development of delusions, is the role of social and psychological factors earlier in life. It's increasingly clear, the early experience of childhood trauma, as well as migration (Selten et al. 2020), deprivation, racism, and bullying can be linked to the development of psychosis and delusions. For example, bullying predicted both the onset and persistence of persecutory ideation (Catone et al. 2015), and how such experiences connected with anxiety, drug use, and sleep problems lead to delusions, hallucinations, and psychosis as a disorder (Moffa et al. 2017). Furthermore, in terms of childhood trauma, delusions have been conceptualized as developing as a result of trauma via biased threat beliefs, stemming from trauma-related negative beliefs about the self and others (Garety et al. 2001). A more specific version of this theory posits that persecutory delusions develop because of early parental neglect, which impacts attachment, and leads to mistrust of others (Baer and Martinez 2006; Bentall et al. 2014). These models have some empirical support (Bentall et al. 2012).

### 4.2.2   *Biological factors*

Dopamine has long been thought of as the key neurotransmitter involved in schizophrenia, and hence delusions. As discussed in this chapter, this was initially argued for via indirect empirical evidence, but now via advances in neurochemical imaging and the use of positron emission tomography (PET) changes in dopamine can be examined *in vivo* and at different stages of psychosis, from those in prodromal phases to chronic refractory illness. The key idea is that dysregulation and overactivity of dopamine in the mesolimbic cortex of the brain is linked to the production of the positive symptoms of psychosis, such as delusions and hallucinations. An important additional step was linking these neurochemical changes to the clinical experience and symptoms of psychosis via the idea of salience. However, if salience dysregulation is the proximal cause of psychosis and dopamine a key element of the final common pathway (Howes and Kapur 2009), a more complicated story needs to be told about a range of distal causes, including potentially genetic vulnerabilities, developmental trajectories, traumatic events, social isolation, migration, and substance abuse. Neuroscience can only take us so far and, to encompass all these factors, an interdisciplinary approach is needed (Broome et al. 2005). However, there are concerns about the ambiguities of terms like *salience* and *affordance*, and a call for the recognition of the many subtly but importantly different ways in which human experience is permeated by a sense of the possible (Ratcliffe and Broome 2022). Further, although dopamine is no doubt important in the pathophysiology of delusions and psychosis more generally, and a key element of treatment is how antipsychotic medications block dopamine, other neurotransmitters are also likely important. For example, glutamate is thought to be key in predicting those who may fail to respond to the usual antipsychotics, and who become treatment-resistant, requiring clozapine, as well as the role of GABA and wider excitatory-inhibition balance.

## 5. Conclusion

Delusions are a key part of the definition and diagnosis of psychotic disorders such as schizophrenia. Within this clinical representation, they can be grouped in various ways, such as by theme, primary or secondary delusion, bizarre or non-bizarre, Schneiderian or non-Schneiderian, as well as in terms of aberrations of world and self-relations or cognitive and prediction errors. Each of these ways either describes certain characteristics of delusions, or/and assumes underlying causes. Thus, we know a lot about different forms that delusions can take and how they might be maintained, however, especially in terms of the etiology of delusions, different individuals may have different mechanisms and underlying causes.

In terms of how we gain more knowledge about delusions in psychosis, current research focuses mainly but separately on both, cognitive and especially prediction error accounts, as well as first-person accounts and phenomenology, highlighting function and meaning. There are attempts to combine prediction error and phenomenology, however, as shown in this chapter as well as in Broeker and Broome (2023), based on the strong deviations of underlying etiological and mechanistic assumptions, phenomenology and mechanistic, formalized, and generalized accounts are extremely difficult to combine.

Furthermore, in this chapter, we have shown that etiology and assumed underlying dysfunctions and aberrations give rise to different treatment approaches.

Lastly, it is important to emphasize that although the deficit account of delusions in psychosis still prevails, meaning, adaptiveness or even madness-as-strategy are old but rediscovered as well as contemporary alternatives to the harmful-dysfunction approach.

## References

American Psychiatric Association (APA) (1994). *Diagnostic criteria from DSM-IV*. 4th ed. Washington, DC: American Psychiatric Association.

American Psychiatric Association (APA) (2000). *Diagnostic and statistical manual of mental disorders: DSM-IV-TR*. 4th ed. Washington, DC: American Psychiatric Association.

American Psychiatric Association (APA) (2013). *Diagnostic and statistical manual of mental disorders*. 5th ed. Washington, DC: American Psychiatric Association. doi:10.1176/appi.books.9780890425596.

Baer, J.C. and Martinez, C.D. (2006). Child maltreatment and insecure attachment: a meta-analysis. *Journal of Reproductive and Infant Psychology*, 24(3), pp.187–197. doi:10.1080/02646830600821231.

Bayne, T. (2017). Delusion and the norms of rationality. In T.-W. Hung & T. J. Lane (Eds.), *Rationality alliance in early psychosis*. Amsterdam Netherlands: Acta Psychiatrica Scandinavica, 106, pp.69–106.

Bell, V., Raihani, N. and Wilkinson, S. (2020). Derationalizing delusions. *Clinical Psychological Science*, 9(1), pp.24–37. doi:10.1177/2167702620951553.

Bentall, R.P., Wickham, S., Shevlin, M. and Varese, F. (2012). Do specific early-life adversities lead to specific symptoms of psychosis? A study from the 2007 the adult psychiatric morbidity survey. *Schizophrenia Bulletin*, 38(4), pp.734–740. doi:10.1093/schbul/sbs049.

Bentall, R.P., de Sousa, P., Varese, F., Wickham, S., Sitko, K., Haarmans, M. and Read, J. (2014). From adversity to psychosis: pathways and mechanisms from specific adversities to specific symptoms. *Social Psychiatry and Psychiatric Epidemiology*, 49(7), pp.1011–1022. doi:10.1007/s00127-014-0914-0.

Bergstein, M., Weizman, A. and Solomon, Z. (2008). Sense of coherence among delusional patients: prediction of remission and risk of relapse. *Comprehensive Psychiatry*, 49, pp.288–96.

Bortolotti, L. (2010). *Delusions and other irrational beliefs*. Oxford; New York: Oxford University Press.

Bortolotti, L. (2011). Précis of delusions and other irrational beliefs. *Neuroethics*, 5(1), pp.1–4. doi:10.1007/s12152-011-9128-2.

Broeker, M.D. and Broome, M.R. (2023). Can an algorithm become delusional? Evaluating ontological commitments and methodology of computational psychiatry. *Phenomenology and the Cognitive Sciences*. doi:10.1007/s11097-023-09895-1.

Broome, M.R., Woolley, J.B., Tabraham, P., Johns, L.C., Bramon, E., Murray, G.K., Pariante, C., McGuire, P.K. and Murray, R.M. (2005). What causes the onset of psychosis? *Schizophrenia Research*, 79(1), pp.23–34. doi:10.1016/j.schres.2005.02.007.

Broome, M.R., Johns, L.C., Valli, I., Woolley, J.B., Tabraham, P., Brett, C., Valmaggia, L., Peters, E., Garety, P.A. and McGuire, P.K. (2007). Delusion formation and reasoning biases in those at clinical high risk for psychosis. *British Journal of Psychiatry*, 191(S51), pp.s38–s42. doi:10.1192/bjp.191.51.s38.

Broome, M.R., Day, F., Valli, I., Valmaggia, L., Johns, L.C., Howes, O., Garety, P. and McGuire, P.K. (2012). Delusional ideation, manic symptomatology and working memory in a cohort at clinical high-risk for psychosis: a longitudinal study. *European Psychiatry*, 27(4), pp.258–263. doi:10.1016/j.eurpsy.2010.07.008.

Catone, G., Marwaha, S., Kuipers, E., Lennox, B., Freeman, D., Bebbington, P. and Broome, M. (2015). Bullying victimisation and risk of psychotic phenomena: analyses of British national survey data. *The Lancet Psychiatry* [online], 2(7), pp.618–624. doi:10.1016/s2215-0366(15)00055-3.

Corlett, P.R., Taylor, J.R., Wang, X.-J., Fletcher, P.C. and Krystal, J.H. (2010). Toward a neurobiology of delusions. *Progress in Neurobiology* [online], 92(3), pp.345–369. doi:10.1016/j.pneurobio.2010.06.007.

De Rossi, G. and Georgiades, A. (2022). Thinking biases and their role in persecutory delusions: a systematic review. *Early Intervention in Psychiatry*. doi:10.1111/eip.13292.

Dudley, R., Taylor, P., Wickham, S. and Hutton, P. (2015). Psychosis, delusions and the 'jumping to conclusions' reasoning bias: a systematic review and meta-analysis. *Schizophrenia Bulletin* [online], 42(3), pp.652–665. doi:10.1093/schbul/sbv150.

Fricker, M. (2007). *Epistemic injustice: power and the ethics of knowing*. Oxford: Oxford University Press.

Garety, P.A., Kuipers, E., Fowler, D., Freeman, D. and Bebbington, P.E. (2001). A cognitive model of the positive symptoms of psychosis. *Psychological Medicine* [online], 31(02). doi:10.1017/s0033291701003312.

Gold, I. and Hohwy, J. (2000). Rationality and schizophrenic delusion. *Mind & Language*, 15(1), 146–167. doi:10.1111/1468-0017.00127.

Howes, O.D. and Kapur, S. (2009). The dopamine hypothesis of schizophrenia: version III–the final common pathway. *Schizophrenia Bulletin* [online], 35(3), pp.549–562. doi:10.1093/schbul/sbp006.

Huq, S.F., Garety, P.A. and Hemsley, D.R. (1988). Probabilistic judgements in deluded and non-deluded subjects. *The Quarterly Journal of Experimental Psychology Section A*, 40(4), pp.801–812. doi:10.1080/14640748808402300.

Jaspers, K. (1997). *General psychopathology/2*, Volume Two. Baltimore, MD: The Johns Hopkins Univ. Press.

Kapur, S. (2003). Psychosis as a state of aberrant salience: a framework linking biology, phenomenology, and pharmacology in schizophrenia. *American Journal of Psychiatry*, 160(1), pp.13–23. doi:10.1176/appi.ajp.160.1.13. PMID: 12505794.

Kendell, R. and Jablensky, A. (2003). Distinguishing between the validity and utility of psychiatric diagnoses. *American Journal of Psychiatry*, 160(1), pp.4–12. doi:10.1176/appi.ajp.160.1.4.

Lancellotta, E. and Bortolotti, L. (2019). Are clinical delusions adaptive? *Wiley Interdisciplinary Reviews: Cognitive Science*, p.e1502. doi:10.1002/wcs.1502.

Langdon, R. and Coltheart, M. (2000). The cognitive neuropsychology of delusions. *Mind & Language*, 15(1), 184–218. doi:10.1111/1468-0017.00129.

McLean, B.F., Mattiske, J.K. and Balzan, R.P. (2017). Association of the jumping to conclusions and evidence integration biases with delusions in psychosis: a detailed meta-analysis. *Schizophrenia Bulletin*, 43(2), 344–354. doi:10.1093/schbul/sbw056.

Modinos, G., Allen, P., Zugman, A., Dima, D., Azis, M., Samson, C., Bonoldi, I., Quinn, B., Gifford, G.W.G., Smart, S.E., Antoniades, M., Bossong, M.G., Broome, M.R., Perez, J., Howes, O.D., Stone, J.M., Grace, A.A. and McGuire, P. (2020). Neural circuitry of novelty salience processing in psychosis risk: association with clinical outcome. *Schizophrenia Bulletin*, 46(3), pp.670–679. doi:10.1093/schbul/sbz089.

Moffa, G., Catone, G., Kuipers, J., Kuipers, E., Freeman, D., Marwaha, S., Lennox, B.R., Broome, M.R. and Bebbington, P. (2017). Using directed acyclic graphs in epidemiological research in psychosis: an analysis of the role of bullying in psychosis. *Schizophrenia Bulletin*, 43(6), pp.1273–1279. doi:10.1093/schbul/sbx013.

Oaksford, M. and Chater, N. (2009). Précis of bayesian rationality: the probabilistic approach to human reasoning. *Behavioral and Brain Sciences*, 32(1), pp.69–84. doi:10.1017/s0140525x09000284.

Pienkos, E., Silverstein, S. and Sass, L. (2017). The phenomenology of anomalous world experience in schizophrenia: a qualitative study. *Journal of Phenomenological Psychology*, 48(2), pp.188–213. doi:10.1163/15691624-12341328.

Ratcliffe, M.J. and Broome, M.R. (2022). Beyond "salience" and "affordance": understanding anomalous experiences of significant possibilities. In S. Archer (ed.), *Salience: A philosophical inquiry*. London: Routledge, 50–69.

Ritunnano, R., Broome, M. and Stanghellini, G. (2021a). Charting new phenomenological paths for empirical research on delusions. *JAMA Psychiatry*. doi:10.1001/jamapsychiatry.2021.1587.

Ritunnano, R., Humpston, C. and Broome, M.R. (2021b). Finding order within the disorder: a case study exploring the meaningfulness of delusions. *BJPsych Bulletin*, 46(2), pp.109–115. doi:10.1192/bjb.2020.151.

Ritunnano, R., Kleinman, J., Whyte Oshodi, D., Michail, M., Nelson, B., Humpston, C.S. and Broome, M.R. (2022). Subjective experience and meaning of delusions in psychosis: a systematic review and qualitative evidence synthesis. *The Lancet Psychiatry*, 9(6), pp.458–476. doi:10.1016/s2215-0366(22)00104-3.

Ritunnano, R. (2022). Overcoming hermeneutical injustice in mental health: a role for critical phenomenology. *Journal of the British Society for Phenomenology*, 53(3), pp. 243–260. doi:10.1080/00071773.2022.2031234

Sass, L., Borda, J. P., Madeira, L., Pienkos, E. and Nelson, B. (2018). Varieties of self disorder: a bio- pheno-social model of schizophrenia. *Schizophrenia Bulletin*, 44(4), 720–727. doi:10.1093/schbul/sby001.

Selten, J., Van der Ven, E. and Termorshuizen, F. (2020). Migration and psychosis: a meta-analysis of incidence studies. *Psychological Medicine*, 50(2), pp.303–313. doi:10.1017/S0033291719000035.

So, S.H. et al. (2012) Jumping to conclusions, a lack of belief flexibility and delusional conviction in psychosis: a longitudinal investigation of the structure, frequency, and relatedness of reasoning biases. *Journal of Abnormal Psychology*, 121(1), pp.129–139. doi:10.1037/a0025297.

So, S.H., Chan, A.P., Chong, C.S., Wong, M.H., Lo, W.T., Chung, D.W. and Chan, S.S. (2015). Metacognitive training for delusions (MCTd): effectiveness on data-gathering and belief flexibility in a Chinese sample. *Frontiers in Psychology*, 6, p.730.

Strube, W., Cimpianu, C.L., Ulbrich, M., Öztürk, Ö.F., Schneider-Axmann, T., Falkai, P., Marshall, L., Bestmann, S. and Hasan, A. (2021). Unstable belief formation and slowed decision-making: evidence that the jumping-to-conclusions bias in schizophrenia is not linked to impulsive decision-making. *Schizophrenia Bulletin*, 48(2), pp.347–358. doi:10.1093/schbul/sbab108.

Tripoli, G., Quattrone, D., Ferraro, L., Gayer-Anderson, C., Rodriguez, V., La Cascia, C., La Barbera, D., Sartorio, C., Seminerio, F., Tarricone, I., Berardi, D., Szöke, A., Arango, C., Tortelli, A., Llorca, P.M., de Haan, L., Velthorst, E., Bobes, J., Bernardo, M., Sanjuán, J., …, Di Forti, M. (2021). Jumping to conclusions, general intelligence, and psychosis liability: findings from the multi-\centre EU-GEI case-control study. *Psychological Medicine*, 51(4), 623–633. doi:10.1017/S003329171900357X.

Veling, W., Counotte, J., Pot-Kolder, R., van Os, J. and van der Gaag, M. (2016). Childhood trauma, psychosis liability and social stress reactivity: a virtual reality study. *Psychological Medicine*, 46(16), pp.3339–3348. doi:10.1017/s0033291716002208.

Xenaki, L.A., Stefanatou, P., Ralli, E., Hatzimanolis, A., Dimitrakopoulos, S., Soldatos, R.F., Vlachos, I.I., Selakovic, M., Foteli, S., Kosteletos, I. and Nianiakas, N. (2022). The relationship between early symptom severity, improvement and remission in first episode psychosis with jumping to conclusions. *Schizophrenia Research*, 240, pp.24–30.

# 8
# DELUSIONS IN ANOREXIA NERVOSA

*Stephen Gadsby*

## 1. Introduction

This chapter discusses the relationship between the beliefs associated with anorexia nervosa (AN) and the concepts of *delusion* and *overvalued idea*. I challenge the utility of labelling the beliefs associated with AN as delusions or overvalued ideas and raise some issues with contemporary methods of assessing the delusionality of those diagnosed with AN.

While the renowned clinician Hilde Bruch (1974) characterised AN as involving a 'delusional denial of thinness', in the decades following her work, researchers studiously avoided the term. The refusal to refer to the beliefs associated with AN as delusions stems from two assumptions. First, delusions are exclusively associated with disorders of psychosis; because AN is not classified as such, the label delusion cannot apply (Veale 2002: 385). However, deciding whether a belief is a delusion based on whether the patient is diagnosed with a disorder of psychosis puts the cart before the horse. Delusions are symptoms, and symptoms are independent of the conditions that they are associated with (Clutton and Gadsby 2018; Sakakibara 2016). Sadness, for example, is a symptom of a mood disorder, but it can also occur in the absence of any disorder whatsoever (Horwitz and Wakefield 2007).

The second, related assumption is that the beliefs associated with AN are better thought of as *overvalued ideas*—a distinct category to delusions (P. McKenna 1984). This chapter will focus on this claim and the arguments for it. In fact, there are two ways to conceive of the distinction between delusions and overvalued ideas—emanating from European and American psychiatric traditions, respectively (Veale 2002). According to the American tradition, overvalued ideas and delusional beliefs sit on a continuum and are distinguished by the strength with which they are held. In contrast, the European tradition considers overvalued ideas and delusions conceptually distinct categories of belief. In this chapter, I discuss both ways of characterising the distinction.

There are various attitudes associated with AN that might qualify as delusions. The most recognisable symptom of the disorder is an extreme desire to lose weight (Bruch 1965). Such desires appear pathological because of their extreme nature, their centrality to other symptoms, and the harm they cause (Tan et al. 2006). Nevertheless, pathological desires are not considered delusions, as (at least within scientific research and clinical practice) the

   DOI: 10.4324/9781003296386-11

term exclusively applies to beliefs (or belief-like states) (Clutton 2018; Mullen and Gillett 2014).

AN involves two categories of clinically relevant beliefs: beliefs about body size and the value of thinness (Gadsby 2023a).[1] The former category involves the belief that one is overweight, has an average body size, or is not thin. In standard cases of AN—where the patient has a severely low body mass index (BMI)[2]—such beliefs are not only false but implausible. However, it is worth spelling out where this implausibility stems from. A common misconception is that the body size beliefs associated with AN stem from extreme evaluative standards, i.e., those with AN have such extreme standards for what constitutes thinness that even their bodies don't qualify. However, while those with AN aspire to be thinner than most, their standards for ideal body size are not extreme. In most cases, body size beliefs are inconsistent with patients' own standards for ideal size (Moscone et al. 2017). Instead, those with AN often believe that they aren't thin because they hold false beliefs about the dimensions of their bodies (Gadsby 2023b).

The second category of beliefs associated with AN relate to the value of thinness. Individuals diagnosed with AN often believe that thinness is of paramount importance and associate it with various positive values such as accomplishment, self-worth, and moral superiority (Bruch 1978; Tan et al. 2006; Vitousek 1996; Vitousek, Watson, and Wilson 1998; Wolf and Serpell 1998). While debates over whether AN involves delusions often conflate these two forms of belief, they likely stem from different factors and therefore should be evaluated separately (Gadsby 2023a).

The chapter is structured like so: first, I discuss whether the body size beliefs associated with AN are more like delusions or overvalued ideas, according to the European tradition. While I do not provide a definitive answer to this question, I note that these beliefs bear many characteristics associated with delusions. I also discuss the status of beliefs about the value of thinness and suggest that these bear more similarity to overvalued ideas. Next, I address the American distinction between delusions and overvalued ideas. I review research on the extent of delusional beliefs and overvalued ideas associated with AN, under this definition, and point out some issues this research faces. My more general point is that while it is essential to understand the beliefs associated with AN, the question of whether they qualify as delusions or overvalued ideas (according to one or another psychiatric tradition) is less important.

## 2.  Body size beliefs: delusions or overvalued ideas?

While the *DSM* provides the most well-known definition(s) of delusional beliefs, it has consistently been criticised, as it excludes many beliefs commonly regarded as delusions and includes many beliefs that are not (Davies et al. 2001; Langdon and Bayne 2010). As things stand, there is no widely agreed-upon definition of delusions involving necessary and sufficient criteria, i.e. that includes all appropriate cases and excludes all inappropriate cases. Consequently, we cannot determine whether a belief qualifies as a delusion based exclusively on whether it satisfies a set of definitional criteria.

An alternative approach to evaluating whether a belief qualifies as a delusion is to focus on paradigmatic features of delusions and assess whether and to what extent those are present in the target beliefs. Robyn Langdon and Timothy Bayne (2010) suggest such an approach, focusing on the *cardinal signs* of delusion: incorrigibility, incomprehensibility, and conviction, three characteristics that have a long-standing association with delusionality (in the European psychiatric tradition), emanating from the work of Karl Jaspers (1946) (see also Spitzer 1990). As I will show, the body size beliefs associated with AN often exhibit each of these signs.

First, consider incomprehensibility. Langdon and Bayne distinguish between two kinds: *sheer* incomprehensibility, which holds across contexts, and *contextual* incomprehensibility, which is context sensitive (2010: 321). Body size beliefs do not exhibit sheer incomprehensibility. Unlike other delusions—such as the belief that one has three snakes in their belly or speaks through soul telephones (Hohwy and Rajan 2012)—the belief that one's body is not thin is commonplace; many neurotypical individuals hold beliefs with the same content. Nevertheless, the belief that one is not thin is contextually incomprehensible, that is, it is incomprehensible when held by those who are excessively thin.

Incorrigibility can be defined as 'the persistence of the belief in the face of counter-evidence and rational counterargument' (Langdon and Bayne 2010: 322). Many body size beliefs undeniably exhibit incorrigibility. Indeed, a hallmark feature of AN is its resistance to treatment, which includes attempts to reason with patients or present them with incontrovertible evidence regarding their body size (Fassino and Abbate-Daga 2013). Despite the pleas of doctors, friends, and families, those with AN persist in their beliefs and behaviour, therefore demonstrating incorrigibility.

The standard way to conceive of conviction is in terms of how much certainty is verbally expressed. This form of conviction is a well-noted feature of AN, as one handbook states, 'a striking feature of anorexia nervosa or bulimia nervosa is the person's conviction about the existence (or severity) of the physical defect' (Rosen 1997: 190). Langdon and Bayne, however, suggest an *epistemic* notion. Specifically, they highlight the importance of *unwarranted* conviction 'in light of general knowledge and/or the evidence to hand, either or both of which ought normally to confer doubt' (2010: 336). Again, this is characteristic of the body size beliefs associated with AN. Indeed, any conviction in such beliefs seems entirely out of line with the wealth of evidence contradicting them (e.g., weight scale readings, knowledge of clothes size, and testimony from family and friends) (cf. Gadsby 2023b).

These three cardinal signs are neither necessary nor sufficient for classifying a belief as delusional. Many (seemingly) non-delusional beliefs exhibit each characteristic—such as religious beliefs (David 1999)—and many delusional beliefs miss one or more of these features. For example, some with delusions appear to exhibit low conviction in their beliefs (these are also sometimes referred to as *partial* delusions) (Mullen and Gillett 2014), others don't satisfy the incorrigibility condition, as they can be convinced (albeit temporarily) out of their delusions (Coltheart 2007: 1054). Consequently, the presence (or absence) of these criteria can't ground a definitive argument in favour of (or opposed to) a belief's delusional status. Nevertheless, their presence can constitute evidence in favour of the classification. Given that each criterion is associated with at least some body size beliefs held by patients with AN, this supports classifying these beliefs as delusions.

As noted, one of the most common arguments that body size beliefs in AN are not delusions is that they are better characterised as overvalued ideas. Primarily arising from the work of Carl Wernicke (1906) and Jaspers (1946), an overvalued idea—as it is conceived in the European tradition—can be defined as

> an isolated, preoccupying belief, neither delusional nor obsessional in nature, which comes to dominate the sufferer's life, often indefinitely. In many cases it seems to develop, to some extent comprehensibly, out of a previously abnormal personality,

but it can equally be a sign of emerging psychosis or organic disorder. The concept
has a reputable, but neglected tradition and carries an air of being of limited clinical
relevance.

*(P. McKenna 1984: 579)*

An essential feature of this definition is that overvalued ideas are distinct from and in contrast to delusions. Nevertheless, as with delusions, there is no definition of an overvalued
idea in terms of necessary and sufficient criteria.

There is a close theoretical link between AN and the European notion of an overvalued
idea. In fact, AN is even used as a motivating factor in retaining the concept; Peter McK-
enna, an early proponent of both overvalued ideas and their association with AN, writes:

Despite being ignored, misunderstood and lost altogether on American psychiatry (it
is difficult to resist the temptation to say undervalued), there seems to be a clear need
for such a second category of abnormal belief [overvalued ideas]. Trying to deny its
existence simply leads to contradictions, of which the nature of the belief in anorexia
nervosa is the most glaring example.

*(2017: 34)*

The arguments for classifying the body size beliefs associated with AN are, however, sparse
and unconvincing. One of the earliest is offered by McKenna himself, who refers to the
*phenomenology* (by which he means characteristics) of body size beliefs in AN:

The anorexic's conviction that she is overweight ... is held with extreme tenacious-
ness, and in the face of the plainest possible evidence to the contrary; it is never,
however, considered delusional. The belief is preoccupying, acted on unquestioningly, and leads the patient to engage in sustained abnormal behaviour. ... The
phenomenology of anorexia nervosa thus shows features that are characteristic of
an overvalued idea

*(P. McKenna 1984: 583)*

In this excerpt, McKenna points to body size beliefs' preoccupying and action-driving
nature—other features of (clinical) belief commonly associated with the European notion
of an overvalued idea. However, these are not sufficient conditions for overvalued ideas
(Veale 2002: 385). Preoccupation is a pervasive aspect of delusions (Sisti et al. 2012), and
those with delusions often act on them (Bourget and Whitehurst 2004). Given that these
features are present in many instances of delusion, more is needed to support the claim that
false body size beliefs in AN are overvalued ideas rather than delusions.

Many proponents of the European distinction between overvalued ideas and delusions
consider aetiology an essential distinguishing factor. Most notably, they emphasise that
overvalued ideas are commonly (though not exclusively) associated with personality traits
(Oyebode 2023: 132). This is echoed by McKenna, who, in arguing for the relationship
between AN and overvalued ideas, notes that 'a prominent aetiological factor in anorexia
nervosa, and the only one that can be identified with certainty, is abnormal personality'
(1984: 583). If the body size beliefs associated with AN stemmed from personality factors,
rather than factors that generally give rise to delusions, this would constitute an argument
in favour of them being considered overvalued ideas.

The aetiology of false body size beliefs in AN remains an open question. While various personality traits are associated with AN and other eating disorders (Lilenfeld et al. 2006), it is not yet clear how features of one's personality could give rise to false beliefs about their bodily dimensions. It has also been argued that body size beliefs bear a striking similarity to the aetiology of delusions. An influential explanation for delusions is that they constitute responses to abnormal experiences (Maher 1974), which themselves stem from cognitive or neurological malfunctions of some form (Coltheart 2007). In a similar vein, it has been argued that the body size beliefs associated with AN arise from abnormal experiences of body size, stemming from malfunctioning mental representations of the body (Gadsby 2017a, 2017b, 2020, 2023b). If this explanation is accurate, the aetiology argument favours labelling body size beliefs as delusions rather than overvalued ideas.

## 3.   Beliefs about the value of thinness

While the body size beliefs associated with AN may have more in common with delusions than overvalued ideas, many arguments for the association between overvalued ideas and AN have a different target in mind, namely, beliefs about the value of thinness (Cooper and Fairburn 1993). Value-based beliefs are not typically considered delusions, partly because (much like desires) they are not straightforwardly truth-evaluable. As David Veale notes, values are 'subjective', 'personal', and 'not subject to empirical testing' (2002: 386), making it difficult to assess their incomprehensibility. The *DSM-5* does, however, allow for the possibility of delusional value-based beliefs, stating: 'When a false belief involves a value judgment, it is regarded as a delusion only when the judgment is so extreme as to defy credibility' (APA 2013: 819; see also Fulford 1991). Consequently, we cannot rule out classifying beliefs about the value of thinness as delusions.

The value of thinness beliefs associated with AN, however, fit the concept of an overvalued idea much better. For example, working from the European tradition, Veale argues that overvalued ideas are best characterised as involving three conditions. First, they are value-based, rather than factual beliefs. Second, they are dominant and idealised. Third, they are excessively identified with the self. According to this definition, factual beliefs about the body cannot qualify as overvalued ideas, but beliefs about the value of thinness are an appropriate match. Such beliefs dominate patients' lives to a considerable degree (Tan et al. 2006) and are strongly associated with their self-identities (Gregertsen, Mandy, and Serpell 2017). Indeed, the way in which those with AN identify with their values regarding thinness is well-recognised as a contributing factor to treatment resistance (Fixsen et al. 2022; Vitousek, Watson, and Wilson 1998). Finally, in terms of aetiology, value of thinness beliefs may bear more similarity to overvalued ideas, as there is a plausible link between such beliefs and personality traits, such as perfectionism (Fairburn, Cooper, and Shafran 2003).

In applying the European concepts of delusion and overvalued idea to the case of AN, body size beliefs bear more resemblance to delusions, while beliefs about the value of thinness bear more resemblance to overvalued ideas. However, as I have reiterated, there is no clear way to distinguish between these categories: each identifying characteristic of one form of belief is sometimes present in the other form. A more critical issue, then, is whether there is any benefit to retaining the distinction. Of course, it is important to research and document the characteristics and aetiologies of the different beliefs that are clinically related to AN. However, beyond doing so, we should question whether applying labels such as 'delusion' or 'overvalued idea' delivers any further explanatory benefit.

## 4. Continuum delusionality and the Brown Assessment of Beliefs Scale

The distinction between overvalued ideas and delusions has been reconceived within the American psychiatric tradition, and this conception has strongly influenced AN research in the past decade. To illustrate the American distinction between delusions and overvalued ideas, consider the *DSM-5*'s definition of an overvalued idea: 'an unreasonable and sustained belief that is maintained with less than delusional intensity (i.e., the person can acknowledge that the belief may not be true)' (APA 2013: 826). In defining delusions, it also states, 'delusional conviction can sometimes be inferred from an overvalued idea (in which case the individual has an unreasonable belief or idea but does not hold it as firmly as is the case with a delusion)' (819). As in the European tradition, an overvalued idea is identified as (somehow) less than delusional. However, there is no emphasis on aetiology or other belief characteristics. Instead, overvalued ideas have the same characteristics as delusions, albeit being held with less strength (Veale 2002: 384). This characterisation rests on the so-called *continuum* view of delusionality, which assumes that pathological beliefs can be rated on a continuum, from delusions to overvalued ideas to beliefs held with good insight (Eisen et al. 1998).

The Brown Assessment of Beliefs Scale (BABS) (Eisen et al. 1998) is the primary diagnostic tool used to assess clinically relevant beliefs under the continuum view. The BABS is a semi-structured interview that begins by establishing relevant belief content with a participant and evaluating the strength with which that belief is held, based on several features. The scale is primarily determined by how much conviction is associated with the belief, which is assessed by asking how convinced the participant is of the relevant statement and how certain they are of its accuracy. To count as delusional, a subject must rate four out of four on the conviction scale and have a total score of 18 or above when combining conviction with five other items: the ability to assess the beliefs of others in regard to one's own belief, the ability to explain the difference between one's own and others' views of the belief, the incorrigibility of the belief, how actively/frequently one tries to disprove or reject the belief and the recognition that the belief has a psychiatric/psychological cause (Konstantakopoulos et al. 2012: 483).

The continuum view of delusionality, as measured by the BABS, faces some conceptual issues. First, it departs considerably from the traditional concept of delusion, as characterised by the cardinal signs. While the BABS incorporates conviction and incorrigibility (two of the cardinal signs), it is unclear why strong conviction is a necessary condition for delusion but not strong incorrigibility. As noted, clinicians often classify those with less conviction as holding at least 'partial' delusions, but the continuum disposes of this category entirely (Mullen 2003: 507). It also leaves out the implausibility of the belief, which is often considered an essential aspect of delusions (Mullen 2003). Instead, it is left to the administering clinician to identify the belief content that is most relevant (see below).

Putting aside conceptual issues with the continuum view, measuring differences in the strength with which pathological beliefs in AN are held is an important task. For example, qualitative research illustrates significant heterogeneity regarding the strength with which body size beliefs are held. Many patients insist they are not underweight and indicate no doubt whatsoever (Espeset et al. 2011; O'Connell et al. 2018). When faced with counter-evidence, these patients often generate (sometimes highly implausible) rationalisations to explain away such evidence. For example, to explain their apparent low weight, some claim that their scales must be broken or that their bones are 'lighter than usual'

(Espeset et al. 2011). Many also adopt beliefs about their biological exceptionality to explain why their bodies can maintain weight and function properly, despite such low caloric intake (O'Connell et al. 2018). As one patient describes, 'my body doesn't treat food like it should…so on that train of logic, I don't need to eat like a normal person' (O'Connell et al. 2018: 5).

Instead of rationalising away counter-evidence, others appreciate the apparent contradictions between their beliefs and their evidence and background knowledge of the world:

> I know logically it doesn't make sense, but I believe it, but I know it's not right. I mean I've done physiology and anatomy, I've got a degree, I know it doesn't make sense, but I can't explain it. I know it all sounds crazy but I know it makes sense in my head even though it doesn't.
>
> *(O'Connell et al. 2018: 6)*

This is similar to many traditional cases of delusions, wherein patients acknowledge the absurdity of their beliefs. As Anthony David (1999: 18) notes, 'A surprising number of deluded patients admit that their belief is strange; some may acknowledge it to be "hard to believe". They may even say they know that it is impossible'. Some who suffer from AN also appear to drop all certainty and suspend judgment about their true body size, for example, claiming 'I don't know how I really look' or 'I've lost my sense of reality' (Espeset et al. 2012: 522).

Several studies have attempted to quantitatively assess these differences in belief strength by employing the BABS, concluding that while some patients exhibit strong enough conviction in their body size beliefs to be considered delusional, most do not hold their beliefs with delusional strength, instead being classified as holding overvalued ideas, or exhibiting good insight (Barton et al. 2022; De Young et al. 2022; Hartmann et al. 2013; Kambanis et al. 2023; Konstantakopoulos et al. 2012, 2020; G. McKenna, Fox, and Haddock 2014; Mountjoy, Farhall, and Rossell 2014; Şenay and Yücel 2022; Steinglass et al. 2007). There are, however, several theoretical issues plaguing this research programme, which I document below.

One issue relates to the content of the beliefs studied. As noted, researchers start by establishing target beliefs with participants. This process begins with a prompt, for example, asking the participant 'what thoughts and beliefs she had about her body weight and shape that might interfere with eating' (Konstantakopoulos et al. 2012: 483; similar prompts were used by: Konstantakopoulos et al. 2020; Şenay and Yücel 2022; Mountjoy et al. 2014). While prompts like this may exclusively identify body size beliefs, no prompt is standardly employed. For example, Joanna Steinglass and colleagues (66) report that 'the dominant belief was elicited by explaining to the patient that the interview aimed to assess beliefs that interfere with eating, even if these beliefs seem irrational'. Other prompts are similarly open ended, for example, 'What ideas or beliefs do you have that are of significant concern to you, specifically about food, eating, or your body shape or weight?' (De Young et al. 2022; Kambanis et al. 2023). Unfortunately, some studies do not report the prompt they used (Barton et al. 2022; Hartmann et al. 2013; McKenna et al. 2014) and only three report the kinds of belief content studied.[3] The lack of standardisation in the prompts used when administering the BABS has led to mixed results, which obscure the true nature of belief strength associated with AN.

The three studies that reported information about the content of the beliefs used open-ended prompts, and their results show considerable diversity in the content of beliefs.

For example, Steinglass and colleagues reported beliefs about losing control ('If I eat [something forbidden], I will lose control'), being full ('If I eat, it will stay in my stomach undigested and I'll never feel hungry again'), the immediate effects of eating or feeling full ('If I feel full, I will change shape right away'), and the value of thinness ('If I'm thin enough, I won't get traumatized/attacked again') (68). Evelyna Kambanis and colleagues and Rachel Barton and colleagues also reported diverse belief content. Some beliefs related to the immediate effect of feeling full ('If I feel full, then I am a bad person', 'If I eat anything, I will gain weight'), others to the value of thinness ('I am worthless as a person because my body is disgusting'), and some related to denying thinness or the importance of control. Consistent with the results of qualitative research (O'Connell et al. 2018), some beliefs also related to biological exceptionality (e.g. 'If I eat, I won't be able to go to the bathroom because my body can't process food') (Kambanis et al. 2023).

Apart from these three studies, others who employ the BABs do not supply information about the belief content the scale applied to. Consequently, it is difficult to ascertain the kinds of beliefs each study targeted. It is standard in the literature to compare results from different studies (Phillipou, Mountjoy, and Rossell 2017). However, if different studies measure different kinds of beliefs, then such comparisons are inappropriate. As noted, the various clinically relevant beliefs associated with AN are different in kind. Some are body size beliefs, which may stem from misperception of the body, others, such as beliefs about physical exceptionalism may stem from an attempt to rationalise evidence that contradicts body size beliefs. Beliefs about the value of thinness are also notably different and may be linked to personality traits. These categories of belief should not be treated as equivalent.

Consistent with the assumption that different studies are tapping into different kinds of beliefs, the results from studies employing the BABS are mixed. The percentage of beliefs diagnosed as either delusions or overvalued ideas differs considerably. The mixed nature of these results can partly be explained by variation in samples (i.e., type of treatment facility), as well as small sample sizes, however, it may also be related to heterogeneity in the types of beliefs studied.

This research programme also faces issues related to selection bias. Most participants in these studies were undergoing treatment (either as in- or out-patients) at the time of participating. This suggests that many had already received some level of treatment. Consequently, these samples disproportionately represent those with good insight, given that developing such insight is a key focus in treatment. Indeed, even selecting participants willing to participate in research studies may bias the sample towards those with greater insight, as participating in a study for patients with a disorder requires accepting that one does in fact suffer from a disorder, which many deny (see below).

This is, of course, not the fault of the experimenters. Testing participants currently receiving treatment is standard practice in eating disorder research. However, it does raise questions about the reliability of the inferences drawn from this research. Before clinical intervention, those with AN generally exhibit poor insight and firm conviction in their body size beliefs, insisting they are not too thin and that nothing is wrong (Kaplan and Garfinkel 1999; Noordenbos 1992; Vitousek, Watson, and Wilson 1998). We ought to, therefore, be careful in assuming that these samples accurately represent the broader population of those who suffer from AN. Given that many with AN exhibit poor insight and high belief conviction prior to clinical intervention, it might be that a more significant proportion of

AN sufferers hold their beliefs with delusional strength, despite only a minority maintaining that strength after receiving treatment. This speaks to the importance of conducting these studies on community samples, though such a task may be practically difficult.

There is undoubtedly considerable diversity among the strength with which clinically relevant beliefs are held in AN. Measuring this diversity and studying the relationship between belief strength and measures of clinical severity is an important task. However, a more careful approach to such research is needed; specifically, studies must clarify, limit, and report the kinds of belief content that they focus on. Research into the strength of clinically relevant beliefs (in AN or any other disorder) can also proceed without labelling the relevant beliefs as delusions or overvalued ideas, based exclusively on the strength with which they are held. Just as those working within the European tradition must ask themselves whether there is any explanatory benefit to applying the label 'delusion' or 'overvalued idea' to a mental state whose characteristics we already know, those working within the American tradition should question whether assessing the strength of clinically relevant beliefs benefits from the conceptual baggage associated with those terms.

## 5.  Conclusion

I surveyed the conceptual landscape related to beliefs associated with AN and the distinction between delusions and overvalued ideas, as conceived within European and American psychiatric traditions. I identified two categories of clinically relevant beliefs: body size beliefs and beliefs about the value of thinness. According to the European tradition, beliefs about body size bear more resemblance to delusions, while beliefs about the value of thinness bear more resemblance to overvalued ideas. According to the American tradition, delusional beliefs and overvalued ideas lie on a continuum, distinguished exclusively in terms of the strength with which they are held. Consequently, both body size beliefs and beliefs about the value of thinness could qualify as delusions, overvalued ideas, or neither, depending on the patient.

The American tradition emphasises the importance of assessing the strength with which clinically relevant beliefs are held. The European tradition emphasises the importance of evaluating various belief characteristics (e.g. preoccupation, action-driving nature, association with self-identity), as well as aetiology. Both these goals are worthwhile. However, they are distinct from applying the labels 'delusion' or 'overvalued idea'. Given the conceptual confusion surrounding those terms, it may be better for AN researchers to focus exclusively on understanding body size beliefs and beliefs about the value of thinness, putting the task of labelling aside. Once these beliefs' characteristics, aetiology, and strength are properly understood and documented, labelling them as delusions or overvalued ideas likely delivers no further explanatory benefit.

## Notes

1 While this chapter focuses on AN, many of the same beliefs are held by those with a diagnosis of Bulimia Nervosa or Other Specified Feeding and Eating Disorder (OSFED), thus the same arguments may hold for those with these related diagnoses.
2 BMI is calculated by dividing a person's weight by the square of their height.
3 Konstantakopoulos and colleagues (2012) provide three examples of the relevant beliefs, though it isn't clear whether and to what extent these examples were characteristic of their entire sample.

# References

APA. (2013). *Diagnostic and statistical manual of mental disorders: DSM-5* (5th ed.). Washington, DC: American Psychiatric Association.

Barton, R., Aouad, P., Hay, P., Buckett, G., Russell, J., Sheridan, M., ..., Touyz, S. (2022). Distinguishing delusional beliefs from overvalued ideas in Anorexia Nervosa: An exploratory pilot study. *Journal of Eating Disorders, 10*(1), 1–10.

Bourget, D., & Whitehurst, L. (2004). Capgras syndrome: A review of the neurophysiological correlates and presenting clinical features in cases involving physical violence. *Canadian Journal of Psychiatry, 49*(11), 719–725.

Bruch, H. (1965). Anorexia nervosa and its differential diagnosis. *The Journal of Nervous and Mental Disease, 141*(5), 555–566.

Bruch, H. (1974). *Eating disorders: Obesity, anorexia nervosa, and the person within.* London: Routledge & Kegan Paul.

Bruch, H. (1978). *The golden cage: The enigma of anorexia nervosa.* Harvard University Press.

Clutton, P. (2018). A new defence of doxasticism about delusions: The cognitive phenomenological defence. *Mind & Language, 33*(2), 198–217.

Clutton, P., & Gadsby, S. (2018). Delusions, harmful dysfunctions, and treatable conditions. *Neuroethics, 11*(2), 167–181.

Coltheart, M. (2007). The 33rd Sir Frederick Bartlett Lecture: Cognitive neuropsychiatry and delusional belief. *The Quarterly Journal of Experimental Psychology, 60*(8), 1041–1062.

Cooper, P. J., & Fairburn, C. G. (1993). Confusion over the core psychopathology of bulimia nervosa. *International Journal of Eating Disorders, 13*(4), 385–389.

David, A. S. (1999). On the impossibility of defining delusions. *Philosophy, Psychiatry, & Psychology, 6*(1), 17–20.

Davies, M., Coltheart, M., Langdon, R., & Breen, N. (2001). Monothematic delusions: Towards a two-factor account. *Philosophy, Psychiatry, & Psychology, 8*(2), 133–158.

De Young, K., Bottera, A., Kambanis, E., Mancuso, C., Cass, K., Lohse, K., ..., Johnson, C. (2022). Delusional intensity as a prognostic indicator among individuals with severe to extreme anorexia nervosa hospitalized at an acute medical stabilization program. *International Journal of Eating Disorders, 55*(2), 215–222.

Eisen, J. L., Phillips, K. A., Baer, L., Beer, D. A., Atala, K. D., & Rasmussen, S. A. (1998). The brown assessment of beliefs scale: Reliability and validity. *American Journal of Psychiatry, 155*(1), 102–108.

Espeset, E. M., Gulliksen, K. S., Nordbø, R. H., Skårderud, F., & Holte, A. (2012). Fluctuations of body images in anorexia nervosa: Patients' perception of contextual triggers. *Clinical Psychology & Psychotherapy, 19*(6), 518–530.

Espeset, E. M., Nordbø, R. H., Gulliksen, K. S., Skårderud, F., Geller, J., & Holte, A. (2011). The concept of body image disturbance in anorexia nervosa: An empirical inquiry utilizing patients' subjective experiences. *Eating Disorders, 19*(2), 175–193.

Fairburn, C. G., Cooper, Z., & Shafran, R. (2003). Cognitive behaviour therapy for eating disorders: A "transdiagnostic" theory and treatment. *Behaviour Research and Therapy, 41*(5), 509–528.

Fassino, S., & Abbate-Daga, G. (2013). Resistance to treatment in eating disorders: A critical challenge. *BMC Psychiatry, 13*, 1–4.

Fixsen, A., Ridge, D., Ponsford, O., Holder, M., & Saran, G. (2022). Battles over 'unruly bodies': Practitioners' interpretations of eating disorders and the utility of psychiatric labelling. *Sociology of Health & Illness, 45*(3), 560–579.

Fulford, K. (1991). Evaluative delusions: Their significance for philosophy and psychiatry. *The British Journal of Psychiatry, 159*(S14), 108–112.

Gadsby, S. (2017a). Anorexia nervosa and oversized experiences. *Philosophical Psychology, 30*(5), 594–615.

Gadsby, S. (2017b). Explaining body size beliefs in anorexia. *Cognitive Neuropsychiatry, 22*(6), 495–507.

Gadsby, S. (2020). Self-deception and the second factor: How desire causes delusion in Anorexia nervosa. *Erkenntnis, 85*(3), 609–626.

Gadsby, S. (2023a). Anorexia nervosa, body dissatisfaction, and problematic beliefs. *Review of Philosophy and Psychology, 1–20.*

Gadsby, S. (2023b). The rationality of eating disorders. *Mind & Language, 38*(3), 732–749.

Gregertsen, E. C., Mandy, W., & Serpell, L. (2017). The egosyntonic nature of anorexia: An impediment to recovery in anorexia nervosa treatment. *Frontiers in Psychology, 8*, 2273.

Hartmann, A. S., Thomas, J. J., Wilson, A. C., & Wilhelm, S. (2013). Insight impairment in body image disorders: Delusionality and overvalued ideas in anorexia nervosa versus body dysmorphic disorder. *Psychiatry Research, 210*(3), 1129–1135.

Hohwy, J., & Rajan, V. (2012). Delusions as forensically disturbing perceptual inferences. *Neuroethics, 5*(1), 5–11.

Horwitz, A. V., & Wakefield, J. C. (2007). *The loss of sadness: How psychiatry transformed normal sorrow into depressive disorder*. New York: Oxford University Press.

Jaspers, K. (1946/1963). *General psychopathology* (J. Hoenig & M. W. Hamilton, Trans.). Manchester, UK: Manchester University Press.

Kambanis, P. E., Bottera, A. R., Mancuso, C. J., Cass, K., Lohse, K., Benabe, J., ..., Mehler, P. (2023). Delusionality of beliefs among 50 adult females with severe and extreme anorexia nervosa upon admission to an acute medical stabilization facility. *Eating Disorders, 31*(4), 353–361.

Kaplan, A. S., & Garfinkel, P. E. (1999). Difficulties in treating patients with eating disorders: A review of patient and clinician variables. *The Canadian Journal of Psychiatry, 44*(7), 665–670.

Konstantakopoulos, G., Ioannidi, N., Patrikelis, P., & Gonidakis, F. (2020). The impact of theory of mind and neurocognition on delusionality in anorexia nervosa. *Journal of Clinical and Experimental Neuropsychology, 42*(6), 611–621.

Konstantakopoulos, G., Varsou, E., Dikeos, D., Ioannidi, N., Gonidakis, F., Papadimitriou, G., & Oulis, P. (2012). Delusionality of body image beliefs in eating disorders. *Psychiatry Research, 200*(2–3), 482–488.

Langdon, R., & Bayne, T. (2010). Delusion and confabulation: Mistakes of perceiving, remembering and believing. *Cognitive Neuropsychiatry, 15*(1–3), 319–345. doi:10.1080/13546800903000229

Lilenfeld, L. R., Wonderlich, S., Riso, L. P., Crosby, R., & Mitchell, J. (2006). Eating disorders and personality: A methodological and empirical review. *Clinical Psychology Review, 26*(3), 299–320.

Maher, B. A. (1974). Delusional thinking and perceptual disorder. *Journal of Individual Psychology, 30*(1), 98.

McKenna, G., Fox, J. R., & Haddock, G. (2014). Investigating the 'jumping to conclusions' bias in people with anorexia nervosa. *European Eating Disorders Review, 22*(5), 352–359.

McKenna, P. (1984). Disorders with overvalued ideas. *The British Journal of Psychiatry: The Journal of Mental Science, 145*, 579.

McKenna, P. (2017). *Delusions: Understanding the un-understandable*. Cambridge: Cambridge University Press.

Moscone, A.-L., Amorim, M.-A., Le Scanff, C., & Leconte, P. (2017). A model-driven approach to studying dissociations between body size mental representations in anorexia nervosa. *Body Image, 20*, 40–48.

Mountjoy, R. L., Farhall, J. F., & Rossell, S. L. (2014). A phenomenological investigation of overvalued ideas and delusions in clinical and subclinical anorexia nervosa. *Psychiatry Research, 220*(1–2), 507–512.

Mullen, R. (2003). Delusions: the continuum versus category debate. *Australian & New Zealand Journal of Psychiatry, 37*(5), 505–511.

Mullen, R., & Gillett, G. (2014). Delusions: A different kind of belief? *Philosophy, Psychiatry, & Psychology, 21*(1), 27–37.

Noordenbos, G. (1992). Important factors in the process of recovery according to patients with anorexia nervosa. In W. Herzog, H. C. Deter, & W. Vandereycken (eds). *The course of eating disorders* (pp. 304–322). Berlin: Springer.

O'Connell, J. E., Bendall, S., Morley, E., Huang, C., & Krug, I. (2018). Delusion-like beliefs in anorexia nervosa: An interpretative phenomenological analysis. *Clinical Psychologist, 22*(3), 317–326.

Oyebode, F. (2023). *Sims' symptoms in the mind: Textbook of descriptive psychopathology* (7th Edition). Elsevier Health Sciences.

Phillipou, A., Mountjoy, R. L., & Rossell, S. L. (2017). Overvalued ideas or delusions in anorexia nervosa? *Australian & New Zealand Journal of Psychiatry, 51*(6), 563–564.

Rosen, J. C. (1997). Cognitive-behavioral body image therapy. In D. M. Garner & P. E. Garfinkel (Eds.), *Handbook of treatment for eating disorders* (pp. 188–201). New York: The Guilford Press.

Sakakibara, E. (2016). Irrationality and pathology of beliefs. *Neuroethics, 9*(2), 147–157.

Şenay, O., & Yücel, B. (2022). Evaluation of insight, self-esteem, and body satisfaction in eating disorders. *The Journal of Nervous and Mental Disease, 10,* 1097.

Sisti, D., Rocchi, M. B., Siddi, S., Mura, T., Manca, S., Preti, A., & Petretto, D. R. (2012). Preoccupation and distress are relevant dimensions in delusional beliefs. *Comprehensive Psychiatry, 53*(7), 1039–1043.

Spitzer, M. (1990). On defining delusions. *Comprehensive Psychiatry, 31*(5), 377–397.

Steinglass, J. E., Eisen, J. L., Attia, E., Mayer, L., & Walsh, B. T. (2007). Is anorexia nervosa a delusional disorder? An assessment of eating beliefs in anorexia nervosa. *Journal of Psychiatric Practice, 13*(2), 65–71.

Tan, J. O., Hope, T., Stewart, A., & Fitzpatrick, R. (2006). Competence to make treatment decisions in anorexia nervosa: Thinking processes and values. *Philosophy, Psychiatry, & Psychology, 13*(4), 267.

Veale, D. (2002). Over-valued ideas: A conceptual analysis. *Behaviour Research and Therapy, 40*(4), 383–400.

Vitousek, K. M. (1996). The current status of cognitive-behavioral models of anorexia nervosa and bulimia nervosa. In P. Salkovskis (Ed.), *Frontiers of cognitive therapy* (pp. 383–418). New York: The Guilford Press.

Vitousek, K., Watson, S., & Wilson, G. T. (1998). Enhancing motivation for change in treatment-resistant eating disorders. *Clinical Psychology Review, 18*(4), 391–420.

Wernicke, C. (1906). *Grundriss der psychiatrie in klinischen vorlesungen.* Thieme.

Wolf, G., & Serpell, L. (1998). A cognitive model and treatment strategies for anorexia nervosa. In H. Hoek, J. Treasure, & M. Katzman (Eds.), *Neurobiology in the treatment of eating disorders* (pp. 407–429). Chichester: Wiley.

9

# DELUSIONS IN OBSESSIVE-COMPULSIVE DISORDER

*Judit Szalai*

## 1. Introduction

Persons with obsessive-compulsive disorder (OCD) have recurrent thoughts that are firmly held, ungrounded, resistant to contrary evidence, and in most cases 'bizarre' or incomprehensible to others. This corresponds to the definition of delusion in *DSM-5*, according to which delusions are 'fixed beliefs that are not amenable to change in light of conflicting evidence […] Delusions are deemed bizarre if they are clearly implausible and not understandable to same-culture peers and do not derive from ordinary life experiences' (American Psychiatric Association (APA) (2013): 87). OCD subjects may worry that their left foot will be cut off by a tram unless they emit a particular sound ten times; that their life will fall apart unless they preserve their supernatural power, manifested in a black dot they see and regularly check in the air, to stave off evil; that their house will be burgled unless they repeat closing the door 20 times while touching the frame with their elbows. Having such thoughts, frequently combined with poor insight (de Avila et al. 2019), persons with OCD appear to be obvious candidates for subjects with delusions.[1]

This chapter identifies the content and special characteristics of obsessive-compulsive delusions, with an emphasis on epistemic features related to experience and evidence. With the character of these delusional beliefs spelled out, a motivational explanation will be offered. The account of OCD delusions proposed here relies on recent theories that make use of empirical data regarding dysfunctional action monitoring in this condition.

I start with a discussion of the cognitive components of OCD, in order to identify those that potentially qualify as delusional (obsessions being part of, but not exhausting, the cognitive profile of OCD). In the second section, the most prominent approaches to this condition are presented, with an emphasis on those theories that accommodate recent findings concerning predictive processing errors in OCD, which will be used in the explanation of OCD-related delusions. In the third section, a motivational account of obsessive delusions is offered, one that is in line with such approaches. It will be also claimed that certain epistemic peculiarities of OCD-related delusions are specifically connected to abnormal action monitoring.

147

DOI: 10.4324/9781003296386-12

## 2.   The cognitive profile of obsessive-compulsive disorder

While sharing in proneness to obsessions, persons with OCD have a common cognitive background profile as well, elements of which are perfectionism, the so-called thought/action and thought/reality fusions, and certain beliefs concerning their own power and responsibility ('magical thinking'). I will address these from the perspective of their potential involvement with delusional beliefs.

A typical formulation of OCD perfectionism is that 'making mistakes or failing to live up to one's perfectionistic ideals should result in punishment or condemnation' (McFall and Wollersheim 1979). Mistakes are seen as failures, unacceptable to oneself or one's social environment (Frost and diBartolo 2002). Such ideas may be due to parental expectations or standards set for oneself. In the literature, these general beliefs about achievement and failure often blend into exacting convictions concerning the execution of *particular actions*, sometimes seen as an independent dimension of perfectionism (Frost and diBartolo 2002: 341).

Do perfectionistic beliefs in either of these senses qualify as delusional? Uncommonly, or even extremely, high general standards regarding thought or action (the first sense of 'perfectionism') would not fit the bill, as long as these standards or expectations do not come with factual content that is systematically distorted in the way *DSM-5* would require: ungrounded, irresponsive to evidence, and–as a rule–bizarre. The belief that 'You should exercise four hours every day' is extreme, but being normative rather than a formulation of a truth claim, it is not delusional. If, in contrast, it is augmented to involve a factual claim that meets our criteria, e.g., 'If you don't exercise four hours every day, your muscles will suffer atrophy', the hypothetical statement can count as delusional. Indeed, obsessive-compulsive delusions will be similar to such statements or beliefs.

The second sense of perfectionism as related to OCD relies on error signal misfunction during the process of executing particular movements. I will address these processing errors in the next section. For now, it is sufficient to summarily point out that the beliefs involved are in a sense not 'ungrounded' but have an experiential basis in sensorimotoric mechanisms. The subject feels that something is 'not just right', the action hasn't quite reached its goal, therefore should be repeated. Persons without difficulties in predictive processing would not come to the same practical conclusion, not sharing the experiences of someone with OCD. These beliefs, besides not being ungrounded (in the sense that they are based in the experience of the subject), also fail to be incomprehensible, thus it wouldn't be justified to categorize them as bizarre delusions; at the same time, complemented in certain ways, they can turn into such beliefs. The belief that 'This door is not closed right; the closing should be repeated' is a misbelief grounded in defective experience. In contrast, as expanded to 'This door is not closed right; unless the closing is repeated ten times, burglars will kill my mother', it appears to qualify as a bizarre delusion: it is highly unlikely that the state of affairs it refers to would be realized, completely out of line with ordinary experience, and there is no evidence to point in its direction. As in the previous case, the element of 'perfectionism' is involved in the delusional version of the belief about closing the door, which, however, would not by itself make for delusional content, even when extreme.

The second element of the OCD cognitive profile is the so-called thought/action and thought/reality fusions. These consist in certain general, implicit assumptions persons with OCD tend to share about the relationship of their thoughts to their actions and to what happens in the world outside. Subjects attach unreasonable degrees of likelihood to future actions and events once those appear in their thoughts, the significance of which they subjectively exaggerate. For instance, they tend to consider the thought of harming a loved one, which may occur to them, as problematic as committing the action itself (thought/action fusion); they tend to regard the thought as indicating that its content will be realized (thought/reality fusion).

How ungrounded and resistant to contrary evidence are these assumptions? Thought/action fusion appears to be the more reasonable of the two: if the subject is focused on a particular action tendency she believes she has, this is at least likely to trigger the thought of that action in the appropriate circumstances. If she is in addition convinced of her inability to avoid performing the action, this seems to indeed raise the chances of committing it. Thus, the thought itself can have causal significance, and thus potential moral weight, since the persistence of the thought might indeed contribute to the action, providing the idea of thought/action fusion with some basis.

For thought/reality fusion, there is no explanation without reference to irrational thinking. Such an assumption is not simply wrong-headed but operates with subjective probabilities that are highly idiosyncratic. OCD subjects overestimate the importance of thoughts the content of which are events they have no impact on and consider those thoughts as *signs* indicative of future events. For instance, a person with OCD would believe that her mental images of getting infected with a dangerous virus are an indication that this will actually happen. When based on evidence, naturally, it may be reasonable to think that such an infection will occur: if all other persons in our household are currently positive for COVID-19, it's not far-fetched to think that we will catch it from them. What the OCD subject takes as evidence in these cases is different, however. What counts as evidence for them is the thought itself, and this is not plausibly connected to the event by any causal mechanism; the thought of an accident 'presaging' the actual occurrence, as it were, without any grounds to causally link the two.

Would it be justified to label these assumptions delusional? Due to anxiety, the subject is focused on a particular idea or image. That focus places the idea or image in the foreground of his thinking, making it readily available for further processing, for using it in reasoning, verbal behaviour, etc. The mechanism seems similar to the operation of other anxious thoughts, e.g., the way in which the contingently triggered idea of, say, unfaithfulness on the part of a spouse could raise its perceived likelihood. This mechanism, unto itself, doesn't make for delusional thought: it's not only that the cognitions involved don't need to be bizarre (which would still leave room for non-bizarre delusions), but this thought/reality fusion doesn't need to be stubbornly resistant to evidence. It might be a fleeting idea that the unbidden mental image of a particular person making its appearance twice on a particular day, for instance, is ominous, indicating that the person will appear in real life and, say, behave in an aggressive way. A subject might even be permanently prone to having such ideas. In normal circumstances, however, finding out, e.g., that the person who was the intentional object of those thoughts has deceased, that is, receiving evidence to the effect that the content of the related fears will not be realized, removes the thought, together with the assumption of its realization. The subject will not work around the evidence in the way OCD subjects are prone to. If the person whose presence they think of as threatening has died, persons with OCD may well modify their convictions and believe that he is still going to harm them from beyond the grave, or that he passed on the task of harming them to someone who is still living.

Another candidate for delusional OCD-related thinking is the obsessional thought itself, which presents the negatively valued event the subject is trying to prevent from happening by performing the compulsive act. Such obsessive thoughts could be the house burning down; a lethal disease getting contracted; the subject indecently exposing themselves in public due to a sudden urge.

An argument advanced against conceiving obsessions as delusions is that, in contrast to delusions, obsessive thoughts are experienced as unwanted: 'In delusions the patient thinks *with* the delusion, in obsessive-compulsive disorder, the patient thinks *against* the obsession' (Denys 2011: 6). Damiaan Denys claims that delusions cannot be either egosyntonic or egodystonic. His argument relies on the controversial premise that the egosyntonic/egodystonic character of thoughts takes *reflection*. Obsessive thoughts are egodystonic (in a reflected way); delusions, in contrast, are pre-reflective, thus neither egosyntonic nor egodystonic, since the 'patient does not have the ability to reflect upon the delusion' (Denys 2011: 6). On a minimalistic understanding of egosyntonicity/egodystonicity, however, the distinction refers to thought or behaviour aligning or failing to align with one's self-image or personal goals, regardless of reflection or lack thereof. It is not implausible to understand delusions as capable of being egosyntonic or egodystonic, and some authors understand them in that way. Particular delusions certainly seem to be endorsed or not endorsed by the subject. Persons with grandiose delusion, for instance, often do not want to assume the role their delusion dictates, such as that of a prophet (Zislin, Kuperman, and Durst 2011: 115, 118). Thus, the objection that, as opposed to obsessions, delusions are incapable of being endorsed or repudiated on reflection seems to be ill-grounded.

Another, more convincing argument against understanding obsessions as delusions is that, as some point out, unlike delusions, obsessions are not beliefs, but rather 'thoughts, impulses, or images' (Oulis et al. 2013: 51). While the subject overestimates the probabilities of certain occurrences, or at least has intrusive thoughts about dreaded future events, there is no *belief* in the way a person with grandiose delusion believes themselves to be a prophet, the Messiah or Satan, or someone with persecutory delusion believes being watched and followed.

What authors do consider delusional *beliefs* in OCD, ones that are resistant to contrary evidence and usually incomprehensible and bizarre, have the content that 'their rituals prevent[...] the occurrence of the feared consequence' (Fear, Sharp, and Healy 2000: 56). We can conceive the content of OCD delusions as hypothetical statements: 'If I don't prevent it from happening by clicking my tongue 30 times, I will be run over by a car'; 'If I don't check that the gas is turned off every half hour, the house will burn down'. These satisfy the requirements for delusional beliefs: they concern factual matters rather than express mere prescriptions; the subject would not accept evidence on the basis of which they could be discarded; additionally, they are 'bizarre' or hard to endorse by anyone other than individuals with high OC symptoms.

The peculiar relationship to evidence, although mostly attributable to factors related to the subject, also has to do with the content of these beliefs, specifically, the future-oriented character of most OCD delusions. It is a standard general feature of delusions that they 'are not amenable to change in light of conflicting evidence' (American Psychiatric Association (APA) (2013): 87, for more on delusion and evidence see Flores, Chapter 12). What would count as conflicting evidence, though, in the case of future events? If a subject claims that 'Unless I click with my tongue 50 times a day, a horrible accident will happen', it is hard to declare her *wrong*, since as yet there is no truth to the matter of whether the dreaded event will occur or not. Current evidence for the future states of affairs that are the content of such obsessions is certainly lacking; however, due to their future character, there is no conclusive evidence *against* them, either. The subject may even cite their special intuition, inaccessible to others, concerning the relevant future facts. They cannot account for their epistemic sources[2]: the 'task', i.e., what they are supposed to do to prevent the frightful event from happening and to keep the thought or image of the event at bay is experienced as simply 'coming to them'. They don't have a sense of imagining or conjuring up these images, nor can they identify an external source. Despite their obscure origins and their content being incapable of getting verified or falsified, these thoughts are associated with a high level conviction: the subject not only has a vision or image of the feared event occurring, but has a firm, unshakeable belief concerning it.

## 3.   Integrating action monitoring dysfunction into the explanation of obsessive-compulsive disorder

OCD has been historically accounted for in a variety of ways: it has been considered a disorder of emotional regulation (due to the role of anxiety), of the will (the subject being allegedly incapable of resisting certain impulses), and of cognition (owing to certain meta-cognitive and object-level beliefs). In present-day theories, affective, volitional, and cognitive elements tend to be all acknowledged in the etiology of OCD, although still with different emphases. The idea of 'surrendering' to irresistible urges, also taken up by philosophers (Watson 1977: 332; Churchland 2002: 208), has been less popular; cognitive-behavioural and metacognitive accounts have dominated the discussion. In the latter, thought/action fusion and perfectionistic beliefs (as above), as well as a sense of inflated responsibility (the subject believing that they can prevent catastrophic events by rituals) have been central.

Miles McFall and Janet Wollersheim understand the mechanism of OCD in terms of primary and secondary threat appraisals, the former being 'whereby the individual esti-mates the danger of an event relative to his perceived resources to cope with it' (McFall and Wollersheim 1979: 334), while the content of the latter are the consequences of the subject's efforts to cope with the threat. Primary appraisals involve the overestimated dan-ger and probability of the feared event occurring; secondary ones involve the subject's self-perception of her low capability of coping with those dangers. Paul Salkovskis adds cognitions to this picture concerning the subject's own responsibility regarding the nega-tively valued future events (Salkovskis 1985, 1999). Such cognitions include the idea, as above, that thoughts about the action are as problematic as actually performing the action itself and make it more likely or should be considered as a sign that the catastrophic event will occur. Due to this distorted significance attached to thoughts, they are perceived as in need of being kept in check, which is the subject's responsibility. Hence the effort to sup-press or neutralize the content of these thoughts by compulsive thinking or behaviour.

To briefly mention alternative, volitional accounts of OCD: Kevin Zaragosa (2006) argues that obsessive-compulsive subjects temporarily lose the capacity of self-control and become 'ego-depleted' when acting compulsively. Being constantly subjected to powerful impulses to execute particular actions, resistance becomes too taxing and persons run out of resources to do so. The inhibitory mechanisms that prevent them from performing the action fail, and they 'give in' to the urge.

While cognitive accounts don't seem to do justice to the element of tension regarding the execution of the action, the way in which such volitional accounts present the subject, viz. as trying not to commit the compulsive act, but ultimately failing, also seem implausible. In reality, the subject is convinced that they *should* perform the act (in order to avert some catastrophe, as above) and concentrates on doing so in the right way, down to minute details. They endorse the action, though not for itself but for its consequences for the future they are trying to influence (Szalai 2016); thus, the compulsive act is not mere tension release, but rather purposeful and effortful behaviour.

Both cognitivist/metacognitivist and volition-based accounts miss certain characteristics essential to compulsions: their repetitive nature and the sense of incompleteness or 'not-just-right' feeling attached to the action. Neither the perceived significance of thought, magical thinking, and an overinflated sense of responsibility (believing that one is capable of influencing events in the world by specific behaviours that are apparently unrelated to them) nor alleged irresistible urges can account for the number of repetitions the obsessive-compulsive subject regards necessary, acting in a ritualistic manner.

Recent empirical findings help illuminate this feature of compulsions, though. According to these, OCD is associated with certain sensorimotor deficits connected with action monitoring. Predictive processing is altered in OCD: forward model mechanisms are compromised by the over-production of error signals, creating a mismatch between desired and actual, as well as actual and perceived outcomes. A lack of fit is more often detected between desired states and actual consequences of the action than in the absence of this condition, and generated error signals are larger and longer (Gehring, Himle, and Nisenson 2000). Due to defective forward model mechanisms, the sensory attenuation characteristic of self-initiated action is also reduced, as the outcomes of the action do not correspond to motor predictions (Gentsch et al. 2012). These processes are responsible for the feeling of the incomplete or 'not-just-right' character of the action (for instance, the sense that the subject has failed to close the door or cleaned their hands properly).

This empirical research has been used in explanations of OCD that attempt to accommodate both the cognitive/metacognitive profile and sensorimotor features of OCD (Szalai 2019; Schmidt et al. 2021; Poletti, Gebhardt, and Raballo 2022). The present account of delusions in OCD is in line with this integrated understanding: the bizarre thoughts that underlie compulsive acts are to be accounted for in part by cognitive factors (especially rigid thinking and resistance to generally recognized evidence) and in part by sensorimotoric deficits that issue in a felt need for repetition and rationalization of repeated action by ritualization. I will also attempt to connect these two factors in the generation of OCD delusions.

## 4. A motivational explanation of delusions in OCD, based on integrative, cognitive-sensomotoric accounts

Towards the end of the previous section, I sketched out action monitoring deficits associated with OCD. Predictive errors have been used in the explanation of delusions in general, or in the context of different specific delusions, by other authors. Philip Corlett, Garry Honey, and Paul Fletcher, for instance, consider delusions the result of a learning process associated with the disruption of prediction-error signalling (Corlett, Honey, and Fletcher 2007). The mechanism of delusion formation is that 'the experience of mismatch when there is none drives an individual to invent bizarre causal structures to explain away their experiences, these are manifest clinically as delusions' (Corlett, Honey, and Fletcher 2007: 238). This approach has been taken, e.g., concerning schizophrenic delusions (Corlett, Honey, and Fletcher 2007: 238) and the Capgras delusion (for more on delusion and prediction error, see Corlett, Chapter 30). In the latter case, the discrepancy between the expected and actual perception of a loved one's face induces the belief that the person has been replaced by a replica (Lancellotta and Bortolotti 2019). While there is no pressure to find a single type of explanation for delusions that applies across the board (cf. Radden 2011), I would like to propose a motivational explanation of delusions in OCD that also relies on anomalous predictive processing.

Motivational accounts of delusions in OCD have already been proposed. For instance, Eugenia Lancelotta and Lisa Bortolotti argue that the belief that the house will otherwise burn down and the desire to avoid this can motivate the delusional belief that the stove needs to be checked 30 times–which, in the light of such belief-desire pairs, can even be considered playing an adaptive role. This account does justice to several features of OCD mentality, including anxiety and magical, ritualistic thinking, as well as the felt need to execute the compulsive act. I would like to complement such approaches by describing how error signals and, relatedly, the handling of evidence can also play an illuminating role.

As was already mentioned above, obsessive-compulsive delusions have been described as subjects believing that 'their rituals prevent[...] the occurrence of the feared consequence' (Fear, Sharp, and Healy 2000), e.g., 'If I don't prevent it by clicking my tongue thirty times, an accident will befall me'. Now people execute rituals in non-pathological, everyday cases as well, based on such implicit hypotheticals as 'If I don't take my old plush bunny to the exam, I won't get an A'. Such rituals also have the purpose of 'magically' influencing the future: 'lucky plushes' influence the outcome of exams; blowing out birthday candles in one breath makes wishes come true. These rituals do not demand *repetition* a particular number of times, however. Why does the OCD subject feel the need for repetition—especially considering that, in some cases, repetition nullifies the results of the previous actions, e.g., closing the door ten times involves reopening it nine times after nine closings?

The predictive processing abnormalities described in the second section cause persons with OCD experiencing manual actions as 'not just right'; they 'need to ritualize until they quiet these sensations' (Coles et al. 2003: 681). These experiences are specifically associated with OCD as opposed to other psychopathologies and, within OCD, are especially strongly related to manual activities such as ordering and (certain forms of) checking. As I have argued elsewhere, although most of the phenomenology of OCD can be explained via cognitive/metacognitive and affective processes, repetition (ritualization) can only be accounted for by reference to error signals (Szalai 2019).

In line with accounts of OCD that integrate predictive processing, the understanding of OCD delusions I propose is the following. The content of the delusion that particular movements have to be performed in order to prevent a catastrophe from happening can be broken down into the components of a nagging worry concerning the future that is very hard to cognitively penetrate (e.g., the experience that the feared event did not occur in the past in similar situations doesn't undermine the belief of the subject[3]) and ideation concerning action that could prevent that occurrence. The action is (usually) conceived as repetitive: it has to be performed a particular number of times and precisely the right way. (This latter feature has been put into focus by the idea of 'low-level agency': the OCD subject focuses on the [low-level, instrumental] details of executing the action rather than the [higher-level] representation of the action's goal [Balconi 2010].)

Both the need for repetition and for 'precision' in execution can be explained through the feelings of incompleteness persons with OCD experience due to the processing errors discussed above. OCD delusions are partly rooted in, and tend to be tied to, sensomotoric activity. (This is also confirmed by the fact that so-called 'pure obsessions', which are not followed by compulsive acts, do not have to be neutralized in a repetitive manner. Mental neutralization can come in the form of mental reviewing of events, self-reassurance, replacing 'bad' thoughts with 'good' ones, counting, etc.; repeating words is just one possibility.) The tendency to repetition gets rationalized through the 'tasks' the subject gives themselves, ones that they are supposed to perform either a determinate number of times, or until the action feels 'completed'. That performing these tasks is necessary in order to prevent a future catastrophy is the content of the delusion. Thus, dysfunctional action monitoring feeds into to the kind of delusions persons with OCD are prone to having: being uncertain about the results of their actions due to lack of a match between expectations and sensory outcomes, they deem more attempts to secure the right outcomes necessary. Being unaware of this sensomotoric deficiency, they rationalize repetition by ritualization.

Why aren't these beliefs responsive to new evidence, though? Here, we are putting aside the consideration above as to lack of present evidence concerning future states, which also contributes to the difficulty of rejecting delusionsal beliefs in OCD, and focusing on the subject's attitude to evidence gathering and use. In many cases, publicly available evidence makes it very unlikely that the dreaded future state would be realized, or at least it appears very clear that there is no publicly available evidence to connect present compulsive acts to those future states. No one without obsessive-compulsive tendencies would find the idea of preventing tram accidents by repetitively emitting idiosyncratic oral sounds plausible. What prevents OCD subjects from revising such beliefs?

Prediction errors and distrusting evidence, including those concerning the future, are plausibly connected with each other. It comes as no surprise that OCD has been called a 'disorder of doubt'. Persons with OCD are used to regarding their experience unreliable: they doubt whether the door that appears to be closed is in fact closed properly, whether their hands are thoroughly washed, whether there are still dangerous germs in their freshly cleaned apartment. Low confidence extends to the deliverances of perception and memory (Cougle, Salkovkis, and Wahl 2007; Hermans et al. 2008) and adversely influences belief updating processes. Probably in part due to feeling less certainty about the content of their experiences, obsessive-compulsive subjects are more reluctant to revise their beliefs and feel the need to collect more evidence than their peers without OCD. Using reversal learning tasks it has been found that individuals with higher OC symptoms exhibit more uncertainty and a 'pattern of behavior potentially indicative of a difficulty in relying on learned contingencies' when circumstances were shifting (Fradkin et al. 2020: 1). (This influences their decision-making skills as well: they take longer and collect more evidence than their peers: Chen et al. 2022.)

Since persons with OCD have difficulties revising their beliefs on the basis of experience, they are more prone to the kind of cognitive rigidity characteristic of delusions. Cognitive rigidity, and negative evaluation of situations that would require cognitive flexibility, have been identified as a notable feature of OCD (Sternheim et al. 2014). This clearly helps the maintenance of delusions publicly available evidence (even if circumstantial and probabilistic) would contradict. The precise relationship between prediction errors and learning from experience is in need of further empirical research, however. It is intuitively plausible that systematic failure to make correct sensory predictions and uncertainty regarding perceptual deliverances (e.g., whether the door is properly closed) due to deficient predictive processing makes for slower updating or revising of beliefs in general. Some researchers hypothesize the causal order to be the reverse, though: excessive uncertainty in accommodating new circumstances (a 'computational impairment') results in a 'reduced ability to use the past to predict the present and future, and to oversensitivity to feedback (i.e. prediction errors)' (Fradkin et al. 2020: 1). Although impossible to clarify without further (empirical) research, the relationship between prediction errors and updating in learning seems to be there. Continued research on OCD predictive processing and agency (e.g. Schmidt et al. 2021) holds out the promise of contributing to the clarification of this mechanism.

## 5. Conclusion

This chapter has looked at OCD from the perspective of delusional cognitions it may involve. Rejecting some candidates as not meeting the criteria for delusions, certain hypotheticals are settled on as the typical format of OCD delusions (in line with their standard interpretation). It is demonstrated that in addition to the explanatory power of some of their epistemic characteristics (being about the future, they cannot be verified or falsified in the present), the emergence and persistence of obsessive-compulsive delusions can be given a motivational account that relies on predictive processing errors.

## Notes

1 'Bizarreness' is not a universal requirement concerning delusions. *DSM-V* differentiates between bizarre and non-bizarre delusions:

> Delusions are deemed bizarre if they are clearly implausible and not understandable to same-culture peers and do not derive from ordinary life experiences. An example of a bizarre delusion is the belief that an outside force has removed his or her internal organs and replaced them with someone else's organs without leaving any wounds or scars. An example of a nonbizarre delusion is the belief that one is under surveillance by the police, despite a lack of convincing evidence.
> *(American Psychiatric Association (APA) (2013): 87)*

  OCD delusions, although often not involving events that could not be part of ordinary life experiences (such as one's internal organs being removed by alien forces, or their actions being executed by outside agents), are usually about causal connections that could not hold under any circumstances, e.g. making certain sounds preventing traffic accidents or certain ritualistic hand gestures keeping away diseases. Therefore, I will consider OCD delusions as normally bizarre, even though in fringe cases there could be an actual causal connection between, e.g., washing hands multiple times and not contracting a disease.
2 OCD subjects 'cannot explain why they view their beliefs as true, or give unconvincing evidence as the basis of their belief' (Brakoulias and Starcevic 2011: 153).
3 For people with standard epistemic attitudes, a conditional belief like 'If I don't click my fingers fifty times every time I leave my apartment, I will have a tram accident that day' can be disproved by sufficient experience with no accident happening when the compulsive action is not executed. There may be circumstances working against such a disproof (e.g., the trams may not run that day); but the believed link between the action and the alleged consequences is normatively required to get weaker with every instance when those consequences fail to materialize. Again, as the belief is about the future, it cannot be excluded that the accident happens one day, which the OCD subject will attribute to the action not having been performed, or, if it was, not having been performed in the right way. But maintaining the belief in the face of overwhelming (circumstantial, probabilistic) evidence to the contrary goes against basic epistemic norms.

# References


American Psychiatric Association (APA) (2013) *Diagnostic and statistical manual of mental disorders* (5th ed.). Washington, DC: Author (DSM-5).

Balconi M. (2010) "Disruption of the sense of agency: From perception to self-knowledge," in: *Neuropsychology of the sense of agency*, M. Balconi (ed.), 125–144. Dordrecht: Springer.

Brakoulias V., Starcevic V. (2011) "The characterization of beliefs in obsessive-compulsive disorder," *Psychiatric Quarterly* 82(2): 151–161.

Chen Y., Liu Y., Wang Z., Yang T., Fan Q. (2022) "Accumulation of evidence during decision making in OCD patients," *Frontiers in Psychiatry* 13: 980905.

Churchland P.S. (2002) *Brain-wise: Studies in neurophilosophy*. Cambridge: MIT Press.

Coles M.E., Frost R.O., Heimberg R.G., Rhéaume J. (2003) "Not just right experiences: Perfectionism, obsessive-compulsive features and general psychopathology," *Behaviour Research and Therapy* 41(6): 681–700.

Corlett P.R., Honey G.D., Fletcher P.C. (2007) "From prediction error to psychosis: ketamine as a pharmacological model of delusions," *Journal of Psychopharmacology* 21(3): 238-52.

Cougle J.R., Salkovskis P.M., Wahl K. (2007) "Perception of memory ability and confidence in recollections in obsessive-compulsive checking," *Journal of Anxiety Disorders* 21: 118–130.

de Avila R.C.S., do Nascimento L.G., Porto R.L.M., Fontenelle L, Filho E.C.M., Brakoulias V, Ferrão Y.A. (2019) "Level of insight in patients with obsessive-compulsive disorder: An exploratory comparative study between patients with "good insight" and "poor insight"," *Frontiers in Psychiatry* 10: 413.

Denys D. (2011) "Obsessionality & compulsivity: A phenomenology of obsessive-compulsive disorder," *Philosophy, Ethics and Humanities in Medicine* 6: 3.

Fear C., Sharp H., Healy D. (2000) "Obsessive-compulsive disorder with delusions," *Psychopathology* 33(2): 55–61.

Fradkin I., Ludwig C., Eldar E., Huppert J.D. (2020) "Doubting what you already know: Uncertainty regarding state transitions is associated with obsessive compulsive symptoms," *PLoS Computational Biology* 16(2): e1007634.

Frost R.O., DiBartolo P.M. (2002) "Perfectionism, anxiety, and obsessive-compulsive disorder," in: *Perfectionism: Theory, research, and treatment*, G.L. Flett & P.L. Hewitt (eds.), 341–371. Washington: American Psychological Association.

Gehring W.J., Himle J., Nisenson L.G. (2000) "Action-monitoring dysfunction in obsessive-compulsive disorder," *Psychological Science* 11(1): 1–6.

Gentsch A., Schütz-Bosbach S., Endrass T., Kathmann N. (2012) "Dysfunctional forward model mechanisms and aberrant sense of agency in obsessive-compulsive disorder," *Biological Psychiatry* 71(7): 652–659.

Hermans D., Engelen U., Grouwels L., Joos E., Lemmens J., Pieters G. (2008) "Cognitive confidence in obsessive-compulsive disorder: Distrusting perception, attention and memory," *Behaviour Research and Therapy* 46(1): 98–113.

Lancellotta E., Bortolotti L. (2019) "Are clinical delusions adaptive?" *Wiley Interdisciplinary Reviews–Cognitive Science* 10(5): e1502.

McFall M.E., Wollersheim, J.P. (1979) "Obsessive-compulsive neurosis: A cognitive-behavioral formulation and approach to treatment," *Cognitive Therapy and Research* 3(4): 333–348.

Oulis P., Konstantakopoulos G., Lykouras L., Michalopoulou P.G. (2013) "Differential diagnosis of obsessive-compulsive symptoms from delusions in schizophrenia: A phenomenological approach," *World Journal of Psychiatry* 3(3): 50–56.

Poletti M., Gebhardt E., Raballo A. (2022) "Along the fringes of agency: Neurodevelopmental account of the obsessive mind," *CNS Spectrums* 27(5): 557–560.

Radden J. (2011) *On delusion*. Abingdon and New York: Routledge.

Salkovskis P.M. (1985) Obsessive–compulsive problems: A cognitive–behavioural analysis. *Behaviour Research and Therapy* 23: 571–583.

Salkovskis P.M. (1999) "Understanding and treating obsessive-compulsive disorder," *Behaviour Research and Therapy* 37(Suppl1): S29–S59.

Schmidt S., Wagner G., Walter M., Stenner M.P. (2021) "A psychophysical window onto the subjective experience of compulsion," *Brain Sciences* 11(2): 182.

Sternheim L., van der Burgh M., Berkhout L.J., Dekker M.R., Ruiter C. (2014) "Poor cognitive flexibility, and the experience thereof, in a subclinical sample of female students with obsessive-compulsive symptoms," *Scandinavian Journal of Psychology* 55(6): 573–577.

Szalai J. (2016) "Agency and mental states in obsessive-compulsive disorder," *Philosophy, Psychiatry, & Psychology* 23(1): 47–59.

Szalai, J. (2019) "The sense of agency in OCD," *Review of Philosophy and Psychology* 10(2): 363–380.

Watson, G. (1977) "Skepticism about weakness of will," *Philosophical Review* 86: 316–339.

Zaragosa, K. (2006) "What happens when someone acts compulsively?" *Philosophical Studies* 131: 251–268.

Zislin J., Kuperman V., Durst R. (2011) ""Ego-dystonic" delusions as a predictor of dangerous behavior," *Psychiatric Quarterly* 82(2): 113–120.

# 10
# DELUSIONS IN DEPRESSION

*Anna Bortolan*

## 1. Introduction

The experience of delusions in depression is comparatively under-explored in the field of philosophy of psychiatry and philosophical psychopathology. Often, the relevant literature has focused on the exploration of forms of delusional thinking that are associated with diagnoses of schizophrenia spectrum disorders, while depressive delusions have been investigated less frequently. (Antrobus and Bortolotti 2016: 193; Doerr-Zegers 2019: 753).

Despite the relative scarcity of philosophical investigations on the topic, delusions are not a rare occurrence in depression. It has been indicated that psychotic features (i.e. delusions, hallucinations or both) are present in 18.5 per cent of major depressive episodes (Ohayon and Schatzberg 2002), with a higher prevalence among hospitalised patients and lower among outpatients (Gaudiano et al. 2009). Delusions have been shown to be more common than hallucinations in major depression with psychotic features (Parker et al. 1991; Meyers 2014) and this is why this form of depression is also often called 'delusional depression' (Smith et al. 2007).

The aim of this chapter is to explore some of the philosophical insights which have been developed with regard to the experience of depressive delusions, outlining some of the core themes around which research has coalesced, and potential avenues for further investigation. In doing so, I will explore in particular a set of ideas which have been put forward within the field of phenomenological psychopathology, and this choice is motivated by two main reasons.

On the one hand, a key aim of phenomenology is the development of a fine-grained understanding of subjective or first-personal experience (cf. Gallagher and Zahavi 2012: Chapter 1), and this involves, amongst other things, a comprehension of what an experience 'is like' for the subject who undergoes it. This has proved to be a very valuable approach for the exploration of the lived dimension of health and illness (Carel 2016), and is particularly useful when trying to comprehend the diversity and meaningfulness of complex experiences like delusions.

On the other hand, the theoretical and methodological framework of philosophical phenomenology has already informed a significant amount of philosophical and

DOI: 10.4324/9781003296386-13

interdisciplinary research on mental illness (cf. Stanghellini et al. 2019), and an important aspect of this work has been the investigation of delusions, especially in the context of schizophrenia. As such, this approach can offer a range of conceptual tools that could be helpfully drawn upon and expanded when trying to understand other dimensions of mental ill-health.

## 2. Depressive delusions

Both the experience of delusions and that of depression encompass multiple phenomena, and it is thus helpful to clarify exactly what is captured by the notion of depressive delusions.

In the *Diagnostic and Statistical Manual of Mental Disorders (DSM)* (American Psychiatric Association [APA] 2022), the criteria for a diagnosis of depression do not require the presence of delusional symptoms. However, 'psychotic features' are indicated as potential features of a major depressive episode (2022: 183–184), and it is thus recognised that delusions, alongside hallucinations, can be associated with this condition. More specifically, it is indicated that the feelings of worthlessness and guilt which are a diagnostic criterion for a major depressive episode can be 'delusional' (2022: 183), and the diagnosis of major depressive episode includes two delusion-related 'specifiers': 'with mood-congruent' and 'with mood-incongruent' psychotic features (2022: 213).[1]

*Mood-congruence* in this context refers to the existence of a complete alignment between the contents of the delusions (or hallucinations) and the main 'themes' which mark the depressive episode (which are implied to be rooted in particular affective experiences, i.e. 'moods'). These themes can concern 'personal inadequacy, guilt, disease, death, nihilism, or deserved punishment' (APA 2022: 213). On the contrary, when the delusional (or hallucinatory) contents are not consistent with the depressive themes listed above – or only some of these contents are – the relevant psychotic features are considered to be *mood-incongruent*.

Historically, the characterisation of depression involving delusions has been a matter of debate. In particular, scholars have been divided as to whether delusional depression is a severe form of unipolar depression, or rather a distinct type of depressive or psychotic disorder (Antrobus and Bortolotti 2016; Doerr-Zegers 2019).[2]

Those who argue in favour of the idea that delusional depression is a different condition from unipolar depression may do so on various grounds (cf. Smith et al. 2007). For example, some differences have been identified in the symptoms of delusional and non-delusional depression, with the former being more frequently marked by symptoms such as psychomotor disturbances and agitation, as well as being characterised by more severe feelings of guilt, and a weaker diurnal variation of mood (Charney and Nelson 1981; Parker et al. 1991). However, some of these differences have been interpreted as being compatible with the idea that psychotic depression is a severe form of depression (e.g. Lattuada et al. 1999), and other studies have not supported the existence of differences in symptomatology between delusional and non-delusional forms of depression (e.g. Bellini et al. 1992). However, the distinction between the two conditions can also be argued for on the basis of the different response to treatment exhibited by delusional and non-delusional depressive patients (Parker et al. 1991). This is the case because those who experience delusions do not typically improve if treated only with anti-depressants, but rather get better when the latter are paired with other forms of treatment (e.g. anti-psychotic medication) (Antrobus and Bortolotti 2016: 193; Doerr-Zegers 2019: 756–757). Furthermore, delusional depression is associated with a significantly higher suicidal risk than depression without psychotic features (Gournellis et al. 2018; Paljärvi et al. 2023; Doerr-Zegers 2019: 757).

On the other hand, as illustrated by Otto Doerr-Zegers (2019), the idea that delusional depression is a severe type of unipolar depression can be defended through the observation that delusional and non-delusional depressive patients display similar personality traits, and that the emergence of delusions can be seen as deriving from the interaction between these traits and certain biographical events (2019: 758–759). In addition, as observed by Magdalena Antrobus and Lisa Bortolotti (2016), it can be noted that depressive delusions can be differentiated from other types of delusions which are present in psychotic conditions such as schizophrenia (Stanghellini and Raballo 2015), thus corroborating the idea that delusional depression is not a distinct kind of psychosis.

Delusions that are associated with the experience of depression can also be of different kinds: nihilistic delusions, somatic delusions, persecutory delusions, delusions of poverty, delusions of guilt, and delusions of worthlessness have all been associated with forms of psychotic depression (Beck and Alford 2009; Picardi et al. 2018). However, delusions of worthlessness and guilt are particularly frequent in severe depression (Beck and Alford 2009: 34).

Delusions of worthlessness involve false beliefs concerning one's value, as people who experience these delusions may unwarrantedly think of themselves as unwanted, inadequate, or lacking in various ways (Beck and Alford 2009). For example, a patient whose experience is discussed by Aaron Beck and Brad Alford reported the following:

> I must weep myself to death. I cannot live. I cannot die. I have failed so. It would be better if I had not been born. My life has always been a burden … I am the most inferior person in the world … I am subhuman.
>
> *(2009: 36)*

Delusions of guilt concern one's alleged culpability for bad decisions, misdeeds, or crimes, but also negative events or situations outside of an individual person's control, such as world poverty (APA 2022: 186). This connects with delusional convictions focusing on the theme of punishment, when a person believes that they deserve or are about to be severely punished for crimes they have committed (Beck and Alford 2009: 37).

Delusions of worthlessness and delusions of guilt are considered to be mood-congruent delusions, since, as outlined above, they are consistent with some of the main themes that mark the experience of a major depressive episode. For example, the *DSM* indicates that those who are diagnosed with this condition 'often misinterpret neutral or trivial day-to-day events as evidence of personal defects and have an exaggerated sense of responsibility for untoward events' (APA 2022: 186).[3]

Another type of delusions that is considered to be mood-congruent is nihilistic delusions. The *DSM* characterises them as involving 'the conviction that a major catastrophe will occur' (2022: 101), but the notion appears to be used more broadly to refer to delusional beliefs that have to do with the destruction or inexistence of oneself or the world. A type of nihilistic delusion is the Cotard syndrome or delusion,[4] which consists in the subject believing that they are dead, or variations of this idea.

In the rest of this chapter, I will discuss further the Cotard delusion, as well as delusions of guilt and worthlessness to illustrate some of the contributions made by the phenomenological approach to the study of delusional experience. Before that, however, it is important to consider another account of depressive delusions, to which the phenomenological approach itself can be seen as complementary.

## 3.  A cognitive account of delusions in depression

Many approaches to the characterisation and explanation of delusions focus on the role of anomalous cognition in these phenomena.

Delusions are often identified with a particular kind of propositional attitude, i.e. beliefs of a certain type. The *DSM*, for example, describes delusions as 'fixed beliefs that are not amenable to change in light of conflicting evidence' (APA 2022: 101).

A 'doxastic' view (e.g. Bortolotti 2009) is prominent in the characterisation of the nature of delusions, and an emphasis on cognition is present also in various theories which seek to explain how delusions emerge. Various accounts indeed suggest that delusions result from clinical abnormalities in cognitive mechanisms. One-factor theories have it that anomalous experiences are part of the causal story (for more see Sullivan-Bissett, Chapter 28), and two-factor theories accept this but add to the story a clinical abnormality in belief formation or evaluation (for more see Davies and Coltheart, Chapter 29).

As far as depressive delusions are concerned, Antrobus and Bortolotti (2016) have developed an account that also highlights the centrality of cognitive processes. Drawing on both Jean Piaget's account of the equilibration of cognitive structures (1977), and Aaron Beck's cognitive model of depression (1967), they argue that depressive delusions arise from an attempt to eliminate inconsistency between existing mental representations and new information acquired by the person. More specifically, they suggest that the delusions make it possible to eliminate the dissonance between one's 'self-schemata' and acquired information which is in conflict with those schemata.

Beck's model is drawn upon by Antrobus and Bortolotti to illustrate the key role played by negative self-assessments in the experience of depression in general, and how this influences the depressed person's self-representations (2016: 195 ff.). Those who experience this condition indeed often have a negatively biased conception of themselves (e.g. as unworthy or inadequate) and this can have wide-ranging cognitive and practical effects (Beck and Alford 2009: 229 ff.).

Piaget's theory, on the other hand, is used to account for the interaction between one's self-representations and the way in which information that is in contrast with them is processed. As reconstructed by Antrobus and Bortolotti (2016: 194), Piaget's state of equilibrium is one in which 'the person's existing schemata can explain what she experiences', and this relies on the presence of both assimilation and accommodation processes (Piaget 1977: 6 ff.). While assimilation refers to circumstances in which the information that is received is compatible with and can be made sense of within an existing schema, accommodation refers to cases in which an existing schema is not applicable and needs to be modified as a result' (Antrobus and Bortolotti 2016: 195).

Antrobus and Bortolotti claim that depressive delusions originate in a disruption of accommodation processes, whereby, rather than updating a schema that does not fit the information that is received, this information is altered in order to fit the schema. As they explain:

People suffering from depression are not capable of successful accommodation, that is, they cannot modify their negative representations of themselves to match new, contradicting information. Because the new information cannot be assimilated in its original form, people distort its content in order to match their self-schemata, and then they assimilate the distorted content. In this way, they compensate for the missing part of the adaptation process, and avoid dissonance.

*(Antrobus and Bortolotti 2016: 196)*

Disturbances of cognition are thus at the core of the account of depressive delusions developed by Antrobus and Bortolotti (as well as being the cornerstone of a pre-eminent model of depression in the literature), and there appear to be significant benefits in unearthing the centrality of cognitive processes in these conditions. There are indeed multiple connections between cognition and affectivity, and mood disorders like depression do not involve only alterations of the way in which we feel, but also of the way in which we think.

However, it is important not to look at cognitive processes in isolation from the range of experiential changes that are present in depression, and considering these changes can also potentially help us to better characterise the nature of depressive delusions themselves.

The cognitive account presented by Antrobus and Bortolotti draws attention to the rigidity of self-representations in severe depression, and how information that conflicts with them may be distorted so as to avoid cognitive dissonance, thus providing grounds for the development of delusional thinking. However, it seems difficult to exhaustively account for the potential inflexibility of a depressed person's self-concept by appealing only to cognition. In particular, the presence of negative biases concerning the self needs to be explained, especially given their very selective nature. Those who experience depression have indeed been shown to be less biased and more accurate than other people in a range of judgements, some of which also concern the self (Alloy and Abramson 1979; Bortolotti and Antrobus 2015).

In addition, while the presence of some negative biases seems to be common among depressed people, it is necessary to be able to explain why only some persons with depression develop delusions while others do not, and why the delusions have different themes which are sometimes incongruent with the focus of the negative biases.

A fine-grained account of the affective experience of depressed patients can help to illuminate some of these questions, by bringing to the fore, for example, the ways in which moods and beliefs concerning the self can influence each other. Research in the field of phenomenological psychopathology has given various contributions to the understanding of both affectivity and depression (e.g. Ratcliffe 2008, 2015), and in later sections of this chapter, I will draw on some of these views to explore specifically the experience of depressive delusions. Before moving to that, and to further contextualise that aspect of my analysis, however, I will first introduce some influential ideas which have emerged from phenomenological research on delusions more broadly.

## 4.   Phenomenology and delusions

Phenomenological accounts of delusions have been developed primarily in relation to delusions associated with the experience of schizophrenia.

Such accounts tend to converge in the suggestion that delusions cannot be conceived primarily – or at all – as false beliefs, and as the result of cognitive errors (cf. Parnas and Sass 2001; Sass and Parnas 2003; Ratcliffe 2008). Rather, from this perspective, delusions are seen as particular forms of experience involving a range of disturbances, for example bodily, affective, and social (Gallagher 2009).

Phenomenologists also attempt to understand how delusions may be connected to non-delusional symptoms, for example, negative symptoms in schizophrenia spectrum disorders (e.g. Sass and Parnas 2003), thus attempting to provide a holistic understanding of some of the relevant diagnostic categories. As Louis Sass and Elizabeth Pienkos explain (2013: 643):

> What is altered is not an isolated belief or framework proposition but the overall lived background or horizon of the whole life-world, thought-world, and lived body. These formal or structural changes set up the conditions for delusion, and the delusional content will frequently reflect these alterations of form [...].

Furthermore, research in phenomenological psychopathology has emphasised that the emergence of delusions can be best understood when considering the transformations of experience that precede the onset of the psychotic symptoms themselves.

Josef Parnas and Louis Sass (2001), for example, draw attention to the presence in the early stages of schizophrenia of a series of anomalies of self-experience, and argue on this basis that 'disorders of the self' are at the core of schizophrenic delusions. More specifically, Sass and Parnas (2003) highlight how in schizophrenia an experiential shift may occur from a *first-personal* to a *third-personal* perspective on one's own experience, a process integral to which are two main experiential transformations. On the one hand, the authors argue that the person's immediate sense of themselves as 'inhabiting' their own experience is weakened ('diminished self-affection'). On the other, a tendency to experience oneself or one's bodily and mental states in a manner similar to how external objects are experienced ('hyper-reflexivity') arises.

It has been suggested that looking at such transformations of experience can help to better understand certain delusions, in particular those that have been characterised as 'bizarre', such as delusions of control (APA 2022).[5] For example, an increased reflective awareness of one's own bodily and mental states may be associated with an increased sense of detachment from one's experience, and this could facilitate the attribution of agency for such experience to external factors rather than to oneself (cf. Parnas and Sass 2001; Sass and Parnas 2003; Sass and Pienkos 2013).

This and other phenomenological accounts of delusions challenge the idea that these delusions are incomprehensible, in so far as they also aim to show how the delusions can emerge from transformations of kinds of experience with which we are all familiar, and draw attention to the meaningfulness of the delusional symptoms of the experiencer.

It is possible to wonder how, if at all, a phenomenological account of delusions would fit within existing classifications. Theories concerning delusion formation, for example, can be distinguished on the basis of how they conceive of the relationship between anomalous experiences and the adoption of false beliefs, with 'bottom-up' approaches claiming that the former cause the latter (see Bongiorno and Parrott, Chapter 26), and 'top-down' ones arguing the opposite (see Ohlhorst, Chapter 27).

Given the emphasis posed by phenomenological psychopathology on disturbances of experience, it might seem that this account of delusions is an example of a 'bottom-up' model. However, I think that this would be an incorrect characterisation, in so far as the experiential alterations that phenomenologists are concerned with do not tend to have a discrete or circumscribed character. While a bottom-up model would revolve around disruptions of specific perceptual processes – for example, the way in which familiar faces are experienced in the Capgras delusion (Stone and Young 1997) – a phenomenological account would typically focus on broader, and often global, transformations of experience (e.g. transformations to the way in which one perceives oneself and the world).

For the same reason, it can also be misleading to classify the phenomenological views as either one-factor or two-factor accounts, as these categorisations seem to rely on the idea that there is a neat separation between different experiential and cognitive functions, and that these can be selectively disrupted. Without denying the distinction between different mental states and processes, however, phenomenological accounts tend to focus on how different functions, and their disturbances, are intertwined, considering also dimensions of experience that appear to underlie different states and processes (Gallagher 2009).

## 5. A phenomenological perspective on delusions in depression

As mentioned above, phenomenological accounts suggest that a comprehensive understanding of the nature and origins of delusions requires the consideration of a range of experiential transformations which can occur prior to the onset of delusions and/or when these are undergone.

These accounts do not generally deny that alterations of cognitive processes may play a role in the development of delusions. However, they suggest that an exhaustive characterisation of both what delusions are and how they come about rests on the understanding of different dimensions of experience.

As far as depressive delusions are concerned, some of the main phenomenological domains considered by researchers are the experience of the *body* and the experience of a particular kind of *affect*. In the remaining sections of this chapter, I will outline some key investigations and ideas which have emerged from this research, looking also at their potential for further development.

### 5.1 *The body and delusions*

Phenomenologists typically establish a close connection between mental life and bodily experience, drawing attention to the way in which mental processes of different kinds are shaped by the ways in which the body feels and acts. In addition, from this perspective, the mind cannot be understood in isolation from the world in which one is immersed: phenomenology conceives of subjects as essentially 'embodied and embedded' in the environment, and seeks to better understand how these dimensions are intertwined in cognition and consciousness (cf. Gallagher and Zahavi 2012).

In this context, it is argued that there is a basic sense of self which accompanies every conscious experience (cf. Gallagher and Zahavi 2012: 52 ff.) and that this is anchored in various dimensions of bodily phenomenology.

In the first place, the sense of self is taken to be rooted in a perception of the body as the centre (or 'zero point') of our perceptual field (Husserl 1989: 166–167), namely as that in relation to which all the objects that are experienced are located and orientated (Merleau-Ponty 2012: 92 ff.).

Furthermore, the experience of the spatial location and orientation of the body is recognised as being intertwined with a sense of the body as voluminous (Legrand 2011), in so far as we do not experience ourselves as mere points in an abstract frame of reference, but rather as three-dimensional, material bodies. As observed by Dorothée Legrand, 'the experienced spatiality of the world is correlational to the experienced voluminosity-location-orientation of one's body' (2011: 217), and this corroborates the idea that experience of the world and experience of the self are fundamentally linked.

In addition to this, phenomenologists emphasise the role played by the perception of bodily skills and potentialities in the sense of self: from this perspective, we have a 'sense of ability' (Slaby 2012), or 'I can' (Husserl 1960; 1989), that is anchored in our bodily capacities, and that provides us with a constant, implicit sense of our agential possibilities (Merleau-Ponty 2012: 84 ff.).

The 'sense of ability' or 'I can' too is fundamentally entwined with the way in which the external world is experienced. This is the case because phenomenologists recognise that perceptual objects appear to the perceiver as affording specific forms of action or interaction: for example, integral to the perception of the glass I am looking at now is the experience of the glass as something that I can drink from (Ratcliffe 2008: 44 ff.).

Importantly, phenomenologists also conceive of the body as being central to affective experience, and of perception and affectivity as fundamentally shaping each other. This is exemplified by the fact that perceptual objects, for instance, are experienced as possessing a range of evaluative properties (e.g. as beautiful or ugly, pleasant or unpleasant, useful or useless), and evaluation is closely connected to feeling states and emotions experienced in the body (cf. Slaby 2008).

The dimensions of bodily experience outlined so far are key to what phenomenologists call the 'lived' or 'living body', namely the body as it is experienced from a first-person perspective, i.e. the perspective of the subject who has that body (Husserl 1989; Merleau-Ponty 2012). The lived body is differentiated from the 'objective body' (cf. also Gallagher and Zahavi 2012: 154), which refers to an experience of the body analogous to the experience we may have of other objects. This is, for example, the body as it can be experienced when it is the object of medical examination or scientific scrutiny (Gallagher and Zahavi 2012: 154).

The phenomenological exploration of the lived body has informed, and has been extensively informed by, the investigation of the experience of mental illness, and research on depression has been key in this regard.

This research has included the study of some delusions associated with the experience of severe depression, for example the Cotard delusion. This delusion is often characterised as the conviction that one is dead. However, as outlined by Ratcliffe (2008: 165–166), variations to this theme can be present, such as the idea that one is 'emotionally dead' or 'not a real person' (Davies and Coltheart 2000: 31).

Phenomenological research on the Cotard delusion has drawn attention to the centrality of alterations of bodily experience in the condition (Ratcliffe 2008; Doerr-Zegers 2019). In particular, it has been suggested that a general weakening of the bodily feelings which are constitutive of the sense of self and the world may be at the origin of this form of delusional thinking.

Doerr-Zegers (2019: 763), for example, depicts the delusion as originating in a 'loss of sensibility' that is common also among depressed patients that do not display delusional symptoms, but which, in his opinion, becomes especially marked in those who develop the Cotard syndrome. Similarly, Matthew Ratcliffe (2008: 165 ff.) links the origin of the delusion to a transformation of a particular kind of bodily feelings, which are seen as grounding our sense of belonging to the world. From this perspective, as it will be illustrated in more detail in the following section, a general diminishment of bodily responsiveness would lead to a modification of one's felt experience of existing as an embodied subject, from which the delusional utterances would arise.

These ideas are supported through the consideration of specific clinical cases and first-personal testimonies. For example, Doerr-Zegers (2019) discusses the experience of a patient with Cotard delusion, who believed to be 'completely dead' and described a variety of disruptions of bodily experience. For instance, the patient reported that she had lost 'touch, smell, or taste for food', that she could not experience tiredness, and were unable to fall asleep due not being able to feel the 'weight' of her eyes (2019: 760).

As pointed to by Doerr-Zegers, some of the key experiential dimensions of the lived body appear to be altered in the case of this patient. The perception of the body's materiality seems compromised, as both the experience of its voluminousness (an aspect of which is 'weight') and perceptual capacities (through the impoverishment of sensory feelings) are affected.

Alongside the alterations of sensory experience described above, Doerr-Zegers' patient also described transformations in emotional reactivity. As she reported:

> Nothing scares me anymore; neither can I feel anger…I live a life of science fiction, the life of a dead person…When I take my children in the arms, I do not feel them… If my children knew that they love an artificial mom…I do not feel the direct contact with the things, neither with the others….
>
> *(Doerr-Zegers 2019: 760)*

Phenomenologists conceive of affectivity as essentially embodied, often thinking of emotions as involving the presence of specific bodily feelings (Slaby 2008; Fuchs 2013). As such, the weakening of emotional responsiveness can also be linked to a transformation of bodily experience, and in particular to a reduction of the body's capacity to resonate with the stimuli in one's environment.

Similarly to what is the case for Parnas and Sass's account of bodily experience in schizophrenia, Doerr-Zegers's (2019) exploration of the phenomenology of the body in the Cotard syndrome draws attention to a series of bodily disturbances which dramatically re-shape the person's experience of self and world, providing the experiential backdrop for the emergence of delusional symptoms. As mentioned above, in this context, the experience of the body is seen as fundamentally connected to the experience of affects, and phenomenological accounts of the latter can shed further light on the nature of depressive delusions.

## 5.2  *Affectivity and delusions*

Phenomenologists have extensively explored the nature of affective experience and its disruptions in mental ill-health, and have contributed in particular to the investigation of affects in depression (e.g. Ratcliffe 2008, 2015).

The phenomenological account of moods – and mood-like states – has been of significant relevance in this area, and is a key aspect of an account of the relationship between affectivity and cognition that has wide-ranging implications for the understanding of depressive delusions.

Various classical and contemporary phenomenologists have drawn attention to the existence of a set of affective states that do not typically have an intentional structure (i.e. they are not directed at particular objects), but have a profound influence on the intentional mental states that one can entertain, modulating them in specific ways. From this perspective, 'moods' can be characterised as experiential orientations, from which specific cognitive and affective responses can stem.

This idea, which is present in the work of early phenomenologists like Martin Heidegger (1962), has been further developed in the recent literature by Ratcliffe (e.g. 2005, 2008), who has coined the notion of 'existential feelings' to refer to a particular set of mood-like experiences.

Existential feelings are characterised by Ratcliffe as a distinct set of bodily feelings which are not directed at 'specific entities' or 'entities in general', but are rather 'ways of finding oneself in the world' that structure one's experience as a whole (2008: 41). In other terms, according to this account, in addition to the stream of emotions, thoughts, and desires with particular contents that punctuate our conscious life, we constantly experience a range of feelings that act as the experiential background for all intentional mental states.

This means that such feelings are not typically objects of attention or reflection – something that is at the forefront of our awareness – but they are not unconscious experiences either. Existential feelings have a distinct phenomenology, even if it may be difficult to pinpoint or dissect it (cf. Ratcliffe 2008: 129). In addition, while they are not themselves directed at particular things, people, or states of affairs, existential feelings are taken to constrain the manner in which we can relate to the objects of our experience by determining which 'kinds' of mental states we can entertain, a feature which Ratcliffe refers to as the 'pre-intentional' character of existential feelings (2010).

Importantly, Ratcliffe's account of existential feelings also aims to illuminate how we come to inhabit a specific 'possibility space' (2008), which I understand as referring to the felt sense we have of what it is possible for us to experience or achieve at a particular time. The phenomenological framework Ratcliffe draws upon indeed conceives of occurrent experiences as being imbued with a sense of how the experiences themselves could or could not evolve (Ratcliffe 2008: 130 ff.), and this applies to both our perceptual and affective phenomenology. When visually perceiving an object, for instance, I have an inkling that there are alternative perspectives I could take on that object (e.g. I could turn around the object, or look at it from above or below (cf. Husserl 1989: 37–38; Ratcliffe 2008: 130–131)). Similarly, when emoted in certain ways, I do have a sense of there being further affective experiences available or unavailable to me (e.g. when I am angry at someone, I may feel that it is not possible for me to forgive them or forget their misdeeds). Furthermore, perceptual and affective phenomenologies are entwined, as there is a correlation between the way in which objects are perceived and our bodily feelings and potentialities: a glass of iced tea is particularly appealing if I am feeling hot and thirsty, but could be rather uninviting in other circumstances.

In addition to the possibilities that are associated with particular experiences, Ratcliffe (2008: 133) suggests that 'there is a kind of inarticulate background that delimits the possible forms that any experience might take' and existential feelings are what play this experience-shaping role. In other terms, the range of mental states I can entertain is constrained by these background affective orientations.

Ratcliffe's account has been extensively applied to the exploration of disturbances of experience in mental-ill health, and especially in depression. In this context, also the experience of the nihilistic delusions associated with the Cotard syndrome, has been considered, and Ratcliffe has proposed a characterisation that is consistent with, and further expands, the phenomenological understanding of delusional thinking.

At the core of this is the idea that statements frequently shared by Cotard patients such as 'I am dead' or 'I do not exist' (Ratcliffe 2008: 165) should not be understood as expressions of propositional attitudes, or more specifically, beliefs held by the person. On the contrary, as Ratcliffe explains:

> What the patient is expressing is a radically altered existential orientation, rather than a propositional content. A background sense of being part of the world, which most of us take for granted most of the time, is absent.
>
> *(2008: 167)*

In Ratcliffe's view, the existential re-orientation that is expressed through the delusional utterances amounts to a transformation of the person's existential feelings, that is a change in one's felt relationship with the world. More specifically, what is altered in these cases is the person's 'sense of existence', which would, according to Ratcliffe, typically act as the 'background to all experience' (2008: 169). As such, when this is diminished or lost, wide-ranging experiential transformations ensue and existing no longer appears as 'a possibility' for the person (2008: 169).

The lack of a felt sense of there being alternative possibilities to the way in which one experiences oneself in these circumstances would then be at the origin of the Cotard delusion itself, as different ways of conceiving of one's predicament are precluded by the person's existential feelings, providing the grounds for the emergence of delusional thinking.

Ratcliffe's account of existential feelings and their role in the Cotard syndrome provides an example of how alterations of affective experience may drive disturbances of cognitive processes, a dynamic which appears to be in play also in other types of depressive delusions. As previously mentioned, for example, delusions of guilt and delusions of worthlessness are often present in depressive experiences with psychotic features, and it seems that these delusions too may be rooted in the presence of specific existential feelings.

Ratcliffe has argued that it is possible for feelings of guilt to have the structure of existential feelings, suggesting that this is exemplified by the phenomenology of certain forms of severe depression (2010). His account draws on the distinction between intentional and non-intentional forms of guilt. Often, our feelings of guilt have intentional objects (e.g. we feel guilty *about* an omission or an action we have performed). However, Ratcliffe observes that it is possible to feel guilty without there being any particular thing that we are feeling guilty about, and he suggests that forms of guilt that lack intentionality can be further differentiated on the basis of whether they are experienced as 'contingent' or 'irrevocable' (2010: 607). According to this distinction, when a sense of contingency marks the feeling of guilt, one retains a sense of there being a possibility for them not to be culpable. On the other hand, when irrevocable guilt is present, one's culpability is perceived as an essential feature of the self: 'one could not have been otherwise and could therefore never be otherwise' (2010: 607).

Non-intentional feelings of irrevocable guilt can have a significant impact on one's mental life, as Ratcliffe suggests that they have the ability to narrow the range of intentional states that one can entertain. In other terms, these feelings of guilt have a pre-intentional structure, displaying the experience-shaping role that Ratcliffe attributes to existential feelings. Such feelings of guilt also possess a particular 'depth' which, in Ratcliffe's view, refers to the extent or range of mental states that an affective experience can impact on. As he explains:

> Deep guilt involves a loss of the conditions of intelligibility for certain kinds of intentional state, and this is what gives it its depth. There is no hope, no practical

significance, no pleasure, and there cannot be. When you feel guilty about something, you can still contemplate feeling otherwise, and you do not feel guilty about plenty of other things. But, in the case of deep guilt, no alternatives to guilt present themselves.

*(Ratcliffe 2010: 614)*

The presence in severe depression of the existential feelings of irrevocable guilt discussed by Ratcliffe could arguably play a role in the emergence of delusions of guilt. This seems to be the case because the presence of these feelings would make it very difficult, if not impossible, for the experiencer to entertain thoughts, emotions, and desires which conflict with the evaluation of oneself as radically culpable that is integral to the feeling of guilt (Bortolan 2017). As a result of this, the person may struggle to process and use information that would challenge that self-evaluation and may provide unwarranted interpretations of events to make their meaning cohere with their negative self-assessment. When this occurs extensively and systematically, an affective and cognitive re-orientation that is conducive to the emergence of delusions of guilt is established.

Similarly, by drawing on phenomenological research concerning affective experiences of self-worth, we can advance the hypothesis that existential feelings play a role also in delusions of worthlessness.

As illustrated by the example of guilt, some existential feelings have a self-evaluative character: they are a particular kind of appraisal – bodily and affective – of certain aspects of the self (Bortolan 2017). As detailed above, for instance, imbued in an existential feeling of guilt is an evaluation of oneself (and one's relationship with the world) as one characterised by blameworthiness.

Some existential feelings convey broader appraisals than the ones associated with guilt, and in my previous work I suggested that self-esteem itself (or a particular form or dimension of it) is best understood as a particular kind of existential feeling (Bortolan 2018, 2020). More specifically, I have argued that our experiences are shaped by a general, felt sense of ourselves as worthy or unworthy to different degrees, and that this exercises a constraining role on our cognitive, affective and volitional states, impacting not only on self-experience, but also on the experience of others and the world more broadly. This characterisation can be drawn upon to illuminate both the experience of depression and the dynamics that may lead to the emergence to delusions of worthlessness in this condition.

The negative self-evaluations that are associated with depressive episodes (Beck and Alford 2009: 22) do not have only a cognitive character. While a depressed person may endorse a range of beliefs or judgements about their own value (or the value of some of their traits, features, and actions), an integral part of this predicament is the experience of intense feelings of low self-worth (APA 2022: 183). While these feelings may focus on particular aspects of the self, severely depressed people can often have a global sense of themselves as being unworthy, or, in other words they may experience worthlessness as a feature of their self as a whole (cf. Beck and Alford 2009: 229–230).

These experiences can be understood as existential feelings of low self-esteem, and, when they are particularly marked, due to their pre-intentional character, they may limit the person's ability to acquire and draw on information about themselves that is in tension with the negative self-evaluation imbued in the sense of worthlessness. An integral aspect of this process is the tendency to 'explain away' or re-interpret any potential evidence that would challenge one's self-assessment in ways that are consistent with it (cf. Bortolan 2023).

These dynamics may lead to the formation of an epistemic perspective that is impermeable to change, and where self-related affective and cognitive states reinforce and constrain each other in ways that are aligned with the background feeling of low self-esteem. In this context, it would become very difficult to mitigate or challenge such feeling and the emergence of delusions of worthlessness would be facilitated, as these convictions would be consonant with the person's felt appraisal of herself and relationship with the world.

## 6.  Conclusion

In this chapter, I have explored some key aspects of contemporary philosophical research on delusions in depression. I started by providing an outline of questions and debates concerning the nature and explanation of depressive delusions, focusing in particular on the cognitive account put forward by Antrobus and Bortolotti (2016). I then moved to consider how insights developed within philosophical phenomenology and phenomenological psychopathology can contribute to the understanding of what delusions are and how they emerge. In particular, I have looked at how phenomenological accounts of bodily and affective experience can shed light on the structure and development of delusions such as the ones associated with the Cotard syndrome, and delusions of guilt and worthlessness. In so doing, I have shown that a fine-grained understanding of different facets of the phenomenology of the body and affectivity can complement a cognitive account of psychotic depression, drawing attention to the existence of multiple connections between mood disturbances and disturbances of thought.

## Notes

1  As outlined by Steven Dubovsky and colleagues (2021), diagnostic manuals of mental disorders have in various cases characterised psychotic depression as a severe form of depression. In the DSM-IV, for example, the relevant specifier was 'severe with psychotic features' (Maj 2008). In the DSM-5 (2013) and DSM-5-TR (2022), however, severity is no longer included in the specifier concerning psychosis.
2  This debate is also connected to the differentiation between 'neurotic' and 'psychotic' depression, although this distinction has now largely been discarded.
3  However, the characterisation of major depressive episode provided by the DSM allows for the fact that not all experiences of worthlessness and guilt associated with this condition are delusional, that is one can be depressed and have 'excessive or inappropriate' feelings of worthlessness or guilt (2022: 182) without this amounting to delusional thinking.
4  In their exploration of the history of this nosological construct, German Berrios and Rogelio Luque (1995) note that while this is often referred to as a single delusion, the condition originally described by the psychiatrist Jules Cotard involved a wider set of phenomena, as he conceived of it as a 'subtype of depressive illness' (218). As such, the term 'Cotard syndrome' may be more accurate than 'Cotard delusion'; however, due to their common use, in this chapter I employ the two as interchangeable terms to indicate delusions that revolve around the theme of one's death or inexistence.
5  According to the DSM, '[d]elusions are deemed *bizarre* if they are clearly implausible and not understandable to same-culture peers and do not derive from ordinary life experiences', and thought withdrawal, throught insertion, and delusions of control are listed as specific examples of this (APA 2022: 101).

## References

Alloy, L.B., Abramson, L.Y. (1979) "Judgment of Contingency in Depressed and Nondepressed Students: Sadder but Wiser?," *Journal of Experimental Psychology: General* 108(4): 441–485.

American Psychiatric Association (APA) (2013) *Diagnostic and Statistical Manual of Mental Disorders*. Fifth Edition, Washington, DC: American Psychiatric Association.

American Psychiatric Association (APA) (2022) *Diagnostic and Statistical Manual of Mental Disorders*. *Fifth Edition. Text Revision*, Washington, DC: American Psychiatric Association.

Antrobus, M., Bortolotti, L. (2016) "Depressive Delusions," *Filosofia Unisinos* 17(2): 192–201.

Beck, A.T. (1967) *Depression: Causes and Treatment*, Philadelphia: University of Pennsylvania Press.

Beck, A.T., Alford, B.A. (2009) *Depression: Causes and Treatment*. Second Edition, Philadelphia: University of Pennsylvania Press.

Bellini, L., Gatti, F., Gasperini, M., Smeraldi, E. (1992) "A Comparison between Delusional and Non-Delusional Depressives," *Journal of Affective Disorders* 25(2): 129–138.

Berrios, G.E., Luque, R. (1995) "Cotard's Delusion or Syndrome?: A Conceptual History," *Comprehensive Psychiatry* 36(3): 218–223.

Bortolan, A. (2017) "Affectivity and Moral Experience: An Extended Phenomenological Account," *Phenomenology and the Cognitive Sciences* 16(3): 471–490.

Bortolan, A. (2018) "Self-Esteem and Ethics: A Phenomenological View," *Hypatia* 33(1): 56–72.

Bortolan, A. (2020) "Self-Esteem, Pride, Embarrassment and Shyness," in T. Szanto, H. Landweer (Eds.). *The Routledge Handbook of Phenomenology of Emotion*, New York: Routledge: 358–368.

Bortolan, A. (2023) "Good Enough to be Myself? The Fraught Relationship between Self-Esteem and Self-Knowledge," in A. Montes Sánchez, A. Salice (Eds.). *Emotional Self Knowledge*, New York: Routledge: 125–144.

Bortolotti, L. (2009) *Delusions and Other Irrational Beliefs*, Oxford: Oxford University Press.

Bortolotti, L., Antrobus, M. (2015) "Costs and Benefits of Realism and Optimism," *Current Opinion in Psychiatry* 28(2): 194–198.

Carel, H. (2016) *Phenomenology of Illness*, Oxford: Oxford University Press.

Charney, D.S., Nelson, J.C. (1981) "Delusional and Nondelusional Unipolar Depression: Further Evidence for Distinct Subtypes," *The American Journal of Psychiatry* 138(3): 328–333.

Davies, M. and Coltheart, M. (2000) "Introduction: Pathologies of Belief," *Mind & Language* 15: 1–46.

Doerr-Zegers, O. (2019) "Delusion and Mood Disorders," in G. Stanghellini, M.R. Broome, A.V. Fernandez, P. Fusar-Poli, A. Raballo, R. Rosfort (Eds.). *The Oxford Handbook of Phenomenological Psychopathology*, Oxford: Oxford University Press: 753–768.

Dubovsky, S.L., Ghosh, B.M., Serotte, J.C., Cranwell, V. (2021) "Psychotic Depression: Diagnosis, Differential Diagnosis, and Treatment," *Psychotherapy and Psychosomatics* 90(3): 160–177.

Fuchs, T. (2013) "The Phenomenology of Affectivity," in K.W.M. Fulford, M. Davies, R.G.T. Gipps, G. Graham, J.Z. Sadler, G. Stanghellini, T. Thornton (Eds.). *The Oxford Handbook of Philosophy and Psychiatry*, Oxford: Oxford University Press: 612–631.

Gallagher, S. (2009) "Delusional Realities," in M.R. Broome, L.Bortolotti (Eds.). *Psychiatry as Cognitive Neuroscience: Philosophical Perspectives*, Oxford: Oxford University Press: 245–266.

Gallagher, S., Zahavi, D. (2012) *The Phenomenological Mind*. Second Edition, New York: Routledge.

Gaudiano B.A., Dalrymple K.L., Zimmerman M. (2009) "Prevalence and Clinical Characteristics of Psychotic Versus Nonpsychotic Major Depression in a General Psychiatric Outpatient Clinic," *Depression and Anxiety* 26(1): 54–64.

Gournellis, R., Tournikioti, K., Touloumi, G., Thomadakis, C., Michalopoulou, P.G., Christodoulou, C., Papadopoulou, A., Douzenis, A. (2018) "Psychotic (Delusional) Depression and Suicidal Attempts: A Systematic Review and Meta-Analysis," *Acta Psychiatrica Scandinavica* 137(1): 18–29.

Heidegger, M. (1962) Being and Time. Trans. J. Macquarrie and E. Robinson. New York: Harper & Row.

Husserl, E. (1960) *Cartesian Meditations*. Trans. D. Cairns, The Hague: Martinus Nijhoff.

Husserl, E. (1989) *Ideas Pertaining to a Pure Phenomenology and to a Phenomenological Philosophy. Second Book. Studies in the Phenomenology of Constitution*. Trans. R. Rojcewicz and A. Schuwer, Dordrecht: Kluwer Academic Publishers.

Lattuada, E., Serretti, A., Cusin, C., Gasperini, M., Smeraldi, E. (1999) "Symptomatologic Analysis of Psychotic and Non-Psychotic Depression," *Journal of Affective Disorders* 54(1–2): 183–187.

Legrand, D. (2011) "Phenomenological Dimensions of Bodily Self-Consciousness," in S. Gallagher (Ed.). *The Oxford Handbook of the Self*, Oxford: Oxford University Press: 204–227.

Maj, M. (2008) "Delusions in Major Depressive Disorder: Recommendations for the DSM-5," *Psychopathology* 41(1): 1–3.

Merleau-Ponty, M. (2012) *Phenomenology of Perception*. Trans. D. A. Landes, New York: Routledge.

Meyers, B.S. (2014, July 31st) "Psychotic Depression: Underrecognized, Undertreated-and Dangerous," *Psychiatric Times* 31(7). https://www.psychiatrictimes.com/view/psychotic-depression-underrecognized-undertreatedand-dangerous

Ohayon, M.M., Schatzberg A.F. (2002) "Prevalence of Depressive Episodes with Psychotic Features in the General Population," *The American Journal of Psychiatry* 159(11): 1855–1861.

Paljärvi, T., Tiihonen, J., Lähteenvuo, M., Tanskanen, A., Fazel, S., Taipale, H. (2023) "Psychotic Depression and Deaths Due to Suicide," *Journal of Affective Disorders* 321: 28–32.

Parker, G., Hadzi-Pavlovic, D., Hickie, I., Mitchell, P., Wilhelm, K., Brodaty, H., Boyce, P., Eyers, K., Pedic, F. (1991) "Psychotic Depression: A Review and Clinical Experience," *Australian & New Zealand Journal of Psychiatry* 25(2): 169–180.

Parnas, J., Sass, L.A. (2001) "Self, Solipsism, and Schizophrenic Delusions," *Philosophy, Psychiatry, & Psychology* 8(2–3): 101–120.

Piaget, J. (1977) *The Development of Thought: Equilibration of Cognitive Structures*, New York: Viking Press.

Picardi, A., Fonzi, L., Pallagrosi, M., Gigantesco, A., Biondi, M. (2018) "Delusional Themes across Affective and Non-Affective Psychoses," *Frontiers in Psychiatry* 9: 132. https://doi.org/10.3389/fpsyt.2018.00132

Ratcliffe, M. (2005) "The Feeling of Being," *Journal of Consciousness Studies* 12(8–10): 43–60.

Ratcliffe, M. (2008) *Feelings of Being: Phenomenology, Psychiatry and the Sense of Reality*, Oxford: Oxford University Press.

Ratcliffe, M. (2010) "Depression, Guilt and Emotional Depth," Inquiry: An Interdisciplinary Journal of Philosophy 53(6): 602–626.

Ratcliffe, M. (2015) *Experiences of Depression: A Study in Phenomenology*, Oxford: Oxford University Press.

Sass, L.A.A., Parnas, J. (2003) "Schizophrenia, Consciousness, and the Self," *Schizophrenia Bulletin* 29(3): 427–444.

Sass, L. A., Pienkos, E. (2013) "Delusion: The Phenomenological Approach," in K.W.M. Fulford, M. Davies, R.G.T. Gipps, G. Graham, J.Z. Sadler, G. Stanghellini, T. Thornton (Eds.). *The Oxford Handbook of Philosophy and Psychiatry*, Oxford: Oxford University Press: 632–657.

Slaby, J. (2008) "Affective Intentionality and the Feeling Body," *Phenomenology and the Cognitive Sciences* 7(4): 429–444.

Slaby, J. (2012) "Affective Self-Construal and the Sense of Ability," *Emotion Review* 4(2): 151–156.

Smith, E.G., Burke, P.R., Grogan, J.E., Fratoni, S.E., Wogsland, C.S., Rothschild, A.J. (2007) "Psychosis in Major Depression," in D. Fujii, I. Ahmed, (Eds.). *The Spectrum of Psychotic Disorders: Neurobiology, Etiology, and Pathogenesis*, Cambridge: Cambridge University Press: 156–194.

Stanghellini, G., Broome, M.R., Fernandez, A.V., Fusar-Poli, P., Raballo, A., Rosfort, R. (Eds.) (2019) *The Oxford Handbook of Phenomenological Psychopathology*, Oxford: Oxford University Press.

Stanghellini, G., Raballo, A. (2015) "Differential Typology of Delusions in Major Depression and Schizophrenia. A Critique to the Unitary Concept of 'Psychosis'," *Journal of Affective Disorders* 171: 171–178.

Stone, T., Young, A.W. (1997) "Delusions and Brain Injury: The Philosophy and Psychology of Belief," *Mind & Language* 12(3–4): 327–364.

# 11

# DELUSIONS IN THE DISORDERS
# OF OLD AGE

*Julian C. Hughes*

## 1. Introduction

Sometime between 1947 and 1948, the philosopher Ludwig Wittgenstein (1889–1951) said to Maurice O'Connor Drury (1907–1976), who was training in psychiatry at St. Patrick's Hospital in Dublin, 'You must always be puzzled by mental illness'. He continued: 'The thing I would dread most, if I became mentally ill, would be your adopting a common sense attitude; that you could take it for granted that I was deluded' (Drury 1981: 166). Reflecting on these words, Drury wrote:

> I think I understand what he meant, and I think he was referring to an attitude that it is only too easy for those dealing daily with mental illness to fall into. I believe that we must let our psychiatric patients see that we understand that they are in a state of affliction which is not comparable to any bodily pain however severe.
>
> *(Drury 1973: 90)*

He added a little later: 'There will always be in psychiatry the realm of the inexplicable' (Drury 1973: 91).

One thing to note is that Wittgenstein seemed, perhaps, to equate delusions with mental illness. To many, indeed, delusions seem the quintessence of madness. The other thing to note is that Drury, in a manifestation maybe of his modesty, says he only *thinks* he understands what Wittgenstein was getting at. It is certainly not clear what Wittgenstein meant. Did Wittgenstein mean that he would rather clinicians were amazed by delusions and did not merely regard them as mundane? But amazement cuts in two directions: you could be amazed that anyone should hold such bizarre beliefs (in which case you think the person silly in some sense – mad even) or you could be amazed at the phenomenological experience (in which case you think the person is unique and special in some way).

Wittgenstein might more simply have meant, as the first sentence suggests, that we should regard delusions as a puzzle: both a human and an intellectual puzzle. But that is not quite what he says. He would not want Drury to 'take it for granted' or to 'take it as a matter of course' (Drury 1973: 90) that he was deluded. This could mean that he wanted

173        DOI: 10.4324/9781003296386-14

the delusion to be tested, the belief to be shaken to see if it is truly unshakeable. It seems unlikely, however, that he was suggesting how to examine for psychopathology. And yet it does seem likely that he was making a point pertinent, as Drury suggests, to how we *are* as clinicians, or even just as people confronted by mental illness. Wittgenstein does not want us to assume that his experiences would simply be wrong. He wants them to be taken seriously. And to do that requires puzzlement.

I thought of Wittgenstein's comment to Drury when I got to know Professor Hindle, whose story is set out below. (I should say that the vignettes used in this chapter are based on real patients I have met, but the details have been modified and amalgamated to provide anonymity.) The case will lead me to discuss the concept of late paraphrenia as an example of how delusional disorders in old age can have a particular feel to them. Following this, I shall provide an overview of mental disorders that occur in older people, with a focus on their delusional content. This will allow me to mention a variety of syndromes characterized by delusions of one sort or another. From this discussion I shall pick out, in conclusion, four themes of importance in discussing delusions in old age but end with the suggestion that, even if we can highlight potential causes of delusions in old age, it remains true – in keeping with Wittgenstein's caution to Drury – that what it is to have a delusion remains in 'the realm of the inexplicable' (Drury 1973: 91). I take it, mundanely, that a psychotic delusion can be characterized as 'an absolute conviction of the truth of a proposition which is idiosyncratic, ego-involved, incorrigible, and often preoccupying' (Kräupl Taylor 1979: 128).[1]

---

### VIGNETTE 1.   Professor Hindle

*I first met Professor Hindle at a moment of crisis. She had called the police, who had in turn alerted the mental health team. For she believed, with complete conviction, that she was to be murdered that day. She claimed that for months she had been tormented by a gang who lived next door to her. They commented on what she was doing; and the most upsetting part for this shy, somewhat solitary, 76-year-old women, was that they even watched her when she was using the toilet. She could hear them talking about her when she was walking in the park. Despite her scientific background, when I asked her how it was she could hear them even in the park she said, vaguely, it must be something to do with the internet. The gang also threatened her and on the day that we met they had said she would be killed by teatime.*

*Professor Hindle had no previous or family history of mental disorder. She readily accepted, without question, the offer of admission to hospital since she was extremely anxious and saw the ward as a safe place. She readily took antipsychotic medication, reasoning that it would help her anxiety. She quickly settled on the ward, which was something of a surprise to me given her normal slightly reclusive lifestyle. She was pleasant and friendly in a quiet way and would discuss her work with anyone who was inclined to listen. She was strikingly intelligent, showed no evidence of formal thought disorder, and there was no hint of any significant cognitive decline. Gradually, she improved and after some accompanied home visits she felt safe enough to be fully discharged from the ward.*

*When I saw her a full six months after she had left the hospital, following some pleasantries, I asked if there had been any further problems with the people next door (who were in fact ordinary and quite innocuous). It was clear she continued to believe that all of the events she had experienced were true, but she had been able to put them to the back of her mind. She felt that our involvement and that of the police had frightened them off and they were now too scared to attempt anything. In other words, as is common in these conditions, her delusional thoughts were now 'encapsulated'. They no longer intruded, but were still intact.*

*Professor Hindle continued to do well. We lowered the dose of her antipsychotic medication, but without it her thoughts about the people next door became troublesome again. She died after about 18 months from a stroke.*

## 2.   The concept of late paraphrenia

Professor Hindle provided a good example of where the term 'late paraphrenia' might seem applicable. The puzzling thing about her and similar cases is that they feel quite different from the psychotic disorders that afflict younger people. It did not seem correct to give her a diagnosis of schizophrenia, even though she had symptoms which would allow such a diagnosis. For instance, she heard voices commenting on her actions, which is one of Kurt Schneider's (1887–1967) first-rank symptoms of schizophrenia (Schneider 1959). She also had very clear persecutory delusions: they were 'held with unusual conviction', were 'not amenable to logic' and 'The absurdity or erroneousness of their content [was] manifest to other people' (Sims 1988: 84). And yet, her quiet, intelligent and civilized personality remained intact, as did her cognitive function. In these ways, she was quite different from many of the younger people living with schizophrenia whom I have met. Younger people with a diagnosis of schizophrenia can have a good outcome, of course, but the story of a deterioration in terms of their achievements and personalities is sadly common enough; and eventually there can be cognitive decline too. The observed differences between many younger people living with schizophrenia and people presenting like Professor Hindle are what encouraged the view that this was a condition specific to old age.

It was Emil Kraepelin (1856–1926) who first used the term 'paraphrenia', which etymologically suggests being beyond or beside the mind (i.e. 'out of mind'), to highlight a group of people with what he termed 'dementia praecox', but which started after the age of 40 years and tended to be benign in its course (Kraepelin 1920). Later, Eugen Bleuler (1857–1939) was to replace the term 'dementia praecox' with 'schizophrenia' (Fusar-Poli and Politi 2008). So here was a group of older people who appeared to have schizophrenia, but who lacked, for instance, the confusion caused by formal thought disorder and who did well.

This observation did not escape the attention of Martin Roth and John Morrissey (1952). They looked at the case records of 150 patients over the age of 60 years who were admitted to Graylingwell Hospital in 1948. 'Affective psychosis' formed the largest group (54 per cent), followed by 'senile psychosis' (24 per cent). They identified 12 people with schizophrenia, where the symptoms had started after the age of 60 years. The disorder was described as 'paraphrenic' in nature. They found three types of paranoid disorder: (i) those with paranoid delusions in the context of depression, often with 'ideas of guilt and unworthiness and tendencies to self-castigate'; (ii) delusions in the context of 'senile psychosis'; and, then, (iii) those where paraphrenic delusions were prominent: 'They occurred in each case in the setting of a well-preserved intellect and personality, were often "primary" in character, and were usually associated with the passivity failings or other volitional disturbances and hallucinations in clear consciousness pathognomonic of Schizophrenia' (Roth and Morrissey 1952: 75).

In his famous paper, 'The Natural History of Mental Disorder in Old Age', Sir Martin Roth (1917–2006) – as he became – one of the pioneers of old age psychiatry, was able to suggest that 'affective psychosis, late paraphrenia and acute confusion are distinct from the two main causes of progressive dementia in old age; senile and arteriosclerotic psychosis' (Roth 1955: 295). Later, he summarized the features that distinguished 'late paraphrenic and paranoid disorders from schizophrenic psychosis': a marked preponderance of females in late paraphrenia, deterioration of personality is 'very rare', the premorbid personality remains essentially unchanged and hereditary factors seem less relevant; on the other hand, deafness seems to be twice as common in those with late paraphrenia (45 per cent) in comparison with those with late affective disorder (22 per cent) (Roth and Cooper 1992: 27). David Kay and Martin Roth (1961) also emphasized the solitary and isolated nature of people, like Professor Hindle, with late paraphrenia.

The inclination to hang on to the term 'late paraphrenia', because, inter alia, of the striking disparity between the bizarre delusions and the otherwise normality of the person's presentation, persisted and the intellectual debates continued. Felix Post (1913–2001), one of the other great pioneers of old age psychiatry in the United Kingdom, in a group who had presented with paranoid delusions and/or hallucinations, found that a third had Schneiderian first-rank symptoms and would qualify for a diagnosis of schizophrenia; another third were disturbed by their symptoms, but these were not first-rank; and the final third seemed rather calm and undisturbed by their symptoms (Post 1966). Reflecting on this later, Post (1992) wrote that he had not accepted Kay and Roth's (1961) concept of

> senile paraphrenia as a late mode of schizophrenia, but preferred to see the persistent persecutory states of late life as a congery of partial schizophrenias, which in the great majority of cases had been foreshadowed by abnormal, usually 'schizoid' personality characteristics.
>
> *(Post 1992: 44)*

Subsequently, Peter Grahame (1984) concluded

> that late paraphrenia is one of the schizophrenias, but whether or not this condition ought to be termed paraphrenia is another matter. Paraphrenic patients develop clinical changes similar to those of schizophrenia with the passage of time, and may therefore be considered to manifest a partial, incomplete or pre-schizophrenic state.

Contrariwise, Neil Holden (1987: 635) suggested that 'late paraphrenia is a heterogenous syndrome giving the appearance of a spectrum of overlapping conditions with paranoid delusions'.

Robert Howard and colleagues (1994a) examined 101 people with a diagnosis of late paraphrenia using a formal, well-validated questionnaire. They found that, although the group satisfied the description of late paraphrenia, they also had all the symptoms, apart from formal thought disorder, of schizophrenia. Using internationally accepted criteria, they were able to categorize the cohort as having schizophrenia (61.4 per cent), delusional disorder (30.7 per cent), and schizoaffective disorder (7.9 per cent). Nevertheless, they concluded that 'the evidence suggests that late paraphrenics are more alike than different from one another', but continued, 'Such clinical homogeneity apparently masks aetiological heterogeneity' (Howard et al. 1994a: 409). Looking at the nature of the delusions, these researchers found, as they expected, 'high prevalences of delusions of persecution (84.2%), reference (76.3%) and misinterpretation or misidentification (59.4%)' (407). But they also found delusions that were more typical of schizophrenia: 'delusions of control (24.8%), of alien forces penetrating or controlling the subject's body or mind (29.7%) and primary delusions (20.8%)' (Howard et al. 1994a: 407).

In an earlier study, Howard and colleagues (1992: 719) highlighted 'a variety of delusional experience commonly encountered in late-onset schizophrenia and late paraphrenia and only rarely seen in schizophrenics with an early onset.' They were describing the notion of a 'partition delusion', which had been defined as 'The delusion that people, gas, electricity or some other force was entering their homes through the walls from a neighbouring dwelling' (Pearlson et al. 1989: 1568). Howard and colleagues (1992) found partition delusions in 68 per cent of those with a diagnosis of late paraphrenia, in 20 per cent of their group of young people with a diagnosis of schizophrenia, and in 13 per cent of those diagnosed with early-onset schizophrenia who were now over 60 years old.

Howard and colleagues (1993) compared early-onset (44 years old or below) and late-onset (45 years or older) people with the diagnosis of schizophrenia. In the group of 470, they found that, 'positive and negative formal thought disorder, affective symptoms, inappropriate affect, delusions of grandiosity or passivity, primary delusions other than delusional perception, and thought insertion and withdrawal were all more common in early-onset cases' (352); whereas 'persecutory delusions with and without hallucinations, organised delusions, and third-person, running commentary and accusatory or abusive auditory hallucinations were all more common in late-onset cases' (352). They concluded that although there were many similarities between the symptoms of early and late onset schizophrenia, there were also 'sufficient differences ... to suggest that they are not phenotypically homogeneous' (Howard et al. 1993: 352).

### 3.   Late-onset and very late-onset schizophrenia

The point about nosology and late paraphrenia is that the delusions people like Professor Hindle experience both do and do not fit into our usual taxonomies. Paranoid persecutory delusions are common enough in a variety of conditions. What is unusual in late paraphrenia is what surrounds them: no or little formal thought disorder, no deterioration in terms of personality, no marked affective component, no significant cognitive decline, but prominent female gender and a good deal of sensory impairment and isolation.

As far as the nosological questions around schizophrenic-like disorders in old age are concerned, the current orthodoxy is to speak in terms of the diagnoses of late-onset schizophrenia (LOS), very late-onset schizophrenia (VLOS), and delusional disorders. Howard and colleagues (2000) came to a consensus, agreed by an international group, that the epidemiology, symptom profile, and identified pathophysiologies pointed to the diagnoses of LOS (with onset after 40 years of age) and VLOS (onset after 60 years) having face validity and clinical utility. Unfortunately, there has not been enough conformity with these diagnostic categories, so that further research is required (Suen et al. 2019). Carl Cohen and colleagues (2015) have also suggested that comorbidity (other medical and neurological diseases) might affect the appearance of psychosis in older people.

Nevertheless, the VLOS category has proven useful inasmuch as it has been possible to show improvement in symptoms using the antipsychotic amisulpride (Howard et al. 2018). Cohen (2018), commenting on Howard and colleagues (2018), pointed out that there were still questions, for instance, about the stability of the diagnosis of VLOS, for studies have shown that many develop dementia within a few years, as if VLOS might be a prodromal condition for dementia.

## 4.  Delusional disorder

Meanwhile, there is the diagnosis of delusional disorder itself. This is where there are non-bizarre delusions, often monothematic, which last for more than a month and where non-prominent hallucinations are allowed if related to the delusions. There are usually no affective or cognitive symptoms. This would be an alternative diagnosis to VLOS for Professor Hindle. Remember that Howard and colleagues (1994a) had categorized 30.7 per cent of their population as having delusional disorder.

In one Australian study, in those with persecutory delusions in the context of late-life delusional disorder, 20 per cent recovered and over half showed some improvement when treated with an atypical antipsychotic; and only a few went on to develop dementia (Nagendra and Snowdon 2020). In contrast, Kørner and colleagues (2008) had found that 15.2 per cent of their first-contact delusional disorder group developed dementia, as opposed to 2.1 per cent of an osteoarthritis group. The figure for the delusional group was near to that (12 per cent) found by Kay and Roth (1961). Alex Kørner and colleagues (2008) calculated that the people with delusional disorder were at an 8 times higher risk of developing dementia compared to those with osteoarthritis and had 5.5 times the risk of the general population.

González-Rodríguez and colleagues (2022), in a review of the literature, found the main types of delusion were persecutory, in 87.3 per cent, followed by delusions of jealousy in 11 per cent and then somatic delusions in 1.8 per cent. The main theme of the delusions was of parasitosis or delusional infestation. The authors of this study were able to point to brain imaging studies which showed small strokes and loss of brain matter as well as evidence of dysfunction in the cerebellum. But they concluded, 'There is … considerable overlap between the symptoms of [delusional disorder] and other psychoses such as schizophrenia, affective disorders with psychotic features and neurologic diseases with psychotic features' (González-Rodríguez et al. 2022: 11). This not only makes it difficult to identify people with delusional disorder but also limits the ability to identify its unique characteristics. In any case it is rare, with a prevalence of 0.04 per cent in people over 65 years of age (Copeland et al. 1998), which compares to a prevalence of 0.1–0.5 per cent for schizophrenia in older people (Cohen et al. 2015).

## 5.  Delusions in delirium and dementia

Delirium (acute confusion) is common in older people, especially those who are hospitalized and especially in those who have pre-existing dementia. Delusions can form part of the symptomatology of delirium. Typical delusional beliefs might be, for instance, that hospital staff are trying to harm the person. In a population of 100 mostly older people with delirium from a palliative care setting, David Meagher and colleagues (2007) found the overall prevalence of delusions to be 31 per cent.

*Table 11.1* Prevalence of delusions in dementia (adapted
from Cipriani et al. 2014)

| *Type of delusion* | *Prevalence (%)* |
| --- | --- |
| Persecutory | 0.04–43 |
| Infidelity | 1–22 |
| Danger | 9–30 |
| Theft | 20–75 |
| Phantom border | 0.02–41 |
| One's house is not one's home | 7–17 |
| Capgras syndrome | 6–36 |

In dementia, the prevalence of delusions is about 70 per cent over the whole course of the disease (Lapid and Ho 2020), although the literature records a wide range of prevalences: from 2 to 76 per cent (Cipriani et al. 2014). Estimates of point prevalence in Alzheimer's disease, that is the prevalence at any one point in time, vary between 15 and 76 per cent (Cipriani et al. 2014).

The consequences of delusions can be profound, both in terms of the suffering of the person experiencing them – and they often signify an increase in the person's decline – and for the family carers who cannot cope with the behavioural consequences of the delusions – if for instance the person living with dementia develops a paranoid belief about his or her family carer – so that institutionalization occurs as a result. Medhat Bassiony and Constantine Lyketsos (2003), for example, reported that in Alzheimer's disease, people with delusions, as opposed to those without, seemed more aggressive, 'wandered' more (although, since 'wandering' is associated with walking without a purpose, we should be wary of using the word given that 'wandering' covers quite a variety of activities, many of which have a purpose even if we cannot initially discern it), and demonstrated more functional impairment, more asocial behaviour, and worse general health, as well as depression.

Delusions in Alzheimer's disease tend to be associated with greater cognitive decline. Quite a variety of delusions can emerge. Typically these are paranoid persecutory delusions. Thus, in the 1907 paper in which Alois Alzheimer (1864–1915) gave the first detailed description of the disease named after him, his patient, Auguste Deter, became jealous of her husband and 'sometimes she thought somebody was trying to kill her' (Stelzmann et al. 1995). But there has even been a case report of erotomania, or de Clérambault's syndrome (named after Gaëtan Henri Alfred Edouard Léon Marie Gatian de Clérambault [1872–1934]), where there is 'a delusional conviction of an amorous relationship with a socially unobtainable person with whom the subject has had little personal contact' (Drevets and Rubin 1987: 400). Neuropsychological testing shows an association between delusions in Alzheimer's disease and deficits in the frontal and temporal lobes of the brain and neuroimaging suggests correlations with frontal lobe dysfunction (Schneider and Dagerman 2004).

Table 11.1, adapted from a review of the literature by Gabriele Cipriani and colleagues (2014), shows the range of prevalences of types of delusion from different forms of dementia.

The prevalence rates are comparable across dementia types, except that in frontotemporal dementia there are fewer delusions, the prevalence range being between 0 and 23 per cent. In a study by Mario Mendez and colleagues (2008) of 86 people living with frontotemporal dementia, only 2 (2.3 per cent) had delusions. There is a suggestion, however, that closer scrutiny using genetic markers in frontotemporal dementia might reveal that delusions and other psychotic phenomena are more common than is generally appreciated (Hall and Finger 2015).

The phantom border delusion, mentioned in Table 11.1, involves the utter conviction that there is someone in your home, who is usually not seen. For instance, I have met a person with dementia who believed fervently that there was someone living in his attic.

The wide variation in prevalence rates in Table 11.1, along with the different rates found in other reviews (e.g. in Bassiony and Lyketsos 2003), suggest either that there is more work to be done to pin down the rates more accurately, or that delusions really are quite variable. But in a community sample in Cache County, Utah, of 5,092 older residents, which was 90 per cent of the population aged 65 years and older (in other words, this was a very thorough study), when screened for dementia, the prevalence of delusions was 19 per cent (Lyketsos et al. 2001).

Table 11.1 also mentions Capgras syndrome, which takes us to Mrs Crawley.

---

### VIGNETTE 2.   Mrs Crawley

*Mrs Crawley had a diagnosis of moderately severe Alzheimer's disease, but with her husband she coped well at home. Out of the blue, however, there was a crisis because she started to deny that her husband was her husband. She caused a disturbance one night when she went out on to the street because she believed she had a stranger in bed with her. She agreed that he looked like her husband, but she was convinced that he was an imposter. The situation was most disturbing for her and led to the police being called, at which point Mr Crawley had to prove to the police officers that he was in fact who he said he was, but this did not convince his wife. It was possible to improve matters with a low dose of an antipsychotic medication, but she was not always compliant with taking the medication because she did not trust the man, her husband, who was giving it to her. On one memorable occasion when I was visiting, Mr Crawley had to withdraw to another room because his presence was causing his wife so much upset. Fifteen minutes or so later, he came back into the room nonchalantly whistling. Mrs Crawley turned and said to him 'Oh there you are. I've missed you'. Mr Crawley said he'd been to the bank where he used to work. All was sweetness and light, at least until the Capgras delusion returned.*

---

Capgras syndrome is named after Jean Marie Joseph Capgras (1873–1950). It is regarded as a syndrome of delusional misidentification in which the affected person firmly believes someone close to them has been replaced by an imposter who looks exactly the same as the replaced person (Capgras and Reboul-Lachaux 1923). It is said mostly to be found in schizophrenia, but recent research suggests that between 25 and 40 per cent of cases are associated with organic disorders, from dementia to head injury, epilepsy, and stroke disease (Edelstyn and Oyebode 1999). In 151 consecutively diagnosed people with likely Alzheimer's disease in a community sample in Miami, 10 per cent had the Capgras delusion, which was associated with the presence of other delusions, worse cognitive function and a poorer functional status (Harwood et al. 1999). Again, there have been suggestions of dysfunction affecting the frontal and temporal regions, particularly on the right side (Edelstyn and Oyebode 1999).

It has also been suggested that Capgras syndrome is common is dementia with Lewy bodies (DLB), where a strong association with visual hallucinations and anxiety has been found (Thaipisuttikul et al. 2013). Delusions are common in DLB, with a study from Taiwan demonstrating a 51.2 per cent prevalence (Tzeng et al. 2018). Delusions of theft (35.3 per cent) were most common, then delusions of danger (21.3 per cent), delusions that the house was not the person's home (10.8 per cent), that the spouse was having an affair (7.2 per cent), that the family planned to abandon the person (4.8 per cent), that there was a phantom border (2.9 per cent) or media people (2.9 per cent) in the house and that people were not who they claimed to be (1.0 per cent) (Tzeng et al. 2018). Others, too, have pointed to the prevalence of delusions in DLB being as high as 60 per cent. Meanwhile, Sho Ochiai and colleagues (2019) reported a case of delusional parasitosis ('a fixed and persistent belief of having a pathogenic infection despite objective evidence to the contrary') in an 89-year-old female who had DLB, where the symptoms resolved with a mixture of a cholinesterase inhibitor and an antipsychotic.

Delusions in vascular dementia have received relatively little attention, but prevalence rates of delusions are judged to be between 15 and 36 per cent; persecutory delusions, in 25 per cent, are the most common (Cipriani et al. 2014), followed by phantom border delusions in 21 per cent (Ballard et al. 2000).

## 6. Delusions in affective disorders

Depression is common in older people and bipolar disorder is not uncommon. Schizoaffective disorder in older people is not as well recognized and many cases may be subsumed by the diagnosis of schizophrenia (Lee et al. 2021: 678–679). Delusions tend to be mood-congruent and often somatic in depressive episodes, but grandiose in mania. Major depressive disorder with psychotic features occurs in older people: about 18.5 per cent of older people who experience major depression report distorted perceptions, delusions, and hallucinations (Lapid and Ho 2020). In psychotic major depression in older people, paranoid and somatic delusions are most common, followed by delusions of guilt (Gournellis et al. 2014).

---

### VIGNETTE 3.   Miss Lake

*Having reached her 70th birthday, Miss Lake, who had been a schoolteacher, began to regret that perhaps she had been too harsh with her pupils. Her mood became very low. She was anxious and unable to enjoy anything. She stopped going out to visit friends, who became concerned for her, particularly when they saw she was losing weight. She developed the belief that she could not work her legs because they had wires wrapped around them forming coils that blocked her nervous system from working. She felt her whole body was ceasing to work and that there was nothing left of her and no reason to go on living. She required electroconvulsive therapy before she made a complete recovery.*

---

Miss Lake demonstrated features of Cotard's syndrome, named after Jules Cotard (1840–1889). '*Cotard's syndrome* contains features typical of psychotic depression in the elderly:

nihilistic and hypochondriacal delusions which are often bizarre, dramatic and tinged with grandiosity; a mood depressed with either agitation or retardation; and a completely negative attitude' (Sims 1988: 99). Cotard's nihilistic delusions, *délire de negations*, can be taken to extremes where everything is negated, where people affected believe their bodily organs do not exist and neither does anything else.

## 7.  Conclusion

Four themes emerge from the literature around delusions in the disorders of old age. First, there are the attempts to differentiate between different psychotic states. Plato's idea, from *Phaedrus*, that it is better to carve nature at its joints is, at first blush, alluring. In other words, it would be helpful if we could divide up psychopathology cleanly into different entities. But life, and psychiatric disorders in old age, are not so obliging. The neat diagnostic packages we have created turn out to be leaky (González-Rodríguez et al. 2022). Psychopathology of the same form, namely delusions, can have the same content too: they can be persecutory and feature in delirium, late paraphrenia, LOS, delusional disorder, Alzheimer's disease, Lewy body dementia, psychotic depression, and so on. Perhaps Kay and Roth (1961) were correct when they said that clear lines of demarcation between groups of cases do not exist. Whilst it is obviously beneficial sometimes to go for categorical diagnoses, e.g. to try to establish effective treatments, it will often be better to accept that the nosological framework should be more dimensional. This is at least because actual people do not like to feel they have merely been put into a pigeonhole. What is more important is that their lived experiences have been taken seriously.

Secondly, there are numerous studies now which point to the organic basis of psychosis and of delusions (e.g. Almeida et al. 1992, Howard et al. 1994b, Edelstyn and Oyebode 1999, Bassiony and Lyketsos 2003, Holt and Albert 2006, González-Rodríguez et al. 2022, Ismail et al. 2022). These are but some of the studies that point in the direction of the underlying neuropathology, increasingly ascribed to the frontal and temporal lobes of the brain. There is the slightly puzzling matter that delusions do not seem to be so common in frontotemporal dementia, although it turns out we might see them more clearly if we look with the aid of genetic markers (Hall and Finger 2015). Michael Shanks and Annalena Venneri (2004) certainly felt that looking at individual delusions in the relatively uncluttered context of early Alzheimer's disease might bring about greater insight into the pathogenesis of these conditions. Perhaps so, although the idea that Alzheimer's disease is straightforwardly one unproblematic condition may itself be naïve.

Thirdly, there is the thought that delusions might be precursors of dementia. Esa Leinonen and colleagues (2004) suggested that older people with major depression and delusional disorder are at an increased risk of subsequent dementia. Corinne Fischer and Luis Agüera-Ortiz (2018) suggested that psychosis in prodromal dementia might be quite common. Hideki Kanemoto and colleagues (2022) found the symptomatology of VLOS seemed to be prodromal for DLB, and so on.

But, fourthly, might not a unifying feature here simply be ageing? Our ageing brains age idiosyncratically, even if patterns emerge. Perhaps, therefore, it should be no surprise if one person has particular experiences that another person with a similar diagnosis does not. And, similarly, it should be no surprise if two quite different people experience very similar delusions. What do we know of the person's detailed narrative, of her genetics, of the environmental factors that shaped her, of her social circle and interests, of her current biochemistry, of her temperament and resilience that might account for why her ageing brain is now working in this way rather than that?

Older people with delusions need to be understood individually. Even so, their symptoms remain intellectually and humanly puzzling. As Drury once wrote, 'Our sanity is at the mercy of a molecule' (Drury 1973: 134). But, in the end, as Drury would have agreed, molecules do not provide us with the phenomenological (lived) experience of sanity or of delusions. It is this experience, now, that should always remain a puzzle, a mystery, and never be taken for granted.

## Note

1 I should acknowledge that no definition of delusions is entirely satisfactory and the exact characterization of delusions is problematic. Greater philosophical attention has been paid to delusions in Thornton (2007: 100–122). Much of the current volume deals with the conceptual complexities of delusions (see Section 1 especially); also, Chapter 14 on delusions and evidence by Carolina Flores, Chapter 16 on delusions and rationality by Adam Bradley and Quinn Hiroshi Gibson, and Chapters 20 and 21 by Paul Noordhof, on delusions and (non-)doxasticism, all provide further insights into the basis of our different understandings of delusions.

## References

Almeida, O.P., Howard, R., Forstl, H. and Levy, R. (1992) "Should the Diagnosis of Late Paraphrenia be Abandoned?" *Psychological Medicine*, 22, 11–14.

Ballard, C., Neill, D., O'Brien, J., McKeith, I.G., Ince, P. and Perry, R. (2000) "Anxiety, Depression and Psychosis in Vascular Dementia: Prevalence and Associations," *Journal of Affective Disorders*, 59, 97–106.

Bassiony, M.M. and Lyketsos, C.G. (2003) "Delusions and Hallucinations in Alzheimer's Disease: Review of the Brain Decade," *Psychosomatics*, 44, 388–401.

Capgras, J. and Reboul-Lachaux, J. (1923) "L'illusion des Sosies dans un Délire Systematique Chronique," *Bulletin de la Societé Clinique de Médecine Mentale*, 11, 6–16.

Cipriani, G., Danti, S., Vedovello, M., Nuti, A. and Lucetti, C. (2014) "Understanding Delusion in Dementia: A Review," *Geriatrics and Gerontology International*, 14, 32–39.

Cohen, C.I. (2018) "Very Late-Onset Schizophrenia-Like Psychosis: Positive Findings but Questions Remain Unanswered," *The Lancet*, Available at: http://dx.doi.org/10.1016/S2215-0366(18)30174-3 (accessed 12 December 2022).

Cohen, C.I., Meesters, P.D. and Zhao, J. (2015) "New Perspectives on Schizophrenia in Later Life: Implications for Treatment, Policy, and Research," *The Lancet Psychiatry*, 2, 340–350.

Copeland, J.R., Dewey, M.E., Scott, A., Gilmore, C., Larkin, B.A., Cleave, N., McCracken, C.F. and McKibbin, P.E. (1998) "Schizophrenia and Delusional Disorder in Older Age: Community Prevalence, Incidence, Comorbidity, and Outcome," *Schizophrenia Bulletin*, 24, 153–161.

Drevets, W.C. and Rubin, E.H. (1987) "Erotomania and Senile Dementia of Alzheimer Type," *British Journal of Psychiatry*, 151, 400–402.

Drury, M.O'C. (1973) *The Danger of Words*, London: Routledge & Kegan Paul.

——— (1981) "Conversations with Wittgenstein," in R. Rhees (ed.) *Ludwig Wittgenstein: Personal Recollections*, Oxford: Basil Blackwell, pp. 112–189.

Edelstyn, N.M.J. and Oyebode, F. (1999) "A Review of the Phenomenology and Cognitive Neuropsychological Origins of the Capgras Syndrome," *International Journal of Geriatric Psychiatry*, 14, 48–59.

Fischer, C.E. and Agüera-Ortiz, L. (2018) "Psychosis and Dementia: Risk Factor, Prodrome, or Cause?" *International Psychogeriatrics*, 30, 209–219.

Fusar-Poli, P. and Politi, P. (2008) "Paul Eugen Bleuler and the Birth of Schizophrenia (1908)," *American Journal of Psychiatry*, 165, 1407.

González-Rodríguez, A., Seeman, M.V., Izquierdo, E., Natividad, M., Guàrdia, A., Román, E. and Monreal, J.A. (2022) "Delusional Disorder in Old Age: A Hypothesis-Driven Review of Recent Work Focusing on Epidemiology, Clinical Aspects, and Outcomes," *International Journal of Environmental Research and Public Health*, 19, 7911. Available at: https://doi.org/10.3390/ijerph19137911 (accessed 28 November 2022).

Gournellis, R., Oulis, P. and Howard, R. (2014) "Psychotic Major Depression in Older People: A Systematic Review," *International Journal of Geriatric Psychiatry*, 29, 784–796.

Grahame, P.S. (1984) "Schizophrenia in Old Age (Late Paraphrenia)," *British Journal of Psychiatry*, 145, 493–495.

Hall, D. and Finger, E.C. (2015) "Psychotic Symptoms in Frontotemporal Dementia," *Current Neurology and Neuroscience Reports*, 15, 46. Available at: https://doi.org/10.1007/s11910-015-0567-8 (accessed 15 December 2022).

Harwood, D.G., Barker, W.W., Ownby, R.L. and Duara, R. (1999) "Prevalence and Correlatives of Capgras Syndrome in Alzheimer's Disease," *International Journal of Geriatric Psychiatry*, 14, 415–420.

Holden, N.L. (1987) "Late Paraphrenia or the Paraphrenias? A Descriptive Study with a 10-Year Follow-up," *British Journal of Psychiatry*, 150, 635–639.

Holt, A.E.M. and Albert, M.L. (2006) "Cognitive Neuroscience of Delusions in Aging," *Neuropsychiatric Disease and Treatment*, 2, 181–189.

Howard, R., Castle, D., O'Brien, J. Almeida, O. and Levy, R. (1992) "Permeable Walls, Floors, Ceilings and Doors. Partition Delusions in Late Paraphrenia," *International Journal of Geriatric Psychiatry*, 7, 719–724.

Howard, R., Castle, D., Wessley, S. and Murray, R. (1993) "A Comparative Study of 470 Cases of Early-Onset and Late-Onset Schizophrenia," *British Journal of Psychiatry*, 163, 352–357.

Howard, R., Almeida, O. and Levy, R. (1994a) "Phenomenology, Demography and Diagnosis in Late Paraphrenia," *Psychological Medicine*, 24, 397–410.

Howard, R., Almeida, O. and Levy, R., Graves, P. and Graves, M. (1994b) "Quantitative Magnetic Resonance Imaging Volumetry Distinguishes Delusional Disorder from Late-Onset Schizophrenia," *British Journal of Psychiatry*, 165, 474–480.

Howard, R., Rabins, P.V., Mary V. Seeman, M.V., Dilip V. Jeste, D.V. and the International Late-Onset Schizophrenia Group (2000) "Late-Onset Schizophrenia and Very-Late-Onset Schizophrenia-Like Psychosis: An International Consensus," *American Journal of Psychiatry*, 157, 172–178.

Howard, R., Cort, E., Bradley, R., Harper, E., Kelly, L., Bentham, P., Ritchie, C., Reeves, S., Fawzi, W., Livingston, G., Sommerlad, A., Oomman, S., Nazir, E., Nilforooshan, R., Barber, R., Fox, C., Macharouthu, A.V., Ramachandra, P., Pattan, V., Sykes, J., Curran, V., Katona, C., Dening, T., Knapp, M., Gray, R. and the ATLAS Trialists Group (2018) "Antipsychotic Treatment of Very Late-Onset Schizophrenia-Like Psychosis (ATLAS): A Randomised, Controlled, Double-Blind Trial," *Lancet Psychiatry*, 5, 553–563.

Ismail, Z., Creese, B., Aarsland, D., Kales, H.C., Lyketsos, C.G., Sweet, R.A. and Ballard, C. (2022) "Psychosis in Alzheimer Disease—Mechanisms, Genetics and Therapeutic Opportunities," *Nature Reviews Neurology*, 18, 131–144.

Kanemoto, H., Satake, Y., Suehiro, T., Taomoto, D., Koizumi, F., Sato, S., Wada, T., Matsunaga, K., Shimosegawa, E., Hashimoto, M., Yoshiyama, K. and Ikeda, M. (2022) "Characteristics of Very Late-Onset Schizophrenia-Like Psychosis as Prodromal Dementia with Lewy Bodies: A Cross-Sectional Study," *Alzheimer's Research & Therapy*, 14, 137. Available at: https://doi.org/10.1186/s13195-022-01080-x (accessed 12 December 2022).

Kay, D.W.K. and Roth, M. (1961) "Environmental and Hereditary Factors in the Schizophrenias of Old Age and Their Bearing on the General Problem of Causation in Schizophrenia," *Journal of Mental Science*, 107(449), 649–686.

Kørner, A., Lopez, A.G., Lauritzen, L., Andersen, P.K. and Kessing, L.V. (2008) "Delusional Disorder in Old Age and the Risk of Developing Dementia–A Nationwide Register-Based Study," *Aging and Mental Health*, 12, 625–629.

Kraepelin, E. (1920) "Die Erscheinungsformen des Irreseins," *Zeitschrift für Gesammte Neurologie und Psychiatrie*, 62, 1–29.

Kräupl Taylor, F. (1979) *Psychopathology: Its Causes and Symptoms*, Sunbury-on-Thames: Quartermaine House Ltd. (first published by Butterworth & Co. in 1966).

Lapid, M.I. and Ho, J.B. (2020) "Challenging Our Beliefs about Delusional Disorder in Late Life," *International Psychogeriatrics*, 32, 423–425.

Lee, E.E., Hou, B., Vahia, I.V. and Jeste, D.V. (2021) "Late-Onset Schizophrenia," in T. Dening, A. Thomas, R. Stewart and J.P. Taylor (eds.) *Oxford Textbook of Old Age Psychiatry*, Oxford: Oxford University Press, pp. 671–693.

Leinonen, E., Santala, M., Hyötylä, T., Santala, H., Eskola, N. and Salokangas, R.K.R. (2004) "Elderly Patients with Major Depressive Disorder and Delusional Disorder Are at Increased Risk of Subsequent Dementia," *Nordic Journal of Psychiatry*, 58, 161–164.

Lyketsos, C.G., Sheppard, J.M., Steinberg, M., Tschanz, J.A., Norton, M.C., Steffens, D.C. and Breitner, J.C. (2001) "Neuropsychiatric Disturbance in Alzheimer's Disease Clusters into Three Groups: The Cache County Study," *International Journal of Geriatric Psychiatry*, 16, 1043–1053.

Meagher, D., Moran, M., Raju, B., Gibbons, D., Donnelly, S., Saunders, J. and Trzepacz, P. (2007) "Phenomenology of Delirium: Assessment of 100 Adult Cases Using Standardised Measures," *British Journal of Psychiatry*, 190, 135–141.

Mendez, M.F., Shapira, J.S., Woods, R.J., Licht, E.A. and Saul, R.E. (2008) "Psychotic Symptoms in Frontotemporal Dementia: Prevalence and Review," *Dementia and Geriatric Cognitive Disorders*, 25, 206–211.

Nagendra, J. and Snowdon, J. (2020) "An Australian Study of Delusional Disorder in Late Life," *International Psychogeriatrics*, 32, 453–462.

Ochiai, S., Sugawara, H., Kajio, Y., Tanaka, H., Ishikawa, T., Fukuhara, R., Jono, T. and Hashimoto, M. (2019) "Delusional Parasitosis in Dementia with Lewy Bodies: A Case Report," *Annals of General Psychiatry*, 18, 29. Available at: https://doi.org/10.1186/s12991-019-0253-3 (accessed 12 December 2022).

Pearlson, G.D., Kreger, L., Rabins, P.V., Chase, G.A., Cohen, B., Wirth, J.B., Schlaepfer, T.B. and Tune, L.E. (1989) "A Chart Review Study of Late-Onset and Early-Onset Schizophrenia," *American Journal of Psychiatry*, 146, 1568–1574.

Post, F. (1966) *Persistent Persecutory States in the Elderly*, Oxford: Pergamon Press.

——— (1992) "Changing Concepts: Persistent Delusions," in C. Katona and R. Levy (eds.) *Delusions and Hallucinations in Old Age*, London: Gaskell, pp. 43–49.

Roth, M. (1955) "The Natural History of Mental Disorder in Old Age," *Journal of Mental Science*, 101, 281–301.

Roth, M. and J. D. Morrissey, J.D. (1952) "Problems in the Diagnosis and Classification of Mental Disorder in Old Age; With a Study of Case Material," *Journal of Mental Science*, 98, 66–80.

Roth, M. and Cooper, A.F. (1992) "A Review of Late Paraphrenia and What Is Known of Its Aetiological Basis," in C. Katona and R. Levy (eds.) *Delusions and Hallucinations in Old Age*, London: Gaskell, pp. 25–42.

Schneider, K. (1959) *Clinical Psychopathology*, 5th edition, trans. M.W. Hamilton, New York and London: Grune & Stratton.

Schneider, L.S. and Dagerman, K.S. (2004) "Psychosis of Alzheimer's Disease: Clinical Characteristics and History," *Journal of Psychiatric Research*, 38, 105–111.

Shanks, M.F. and Venneri, A. (2004) "Thinking Through Delusions in Alzheimer's Disease," *British Journal of Psychiatry*, 184, 193–194.

Sims, A. (1988) *Symptoms in the Mind: An Introduction to Descriptive Psychopathology*, London: Baillière Tindall.

Stelzmann, R.A., Schnitzlein, H.N. and Murtagh, F.R. (1995) "An English Translation of Alzheimer's 1907 Paper, "Über eine eigenartige Erkankung der Hirnrinde"," *Clinical Anatomy*, 8, 429–431.

Suen, Y.N. Wong, S.M.Y., Hui, C.L.M., Chan, S.K.W., Lee, E.H.M., Chang, W.C. and Chen, E.Y.H. (2019) "Late-Onset Psychosis and Very Late-Onset-Schizophrenia-Like-Psychosis: An Updated Systematic Review," *International Review of Psychiatry*, 31, 523–542.

Thaipisuttikul, P., Lobach, I., Zweig, Y., Gurnani, A. and Galvin, J.E. (2013) "Capgras Syndrome in Dementia with Lewy Bodies," *International Psychogeriatrics*, 25, 843–849.

Thornton, T. (2007) *Essential Philosophy of Psychiatry*, Oxford: Oxford University Press.

Tzeng, R.-C., Ching-Fang Tsai, C.-F., Wang, C.-T., Wang, T.-Y. and Chiu, P.-Y. (2018) "Delusions in Patients with Dementia with Lewy Bodies and the Associated Factors," *Behavioural Neurology*, Article ID 6707291. Available at: https://doi.org/10.1155/2018/6707291 (accessed 12 December 2022).

# PART 3

# Epistemology of delusion

# 12
# DELUSION AND EVIDENCE

*Carolina Flores*

## 1.  Introduction

Delusions are standardly defined as attitudes that are 'not amenable to change in light of conflicting evidence' (DSM-5 2013). But what evidence do people with delusion have for and against it? Do delusions really go against their total evidence? How are the answers affected by different conceptions of evidence?

This chapter focuses on how delusions relate to evidence. This matters for questions about the nature of delusions, such as whether delusions are beliefs (for more on delusion and belief see Noordhof, Chapter 19). On many views, to count as beliefs, delusions must relate to evidence in sufficiently similar ways to ordinary beliefs. The relationship between delusion and evidence is also crucial for what we say about the epistemic rationality of delusions (Bortolotti 2009, Noordhof and Sullivan-Bissett 2023). Finally, it matters for explanations of delusion formation and maintenance, for effective treatment, and for ascriptions of responsibility.

In Section 2, I will discuss the nature of evidence, focusing on the distinction between internalist and externalist conceptions. In Section 3, I will consider what delusions-relevant evidence people with delusions have. I will give some reasons to think that people typically have evidence for their delusions, and that the evidence they have against them is often overstated. In Section 4, I will draw on this discussion to consider whether delusions are evidentially supported and epistemically rational. Finally, I will discuss implications for the nature of delusion, responsibility, and treatment, and suggest directions for future research (Section 5).

## 2.  Evidence: a primer

Depending on which theorist you ask, evidence is what justifies belief, is respected by rational thinkers, guides thinkers towards truth, or functions as a neutral arbiter that allows for objectivity (Kelly 2016). Philosophers arrive at different conceptions of evidence by focusing on some of these theoretical roles over others.

Focusing on the two first roles leads to *internalism*. According to internalists, evidence is what makes beliefs rational or justified, where a rational or justified belief is one that the agent

       DOI: 10.4324/9781003296386-16

cannot be blamed for having. The internalist points out that it seems inappropriate to blame agents for their beliefs when they are in deceptive scenarios that are indistinguishable from non-deceptive ones, as agents deceived by an Evil Demon would be. Their beliefs, on this view, are rational or justified because agents correctly respond to how things seem to them.

This pushes towards the *phenomenal conception of evidence*. On this conception, one's evidence is exhausted by one's subjective, non-factive (i.e. not necessarily true) mental states. Evidence is exhausted by the sense data of which the agent is consciously aware (Ayer 1936, Russell 1912), or perhaps by the agent's conscious mental states (Conee and Feldman 2004).

In contrast, *externalists* prioritize the role of evidence as a guide to truth and neutral arbiter. As Evil Demon scenarios illustrate, one's subjective mental states might be radically inaccurate, and therefore lead an agent away from the truth.

These considerations lead to the *factive conception of evidence*, on which only true propositions can count as evidence. Factive conceptions might equate an agent's total evidence with the propositions they know (Williamson 2002) or the facts they are in a position to know (Simion 2021). Hallucinations and other deceptive appearances do not yield evidence about the world. At best, if agents reflect on their own mind, they have introspective evidence that they are having a certain experience (Williamson 2002).[1]

One aim of this chapter is to show that the internalism–externalism distinction makes a difference to the epistemology of delusion. To do so, I will rely on the following (fairly uncontroversial) claims about evidence.

First, agents can acquire evidence through perception, introspection, and testimony. Second, minimally, for a particular mental state or proposition to be evidence for some hypothesis, it must probabilify the truth of the hypothesis. Third, whether a hypothesis is evidentially supported is a matter of whether it is supported by the agent's total evidence, not just by a proper subset of it; when an individual receives evidence that supports a hypothesis, this does not mean by default that they now ought to endorse that hypothesis. Finally, the extent of support a hypothesis receives depends on the hypotheses that the agent considers (Kelly 2016).

## 3.  What evidence do people with delusions have?

People with delusions are often thought to have plenty of evidence against their delusion, and not much in its favour. In this section, I will discuss this view and then consider some reasons against it.

### 3.1  *The orthodox view*

People with delusions appear to have plenty of evidence against their delusions, no matter how one thinks of evidence.

First, they have background beliefs and knowledge that are counter-evidence to the delusion. Consider this post-remission testimony from a person who had Capgras delusion (the delusion that someone the subject knows well [e.g., a romantic partner] has been replaced by an identical-looking impostor [Pandis et al. 2019]).

I've started going through it, and seeing what could possibly happen and what couldn't happen… Mary couldn't suddenly disappear from the room, so there must

be an explanation for it. The lady knows me way back. She could say things that happened 40 years go, and I wonder where she gets them from. … And then I worked it
out and I've wondered if it's Mary all the time. It's nobody else.

*(Turner and Coltheart 2010: 371)*

This person had plenty of beliefs that were in tension with the delusion, though he was
not bringing them together with the delusion. This suggests that subjects may often have
counter-evidence to their delusions but fail to access it due to belief fragmentation (Davies
and Egan 2013).

Second, people with delusions often receive testimonial counter-evidence to their delusions. For instance, the supposed impostor in Capgras might deny being an impostor, and
other people will endorse this. People with delusions may also hear arguments against
the claim that the person is an impostor. They might even be told that they are delusional
(which amounts to receiving higher-order evidence against the delusion).[2]

Do subjects have evidence for the delusion? Here, there is disagreement—though the
orthodox view is that, even if subjects have such evidence, it is much weaker than evidence
they have against the delusion. For now, I will discuss views on which subjects have *no*
evidence for the delusion.

The case for this claim is strongest for delusions which appear to be formed without
alterations in the subject's experience of the world, such as erotomania (where the subject claims that a high-status individual, e.g., a celebrity, is in love with them [Jordan and
Howe 1980]). In such cases, it is hard to find anything that could count as evidence for the
delusion.

More commonly, there are alterations to people's experience of the world when they
have delusions. For instance, people with Capgras have a deficit in the visual processing
of faces. Their facial recognition systems are intact, but they lack the usual autonomic
responses to loved ones, as measured by skin conductance tests (Ellis and Lewis 2001, Ellis
and Young 1990). Similar mechanisms have been hypothesized and studied for other circumscribed, monothematic delusions.

Such alterations in perceptual processing yield what may count as relevant evidence. But
one can resist that view.

For instance, Max Coltheart and colleagues (2010) argue that the lack of an autonomic
response does not amount to a conscious experience. They claim that everything leading
from perceptual input to the occurrent thought 'This is not my partner' is unconscious.
Consequently, people with Capgras lack relevant phenomenal evidence, as such evidence
requires that things appear a certain way to the subject. They also lack introspective evidence, as you cannot introspect unconscious phenomena.

Alternatively, some theorists hold that the resulting altered experience is a best characterized as an alteration to the subject's feelings (McLaughlin 2010), perhaps as a result of
miscalibrated prediction error (Corlett et al. 2010, see also Corlett, Chapter 30). Specifically, because the feeling of familiarity that the subject expects is absent, the subject comes
to have a feeling of unfamiliarity.

Further, one might think that feelings lack representational content (Deonna and Teroni
2012, Tomkins 2008). On such views, it is hard to see how feelings provide phenomenal
evidence, which is typically equated with the representational contents of experience. At
best, they provide weak introspective evidence for the delusion, insofar as having a strange
bodily feeling can offer support to the impostor hypothesis.

If delusions are formed in response to mere feelings (or don't even involve conscious experience), then subjects' experience does not yield evidence for their delusion. Importantly, many delusions in schizophrenia seem to be formed in response to mental episodes best described as feelings: depressive or anxious moods, feelings of strangeness and tension, fear and a sense of threat, alienating introspection, a disempowering state of confusion and disorientation, and intense emotions of exaltation and manic-like euphoria.[34] If mere feelings do not provide evidence, then people with delusions in schizophrenia lack evidence for their delusions.

### 3.2  Some reasons against the orthodox view about delusion-relevant evidence

There are reasons to think that delusions are not quite so divorced from the evidence. To begin, many theorists grant that people with delusions have at least some evidence for their delusion.

Against the view of feelings discussed above, feelings might provide evidence. On evaluative perception theories, feelings are analogous to perceptual states. They function to represent evaluative properties (Roberts 2003, Tappolet 2016) such as unfamiliarity. On noetic or metacognitive views (Proust 2013), these feelings function to indicate facts about one's cognitive processing. All the same, their content includes ascribing unfamiliarity. On both views, feelings provide evidence: phenomenal evidence that the person is unfamiliar, and factive introspective evidence that one is experiencing unfamiliarity.

A similar conclusion applies if we think of these feelings as seemings, *sui generis* attitudes with an assertive phenomenological character that leads to a felt inclination to believe their content. Much as, in the Müller-Lyer illusion, the two identical lines *seem* to be of different lengths, the person with whom the subject with Capgras is interacting just *seems* unfamiliar. Proponents of seemings usually think that they constitute (phenomenal) evidence for the corresponding belief (Huemer 2013, Pryor 2000). If this is right, people with delusions have some evidence for their delusions.[4]

Even if delusional experiences are best characterized as feelings, they might yield evidence, then. Moreover, the standard take since Brendan Maher (1974) is that the representational content of the subject's perceptual experience is altered in Capgras and similar cases. Such contents plausibly constitute evidence for the delusion.

Endorsement theorists think that the experience has rich content ('This person is not my partner' [Pacherie 2009, Wilkinson 2016] or 'This person is an impostor' [Bongiorno 2020]) and that the delusion is formed simply by endorsing such content. It follows that people with Capgras have strong phenomenal evidence for their delusion. Because the experience is illusory, this is not factive evidence. However, if the subject introspects their experience, they will have factive evidence 'I am having an experience as of this person not being my partner/being an impostor'. The probability that one's partner is an impostor is higher if one has such an experience than if one does not.[5] Therefore, this is also evidence for the delusional hypothesis. So, on the endorsement view, externalists and internalists agree that the subject has evidence for their delusion, albeit of different kinds and strengths.

Endorsement accounts require perception to have rich contents, which is controversial (Davies and Egan 2013). Most theorists hold that the subject's perceptual experience has thinner content, with the subject forming a delusional belief to *explain* such content (for more on empiricist approaches see Bongiorno and Parrott, Chapter 26). For instance, maybe the content predicates unfamiliarity of the person perceived, or perhaps it simply fails to distinguish between familiar and unfamiliar faces (Davies and Egan 2013). This still provides evidence for the delusion, albeit weaker evidence (i.e., evidence that probabilifies the delusion to a lesser extent). The same points about phenomenal and factive introspective evidence apply.[6]

Overall, then, internalism suggests that experience yields substantive phenomenal evidence for the delusion, and externalism that it yields some introspective evidence that supports the delusions. Further, subjects have many repeated experiences of unfamiliarity. Given that these are experiences of interacting in different contexts and ways, each of these experiences arguably provides them with additional evidence for their delusion. As the evidence accrues, the evidential weight behind the delusion grows.

As Paul Noordhof and Ema Sullivan-Bissett (2021) note, most circumscribed monothematic delusions 'are accompanied by some highly distinctive anomalous experiences which, themselves, constitute an at least apparent source of evidence in their own right for the beliefs in question' (Noordhof and Sullivan-Bissett 2021: 10280). For instance, mirrored self-misidentification is accompanied by experiencing images in mirrors as if through a window (Coltheart 2011), and Cotard delusion (the delusion that one is dead or has ceased to exist; Young and Leafhead 1996) by a generalized lack of affective response. If this discussion is right, we should think that such experiences provide genuine (phenomenal and factive introspective) evidence for the delusion, though work needs to be done to spell out exactly what evidence such experiences provide in each case.

Further, in a range of cases of schizophrenia, delusions arise in response to hallucinatory visual and auditory experiences, not to mere feelings. For instance, people with schizophrenia might hear voices (Cho and Wu 2013). Such hallucinatory experiences also provide phenomenal and introspective evidence for delusions.

It is plausible, then, that many people with delusions have some evidence for their delusion. At the same time, the kind and strength of such evidence varies and cannot be determined independently of commitments about the nature of evidence and about the experience at play in delusions.

Let's return to the counter-evidence people with delusions have. Here, there is room to question how much counter-evidence they get from their own background beliefs and from testimony.

First, on many internalist views of evidence, the agent only has evidence that consciously occurs to them (e.g. Ayer 1936, Conee and Feldman 2004, Russell 1912). Agents who have non-accessed beliefs in tension with the delusion do not count as having the corresponding evidence.

Second, the delusion might lead people to lose such beliefs. Their repeated strange experiences might make them doubt their own memory or sense of reality. As one person put it,

> You can't trust anything anymore. Is this a table? It might seem so, but is it really the case? Probably not (laughs). These people are sitting here, but are they really people or is it my imagination, or…? Everything is possible…everything is possible.
>
> *(Sips et al. 2021: 6)*

If subjects cease to have relevant background beliefs, then they will not have the corresponding counter-evidence. If knowledge requires belief, they will also cease to have factive counter-evidence they previously had.

Third, even if the subject accesses some of this counter-evidence, they are like to feel motivated to explain it away. On plausible ways of thinking about *explaining away*, their overall body of evidence will change to neutralize the initial counter-evidence. Let me explain.

There are compelling reasons to think that subjects are generally motivated to hold on to their delusions, and therefore to try to explain away counter-evidence. Some delusions (such as grandiose delusions or erotomania) have positive content that the subject would like to be true. Even when they don't have positive content, delusions provide an explanation for strange and unsettling experiences. Without such an explanation, the subject would feel at sea in the world, whereas once they devise an explanation, they might feel a deeply satisfying sense of clarity at 'the pieces of the puzzle falling in place' (Sips et al. 2021: 4). In contrast, admitting that one is severely mentally ill is exactly the kind of conclusion that most of us (including people with delusions) would like to avoid.

For these reasons, we should expect subjects to expend significant effort at generating alternative explanations for counter-evidence to their delusions.[7] Their overall belief set changes as a result. If we think of evidence as including or consisting in one's set of beliefs or occurrent beliefs, the result of this is that subjects end up with a different body of evidence from a neutral observer.[8]

For instance, assume the person with Capgras notices that the supposed impostor remembers things from 40 years ago. They might hypothesize, and come to believe, that the impostor abducted their partner and learned about their life together in great detail. This is now part of the body of (non-factive) evidence that the person with Capgras has. Such reasoning leads the subject's overall belief set (i.e., evidence, on internalist views) to be one that supports the delusional belief.[9]

In the case of schizophrenia, this process is aided by the liberal acceptance bias (Moritz and Woodward 2004), i.e., the disposition to entertain explanations that common sense or prior knowledge of the world would lead control subjects to exclude. As a result, their total evidence comes to incorporate far-fetched explanations for counter-evidence, thus less strongly supporting abandoning the delusion.[10]

In sum, though the subject's background beliefs might include counter-evidence, they might lack access to those beliefs, lose them as the result of delusional experiences, or incorporate them in a wider belief set which is not in tension with the delusion. For these reasons, it is not clear that background beliefs provide strong counter-evidence to the delusion.

There are also reasons to think that the subject acquires less decisive counter-evidence from testimony than it might initially appear. For instance, 'I am not an impostor' is just what an impostor would say. As such, it is not counter-evidence to the delusion. Similarly, if the impostor is indeed identical-looking, as the person with Capgras thinks, then it will be no surprise that others don't realize that they are interacting with an impostor. The fact that others say they are not an impostor at most provides weak counter-evidence to the delusion (Davies and Egan 2013).

As for arguments against the delusion that others offer, the person with a delusion is likely to interact with these in the same way as they interact with recalled counter-evidence. In particular, they are likely to explain away such claims, leading their overall evidence to no longer be decisive against the delusion.

When it comes to testimonial evidence, there are additional difficulties surrounding trust. Kengo Miyazono and Alessandro Salice (2021) have argued that people with delusions in schizophrenia are likely not to trust others due to underestimating their sincerity (if they have paranoid feelings) or competence (if they have grandiose feelings). Even without such feelings, people with schizophrenia often experience failures of group identification, which has been hypothesized to lead to generalized distrust (Miyazono and

Salice 2021). Additionally, subjects might come to distrust others as a result of feeling deeply misunderstood, dismissed, and treated with contempt (Ritunnano et al. 2022).

If subjects do not trust a testifier, they will not acquire the evidence the testifier intends to transmit (the content of their assertion, $p$). Instead, the evidence they acquire is of the form '$X$ said that $p$'. Given that they don't trust $X$, this gives them at best weak evidence for the truth of $p$.[11]

One might worry that this discussion focuses excessively on possessed evidence as opposed to *available* evidence. Indeed, many discussions of evidence-resistance in delusions talk of available evidence (e.g. Bortolotti 2009), focusing on the claim that delusions are beliefs that reality has failed to constrain (McKay et al. 2005), not that they are beliefs that the subject's evidence fails to support.

It is true that there is available counter-evidence that the subject does not gather. First, motivation to hold on to one's beliefs leads agents to avoid gathering counter- evidence. As Esme Weijun Wang writes about her stint with Cotard delusion:

> Being dead butted up against the so-called evidence of being alive, and so I grew to avoid that evidence because proof was not a comfort; instead, it pointed to my insanity.
>
> *(Wang 2019: 157)*

Second, it is well-documented that people with schizophrenia display a data-gathering bias, tending to collect less information before settling on a belief than control subjects do.[12] Third, people with schizophrenia are often testimonially isolated (Miyazono and Salice 2021). For this reason, they are likely to receive less testimony against their delusion than control subjects would.

As a result, the subject's delusion is out of sync with the available evidence. At the same time, if the subject were to gather this additional evidence, it might not make much of a difference. Even if they were to receive more testimony, they may still fail to trust these testifiers. And even if they trusted them, they would still be motivated to explain away the additional counter-evidence, leading to a body of evidence that is not radically contrary to the delusion.

In this section, we have seen a range of different takes on what evidence people with delusions have. There is no uniform answer: the evidence they have depends on the cause of the delusion, as well as on the subject's patterns of trust and how they reason. In general, cases can be made for views ranging from 'People with delusions have a lot of counter-evidence and no evidence for the delusion' to 'They have strong evidence for the delusion and little or no evidence against it'. Further, where one falls along this spectrum depends on one's take on the nature of evidence, as well as on epistemic issues surrounding trust, rationalization, and the epistemic significance of feelings.

## 4.  Overall evidential support and epistemic rationality

Taking into account the total evidence subjects have, are delusions evidentially supported? And, in light of the answer to that question, are delusions epistemically rational (or justified)?[15] Whether one is an internalist or externalist about evidence, as well as about rationality, makes a difference to how one answers these questions.

Internalists who find the discussion in Section 3.2 persuasive will say that the subject's delusion is evidentially supported. According to the extreme internalist, the subject's evidence is the set of their occurrent mental states (Conee and Feldman 2004). The subject's evidence includes phenomenal evidence from their repeated experiences; delusion-relevant beliefs they bring to mind; and testimony against the delusion they receive from sources they trust, jointly with other beliefs they arrive at by reasoning about that evidence (more on delusion and rationality, see Bradley and Gibson, Chapter 14).[13]

On this view, subjects have strong phenomenal evidence in favour of their delusion. If the discussion in Section 3.2 is along the right lines, their occurrent mental states do not include much strong evidence against the delusion. The delusion is evidentially well-supported.

In contrast, even accepting the discussion in Section 3.2, externalism yields a less generous verdict about the balance of the subject's evidence. Suppose you equate evidence with the agent's knowledge (Williamson 2002). The subject's evidence now includes introspective evidence about their own strange experiences, which favours the delusion. On the other hand, it includes background knowledge that is in tension with the delusion, true testimony they accept, and knowledge they acquired by reflecting on these materials—but *not* false beliefs they arrive at in these ways. Arguably, the introspective evidence is defeated by past knowledge and testimony, so that the delusional hypothesis comes out evidentially unsupported.

Significantly, then, what we say about whether delusions are evidentially supported depends on our background views about the nature of evidence. The same is true when we turn to asking about their epistemic rationality.

Consider the following *evidentialist thesis*:

> For any person $S$, time $t$, and proposition $p$, if $S$ has any doxastic attitude at all toward $p$ at $t$ and $S$'s evidence at $t$ supports $p$, then $S$ epistemically ought to have the attitude toward $p$ supported by $S$'s evidence at $t$.
>
> *(Feldman 2000: 679)*

If you couple this thesis with extreme internalism about evidence, the result is arguably that the subject ought to have the delusional belief. After all, it is supported by their evidence.[14]

One might worry that the delusional hypothesis remains unlikely, even given the evidence. As Cordelia Fine and colleagues (2005) note, the hypotheses that people with delusions entertain seem to be 'explanatory nonstarters', so unlikely that subjects should not even consider them. Instead, they should consider the hypothesis that something has gone seriously wrong with their minds.

This might be right. As Matthew Parrott (2021) argues, if we are looking for sources of abnormality in delusions, we should focus on hypothesis generation. However, for the internalist evidentialist, doing poorly at hypothesis generation is irrelevant to epistemic rationality. Assessing epistemic rationality relies only on whether the delusion is the most evidentially supported of the hypotheses that the subject considers, by their lights, given their mental states.

The claim that delusions can be epistemically rational is extremely counterintuitive. Indeed, one could use this discussion as an argument against this version of internalist evidentialism. At the same time, this verdict fits with what internalists say about other cases. Internalists want to secure a connection between epistemic rationality and blamelessness, so that an agent radically deceived by an evil demon comes out as having rational beliefs. People with delusions are not deceived by an evil demon, but they are hostage to deceptive perceptual and emotional experiences. Once those are taken into account, people with delusions may turn out to be as blameless in how they interact with their evidence as agents in Evil Demon cases.

Other epistemologists deny that evidential support is sufficient for rationality or justification. They point out that one's evidence may be bad, especially if it is the result of cognitive penetration (Siegel 2012) or of vicious attention and evidence-gathering (Hughes 2021). They suggest that positive epistemic statuses require good epistemic dispositions (Lasonen-Aarnio 2020), virtues (Sosa 2007), or a reliable connection to the external world (Goldman 1979). On all these views, even if the delusion is evidentially supported, it is likely to be irrational. This is because the evidence for the delusion at least partly depends on bad patterns of attention and evidence-gathering, and perhaps on cognitive penetration.

The result that delusions are irrational fits with the central motivation for such pictures of epistemic assessment, namely, the idea that rationality requires that our beliefs be constrained by the world. Delusions emerge as irrational, for the subject's perceptual access to the world leaves them unmoored from reality.

## 5. Implications and further directions of research

I have considered the evidence that people with delusions have, and sketched how they interact with it.

One important upshot is that delusions resemble standard beliefs in their relationship with evidence. Elsewhere, I have argued that delusions are underwritten by capacities to rationally respond to counter-evidence (Flores 2021b). I used this claim to argue that we can both subscribe to a rationality constraint on belief and claim that delusions are beliefs. In showing that there is room to hold that delusions are not deeply irrational (exemplifying, perhaps, mere 'everyday irrationality' [Noordhof and Sullivan-Bissett 2023]), the discussion here bolsters that conclusion.

Further, this discussion suggests that one-factor theories of delusion deserve more exploration (concurring with Noordhof and Sullivan-Bissett [2021], see also Sullivan-Bissett, Chapter 28). Subjects have evidence that supports the delusion, and, if the discussion above is right, they interact with evidence in ways that are similar to those of ordinary believers. For this reason, we might not need to appeal to a clinical abnormality or deep irrationality at the level of reasoning to explain delusion formation and maintenance, as two-factor theories do (Davies et al. 2001, see also Davies and Coltheart, Chapter 29).

The discussion also has implications for treatment. Treatment needs to take into account the fact that, due to experiential disturbances, the subject has plenty of evidence for their delusion (or, at least, that it looks like they have such evidence from their perspective). Practitioners also need to consider the conditions under which counter-evidence is offered: are persuasion-enabling trust, motivation, and emotions at play? If we offer counter-evidence without considering such factors, we run the risk of further entrenching the delusion.

There are also applications to thinking about responsibility. Insofar as delusions are evidence-responsive in ways that resemble ordinary beliefs, subjects may meet conditions for epistemic responsibility (McHugh 2013) for their delusions. Determining whether this is the case requires careful attention to different proposals concerning epistemic responsibility and delusion maintenance—a line of inquiry that deserves more exploration.

Finally, I hope that this discussion leads to new, more ecumenical approaches to delusions. Those who are interested in cognitive explanations of delusions and in assessing their rationality would benefit from paying more attention to phenomenological approaches. In highlighting the subject's experience, phenomenological approaches give us valuable information about the evidence people with delusions have. Myopically ignoring this information exaggerates the appearance of irrationality at the level of reasoning. Similarly, theorists of delusion would do well to incorporate the tools of epistemology, in particular, well-developed theories of evidence and epistemic rationality.

In the reverse direction, epistemologists should use delusions to constrain the notion of evidence, much as they have used delusions to constrain the notion of belief. Along these lines, for instance, one might reject an internalist conception of evidence on the grounds that it makes some delusions come out as evidentially supported. This is a promising avenue of research, especially if we care about having epistemic concepts that are useful for describing and regulating real-world epistemic agents.

Finally, I have here focused on the evidence the agent *has* and whether it is reflected in beliefs. This leaves open questions about the epistemic significance of salience and mood, which are altered in many delusions. It also leaves room for investigating cognitive dispositions and epistemic styles (Flores 2021a) in different delusional contexts. And it leaves room for broadening the epistemology of delusions beyond epistemology's traditional focus on what agents do with the materials in their minds (Flores and Woodard 2023). This would build on epistemology's ongoing turn towards inquiry (Friedman forthcoming) and on recent work on inquiry in other psychiatric conditions, such as Obsessive-compulsive disorder (OCD) (Haerle 2023). Such an expansion is crucial for understanding delusion maintenance and its (ir)rationality.

## 6. Conclusion

I have surveyed what relevant evidence subjects with delusions have, on different conceptions of evidence, and explored implications for the epistemic rationality of delusions. It emerged that what we should say about the epistemic standing of delusions depends substantively on our positions in epistemology, in particular, on the debate between internalists and externalists about evidence. If we want clarity on the epistemic standing of delusions, we need to incorporate more sophisticated tools from epistemology.

## Acknowledgements

Thanks to Ema Sullivan-Bisset and Dan Williams for comments on a previous version.

## Notes

1 Ecumenically, one can grant that both factive and phenomenal evidence are evidence, with subjects who have factive evidence as opposed to merely phenomenal evidence having more evidence for the relevant belief (Schellenberg 2018).

2 Higher-order evidence is evidence that bears on a thinker's rational capacities, performance, or evidential situation, without directly bearing on their beliefs (Horowitz 2022).

3 See Rosa Ritunanno and colleagues 2022 for an excellent overview.

4 The externalist would say that the evidence available is something like 'It seems to me that this person is unfamiliar'.

5 Equivalently: the probability that one has this strange experience if the person is indeed an impostor is higher than the probability of having this experience if they are not an impostor. This does not mean that the subject ought to endorse the delusional hypothesis. That depends on whether that hypothesis is best supported by the subject's total evidence. In Bayesian terms, accepting a hypothesis just because it is probabilified by evidence amounts to ignoring the prior probability of

that hypothesis, i.e., displaying a bias towards explanatory adequacy. According to Ryan McKay (2012), this is exactly what people with delusions do.

6  If, as top-down accounts of delusion formation claim (Campbell 2001, see also Ohlhorst, Chapter 27), the experiences at play in delusion are the result of cognitive penetration (i.e., of the subject's beliefs leading them to experience their partner as impostor-like), then experience might not constitute evidence for the belief. However, there is a lively debate about (1) whether cognitive penetration of content happens (Firestone and Scholl 2016), and (2) whether subjects get evidence in such cases, even if only phenomenal evidence (see Siegel 2016 for discussion). This issue merits more attention in the context of the epistemology of delusions.

7  Indeed, even if people with delusions are not especially motivated to hold on to them, they will more closely scrutinize counter-evidence than supporting evidence. In general, we devote more energy to understanding things that violate our expectations.

8  See Kelly 2008 for detailed discussion.

9  If we think of evidence as the agent's factive mental states, this only applies when the claims agents appeal to for their explanations are true. Note, also, that this is not yet to make any claims about the rationality of the delusion: one might hold that the delusion is supported by the evidence the subject arrives at, but is irrational because the subject arrives at that evidence through a bad process.

10  The well-documented bias against disconfirming evidence (Woodward et al. 2006) (i.e. tendency to update more slowly away from an endorsed hypothesis in light of counter-evidence) in schizophrenia may be the result of liberal acceptance. In leading subjects to consider additional explanations for the counter-evidence, liberal acceptance reduce the epistemic force of that counter-evidence.

11  Plausibly, such allocations of trust violate epistemic norms. But, once subjects have allocated their trust in these ways, they get less evidence than they would otherwise.

12  I.e., they display a *jumping to conclusions bias* (Dudley et al. 2016).

13  Internalists who disagree with the points in Section 3.2 have room to argue that the subject's delusion is not evidentially supported.

14  See Jeppsson 2022 for more discussion of evidentialism as it applies to psychosis.


# References


Alfred Jules Ayer. *Language, Truth and Logic*. London: V. Gollancz, 1936.

Federico Bongiorno. Is the Capgras delusion an endorsement of experience? *Mind & Language*, 35(3):293–312, 2020.

Lisa Bortolotti. *Delusions and Other Irrational Beliefs*. Oxford University Press, 2009.

John Campbell. Rationality, meaning, and the analysis of delusion. *Philosophy, Psychiatry, & Psychology*, 8(2):89–100, 2001.

Raymond Cho and Wayne Wu. Mechanisms of auditory verbal hallucination in schizophrenia. *Frontiers in Psychiatry*, 4:155, 2013.

Max Coltheart. The mirrored-self misidentification delusion. *Neuropsychiatry*, 1(6): 521, 2011.

Max Coltheart, Peter Menzies, and John Sutton. Abductive inference and delusional belief. *Cognitive Neuropsychiatry*, 15(1–3):261–287, 2010.

Earl Conee and Richard Feldman. *Evidentialism: Essays in Epistemology*. Oxford: Oxford University Press, 2004.

Phil R. Corlett, J.R. Taylor, X.-J. Wang, P.C. Fletcher, and J.H. Krystal. Toward a neurobiology of delusions. *Progress in Neurobiology*, 92(3):345–369, 2010.

Martin Davies, Max Coltheart, Robyn Langdon, and Nora Breen. Monothematic delusions: Towards a two-factor account. *Philosophy, Psychiatry, & Psychology*, 8(2):133–158, 2001.

Martin Davies and Andy Egan. Delusion: Cognitive approaches–Bayesian inference and compartmentalization. In K.W.M. Fulford, M. Davies, R. Gipps, G. Graham, J. Sadler, G. Stanghellini, and T. Thornton, editors, *The Oxford Handbook of Philosophy and Psychiatry*, pages 689–727, Oxford: Oxford University Press, 2013.

Julien Deonna and Fabrice Teroni. *The Emotions: A Philosophical Introduction*. Oxford: Routledge, 2012.

DSM-5. *Diagnostic and Statistical Manual of Mental Disorders (DSM-5®)*. American Psychiatric Pub, 2013.

Robert Dudley, Peter Taylor, Sophie Wickham, and Paul Hutton. Psychosis, delusions and the "jumping to conclusions" reasoning bias: A systematic review and meta-analysis. *Schizophrenia Bulletin*, 42(3):652–665, 2016.

Hadyn D. Ellis and Michael B. Lewis. Capgras delusion: A window on face recognition. *Trends in Cognitive Sciences*, 5(4):149–156, 2001.

Hadyn D. Ellis and Andrew W. Young. Accounting for delusional misidentifications. *The British Journal of Psychiatry*, 157(2):239–248, 1990.

Richard Feldman. The ethics of belief. *Philosophy and Phenomenological Research*, 60(3):667–695, 2000. doi: 10.2307/2653823.

Cordelia Fine, Jillian Craigie, and Ian Gold. Damned if you do; damned if you don't: The impasse in cognitive accounts of the Capgras delusion. *Philosophy, Psychiatry, & Psychology*, 12(2):143–151, 2005.

Chaz Firestone and Brian J. Scholl. Cognition does not affect perception: Evaluating the evidence for "top-down" effects. *Behavioral and Brain Sciences*, 39: e229, 2016.

Carolina Flores. Epistemic style. *Philosophical Topics*, 49(2):35–55, 2021a.

Carolina Flores. Delusional evidence-responsiveness. *Synthese*, 199(3):6299–6330, 2021b.

Carolina Flores and Elise Woodard. Epistemic norms on evidence-gathering. *Philosophical Studies*, 180:2547–2571, 2023.

Jane Friedman. forthcoming Zetetic epistemology. In Baron Reed and A.K. Flowerree, editors, *Towards an Expansive Epistemology: Norms, Action, and the Social Sphere*. Oxford: Routledge, forthcoming.

Alvin I. Goldman. What is justified belief? In George Pappas, editor, *Justification and Knowledge*, pages 1–23. Dordretch: Springer Netherlands, 1979.

Pablo Hubacher Haerle. Is OCD epistemically irrational? *Philosophy, Psychiatry, and Psychology*, 30(2):133–146, 2023.

Sophie Horowitz. Higher-order evidence. In Edward N. Zalta and Uri Nodelman, editors, *The Stanford Encyclopedia of Philosophy*. Metaphysics Research Lab, Stanford University, Fall, 2022 edition, 2022.

Michael Huemer. Phenomenal conservatism über alles. In Chris Tucker, editor, *Seemings and Justification: New Essays on Dogmatism and Phenomenal Conservatism*, pages 328–350, New York: Oxford University Press2013.

Nick Hughes. Epistemic feedback loops (or: How not to get evidence). *Philosophy and Phenomenological Research*, 106.(2):368–393, 2023.

Sofia Jeppsson. Radical psychotic doubt and epistemology. *Philosophical Psychology*, 36(8): 1482–1506, 2023.

Harold W. Jordan and Gray Howe. De Clerambault syndrome (erotomania): A review and case presentation. *Journal of the National Medical Association*, 72(10):1980.

Thomas Kelly. Disagreement, dogmatism, and belief polarization. *The Journal of Philosophy*, 105(10):611–633, 2008.

Thomas Kelly. Evidence. In Edward N. Zalta, editor, *The Stanford Encyclopedia of Philosophy*. Metaphysics Research Lab, Stanford University, Winter, 2016 edition, 2016.

Maria Lasonen-Aarnio. Perspectives and good dispositions. *Philosophy and Phenomenological Research*, 2024.

Brendan A. Maher. Delusional thinking and perceptual disorder. *Journal of Individual Psychology*, 30(1):98, 1974.

Conor McHugh. Epistemic responsibility and doxastic agency. *Philosophical Issues*, 23:132–157, 2013.

Ryan McKay. Delusional inference. *Mind & Language*, 27(3):330–355, 2012.

Ryan McKay, Robyn Langdon, and Max Coltheart. "Sleights of mind": Delusions, defences, and self-deception. *Cognitive Neuropsychiatry*, 10(4):305–326, 2005.

Brian P. McLaughlin. Monothematic delusions and existential feelings. In Tim Bayne and Jordi Fernández, editors, *Delusion and Self-Deception: Affective and Motivational Influences on Belief Formation*, pages 139–164, New York: Psychology Press, 2010.

Kengo Miyazono and Alessandro Salice. Social epistemological conception of delusion. *Synthese*, 199(1):1831–1851, 2021.

Steffen Moritz and Todd S. Woodward. Plausibility judgment in schizophrenic patients: Evidence for a liberal acceptance bias. *German Journal of Psychiatry*, 7(4):66–74, 2004.

Paul Noordhof and Ema Sullivan-Bissett. The clinical significance of anomalous experience in the explanation of monothematic delusions. *Synthese*, 199(3):10277–10309, 2021.

Paul Noordhof and Ema Sullivan-Bissett. The everyday irrationality of monothematic delusion. In Paul Henne and Samuel Murray, editors, *Advances in Experimental Philosophy of Action*, pages. 87–111. London: Bloomsbury, 2023.

Elisabeth Pacherie. Perception, emotions, and delusions: The case of the Capgras delusion. In Bayne, Tim Bayne and Jordi Fernández, editors, *Delusion and Self-Deception: Affective and Motivational Influences on Belief Formation*, pages 107–125, New York: Psychology Press, 2009.

Charalampos Pandis, Niruj Agrawal, and Norman Poole. Capgras' delusion: A systematic review of 255 published cases. *Psychopathology*, 52:1–13, 2019. doi: 10.1159/000500474.

Matthew Parrott. Delusional predictions and explanations. *The British Journal for the Philosophy of Science*, 72(1):325–353 2021.

Joëlle Proust. *The Philosophy of Metacognition: Mental Agency and Self-Awareness*. Oxford: Oxford University Press, 2013.

James Pryor. The skeptic and the dogmatist. *Noûs*, 34(4):517–549, 2000.

Rosa Ritunnano, Joshua Kleinman, Danniella Whyte Oshodi, Maria Michail, Barnaby Nelson, Clara S. Humpston, and Matthew R. Broome. Subjective experience and meaning of delusions in psychosis: A systematic review and qualitative evidence synthesis. *The Lancet Psychiatry*, 9(6):458–476, 2022.

Robert C. Roberts. *Emotions: An Essay in Aid of Moral Psychology*. Cambridge: Cambridge University Press, 2003.

Bertrand Russell. *The Problems of Philosophy*. Home University Library, 1912.

Susanna Schellenberg. *The Unity of Perception: Content, Consciousness, Evidence*. Oxford University Press, 2018.

Susanna Siegel. Congnitive penetrability and perceptual justification. *Noûs*, 46(2): 201–222, 2012.

Susanna Siegel. *The Rationality of Perception*. Oxford University Press, 2016.

Mona Simion. Resistance to evidence and the duty to believe. *Philosophy and Phenomenological Research*, 108(1):203–216, 2024.

Rob Sips, Zeno Van Duppen, Zuzana Kasanova, Lena De Thurah, Ana Teixeira, Jasper Feyaerts, and Inez Myin-Germeys. Psychosis as a dialectic of aha- and anti-aha-experiences: A qualitative study. *Psychosis*, 13(1):47–57, 2021.

Ernest Sosa. *A Virtue Epistemology: Apt Belief and Reflective Knowledge*, volume 1. Oxford: Oxford University Press, 2007.

Christine Tappolet. *Emotions, Values, and Agency*. Oxford: Oxford University Press, 2016.

Silvan S. Tomkins. *Affect Imagery Consciousness: The Complete Edition: Two Volumes*. Springer Publishing Company, 2008.

Martha Turner and Max Coltheart. Confabulation and delusion: A common monitoring framework. *Cognitive Neuropsychiatry*, 15:346–376, 2010.

Esmé Weijun Wang. *The Collected Schizophrenias*. Minneapolis: Graywolf Press, 2019.

Sam Wilkinson. A mental files approach to delusional misidentification. *Review of Philosophy and Psychology*, 7(2):389–404, 2016.

Timothy Williamson. *Knowledge and Its Limits*. Oxford: Oxford University Press, 2002.

Todd S. Woodward, Steffen Moritz, Carrie Cuttler, and Jennifer C. Whitman. The contribution of a cognitive bias against disconfirmatory evidence (bade) to delusions in schizophrenia. *Journal of Clinical and Experimental Neuropsychology*, 28(4):605–617, 2006.

Andrew Young and Kate Leafhead. Betwixt life and death: Case studies of the Cotard delusion. In Peter Halligan and John Marshall, editors, *Method in Madness: Case Studies in Cognitive Neuropsychiatry*, pages 147–171, New York: Psychology Press, 1996.

# 13

# DELUSION AND DOUBLE BOOKKEEPING

*José Eduardo Porcher*

## 1. Introduction

Eugen Bleuler forged the notion of *double bookkeeping* in his monograph *Dementia Praecox or the Group of Schizophrenias* (1911/1950) and his subsequent *Textbook of Psychiatry* (1916/1924), referring to patients' ability to separate their delusional world from the everyday socially shared world. Bleuler observed that his patients frequently failed to act according to their delusions, for instance, to bark like a dog when they professed to be a dog (1916/1924: 144): 'Kings and emperors, popes and redeemers engage, for the most part, in quite banal work.... None of our generals has ever attempted to act in accordance with his imaginary rank and station' (1911/1950: 129).

Bleuler introduces the concept of 'double-entry bookkeeping' at the beginning of his book, in the section on 'intact simple functions', where he contends that schizophrenia is not a deficit of cognitive capacities. He observed that even when patients are absorbed in their psychotic experiences and nearly impossible to interact with, they are acutely aware of what is happening in the shared world. Louis Sass, who is responsible for the revival of interest in double bookkeeping, notes that this kind of ambivalence is widespread in patients with schizophrenia. While deeply engaged in their delusions, some treat them with distance or irony, even during heightened psychotic periods. 'Rather than mistaking the imaginary for the real, they often appear to be living in two parallel but separate worlds: consensual reality and the realm of their hallucinations and delusions' (Sass 1994: 21).

Some patients describe this duality with illuminating precision:

I often feel that many of my aberrant pseudo-perceptions feel the way they do because I am actually perceiving them taking place in a parallel reality that only partially overlaps with this one.

*(Patient quoted in Sass 2014)*

There are two worlds. There is the unreal world, which is the world I am in and we are in. And then there is the real world. The only thing that is real in the unreal world is my own self. Everything else—buildings, trees, houses—is unreal. All other humans are extras. My body is part of the charade. There is a real world somewhere and from there someone or something is trying to control me by putting thoughts into my head or by creating ... screaming voices inside my head.

*(Patient quoted in Parnas and Henriksen 2016)*

It was at this point, I think, that my life truly began to operate as though it were being lived on two trains, their tracks side by side. On one track, the train held the things of the 'real world'—my academic schedule and responsibilities, my books, my connection to my family. ... On the other track: the increasingly confusing and even frightening inner workings of my mind. The struggle was to keep the trains parallel on their tracks, and not have them suddenly and violently collide with each other.

*(Saks 2007)*

Even though the phenomenon is well-known to most experienced clinicians, contemporary mainstream psychiatry has failed to address it (Parnas and Henriksen 2016). Nevertheless, in the last decade or so, there has been emerging interest in double bookkeeping (Gallagher 2009; Sass 2014; Cermolacce et al. 2018; Porcher 2019a). These contributions deal mainly with theoretical issues concerning delusion and draw from first-person accounts of schizophrenia. In contrast to mainstream psychiatry, the basic idea in these latter studies is that the patient's experience of the world must not simply be mistaken but altered or transformed globally.

Sass maintains that keeping two separate sets of mental 'books' safeguards the patient's thoughts' relative internal coherence. In the first book, the one used for everyday life and social interaction and the one which nondelusional subjects share, the patient's thoughts are treated as empirical beliefs subject to reality testing by intersubjective standards of confirmation. Moreover, as empirical beliefs, these thoughts will have the appropriate, stereotypical connections to reasoning, action, and affect. Of course, this represents the vast majority of even the most floridly delusional patient's beliefs.

In the second book, intersubjective standards of confirmation are suspended, as are the usual connections to the patient's other mental states, actions, and emotions. In this book, thoughts are treated in a highly subjective way. As Jennifer Radden (2011: 9) notes, Immanuel Kant anticipates this view in his *Anthropology from a Pragmatic Point of View*, where he describes delusional states as 'a play of thoughts in which he sees, acts, and judges, not in a common world, but rather in his own world (as in dreaming)' (Kant 1798/2006: 114).

Philip Gerrans (2013) provides a helpful illustration regarding how the dynamics of double bookkeeping might work. A violent headache might trigger the thought, 'I have a brain tumour'. Suppose someone enters this thought in the first (intersubjective) book. That thought is quickly canceled because one will consider alternative causes (e.g., 'I received a blow to the head in boxing practice earlier today'). However, in the case of someone who enters this thought in the second (subjective) book, the absence of a commitment towards revising or replacing the thought (if another has better epistemic credentials) will result in its adoption. As Gerrans observes, double bookkeeping 'represents a psychology trying to maintain an unstable solipsistic attitude, which is why the patient has to keep two sets of books but constantly struggles to reconcile them' (Gerrans 2013: 86).

This chapter connects the phenomenon of double bookkeeping to two critical debates in the philosophy of delusion: one from the analytic tradition and one from the phenomenological tradition. First, I will show how the failure of action guidance on the part of some delusions suggests an argument against the standard view that delusions are beliefs (doxasticism about delusion) and how its proponents have countered it by ascribing behavioral inertia to avolition, emotional disturbances, or a failure of the surrounding environment in supporting the agent's motivation to act. Second, I will show how the mismatch between the experience of double bookkeeping and that of having the usual propositional attitudes of folk psychology suggests another, more recalcitrant argument not only against doxasticism but against the very attempt to fit delusion into folk psychology (Porcher 2019b). Third, I will show how phenomenologically inspired theories of delusion, such as the multiple realities hypothesis, bypass the debates above and focus on describing and understanding the disturbances in the structure of experience undergone by patients. I conclude that the philosophical discussions ensuing from an appreciation of double book-keeping show some of the limitations of the analytic philosophical approach to delusion.

## 2. Belief and action

Clinicians, theorists, and the general population commonly think of and characterize delusions as beliefs (Rose, Buckwalter, and Turri 2014). The definition of delusion in the Glossary of Technical Terms of the *Diagnostic and Statistical Manual of Mental Disorders* (*DSM-5*) reflects that popular intuition:

> A false belief based on incorrect inference about external reality that is firmly held despite what almost everyone else believes and despite what constitutes incontrovertible and obvious proof or evidence to the contrary. The belief is not one ordinarily accepted by other members of the person's culture or subculture (e.g., it is not an article of religious faith).
>
> *(American Psychiatric Association 2013: 819)*

The behavioural inertia of some delusional patients motivates one of the main arguments against doxasticism about delusion, namely, the argument from action guidance. It shares its structure with other arguments indicating that delusion's functional role departs from that of belief. Consequently, one can restate the general argument by pointing to other disparities between the functional role of delusion and that expected of belief (e.g., inferential, affective, phenomenological, etc.). Regarding the argument from action guidance, what matters is that, as we have seen, some patients who seem convinced of their delusions nevertheless act as if they were either untrue or irrelevant (see Tumulty, Chapter 18, for more on delusion and action).

The argument's major premise is a broad functionalism about belief, i.e., the idea that what it takes for a mental state to be a belief is for it to play a specific functional role. Such a functionalist view is assumed throughout the literature, so I will not take issue with it here. The argument's minor premise, drawing on clinical experience, denies that delusion plays the expected functional role concerning action guidance. Therefore, the argument goes, those patients do not believe the content of their delusions (cf. Miyazono and Bortolotti 2015 for a critical response to the argument).

There are at least two problems with this line of argument. The first problem is that various factors may explain why patients fail to behave as expected, even in the grip of a delusional belief. Action is not caused by cognitive states alone but by cognitive states in conjunction with motivational states. The motivation to act may not be acquired or sustained in some cases. Hence, to conclude from the fact that some delusional patients fail to act in the expected ways that they do not believe the content of their delusions is to ignore that the patient's state involves less than ideal conditions for belief to influence action (Bayne and Pacherie 2005).

Behavioural inertia may be due to several cognitive and affective internal causes. On the cognitive side, failures in the metarepresentational capacities involved in accessing one's goals may account for the inability to produce self-willed as opposed to stimulus-elicited action (Frith 1992). On the affective side, Lisa Bortolotti (2011) cites three possible causes. First, flattened affect, which Bleuler identified with schizophrenia: 'Indifference seems to be the external sign of their state.... The patients appear lazy and negligent because they no longer have the urge to do anything either of their own initiative or at the bidding of another' (1911/1950: 70). Second, avolition, a failure to convert experience into goal-directed action, which Emil Kraepelin likewise identified with schizophrenia (Foussias and Remington 2010). Third, a deficit in the ability to couple behavior to the motivational properties of a stimulus despite equivalent subjective in-the-moment pleasantness and arousal ratings for these stimuli compared with healthy controls (Heerey and Gold 2007).

Yet another possible cause undermining motivation is the presence of emotional disturbances and developmental and epidemiological factors influencing the onset of psychosis. People at high risk of psychosis experience distress, decreased motivation, and poor socialization from an early age (Broome et al. 2005). Due to the widespread comorbidity between schizophrenia and depression, hopelessness and pessimism may explain why some delusional patients may find it hard to acquire or sustain a motivation to act.

Besides the cognitive and affective aspects of schizophrenia and delusional disorders, the surrounding environment in which delusion (or the patient's perception of it) manifests may also not support the agent's motivation to act. For instance, because some patients may know that acting on their beliefs might result in hospitalization, a fear of involuntary commitment may account for the failure of patients to act accordingly (Bayne and Pacherie 2005: 185).

The second problem with the argument from action guidance is that the behavioural circumscription working as its minor premise, though observed in many cases of delusion, is by no means a general feature. Consequently, some cases will support the attribution of belief (Bayne and Pacherie 2005). A large study reported that 77 per cent of delusional patients acted on their delusions the month before admission (Wessely *et al.* 1993). A review of 260 cases of delusional misidentification found that physical violence occurred in 18 per cent of cases (Förstl *et al.* 1991). It is well known, for instance, that some erotomania patients often act violently based on their delusions (O'Dwyer 1990) and that some Cotard delusion patients display congruent behaviors, such as refusing to move, eat, or shower (Young and Leafhead 1996). Hence, the argument from action guidance has, at best, the power to undermine the generality of a doxastic account of delusions without thereby establishing the generality of an alternative characterization. Not only that, Bortolotti (2009) notes that all sorts of beliefs fail to be appropriately hooked up to action without us questioning their doxastic status.

Moreover, the empirical evidence just mentioned fits the doxastic model better than imagination-based metacognitive accounts (e.g., Currie 2000). If doxasticism cannot provide a general enough account because it fails to include the cases to which its detractors allude, the reverse is also true: the cases that more naturally are explainable by doxasticism resist explanation by non-doxasticism. Thus, no sweeping positive morals are forthcoming from the debate on action guidance. On the contrary, the heterogeneity of delusions puts pressure on anyone ever arriving at a characterization that is at once general and precise (Porcher 2018).

## 3.  Belief and experience

While the behavioral output of double bookkeeping cannot conclusively undermine doxasticism about delusion, the experience of double bookkeeping seems to depart so starkly from the typical experience of believing that it motivates another argument against doxasticism (Radden 2011; Gerrans 2013). While the major premise of the argument from action guidance states that to be a belief is to play a functional role, the argument from experience presupposes, at a minimum, that there is something it is like to have a belief. Like the minor premise in the argument from action guidance, the argument from experience denies that cases of double bookkeeping match the phenomenology of believing. Therefore, such cases, at least, are not instances of believing.

In his account of double bookkeeping, Sass focuses on the most famous case in psychiatric history, namely that of Daniel Paul Schreber, an appellate judge in the kingdom of Saxony who spent 13 years in mental asylums. Schreber wrote vividly and lucidly of his experiences with schizophrenia in *Memoirs of My Nervous Illness*. His account was the subject of significant attention by the foremost psychiatrists of the time (Freud 1911; Bleuler 1912; Jaspers 1913). The core of Schreber's delusional system was the conviction that he had a mission to redeem the world and restore humanity to its lost state of bliss. For this to happen, divine forces were preparing him for a sexual union with God by changing him into a woman so he could give birth to a new race free from original sin.

Over the years, many have interpreted Schreber's delusions as instances of poor reality testing. In a legal brief, the superintendent of his asylum wrote of Schreber, 'What objectively seen appears as delusions and hallucinations is to him (a) unassailable truth and (b) adequate motive for action' (Schreber 1903/1988: 301). It is thus remarkable that Schreber himself rejects the superintendent's characterization in the same legal document:

> I have to confirm . . . that my so-called delusional system is unshakeable certainty, with the same decisive 'yes' as I have to counter . . . that my delusions are adequate motives for action, with the strongest possible 'no.' I could even say with Jesus Christ: 'My Kingdom is not of this world,' my so-called delusions are concerned solely with God and the beyond, they can therefore never in any way influence my behavior in any worldly matter ...
>
> *(Schreber 1903/1988: 301–302)*

As we can see in Schreber's testimony, double bookkeeping gives rise to first-person reports that point to the ineffability of the experience, often expressed in figurative and metaphorical language: 'To make myself at least somewhat comprehensible', Schreber says, 'I shall have to speak much in images and similes, which may at times perhaps be only *approximately* correct' (1903/1988: 41). While describing how he was affected during his experiences, Schreber may seem to have referred to the neurology of his time, but his 'nerves' are not affected physically but spiritually through the mediation of supernatural 'rays'

(Radden 2011: 50). As he explains in the following passage, we are used to thinking of all impressions we receive from the external world as derived from the five senses. However:

> in the case of a human being who like myself has entered into contact with rays and whose head is in consequence so to speak illuminated by rays, this is not so at all. I receive light and sound sensations which are projected directly on to my inner nervous system by the rays; for their reception the external organs of seeing and hearing are not necessary.
>
> *(Schreber 1903/1988: 117)*

As Sass (2014: 132) notes, the non-literal nature of Schreber's delusion is apparent in his account of being transformed into a woman. According to Schreber, this event occurred when he stood in front of a mirror looking at himself while stripped to the waist wearing jewelry: 'my breast gives the impression of a pretty well-developed female bosom' (Schreber 1903/1988: 207). Schreber is not describing an actual anatomical change but a way of seeing or construing physical reality.

The high frequency of subjunctification betrays the seeming ineffability of some delusional experiences, and we find it peppered throughout first-person accounts of double bookkeeping. A subjunctifier is 'anything that gives a sign that a subject's utterance is not to be confidently understood as a straightforward description of momentary experience' (Hurlburt 2011: 116). Subjunctifier phrases such as 'I think,' 'It's like a . . .,' 'kind of,' and 'that's the best way I can think to describe it' are qualifications, shifting descriptions, and explicitly voiced doubts and uncertainties that accompany introspective reports.

Consider mathematician John Nash's assertion to an interviewer in the PBS documentary *A Brilliant Madness* that his delusions are 'kind of like a dream'. Or the patient who, when describing what the subjective, lived dimension of his delusion is like, states that 'I feel that I'm concocting a story' (Alexander, Stuss, and Benson 1979: 335). While not all patients report feeling the same kind of atmosphere, reports of feelings are commonplace when experience seems to beggar description in straightforward doxastic terminology. Consider, for example, the following remarks by a highly ambivalent patient:

> I've never rigidly held my beliefs about Pepperidge Farm [an American brand of baked foods] and microwaves, but they've always involved a strong feeling of fear and aversion, related to my feeling that nothing exists—however, I have acted consistently, over long periods of time, as if these beliefs were unquestionably true... but I've always had a dimension of doubt about these beliefs, and, of course, I realize how profoundly irrational they sound to other people... I would much prefer to believe that I am delusional rather than that all these magical events and processes are real.
>
> *(Patient quoted in Sass 2004: 79)*

The difficulty in pigeonholing delusions, whether in the category of belief or as imaginative states misidentified as beliefs, leads to the recognition that the subject may have an ambiguous relationship with the content of the delusion. Accordingly, it may be that such delusions play a functional role somewhere in between that of a belief and an imagining (Currie 2000: 174). This is sometimes called the *continuum hypothesis* (Kind, 2024). We may conceive belief and imagination as a many-dimensional cognitive space with two main clusters and various outliers. In this vein, Andy Egan (2009) has proposed blurring the boundaries between belief and imagination by introducing a hybrid propositional attitude he calls 'bimagination', speculating that this type of attitude has some of the features of belief and some of the features of imagination.

While it seems correct that a definite distinction between belief and imagination is not forthcoming since both are vague folk psychological concepts, replacing belief or imagination with bimagination does not solve the problem of accurately characterizing the mental state of delusional patients—especially those who manifest double bookkeeping. While the functional role and phenomenology of belief do not match up with some cases of delusion, little or nothing is to be gained by a redescription in terms of hybrid attitudes (Porcher 2018). Indeed, first-person testimonies do not raise the question: Does the patient believe such and such? Instead, they raise etiological and explanatory questions: what gives rise to the patient's experiences? Why does the patient interpret them the way they do?

Even if the concept of belief or other folk psychological attitudes were sufficiently precise, it is a further question as to why we should care about whether delusions are anomalous beliefs, cognitive hallucinations, or some hybrid state. Is the language of folk psychology apt to play a prominent role in explaining delusion (Porcher 2016, see also Murphy, Chapter 25)? Although a valuable tool for conceptualizing and dealing with ourselves and others, the vocabulary of folk psychology abstracts entirely from cognitive and neural processes and may thereby jeopardize the prospect of an explanation of the phenomena that integrates multiple levels of description (Gerrans 2014).

## 4. Phenomenology

In his monumental *General Psychopathology*, Karl Jaspers argues that simply saying that a delusion is an incorrigible, firmly held misconception held by the patient is only a superficial description. Indeed, in light of the preceding discussion, the definition of delusion as 'a false belief … about external reality' (American Psychiatric Association [APA] 2013: 819) seems like an impoverished one to contemplate their intricate complexity. We can say confidently that at least schizophrenic delusions involving double bookkeeping are more than just erroneous beliefs. For this reason, Jaspers (1913/1963: 93–94) is adamant that we must understand them as arising in the context of shifts in the sense of reality and belonging since they involve a transformation in one's total awareness of reality.

A fundamental notion developed by Jaspers in connection with delusion is that of the delusional 'atmosphere'. The formation of what he and Kurt Schneider called 'primary' delusions happens as a felt experience, and hints of subthreshold psychotic experiences frequently announce it. Jaspers describes this instability in the foundation of the field of experience as an 'abnormal awareness of significance', and it has been variously designated as predelusional, prodromal, or micropsychotic. As Mads Henriksen and Josef Parnas explain:

> A crystallization of a primary delusion is not based on an *inferential error* about empirical matters in the public world but on the *affection of and within* the subjectivity itself by a revelation of delusional meaning, often carrying with it a sense of 'absolute', 'apodictic' certainty, not completely unlike the certainty of experiencing a sensation (a so-called 'egological conviction', like the certitude of having a toothache).
>
> *(Henriksen and Parnas 2014: 545)*

In schizophrenia spectrum disorders, delusional atmosphere often elicits a distinctive hyper-reflexive attitude in which patients become intensely absorbed with the felt qualities of subjective experience (Feyaerts et al. 2021). As double bookkeeping underscores, rather than mistaking their delusions for reality, patients regularly point out how they pertain to a different quasi-solipsistic realm (Sass 1994). Thus, they lack the complete actuality, practical consequences, and availability to others that accompany real-world experience. On the other hand, this altered sense of reality does not render such delusions merely subjective. As Schreber's case elucidates, for some patients, the salience and relevance of delusional experience can considerably exceed the banality of everyday life.

The things said and done by the person with schizophrenic delusions will remain mysterious if we do not understand their existential context (Laing 1960: 15). That is why Sass and Parnas (2007: 65) insist that we must interpret the symptoms of schizophrenia as alterations in the overall structure of experience. A phenomenological understanding may allow us to make sense of actions or beliefs that might initially seem incomprehensible. As Matthew Ratcliffe forcefully argues:

> It is not that they take the real to be unreal or vice versa. Rather, the overall structure of experience has changed and the patient no longer experiences or believes anything in quite the same way anymore. It follows that her experience cannot be adequately interpreted if it is assumed from the outset that she occupies the same background 'natural attitude' as oneself. One has to cease presupposing the usual sense of reality and recognize that her existential orientation has shifted, sometimes radically. Phenomenology therefore plays an indispensable interpretive role.
>
> *(Ratcliffe 2009: 228)*

As many of the experiential changes reported in psychiatric illness involve alterations of the sense of reality and belonging, Ratcliffe (2009: 227) argues that we must adopt a *phenomenological stance* to endeavor to understand such existential changes. He insists that such a stance does not mean a radical transformation of all experience, where one becomes, as Edmund Husserl put it, a 'non-participating observer'. Minimally, it is a methodological shift by which one comes to appreciate that any point of view that takes the sense of reality for granted will be insufficient to deal with profound experiential alterations. That would include alterations like double bookkeeping and other changes in the structures of experience, such as those manifesting in depressive disorders.

In recognizing an experientially constituted sense of reality and belonging and committing to investigate and describe this and other aspects of experience, phenomenologically informed theorists have provided frameworks that have enriched our understanding of psychosis. Concerning double bookkeeping, in particular, the idea of *multiple realities* due to Alfred Schütz (1945)—via the 'sub-universes' of William James (1890: 291–306)—may be particularly enlightening.

As Shaun Gallagher (2009: 254ff.) explains, the experiencing subject does not live in a unified world of meaning that is objectively defined but in finite provinces of meaning. James and Schütz agree that there is an ultimate reality, the reality of shared everyday life in which we usually engage, work, socialize, etc. But several other realities take us away from everyday reality. When we read fiction, watch a play or film, or play a video game, we spend time inhabiting a different reality that unfolds on the page, the stage, or the screen. In such realities, we may not have a role to play and may identify with one or more characters. In dreams and various fantasies, we may play a more active role as ourselves or as a modified version of ourselves, but not the one we play in our everyday reality.

As Sass observes, the delusional subject 'inhabits a world radically alien to that of common sense' (1992: 109). Accordingly, Gallagher hypothesizes that when a subject enters a delusional state, they enter an alternative reality. Unlike other realities, however, this one may be 'firmly sustained' and 'not one ordinarily accepted by other members of the person's culture or subculture.' The degree with which it is sustained will, of course, vary:

> A dream is something that ends and too quickly dissipates as we wake up ... a drama comes to an end when the theatre lights come on. One can slip in and out of a delusional reality. Some delusions, however, may progress to the point where they are more like being in a theatre where the lights fail to come on. Thus delusional patients sometime report pervasive feelings of strangeness, where everything seems somehow unreal or unfamiliar ... Furthermore, and importantly, realities created in theatre, film, novels, and games are socially constructed realities, they are for others, and by definition are understandable to many people. Some delusions are more like dreams; they are in some regards idiosyncratic ... although they may share certain themes, such as being controlled by others, seeing others as impostors, and so forth. Thus, although delusions are not 'for others' they do not exclude others from appearing within the delusional reality.
>
> *(Gallagher 2009: 256)*

To consider a delusion an alternative reality, as defined by Schütz, requires that we see it neither as a set of false beliefs about the everyday world nor a mere collection of odd beliefs about an alternative world. Instead, it is primarily something experiential. It honours Jaspers' insistence that we should not try to abstract it from that through which the subject lives. However, if Gallagher is correct, the mistake of those who reduce delusion to a belief about everyday reality is not only to remain 'too cognitive,' but to *target the wrong world* (2009: 257, my emphasis). Suppose the delusion is not about external or everyday reality but concerns an alternative reality in the same way that events that occur in a play are tied to a fictional reality. In that case, this fact has not only theoretical but clinical significance.

Gallagher (2009: 260) argues that the multiple realities hypothesis throws light onto the paradox of double bookkeeping because it predicts the possibility of the subjects taking an ironic attitude towards the delusion. They may be unable to maintain distance as they are caught up in the delusional reality. Still, to the extent that they can shift back to everyday reality, they may be able to appreciate the strangeness of the delusion. Consider, for example, the following excerpt of an interview with a patient who showed symptoms of both Capgras delusion and reduplicative paramnesia. The patient maintained that his house and family had been replaced by duplicates:

E:  *Isn't that [two families] unusual?*
S:  *It was unbelievable!*
E:  *How do you account for it?*
S:  *I don't know. I try to understand it myself, and it was virtually impossible.*
E:  *What if I told you I don't believe it?*
S:  *That's perfectly understandable. In fact, when I tell the story, I feel that I'm concocting a story . . . It's not quite right. Something is wrong.*

*E:   If someone told you the story, what would you think?*
*S:    I would find it extremely hard to believe. I should be defending myself.*
(Alexander, Stuss, and Benson 1979: 335)

Such shifting back and forth may also explain why the patient viewed his wife as an impostor (in delusional reality) but happily ate the food she gave him (in everyday reality). For this hypothesis to be empirically helpful, Gallagher recommends the investigation of the frequency and degree to which patients can shift between multiple realities as they move in and out of delusional states, the nature of the transitions, whether shifting is more frequent in prodromal cases, or cases of partial remission, and so on (Gallagher 2009: 260).

Michel Cermolacce and colleagues see therapeutical potential in the multiple realities hypothesis. They argue that in cases of double bookkeeping, shared reality and delusional reality, although exclusive to one another, are not incompatible but *compossible*. They may therefore be articulated under some third-party reality, or what they call 'hybrid objects', the existence of which reveals the possibility of being part of several realities at the same time and for a subject to be set free of a particular reality via their interplay. 'So can we both account for the flexibility of delusion and for the possible conditions for a verbal treatment of it' (Cermolacce *et al.* 2018: 5).

Whatever the merits of this particular framework, psychiatry should strive to understand disordered human experience besides evaluating, diagnosing, and classifying it. In offering tools to make sense of mental distress, phenomenological psychopathology pivots the focus on diagnosis and symptoms to include the complexity and diversity of people's experiences. Furthermore, it embraces scrutiny of what is significant from the patient's point of view, potentially revealing how a patient's vulnerability and distress are distinctly personal. Instead of correcting 'errors of judgment', phenomenologically informed approaches explore patients' experiences as relevant sources of meaning for them (Henriksen and Parnas 2014). This is essential since giving them a voice is a precondition for understanding their wounded existence and opening themselves up to discovering new psychopathological knowledge.

## 5.   Conclusion

In this chapter, I have given a brief but opinionated overview of philosophical treatments of the phenomenon of double bookkeeping. Its paradigmatic cases suggest that schizophrenic delusions, although they linguistically resemble epistemic claims about worldly matters, are actually attempts to frame and verbalize anomalous experiences of an already altered subjectivity (Škodlar *et al.* 2013). As we have seen, patients with schizophrenic delusions can sometimes cope with everyday reality despite their delusions' seeming incomprehensibility and incorrigibility, as though they were untrue or irrelevant, and the coexistence of delusional and everyday realms implies the inconsequentiality of delusional experience we have touched upon (Poupart *et al.* 2021). Moreover, double bookkeeping points to the fact that the medical notions of symptoms and signs cannot adequately address the psychopathological manifestations of schizophrenia (Parnas, Urfer-Parnas, and Stephensen 2021). Finally, double bookkeeping may also partly explain why current research on insight, ignoring the possible coexistence of multiple realities, may fail to give a consistent and specific model of schizophrenic delusion (Henriksen and Parnas 2014).

Besides being of interest in itself, double bookkeeping sheds light on the reach of analytic philosophical vs. phenomenological ways of attending to psychiatric illness (Sass 2004). However, this divide is thankfully becoming increasingly blurred. In analytic philosophy of psychiatry, it has inspired debates about whether or not delusions are beliefs, and if they are, how we are to explain their deviations from the stereotypical functional role of belief. These discussions have shed light on the role and applicability of folk psychological categories and led to significant conclusions on delusional action guidance. For this, they are welcome additions to the literature. However, I have noted that they often bypass the more essential questions regarding the patients' experiences with double bookkeeping and how we should understand such alterations. In the phenomenological philosophy of psychiatry, double bookkeeping has inspired a wealth of analyses, interpretations, and theories to account for this most puzzling of human experiences. Hopefully, these will gain even more traction in main psychiatry in the next years and increasingly inform empirical research and psychotherapeutic approaches.

# References


Alexander, M. P., Stuss, D. T., & Benson, D. F. (1979). Capgras syndrome: A reduplicative phenomenon. *Neurology* 29(3): 334–339.

American Psychiatric Association (2013). *Diagnostic and Statistical Manual of Mental Disorders* (5th ed.). Washington, DC: American Psychiatric Publishing.

Bayne, T. & Pacherie, E. (2005). In defence of the doxastic conception of delusions. *Mind & Language* 20: 163–188.

Bleuler, E. (1911/1950). *Dementia Praecox or the Group of Schizophrenias* (J. Zinkin, Trans.). New York: New York International Universities Press.

Bleuler, E. (1912). Freud, Psychoanalytische Bemerkungen über einen autobiographisch beschriebenen Fall von Paranoia (Dementia paranoides). Jahrbuch für psychoanalytische und psychopathologische Forschungen, Bd. III. *Zentralblatt für Psychoanalyse* 2: 343–348.

Bleuler, E. (1916/1924). *Textbook of Psychiatry* (A. A. Brill, Trans.). New York: Macmillan.

Bortolotti, L. (2009). *Delusions and Other Irrational Beliefs*. Oxford: Oxford University Press.

Bortolotti, L. (2011). Double bookkeeping in delusions: Explaining the gap between saying and doing. In J. H. Aguilar, A. A. Buckareff, & K. Frankish (Eds.) *New Waves in Philosophy of Action*. New York: Palgrave Macmillan: 237–256.

Broome, M. R., Woolley, J. B., Tabraham, P., Johns, L. C., Bramon, E., Murray, G. K., Pariante, C., McGuire, P. K., & Murray, R. M. (2005). What causes the onset of psychosis? *Schizophrenia Research* 79(1): 23–34.

Cermolacce, M., Despax, K., Richieri, R., & Naudin, J. (2018). Multiple realities and hybrid objects: A creative approach of schizophrenic delusion. *Frontiers in Psychology* 9: 107.

Currie, G. (2000). Imagination, delusion and hallucinations. *Mind & Language* 15(1): 168–183.

Egan, A. (2009). Imagination, delusion, and self-deception. In T. Bayne & J. Fernandez (Eds.) *Delusion and Self-Deception: Affective and Motivational Influences on Belief Formation*. New York: Psychology Press: 263–280.

Feyaerts, J., Henriksen, M. G., Vanheule, S., Myin-Germeys, I., & Sass, L. A. (2021). Delusions beyond beliefs: A critical overview of diagnostic, aetiological, and therapeutic schizophrenia research from a clinical-phenomenological perspective. *The Lancet Psychiatry* 8(3): 237–249.

Förstl, H., Almeida, O. P., Owen, A. M., Burns, A., & Howard, R. (1991). Psychiatric, neurological and medical aspects of misidentification syndromes: A review of 260 cases. *Psychological Medicine* 21: 905–910.

Foussias, G. & Remington, G. (2010). Negative symptoms in schizophrenia: Avolition and Occam's razor. *Schizophrenia Bulletin* 36(2): 359–369.

Freud, S. (1911/2003). *The Schreber Case* (A. Webber, Trans.). New York: Penguin Classics.

Frith, C. D. (1992). *The Cognitive Neuropsychology of Schizophrenia*. Hove: Psychology Press.

Gallagher, S. (2009). Delusional realities. In M. Broome & L. Bortolotti (Eds.) *Psychiatry as Cognitive Neuroscience: Philosophical Perspectives*. New York: Oxford University Press: 245–266.

Gerrans, P. (2013). Delusional attitudes and default thinking. *Mind & Language* 28(1): 83–102.

Gerrans, P. (2014). *The Measure of Madness: Philosophy of Mind, Cognitive Neuroscience, and Delusional Thought*. Cambridge: The MIT Press.

Heerey, E. A. & Gold, J. M. (2007). Patients with schizophrenia demonstrate dissociation between affective experience and motivated behavior. *Journal of Abnormal Psychology* 116(2): 268–278.

Henriksen, M. G. & Parnas, J. (2014). Self-disorders and schizophrenia: A phenomenological reappraisal of poor insight and noncompliance. *Schizophrenia Bulletin* 40(3): 542–547.

Hurlburt, R. T. (2011). *Investigating Pristine Inner Experience: Moments of Truth*. Cambridge: Cambridge University Press.

James, W. (1890). *The Principles of Psychology* (Vol. 2). New York: Henry Holt and Company.

Jaspers, K. (1913/1963). *General Psychopathology* (J. Hoenig & M. W. Hamilton, Trans.). Manchester: Manchester University Press.

Kant, I. (1798/2006). *Anthropology from a Pragmatic Point of View* (R. B. Louden, Trans.). Cambridge: Cambridge University Press.

Kind, A. (2024). Contrast or continuum? The case of belief and imagination. In E. Sullivan-Bissett (Ed.) *Belief, Imagination, and Delusion*. Oxford: Oxford University Press: 42–59.

Laing, R. D. (1960). *The Divided Self: A Study of Sanity and Madness*. London: Tavistock Publications.

Miyazono, K. & Bortolotti, L. (2015). The causal role argument against doxasticism about delusions. *Avant* 5(3): 30–50.

O'Dwyer, J. M. (1990). Coexistence of the Capgras and de Clerambault's syndromes. *British Journal of Psychiatry* 156: 575–577.

Parnas, J. & Henriksen, M. G. (2016). Mysticism and schizophrenia: A phenomenological exploration of the structure of consciousness in the schizophrenia spectrum disorders. *Consciousness and Cognition* 43: 75–88.

Parnas, J., Urfer-Parnas, A., & Stephensen, H. (2021). Double bookkeeping and schizophrenia spectrum: Divided unified phenomenal consciousness. *European Archives of Psychiatry and Clinical Neuroscience* 271(8): 1513–1523.

Porcher, J. E. (2016). Delusion as a folk psychological kind. *Filosofia Unisinos* 17(2): 212–226.

Porcher, J. E. (2018). The doxastic status of delusion and the limits of folk psychology. In I. Hipólito, J. Gonçalves, & J. Pereira (Eds.) *Schizophrenia and Common Sense*. Cham: Springer: 175–90.

Porcher, J. E. (2019a). Double bookkeeping and doxasticism about delusion. *Philosophy, Psychiatry, & Psychology* 26(2): 111–119.

Porcher, J. E. (2019b). Delusion, folk psychology, and the scientific image. *Philosophy, Psychiatry, & Psychology* 26(2): 129–131.

Poupart, F., Bouscail, M., Sturm, G., Bensoussan, A., Galliot, G., & Gozé, T. (2021). Acting on delusion and delusional inconsequentiality: A review. *Comprehensive Psychiatry* 106: 152230.

Radden, J. (2011). *On Delusion*. London: Routledge.

Ratcliffe, M. (2009). Understanding existential changes in psychiatric illness: The indispensability of phenomenology. In M. Broome & L. Bortolotti (Eds.) *Psychiatry as Cognitive Neuroscience: Philosophical Perspectives*. New York: Oxford University Press: 221–244.

Rose, D., Buckwalter, W., & Turri, J. (2014). When words speak louder than actions: Delusion, belief, and the power of assertion. *Australasian Journal of Philosophy* 92(4): 683–700.

Saks, E. R. (2007). *The Center Cannot Hold*. New York: Hyperion.

Sass, L. A. (1992). Heidegger, schizophrenia and the ontological difference. *Philosophical Psychology* 5: 109–132.

Sass, L. A. (1994). *The Paradoxes of Delusion: Wittgenstein, Schreber, and the Schizophrenic mind*. New York: Cornell University Press.

Sass, L. A. (2004). Some reflections on the (analytic) philosophical approach to delusion. *Philosophy, Psychiatry, & Psychology* 11(1): 71–80.

Sass, L. A. (2014). Delusion and double bookkeeping. In T. Fuchs, T. Breyer & C. Mundt C (Eds.) *Karl Jaspers' Philosophy and Psychopathology*. New York: Springer: 125–247.

Sass, L. A., & Parnas, J. (2007). Explaining schizophrenia: The relevance of phenomenology. In M. C. Chung, K. W. M. (B.) Fulford, & G. Graham (Eds.) *Reconceiving Schizophrenia*. Oxford: Oxford University Press: 63–95.

Schreber, D. P. (1903/1988). *Memoirs of My Nervous Illness* (I. Macalpine & R. A. Hunter, Trans.). Cambridge, MA: Harvard University Press.

Schütz, A. (1945). On multiple realities. *Philosophy and Phenomenological Research* 5: 533–576.

Škodlar, B., Henriksen, M. G., Sass, L. A., Nelson, B., & Parnas, J. (2013). Cognitive-behavioral therapy for schizophrenia: A critical evaluation of its theoretical framework from a clinical-phenomenological perspective. *Psychopathology* 46(4): 249–265.

Wessely, S., Buchanan, A., Reed, A., Cutting, J., Everitt, B., Garety, P., & Taylor, P. J. (1993). Acting on delusions. I: Prevalence. *British Journal of Psychiatry* 163: 69–76.

Young, A. W. & Leafhead, K. (1996). Betwixt life and death: Case studies of the Cotard delusion. In P. Halligan & J. Marshall (Eds.) *Method in Madness*. New York: Psychology Press: 147–171.

# 14
# DELUSION AND RATIONALITY

*Quinn Hiroshi Gibson and Adam Bradley*

## 1. Introduction

Delusional beliefs are paradigmatic examples of deeply irrational states of mind. For example, a subject suffering from Capgras delusion will assert—and appear to believe—that someone close to them has been replaced by an impostor (Capgras and Rebould-Lechaux 1923). A subject with Cotard delusion will assert that they are dead or do not exist (Cotard 1882). A subject with somatoparaphrenia will assert that a paralyzed limb belongs to someone else (Vallar and Ronchi 2009). On the face of it, these states of mind are highly irrational. Yet as soon as we inquire into the relationship between delusions and rationality, we find ourselves in a maze of questions and puzzles. In this chapter we try to work our way through this maze.

Throughout we mostly discuss *monothematic delusions* like Capgras and Cotard, which tend to be circumscribed to only one subject matter, such as the identity of one's spouse. Monothematic delusions often arise in patients as a result of neurological damage and subjects with monothematic delusions may have no other noticeable pathologies or abnormalities of belief. Monothematic delusions contrast with *polythematic delusions*, which concern many different subjects, are often highly elaborated, and tend to occur in the context of other psychiatric disorders, schizophrenia in particular (Davies et al. 2001: 135). We will follow the trend in recent work in the philosophy of psychiatry by focusing on monothematic delusions.[1]

Here is the outline. First, we make the case that delusions are abnormal irrational beliefs. This requires establishing that delusions are beliefs. We then argue that delusions are *abnormally irrational* beliefs, considering and rejecting several views which deny this. We next turn to the prominent two-factor model of delusion and consider where in the course of a delusional syndrome to locate irrationality.

## 2. Delusions as beliefs

The question of the rationality of delusions is inseparable from the question of what type of mental state they are, as only some mental states are subject to rational constraints.



DOI: 10.4324/9781003296386-18

A subject is irrational in simultaneously believing $p$ and $\sim p$, but not in simultaneously supposing $p$ and $\sim p$ while doing their logic homework. So before we can investigate the rational status of delusions, we need to establish what type of mental state they are. Here we will adopt the view that delusions are beliefs. This view—*doxasticism*—is widely held. For instance, doxasticism is built into the characterization of delusions found in the *DSM-5*: 'Delusions are fixed beliefs that are not amenable to change in light of conflicting evidence' (APA 2013: 87). It is defended by researchers such as Tim Bayne and Elisabeth Pacherie (2005) and Lisa Bortolotti (2009) (for more see Noordhof, Chapter 19).

One may reasonably ask: Why is the doxastic conception of delusions widely held? In short, because delusions appear to have many properties of beliefs. Without articulating a full theory of belief, we can take beliefs to be states of mind that are characteristically truth-directed and which typically play a certain role in guiding speech, inference, and action (Schwitzgebel 2019). For example, a subject with the belief that *it is raining* will characteristically say, infer, and do things consistent with that belief (like carrying an umbrella) and will be sensitive to new evidence on the question (if she looks outside and sees clear skies, she will update her belief).

Monothematic delusions appear to play a similar role in subjects' minds and hence to constitute beliefs. For example, a subject with Capgras delusion will make the apparently sincere assertion that their partner has been replaced by an imposter. Their delusion may also interface with their other mental states in belief-like ways. A subject with this delusion may infer that their real spouse is missing, or take actions to avoid the alleged imposter. Prompting inferences and motivating actions are characteristic features of beliefs. To the extent that delusions do these things, they ought to be regarded as beliefs (for more on delusion and action see Tumulty, Chapter 18).

It should be acknowledged, however, that delusions do not always fit squarely into the category of belief, and that many researchers reject doxasticism (Currie 2000; Currie and Jureidini 2001; Egan 2009; Sass and Pienkos 2013). Opponents of doxasticism emphasize the apparent differences between delusions and paradigmatic beliefs. For example, beliefs are characteristically sensitive to evidence. But delusions are infamously recalcitrant to conflicting evidence: a subject with Cotard delusion will claim that they are dead, ignoring the fact that they are breathing, that their heart is beating, etc. (for more on delusion and evidence see Flores 2021, and Chapter 12). Similarly, beliefs ramify throughout a subject's mind: a new belief influences a subject's other beliefs, and subjects attempt to resolve contradictions that emerge in their belief system. But monothematic delusions are often circumscribed: they are not well-integrated with the delusional subject's wider belief set (a phenomenon known as 'double-bookkeeping' in the literature). For instance, a subject with Capgras delusion may assert that their spouse has been replaced by an imposter, ignoring overwhelming evidence that this is not true. They may continue living with the person claiming to be their spouse, may not call the police to report their missing spouse, and so on. To put it mildly, these do not seem like the actions of someone who genuinely believes that their spouse has been replaced by an uncanny imposter (for more on delusion and double bookkeeping see Porcher, Chapter 13).

There is, therefore, a basic tension in our thinking about delusions: in some ways they resemble beliefs, in others they do not. Indeed, this basic tension animates much of the interest in delusions from psychiatric and philosophical researchers. This tension, however, does not demonstrate that delusions are not beliefs. For one thing, ordinary beliefs themselves often deviate from the ideals of rationality, meaning that the difference between ordinary and delusional beliefs may only be a difference of degree rather than kind (Bortolotti 2009, 2012). For another, non-doxastic views face pressure to explain the belief-like aspects of delusions. One option here is to split the difference in some way by claiming that delusions are 'in-between' beliefs (Schwitzgebel 2012) or some other belief-like state such as aliefs (Gendler 2011) or bimaginings (Egan 2008). For purposes of this chapter, we are setting aside these alternatives and working with the consensus view that delusions are a type of belief (for more on delusion and non-doxasticism see Noordhof, Chapter 20).

## 3.  Delusions as abnormal irrational beliefs

Having settled on the view that delusions are beliefs, we can now turn to the issue of their rationality. As we have discussed, certain rational principles are widely held to be constitutive of belief. Indeed, somewhat paradoxically, a strong (though defeasible) reason for thinking that delusions are beliefs is precisely that they are ordinarily judged seriously irrational. This is because only beliefs appear to have the right normative profile for the issue of rationality to even arise. For instance, if delusions are imaginings (as per Currie), it is hard to say what is irrational about them, since imaginings are not subject to the norms of coherence, evidence sensitivity, and so on, that plausibly characterize belief.[2] It may be odd to routinely imagine that your spouse has been replaced by an imposter, but it is not irrational. So the very fact that we hold delusions to the rational standard of belief suggests that they are beliefs, albeit irrational ones.

As a first pass—and without excluding the possibility that delusions are irrational in other senses—it is very plausible that delusions are *epistemically irrational*. Epistemic rationality is typically characterized in terms of a subject's responsiveness to the evidence that is available to them. A rational subject is a subject who forms beliefs that are appropriate in light of the evidence available to them. An irrational subject is a subject who does not form the beliefs that are appropriate in light of the evidence available to them. For example, a subject who believes that *there is an international cabal of Satanic lizards directing world affairs*, despite having no evidence in support of this claim, is epistemically irrational in virtue of holding this belief.

By this standard, it is plausible that delusional subjects are epistemically irrational. A delusional subject suffering from somatoparaphrenia, for example, will form the belief that *the left arm attached to their body is not, in fact, their own arm but rather belongs to someone else* (Vallar and Ronchi 2009). In one case, a somatoparaphrenic subject attributed their arm to their niece who worked in the hospital (Romano et al. 2014: 216). Suffice it to say, this belief does not square well with the subject's total evidence about the world. Moreover, when you raise dispositive contrary evidence—that the arm is attached to their body, for example—the delusional subject will ignore it or confabulate a reason why it is irrelevant. In short, these subjects do not appear to be rationally responding to the evidence that is available to them.

One complication here is raised by Bortolotti's work on *epistemic innocence* (2015, 2020). Bortolotti argues that while delusions are epistemically irrational, they may still warrant a form of positive epistemic assessment. How can this be? Because delusions, though epistemically irrational, may provide otherwise unobtainable epistemic benefits. For example, consider what Bortolotti calls *motivated delusions*, or delusional beliefs that protect a subject's self-esteem and mental well-being (2015). In a well-known case, a subject developed reverse Othello syndrome—the delusional belief in the persistence of a romantic relationship which has ended—after suffering a traumatic brain injury and having their partner break up with them. The subject's belief in the persistence of their relationship is plainly epistemically irrational. But, plausibly, the delusion plays a role in helping the subject deal with the dual trauma of severe injury and romantic failure. A distinctive epistemic benefit such a delusion might confer is enabling the subject to reason correctly about matters other than the relationship. If the subject has to confront their breakup, they may become too depressed or distraught to properly reason about anything. If so, then this delusional belief would be epistemically irrational, because it conflicts with the subject's wider belief set, but it could nevertheless have a kind of positive epistemic status, in that it enables the subject to engage in better epistemic conduct than they would otherwise be able to. This raises difficult questions about the relation between rationality and positive epistemic assessment generally.

While delusional beliefs appear to be epistemically irrational, they also seem to be irrational in other ways. Epistemic irrationality is a form of *substantive* irrationality: substantively irrational beliefs are poorly justified or fail to be reasonable. But delusional beliefs also seem to violate principles of *structural* rationality. Principles of structural rationality concern how well or poorly one's doxastic attitudes cohere or fit together.[3] Many delusional beliefs appear to violate principles of structural rationality such as consistency. As we have seen, double-bookkeeping is common in delusional subjects, and they sometimes even acknowledge that their delusional beliefs are inconsistent with their other beliefs. For instance, Ryan McKay and Lisa Cipolotti (2007: 353) report the case of LU, who presented with Cotard delusion, but who also 'acknowledged that the fact that she herself was moving and talking was inconsistent with the typical characteristics of dead people'. So, delusional subjects appear to violate principles of structural rationality as well as epistemic rationality.

Finally, we want to emphasize that delusional beliefs are generally irrational in a way that stands out against other beliefs. When we call delusional beliefs 'irrational' in this chapter, we do not merely mean that they are less than fully rational in some idealized sense. Plausibly, few if any of our beliefs satisfy this exacting standard. But even by the rough and ready standards of ordinary cognition, delusions stand out. They strike both ordinary subjects and researchers as outside the norm of human cognition. This leads many researchers to posit some abnormality in the processes of belief formation or maintenance to account for delusional belief. We thus say that delusional beliefs are *abnormally irrational* in order to pick out the fact that they are irrational in a distinctive way, one which calls out for explanation.

This is our initial case for the claim that delusions are abnormally irrational beliefs. There is a remaining question about *scope*: Are all delusions abnormally irrational? Most? Some? We want to say that severe irrationality is a constitutive feature of delusional beliefs, but it is difficult to establish this strong claim. If the idea that delusions are seriously irrational beliefs is meant to be a stipulative definition, then the claim is true but trivial. If, as we intend, the claim is meant to be a generalization about the empirical phenomenon we call 'delusion', then it is questionable whether it is true in all actual delusions let alone all possible delusions. We will now consider a number of positions according to which delusions are not irrational, or at least, not irrational in a distinctive way. By examining these views and their deficiencies, we will not only explore the relationship between delusions and rationality, but also strengthen the case that delusions are indeed irrational.

## 4. Rational after all?

One way of pushing back on the view we have adopted is to claim that while delusions are beliefs, they are not in fact abnormally irrational. Perhaps the clearest example of this approach is the view of Brendan Maher (1974, 1999). Maher holds that delusions are normal cognitive responses to abnormal experiences. In claiming that delusions are reactions to experiences, Maher's view is a paradigmatic version of what John Campbell calls *empiricism* about delusion formation (Campbell 2001). Strictly speaking, Maher's view is not that delusional beliefs are rational per se. Rather, his claim is that delusional beliefs are, as we might say, *ordinarily* rational. This need not imply that the ordinary beliefs we form in our daily lives are rational in any strict sense of the term. Decades of psychological and economic research have shown that human beings are not perfectly rational (if that wasn't already obvious before to any observer of human affairs). This work has charted the ways in which human cognition departs from the ideal of rationality. For example, the base rate fallacy, confirmation bias, anchoring bias, the availability heuristic, and countless other biases have been extremely well investigated (e.g., Tversky and Kahneman 1974; Kahneman et al. 1982).

Maher maintains that the very same epistemic faculties that generate ordinary beliefs in response to ordinary experiences generate delusional beliefs in response to extraordinary experiences. Delusional beliefs are thus no more or less rational than any of our other beliefs. Maher is thus denying that delusions stand out from other beliefs as distinctively irrational. What is true, he acknowledges, is that delusional beliefs strike ordinary subjects as *odd*. But they only seem odd to ordinary subjects because they have not had the sorts of experiences which prompt delusions. If an ordinary subject had the same experiences as a subject with a delusional belief, then they might form the delusion as well.

Despite its appealing simplicity, Maher's view faces what many have taken to be a very basic problem: not every subject who has the type of experience characteristic of a given delusional syndrome goes on to form the corresponding delusional belief. To see this, we will discuss a prominent explanation of Capgras delusion that appeals to a deficit in affective face-processing (Young et al. 1993; Ellis et al. 1997). On this proposal, 'the basis of the Capgras delusion lies in damage to neuro-anatomical pathways responsible for appropriate emotional reactions to familiar visual stimuli' (Young et al. 1993: 698). In short, part of our ordinary processing of visual scenes is to 'tag' visual stimuli with appropriate emotional responses. Visual awareness of a snake prompts a feeling of fear, for example. On this proposal, ordinary visual awareness of a loved one prompts affective responses of warmth and familiarity. But, the theory goes, subjects with Capgras delusion have a neurological impairment to this part of the face-processing system, altering their affective response to loved ones. To account for this mismatch between what they expect to feel when seeing a loved (warmth and familiarity) and what they in fact feel (nothing), these subjects propose that their loved one has been replaced by an imposter as a way of explaining this discrepancy.

So far, this story seems to cohere with Maher's account quite well: a bizarre experience prompts a cognitive response. But is this response appropriate, in the sense that any ordinary subject might reason the same way? Here theorists differ. For instance, Tranel and colleagues (Tranel et al. 1995) found a class of subjects who appear to have the same impairment to visual processing that we find in cases of Capgras delusion, but these subjects did not go on to form the delusional belief. This suggests that a second factor, in addition to the disturbance of experience, is required to explain why some subjects form the Capgras delusion (Langdon and Coltheart 2000). This is not merely an empirical, but rather a conceptual, shortcoming of Maher's view. It is always possible in principle for two subjects to react differently to the same experience. Some second cognitive factor then needs to be invoked in order to explain the different reactions. What is this second factor? Theorists differ in their answer to this question, but most posit some rational defect in cognition to explain the origin of the delusional belief. We will examine the role of this second factor in more depth when we discuss so-called 'two-factor' accounts of delusional belief.

Not all theorists agree, however, that a second factor is needed to explain delusion formation. For one thing, not all theorists agree that the subjects discussed by Tranel and colleagues pose a problem for Maher's view. Both Sam Wilkinson (2015) and Philip Corlett (2019) emphasize that their lesions are in different areas of the brain and that the non-Capgras subjects have more global impairments which lead them to treat intimates and strangers alike. If this is correct, it could undercut the claim that the Capgras and non-Capgas subjects undergo the same types of experience, and hence that a second factor is needed to differentiate them.

Moreover, even if we take the data from Tranel and colleagues at face value, one might question whether it really points to the need for a second factor, and in particular a rational deficit. For instance, Ema Sullivan-Bissett (2022) and Paul Noordhof and Sullivan-Bissett (2021, 2023) argue that even everyday differences in cognition could explain why subjects respond differently to these experiences. After all, this sort of thing is common in everyday life. If a gust of wind blows out a candle, my superstitious aunt might form the belief that a ghost is responsible, while I might think it was merely a draft from the open window. And while my aunt's belief may be superstitious or even eccentric, we would not generally think that is pathological. Rather, it seems to fall within the boundaries of normal human variation. Thus, a Maherian can maintain that an experience of a given type is not sufficient for the generation of a delusional belief.[4] After all, subjects often respond differently to things they experience. There may be no need, therefore, to think that whatever irrationality we find in delusional subjects rises to a pathological level. Hence, there may be no need for a second factor to explain this irrationality (Noordhof and Sullivan-Bissett 2021).

One problem for this proposal is that it seems like monothematic delusions are just categorically different from ordinary irrational beliefs. It's one thing when your stubborn uncle refuses to admit that Donald Trump is unfit for office. It's another when someone claims that the left arm attached to their body isn't their own, or that their spouse has been replaced by an identical-looking robot. Key to the one-factor view is the idea that experience can in some way render these hypotheses intelligible, or else be made intelligible by them. But neither seems likely. What could experience be like such that it has the content that *my spouse is a robot*? Or: What could experience be like such that a good explanation of it is that this hypothesis is true? Empiricist approaches in general presuppose that it makes sense to explain, say, an affective deficit in one's perception of a loved one with an outlandish hypothesis like the one about the robot. But this claim is certainly questionable. After all, such a hypothesis appears to be deeply and inherently irrational. No subject reasoning normally would ever seriously entertain it, let alone believe it. Such a subject might say 'It feels like my spouse is a robot' but they would understand themselves to be speaking metaphorically (Bradley and Gibson 2023: 827). Simply put, these delusions do not appear to fall into the (admittedly vague) boundaries of 'ordinary irrationality'. This is the crux of the disagreement between the one-factor and two-factor theorists. Do these delusions cluster with the everyday irrationality of your aunt and uncle, or do they cluster with the symptoms of severe cognitive pathologies such as schizophrenia?

Stepping back from the debate about the second factor, there is another way of pushing back against the idea that delusions are irrational. One could hold that delusions are in some sense *arational*. This is arguably the view of Campbell (2001), who defends what he calls *rationalism* about delusional belief. In contrast to empiricist views like Maher's, which explain delusion formation in terms of a cognitive reaction to some antecedent experience, Campbell flips the order of explanation. He does not dispute that delusional subjects have strange experiences, but he holds that these strange experiences are the result of top-down 'cognitive loading' of experience by an antecedently formed delusional belief, where the delusional belief is itself the direct result of 'organic malfunction' (2001: 97–98). In other words, brain damage causes a delusional belief *ex nihilo*.

According to Campbell, delusional beliefs play the role of Wittgensteinian 'hinge' or 'framework' propositions. A thorough examination of Wittgensteinian epistemology is beyond the scope of this chapter. For our purposes, what matters is just that such hinge beliefs are supposed to be beyond the bounds of rational evaluation. This is because they 'form the background needed for any inquiry into truth and falsity' (Campbell 2011: 96). To draw an analogy, consider the belief that there are no true contradictions. It is arguably impossible to produce a non-question begging argument for the truth of this claim. And, plausibly, such an assumption forms part of the background of any inquiry one makes into the truth or rationality of any other belief. There is thus a sense in which this belief itself is arational or non-rational—for a subject who holds it, it plays such a central role in their web of beliefs that rational inquiry into its epistemic status is impossible. Campbell's thought is that delusional beliefs have this character for delusional subjects. For them, the belief that their loved one is an imposter is a fundamental feature of how they think about the world. From within their web of belief, it is just as unquestionable as someone else's belief that there are no true contradictions or that there are material objects (for more on rationalism, see Ohlhorst, Chapter 27).

While Campbell's proposal is interesting, it is hard to accept. One basic problem is that it just does not seem like many delusional beliefs are basic enough elements of a subject's belief set to count as 'hinge propositions'. On a Quinean model, on which beliefs can be more or less central parts of our total web of belief, hinge propositions would form the innermost part of the web. Plausibly, beliefs about fundamental logical principles and the existence of an external world occupy this central place. But can very specific delusional beliefs occupy it as well? What makes a given belief 'central' to one's belief set is the role it plays in justifying other things that the subject believes. How does the belief that the arm that is attached to my body is the doctor's arm do this? As we have seen, what is striking about monothematic delusional beliefs is precisely that they tend to be relatively isolated from the rest of a subject's belief set. So these beliefs would appear to lie at the periphery of the web of belief, or even fail to be integrated into it at all.[5]

Having considered these alternatives, we think that the case for the claim that delusions are abnormally irrational beliefs is strong. In part, this claim is a matter of ordinary judgment. Our initial grasp on the phenomenon of rationality comes from judgments about cases and delusions are perhaps the paradigmatic example of irrational beliefs, so much so that colloquial talk of irrationality is often put in the language of delusion. Of course, that we intuitively regard delusions as abnormally irrational is not proof that they are. This claim is certainly open to revision in light of what we learn in philosophy and psychiatry.

But there is a strong presumption in favor of the claim that delusions are pathologically irrational, and none of the views we have considered decisively overturn that presumption.

## 5.   Stages of delusion and the two-factor model

We have so far argued that delusions are abnormally irrational beliefs. But where does irrationality arise in the course of the delusion? We can—perhaps somewhat artificially—divide the process of coming to a delusional belief into three temporal stages: *entertainment, adoption*, and *maintenance* (following Davies and Egan 2013; Parrott 2019). At the entertainment stage, the content of the delusional belief enters the subject's mind, but is not yet believed. After all, a subject may consider the thought that they are dead but reject it—and indeed, this is what happens to non-delusional subjects suffering from conditions like depersonalization (Sierra 2009). Adoption is the stage at which a thought is taken up as a belief. And maintenance is the phase during which the delusion persists after it is formed, often in the face of substantial contrary evidence. In principle, a subject could be irrational at any of these three stages: a subject may be irrational in first thinking the delusional thought, adopting it as a belief, or maintaining it despite evidence of its falsity. And of course a subject may be irrational at more than one of these stages—they are not mutually exclusive.

Distinguishing these different stages is useful for introducing the two-factor model of monothematic delusions (Davies et al. 2001). To set the stage for the two-factor account, recall Maher's view. Maher denies that subjects are any more irrational than non-delusional subjects at any stage of the delusion, since he claims that delusions are normal responses to bizarre experiences. But, as we saw above, Maher's view faces the problem that different subjects seem to respond to these experiences differently. Some subjects with these experiences go on to form delusional beliefs, while others do not. As mentioned above—and *pace* the criticisms mentioned there—for this reason, many theorists who are inspired by Maher have proposed *two-factor* empiricist views, which invoke an additional cognitive factor to explain the occurrence of delusional belief. Maher's view is thus a *one-factor* empiricist view. (For more on one-factor theories, see Sullivan-Bissett, Chapter 28.)

Two-factor empiricist views differ in terms of how they model the relation between the first and second factors. The main dividing line is between so-called *explanationist* and *endorsement* views (Bayne and Pacherie 2004). Explanationist two-factor views hold that subjects adopt delusional beliefs as a means of explaining an otherwise inexplicable experience they are having. Such a view might say that the first factor in the formation of the Capgras delusion is a disturbance in the affective experience of a loved one. But, as we have seen, this experience on its own is insufficient to explain delusional belief. This is where the second factor enters the story. One prominent two-factor view holds that the second factor which contributes to the Capgras delusion is 'a loss of the ability to reject a candidate for belief on the grounds of its implausibility and its inconsistency with everything else that the patient knows' (Davies et al. 2001: 149). Roughly, this view holds that subjects with Capgras delusion entertain the thought 'my loved one has been replaced by an imposter' as a means of explaining their bizarre experiences. But, owing to a further cognitive deficit, these subjects are unable to reject this hypothesis on the basis of its patent absurdity. Hence, Capgras delusion—and other, similar monothematic delusions—are the result of these two factors, a bizarre experience and an abnormal cognitive response.

Endorsement two-factor views, by contrast, hold that subjects adopt delusional beliefs by endorsing the contents of their bizarre experiences (Bongiorno 2019). Like the explanationist, the endorsement theorist typically holds that first factor in the formation of the Capgras delusion is a disturbance in the affective experience of a loved one brought on by the neurological deficit in the face-processing system. But the endorsement theorist further maintains that this experience has a specific representational content: it represents, of the subject's loved one, something like *that person is an imposter*. In this way, the endorsement theorist maintains that the experiences which occur in cases of delusion are just like other visual experiences in having a representational content. A visual experience of a dog, for example, might have the content *that is a dog*. Many philosophers hold that it is rational for subjects to endorse the contents of their experiences: that a visual experience of the content provides prima facie warrant to form a belief with that content—this is *dogmatism* (Pryor 2000). So just as we typically form the belief a dog is before us by endorsing an experience with that content, a subject with an experiential disorder forms the belief that an imposter is before them by endorsing an experience with that content. One problem here is that in many cases, it is difficult for the endorsement theorist to specify the relevant content (Bongiorno 2019; Bradley and Gibson 2023: 821).

So far we have no explanation of what distinguishes delusional vs. non-delusional subjects. What explains why delusional subjects endorse the bizarre contents of their experiences when, rationally, they should not? This is where the second factor comes in for the endorsement account. As Bayne and Pacherie put it, 'deluded patients are not always responsive to tensions between their delusional belief and their other beliefs in the ways in which a rational person should be' (2004: 3). In other words, non-delusional subjects have the ability to resist forming beliefs on the basis of perception when these beliefs conflict with things the subject otherwise believes. This is just what happens in the case of looking at a known illusion: if you look at a visual illusion while knowing that it's an illusion, you will not endorse the content of your visual experience because you know it is false. But delusional subjects, for whatever reason, are unable to do this. They unreflectively endorse the content of their experience and maintain the corresponding belief even when presented with convincing evidence of its falsity.

Let us now return to stages of delusional belief. As we have seen, the second factor in the two-factor account is meant to explain how delusional subjects deviate from rationality. Roughly following Martin Davies and Andy Egan (2013: 693), we can distinguish between views which locate irrationality at the stage of a delusion's adoption or only its maintenance. What we call *adoption two-factor views* hold that subjects are irrational in adopting the delusional belief, and that the second, cognitive factor is needed to explain this departure from rationality. *Maintenance two-factor views*, by contrast, hold that subjects are rational in adopting the delusional belief, and invoke the second, cognitive factor only to explain why subjects irrationally maintain it in the face of contradictory evidence.

To illustrate a maintenance two-factor view, consider Max Coltheart and colleagues' (2010) view on which the Capgras delusion arises from the application of Bayesian reasoning to 'abnormal data'.[6] On this view, the delusional hypothesis that a loved one has been replaced by an imposter is the best available explanation of 'abnormal data' generated by a broken visual system. Why is this the 'best explanation'? Because this hypothesis best explains the abnormal data: if a loved one were replaced by an imposter, that would explain the abnormal visual response, or so the story goes. Hence, in adopting the belief, the subject is behaving rationally, in accordance with the rules of Bayesian inference. However, the subject will 'fail at [the maintenance stage] to accept the exogenous information available to them through their senses and the testimony of others' (Coltheart et al. 2010: 281). In other words, while the hypothesis that their loved one has been replaced by an imposter is the best explanation of the 'abnormal data' from their defective perceptual system, it is not the best explanation of all of the data available to the subject later on, once they receive proof that the person is their loved one. This view is thus a Maintenance Two-Factor view, since it treats the adoption of the delusion as rational, but finds fault with the subject's epistemic conduct in maintaining the belief. Adoption two-factor views, by contrast, locate irrationality at the adoption stage, for instance, by holding that subjects apply an irrationally biased form of Bayesian updating (McKay 2012). The difference is where in the process irrationality enters.

Maintenance two-factor views can be seen as carrying on the legacy of Maher. They hold that in adopting the delusional belief, the subject is behaving normally from a rational point of view. But is this really plausible? To first appearances, the hypothesis that a loved one has been replaced by a lookalike does not appear to be a very good explanation of a missing visual affective response, even by the standards of ordinary cognition. For one thing, if the 'lookalike' really looks *exactly* like a loved one—which they do—then presumably they should cause the very same affective response in my visual system. For another thing, this hypothesis is so bizarre and implausible that the fact that the subject is seriously considering it calls out for explanation. Quoting Cordelia Fine and colleagues (2005: 160):

> The putative explanations of patients with delusions are bad because] they do not [...] really explain the anomalous thought at all—or they explain the anomalous thought in a way that is so far-fetched as to strain the notion of explanation. The explanations produced by patients with delusions to account for their anomalous thoughts are not just incorrect; they are nonstarters. Appealing to the notion of explanation, therefore, does not clarify how the delusional belief comes about in the first place because the explanations of the delusional patients are nothing like explanations as we understand them.

In other words, there is already a question of rational conduct at the entertainment stage, prior to the adoption of the delusional belief. What could lead a subject to even entertain that they are dead or that their left arm is actually the doctor's? We think that serious consideration of this question is crucial to understanding delusional syndromes, since if abnormal cognition is already present in the entertainment of the delusional thought, then we need some explanation of what this initial abnormality consists in (Bradley and Gibson 2023). Of course, this is not to deny that abnormal irrationality is implicated in forming and maintaining the delusion either.

## 6. Conclusion

In this chapter we have surveyed some of the most important issues and views in recent discussions of delusions and rationality. We hope to have given the reader a sense of the difficulties that arise in trying to think rationally about the irrational.

## Acknowledgments

For helpful comments, which greatly improved this chapter, we would like to thank Ema Sullivan-Bissett.

## Notes

1 Why do researchers tend to focus on monothematic delusions? Simply put, schizophrenia is a very complicated disorder and the delusions that arise in it often appear to defy human understanding. Karl Jaspers famously held that certain schizophrenic delusions are not amenable to first-personal or 'empathetic' understanding at all (Jaspers 1968: 1318). For some pushback on this, see Louis Sass (1992).
2 Currie might reply that delusional subjects are doing something irrational, namely mistaking an imagining for a belief. But if these subjects believe that they believe the delusional content, and act as if they believe it, it's hard to see what grounds there are for denying that they do, in fact, believe it.
3 On the distinction between substantive and structural rationality see Scanlon (2007), Worsnip (2021), Fogal and Worsnip (2021).
4 Thanks to Ema Sullivan-Bissett for discussion on this point.
5 For pertinent discussion of delusional belief in the context of fragmented belief sets, see Davies and Egan (2013).
6 For critical discussion of Bayesian approaches to delusion formation, see Parrott (2016).

## References

APA (2013) *Diagnostic and Statistical Manual of Mental Disorders*, 5th edition, Washington, DC: American Psychiatric Association.
Bayne, T. (2010) "Delusions as Doxastic States: Contexts, Compartments and Commitments," *Philosophy, Psychiatry & Psychology* 17(4): 329–336.
Bayne, T. and Pacherie, E. (2004) "Bottom-Up or Top-Down: Campbell's Rationalist Account of Monothematic Delusions," *Philosophy, Psychiatry, & Psychology* 11: 1–11.
Bayne, T. and Pacherie, E. (2005) "In Defence of the Doxastic Conception of Delusions," *Mind & Language* 20(2): 163–188.
Bongiorno, F. (2019) "Is the Capgras Delusion an Endorsement of Experience?" *Mind & Language* 1–20. https://doi.org/10.1111/mila.12239
Bortolotti, L. (2009) *Delusions and Other Irrational Beliefs*, Oxford: Oxford University Press.
Bortolotti, L. (2012) "In Defense of Modest Doxasticism About Delusions," *Neuroethics* 5(1): 39–53.
Bortolotti, L. (2015) "The Epistemic Innocence of Motivated Delusions," *Consciousness and Cognition* 33: 490–499
Bortolotti, L. (2020) *The Epistemic Innocence of Irrational Beliefs*, Oxford: Oxford University Press.
Bradley, A. and Gibson, Q. H. (2023) "Monothematic Delusions and the Limits of Rationality," *The British Journal for the Philosophy of Science* 74(3): 811–835.
Campbell, J. (2001) "Rationality, Meaning, and the Analysis of Delusion," *Philosophy, Psychiatry, & Psychology* 8(2–3): 89–100.
Capgras, J. and Rebould-Lechaux, J. (1923) "L'Illusion des 'Sosies' dans un Délire Systématisé Chronique," *Bulletin de la Société Clinique de Médecine Mentale* 11: 6–16.
Coltheart, M., Menzies, P., and Sutton, J. (2010) "Abductive Inference and Delusional Belief," *Cognitive Neuropsychiatry* 15: 261–287. https://doi.org/10.1080/13546800903439120
Corlett, P. (2019) "Factor One, Familiarity, and the Frontal Cortex," *Cognitive Neuropsychiatry* 24(3): 165–177.
Cotard, J. (1882) "Du Délire des Négations," *Archives de Neurologie* 4: 152–170, 282–295.
Currie, G. (2000) "Imagination, Delusion and Hallucinations," in M. Coltheart & M. Davies (eds.), *Pathologies of Belief*, Oxford: Blackwell, pp. 167–182.
Currie, G. and Jureidini, J. (2001) "Delusions, Rationality, Empathy: Commentary on Davies et al.," *Philosophy, Psychiatry, & Psychology* 8(2–3): 159–162.

Davies, M., Coltheart, M., Langdon, R., and Breen, N. (2001) "Monothematic Delusions: Towards a Two-Factor Account," *Philosophy, Psychiatry, & Psychology* 8(2/3): 133–158. https://doi.org/10.1353/ppp.2001.0007

Davies, M. and Egan, A. (2013) "Delusion: Cognitive Approaches — Bayesian Inference and Compartmentalization," in K. W. M. Fulford, M. Davies, R. Gipps, G. Graham, J. Sadler, G. Stranghellini and T. Thornton (eds.), *The Oxford Handbook of Philosophy and Psychiatry*, Oxford: Clarendon Press, pp. 689–727.

Egan, A. (2008) "Imagination, Delusion, and Self-Deception," in T. Bayne and J. Fernandez (eds.), *Delusions and Self-Deception: Affective and Motivational Influences on Belief Formation*, Hove: Psychology Press, pp. 263–280.

Ellis, H. D., Young, A. W., Quayle, A. H., and De Pauw, K. W. (1997) "Reduced Autonomic Responses to Faces in Capgras Delusion," *Proceedings of the Royal Society B: Biological Sciences* 264(1384): 1085–1092. https://doi.org/10.1098/rspb.1997.0150

Fine, C., Craigie, J., and Gold, I. (2005) "Damned If You Do; Damned If You Don't: The Impasse in Cognitive Accounts of the Capgras Delusion," *Philosophy, Psychiatry, & Psychology* 12: 143–151.

Flores, C. (2021) "Delusional Evidence-Responsiveness," *Synthese* 199 (3–4): 6299–6330.

Fogal, D. and Worsnip, A. (2021) "Which Reasons? Which Rationality?," *Ergo* 8: 11. https://doi.org/10.3998/ergo.1148

Gendler. T. (2011) *Intuition, Imagination, and Philosophical Methodology*. New York: Oxford University Press.

Jaspers, K. (1968) "The Phenomenological Approach in Psychopathology," *British Journal of Psychiatry*, 114: 1313–1324.

Kahneman, D. Slovic, P., and Tversky, A. (1982) *Judgment Under Uncertainty: Heuristics and Biases*, 1st edition, New York: Cambridge University Press.

Langdon, R. and Coltheart, M. (2000) "The Cognitive Neuropsychology of Delusions," *Mind and Language* 15(1): 183–216.

Maher, B. A. (1974) "Delusional Thinking and Perceptual Disorder," *Journal of Individual Psychology* 30: 98–113.

Maher, B. A. (1999) "Anomalous Experience in Everyday Life: Its Significance for Psychopathology," *The Monist* 82: 547–570.

McKay, R. (2012) "Delusional Inference," *Mind and Language* 27: 330–355. https://doi.org/10.1111/j.1468-0017.2012.01447.x

McKay, R. and Cipolotti, L. (2007) "Attributional Style in a Case of Cotard Delusion," *Consciousness and Cognition* 16(2): 349–359.

Noordhof, P. and Sullivan-Bissett, E. (2021) "The Clinical Significance of Anomalous Experience in the Explanation of Monothematic Delusions," *Synthese* 199(3–4): 10277–10309.

Noordhof, P. and Sullivan-Bissett, E. (2023) "The Everyday Irrationality of Monothematic Delusion," in P. Henne and S. Murray (eds.), *Advances in Experimental Philosophy of Action* (forthcoming), London: Bloomsbury Press, pp. 87–111.

Parrott, M. (2016) "Bayesian Models, Delusional Beliefs, and Epistemic Possibilities," *The British Journal for the Philosophy of Science* 67: 271–296.

Parrott, M. (2019) "Delusional Predictions and Explanations," *The British Journal for the Philosophy of Science*. https://doi.org/10.1093/bjps/axz003

Pryor, J. (2000) "The Skeptic and the Dogmatist," *Nous* 34(4): 517–549. https://doi.org/10.1111/0029-4624.00277

Romano, D., Gandola, M., Bottini, G., and Maravita, A. (2014) "Arousal Responses to Noxious Stimuli in Somatoparaphrenia and Anosognosia: Clues to Body Awareness," *Brain* 137(4): 1213–1223. https://doi.org/10.1093/brain/awu009

Sass, L. (1992) *Madness and Modernism: Insanity In The Light Of Modern Art, Literature, and Thought*, New York: Basic Books.

Sass, L. A. and Pienkos, E. (2013) "Delusion: The Phenomenological Approach," in K. W. M. Fulford, M. Davies, R. G. T. Gipps, G. Graham, J. Z. Sadler, G. Stanghellini, and T. Thornton (eds.), *The Oxford Handbook of Philosophy and Psychiatry*, Oxford: Oxford University Press, pp. 632–657.

Scanlon, T. M. (2007) "Structural Irrationality," in G. Brennan, R. Goodin, F. Jackson, and M. Smith (eds.), *Common Minds: Themes from the Philosophy of Philip Pettit*, New York: Oxford University Press, pp. 84–103.

Schwitzgebel, E. (2012) "Mad Belief?", *Neuroethics* 5: 13–17.
Schwitzgebel, E. (2019) "Belief," in Edward N. Zalta (ed.), *The Stanford Encyclopedia of Philosophy* (Winter 2021 Edition), https://plato.stanford.edu/archives/win2021/entries/belief/
Sierra, M. (2009) *Depersonalization: A New Look at a Neglected Syndrome,* Cambridge: Cambridge University Press.
Sullivan-Bissett, E. (2022) "Against a Second Factor," *Asian Journal of Philosophy* 1: 33. https://doi.org/10.1007/s44204-022-00036-0
Tranel, D., Damasio, H., and Damasio, A. R. (1995) "Double Dissociation between Overt and Covert Face Recognition," *Journal of Cognitive Neuroscience* 7(4): 425–432. https://doi.org/10.1162/jocn.1995.7.4.425
Tversky A. and Kahneman, D. (1974) "Judgment Under Uncertainty: Heuristics and Biases," *Science* 185(4157): 1124–1131.
Vallar, G. and Ronchi, R. (2009) "Somatoparaphrenia: A Body Delusion. A Review of the Neuropsychological Literature," *Experimental Brain Research* 192: 533–551. https://doi.org/10.1007/s00221-008-1562-y
Wilkinson, S. (2015) "Delusions, Dreams, and the Nature of Identification," *Philosophical Psychology* 28(2): 203–226.
Worsnip, A. (2021) *Fitting Things Together: Coherence and the Demands of Structural Rationality,* New York: Oxford University Press.
Young, A. W., Reid, I., Wright, S., and Hellawell, D. J. (1993) "Face-Processing Impairments and the Capgras Delusion," *British Journal of Psychiatry* 162: 695–698.

# 15
# DELUSION ATTRIBUTION

*Sam Wilkinson*

We can talk about a thing in the world called 'delusion', and ask various things about it. For example, we can ask whether that thing is a mental state, and whether, if it is, it is a belief or something else (Currie and Jureidini 2001; Bayne and Pacherie 2005; Bortolotti 2009; see chapters in Section IV). We can even ask if it's a natural kind (Samuels 2009, Samuels, Chapter 5).

A very different theoretical approach to delusion puts this aside and starts, not with delusion itself, but with delusion *attribution*. What are we doing when we call someone delusional? What justifies, or motivates, the calling of something a delusion, or someone delusional? Under what conditions is it accurate, or appropriate, to call something a delusion? Implicit in such an approach is the idea that, first and foremost, delusional status is something that we attribute to certain things (e.g. people, claims, and beliefs) and that we can make sense of our practices of doing so.

This might simply be a different approach that is entirely compatible with looking at delusion as a phenomenon in the world. Alternatively, it could embody a more critical view. The idea behind the latter would be as follows: by focusing on our practices of delusion attribution, we see that the phenomena that attract that attribution, though very real in themselves, are heterogeneous. Taking things a step further, we may see that they are so deeply heterogeneous that there is nothing that they all really have in common and, indeed, that once we properly understand delusion attribution, it is misguided to expect there to be. This final step amounts to a critique of attempts to define 'delusion' in favour of a quietist understanding of why that could never be achieved.

Here I start by presenting an orthodox 'descriptivist' view about delusion attribution. I call this 'orthodox' because it is that which is implicit in the canonical context in which delusion presents itself, namely, psychiatric diagnostic practice. I then present and discuss a recent 'expressivist' view that goes against this orthodoxy. Next, I outline an even more recent hybrid approach that integrates both descriptivist and expressivist elements. Finally, I end by presenting some remaining issues and future directions.

## 1. Descriptivism about delusion attribution

In this section, I present what might be called 'descriptivism' about delusion attribution. Put simply, descriptivism takes delusions to be the set of things that satisfy a certain description;

that fit certain criteria. Different versions of this are generated by the proposal of different criteria, and indeed of different *types* of criteria.

### 1.1   Introducing the approach

Since something being a delusion is about it fulfilling certain criteria, what appropriate delusion attribution is, then, is simply the accurate detection of these criteria in the target phenomenon.

This is clearly seen in diagnostic practice in general, and the *DSM* 'definition' of delusion in particular. The purpose of this definition (and the *DSM* more generally) is to enable a clinician to *identify* and hence *attribute* delusion to a potential patient. The definition in the *DSM-IV*, and in the glossary of *DSM-5*, is as follows:

> Delusion. A false belief based on incorrect inference about external reality that is firmly sustained despite what almost everyone else believes and despite what constitutes incontrovertible and obvious proof or evidence to the contrary. The belief is not one ordinarily accepted by other members of the person's culture or subculture (e.g., it is not an article of religious faith). When a false belief involves a value judgment, it is regarded as a delusion only when the judgment is so extreme as to defy credibility.
> *(DSM-5, American Psychiatric Association [APA] 2013, p. 819)*

One thing to note is that the *DSM* definition is problematic as a strict definition. For example, Max Coltheart (2007) puts into question more or less every statement contained within it:

> 1. Couldn't a true belief be a delusion, as long as the believer had no good reason for holding the belief? 2. Do delusions really have to be beliefs – might they not instead be imaginings that are mistaken for beliefs by the imaginer? 3. Must all delusions be based on inference? 4. Aren't there delusions that are not about external reality? 'I have no bodily organs' or 'my thoughts are not mine but are inserted into my mind by others' are beliefs expressed by some people with schizophrenia, yet are not about external reality; aren't these nevertheless still delusional beliefs? 5. Couldn't a belief held by all members of one's community still be delusional?
> *(Coltheart 2007, p. 1043)*

Another thing to note is that, while this definition features in the *DSM*, and so implies that we are talking about a pathological phenomenon, a phenomenon of clinical interest, it is laden with epistemic notions (false belief, evidence, credibility). This points to two different approaches to the criteria: psychiatric approaches, and epistemic approaches. In other words, delusion can be seen as primarily a phenomenon of central psychiatric importance, or fundamentally an epistemic category.

### 1.2   Psychiatric approaches

It is often assumed (if not explicitly stated) that delusion is, by definition, pathological. Indeed, one approach may be to *define* delusion as *pathological belief*, and then to reflect on what it is for a belief to be pathological (see Petrolini, Chapter 1). For example, following Jerome Wakefield (1992), pathology might be harmful dysfunction, and then delusion is simply belief that is pathological in this sense, namely, the belief isn't doing what beliefs are supposed to do (e.g. 'aim at truth'), and it is harmful.[1] On such a view, one might think that many beliefs are false, but they are at least 'trying to be true' (for more on delusion and malfunction see Miyazono, Chapter 4). However, delusions aren't even doing *that*. They aren't failing at the game of truth; they aren't playing it at all. (We will see interesting ways in which this approximates some *prima facie* very different views.)

Is it plausible, however, that delusion is simply pathological belief? If it were, that would entail that *non-pathological delusion* is a contradiction-in-terms. In other words, the discovery that something was not pathological would mandate a retraction of delusion attribution. Some theorists seem to think that this is the case. For example, Anthony David (1999) cites as obstacles to definitions of 'delusion' that some of the proposed definitional features are found in the non-clinical population. For example, 'the irrationality seen in "normal" reasoning, undermines the specificity of these characteristics for delusions' (p. 17). And 'its maladaptiveness generally, again, sometimes equally applicable to other beliefs held by non-psychotic fanatics of one sort or another' (p. 18). The fact that these non-clinical cases are treated as counter-examples, rather than admitted as cases of delusion, suggests that something non-pathological, healthy, cannot be 'delusion'.

In stark contrast to this, philosophers have tended to think that the relationship between delusion and pathology, though potentially causally tight, is not conceptual (Miyazono 2015; Bortolotti 2022). On such a view, delusion is an indicator, but crucially a defeasible one, of underlying pathology, and there is no *conceptual contradiction* in non-pathological delusion, in a healthy person having a delusion. The reason that philosophers think this is because they suspect that delusion is fundamentally an epistemic term. Indeed, one way of thinking of delusion is as diametrically opposed to knowledge. Just as knowledge is epistemically good belief, delusion is epistemically bad belief.[2]

So, what are some of these candidate epistemic criteria?

## *1.3   Epistemic approaches*

Whatever we take delusion to be, one thing that seems fairly obvious is that they (and the subjects who have them) are breaking norms, and, in particular, epistemic norms. It is questionable that falsity will do the trick, since there seems to be the possibility of accidentally true delusion. So, perhaps what we are after is some fleshing out of 'accidentally' (and 'non-accidentally'). This seems to be about the way in which belief is formed, retained, and revised. This is often put in terms of epistemic *rationality*.

Roughly speaking, while practical rationality maximises the chance of you fulfilling your practical goals, given your beliefs, epistemic rationality maximises your chances of achieving epistemic goals with your beliefs, and chief among these: truth. So, what is actually involved in epistemic rationality, such that it is (as epistemologists say) *truth-conducive*?

A combination of things might count. For example, using adequate evidence in the *formation* of a belief, giving due weight to evidence that might cause you to *revise* your belief, not allowing motivational influences to derail your tracking of the truth (i.e. wishful thinking), having a certain degree of consistency among the beliefs that you hold, not compartmentalising information that is inconsistent, and so on. So, can delusion be defined in terms of epistemic irrationality, thus construed? While this seems more promising than mere falsehood, since, while a delusion can be accidentally true, it cannot be the result of a truth-*conducive* process, arguably, this is neither sufficient, nor necessary. Let's address these in turn.

### *1.3.1   Not sufficient: non-delusional irrationality*

According to a definition of delusion in terms of irrationality, we would expect a correlation between rationality and delusionality. In other words, the more irrational you are, the more delusional you should be. The worry is that this correlation may not hold. Stated plainly, Person A might be *more* epistemically *irrational* than Person B, but in fact turn out to be *less delusional*.

Consider, for example (from Nozick 1993, cited in Murphy 2012), a mother whose son has been convicted of murder. We can understand that she will be *highly* resistant to evidence that suggests that he is guilty. We will not, however, be tempted to call her delusional. People in these situations are being deeply epistemically irrational, but they are intuitively not delusional.[3]

### *1.3.2   Not necessary: rational delusion?*

With advancements in cognitive neuropsychiatry, there has been increasing support for the view that some delusions, at least, are in fact formed on the basis of anomalous experiences. As Brendan Maher, puts it, 'The delusional belief is not being held "in the face of evidence strong enough to destroy it," but is being held because evidence is strong enough to support it' (1974, p. 99). The idea is that (at least some) delusions could arise from *correct* use of very bizarre input, instead of from a *misuse* of normal input.

Whether or not this is the case for any delusions is an empirical question, whereas our question here is conceptual: *If* there *were* people who believed these bizarre things on the basis of fully adequate private grounds, and hence are epistemically rational (or at least *as* epistemically rational as 'normal' people) *would* we still rightly consider them to be delusional?[4]

Interestingly, Jennifer Radden (2010) thinks not. As 'reasonable inferences from misleading perceptual experiences, "perceptual delusions" are *not epistemic lapses of the sort by which delusional states are identified*' (2010, p. 28, emphasis added). This would amount to us retrospectively retracting our delusion attributions in light of a *stipulation* that delusions are in fact tied to epistemic irrationality. In other words, it may turn out that some paradigmatic cases of delusion aren't delusional after all. There is nothing incoherent about such a view, but such a revision would need to be well motivated (more on this later).

A contrasting approach asks: *Granting* that these subjects are delusional, how can we explain their delusional state? If it turns out that some of these are epistemically rational, because the experiences on which they are based are so compelling, then that doesn't disqualify them from being delusional. It rather tells us that delusions don't always have to be irrational, and our concept of delusion ought to accommodate that.

## *1.4   Consequences and issues that arise*

To sum up, then, psychiatric approaches struggle to define delusion, finding all manner of delusion-like phenomena in the healthy population. Epistemic approaches, in contrast, see no conceptual obstacle to there being non-pathological delusion (any more than knowledge conceptually assures good health!), but still find themselves subject to counterexamples from accidentally true delusions, rational delusions, and irrational non-delusions.

Here is a more general consequence that applies to both psychiatric and epistemic approaches, insofar as they are forms of *descriptivism*. Descriptivism about delusion attribution assumes that there is a thing in the world called *delusion*, and once we get clear on what that thing is, we can then detect it and attribute it. This becomes especially clear when we reflect on the medical context, and the historical and institutional role of delusion in diagnosis. Somebody comes to you, as a clinician, with a particular medical condition. If you accurately identify or detect that condition, then you attribute it. You have detected the presence of delusion; this person has a delusion; this person is delusional. Other approaches see things rather differently. To attribute delusion is not to respond to something you detect in the world. Indeed, as we'll see, according to some views, delusion attribution has an altogether different 'direction-of-fit': it doesn't simply react to and detect something in the world, but rather projects something onto it.

Another upshot of descriptivism is that it does not allow for, or at least restricts, heterogeneity. This, in turn, exposes any presented view to purported counterexamples. Alternative approaches don't even set the bar so high as to be troubled by counterexample and they would expect heterogeneity.

## 2.   Expressivism about delusion attribution

Expressivism about delusion attribution (Wilkinson 2020) starts with the observation that calling someone delusional is a negative evaluation. Then, in line with some other treatments of evaluative discourse (e.g. Ayer 1952; Hare 1952, etc.) claims that, although it looks like delusion attribution is describing the world, it is actually doing something else (namely, 'expressing' something in a sense that I will make clear shortly).

### 2.1   *Two kinds of evaluation and evaluative discourse*

When we say that people are delusional, we are *evaluating* them negatively. Everyone will agree with this. However, it is vitally important to distinguish descriptive evaluations from what we might call *deep* evaluations. What you do when you *descriptively evaluate* is you describe a benchmark, and say that the thing in question is attaining or failing to attain said benchmark. These benchmarks will often be theoretically informed. For example, theorists in philosophy of biology will provide conditions for biological proper function. Traditional epistemology does the same for knowledge.

In contrast, 'deep' evaluations are not about neatly picking out a benchmark and merely stating that the thing in question either attains of fails to attain that benchmark. They are claims we make when we are evaluating as opposed to describing, namely, in *evaluative* rather than *descriptive* mental states.

Typical candidates of such evaluations are moral evaluations (right and wrong, good and evil). An expressivist about delusion attribution would take the attribution of delusion to be an evaluation in this deep sense. This does not mean that calling someone delusional is negatively evaluating them *morally* (in fact, it often has quite the opposite effect). Rather, what moral discourse and delusion attribution have in common is that they are both evaluative in a way that doesn't allow them to be analysed in factual, non-evaluative terms.

### 2.2   *What is expressivism?*

Expressivism about a certain kind of discourse is a position concerning what we are doing when we are engaged in that discourse. In particular, the idea is that we are expressing our states of mind rather than describing the world, which is what we might appear to be doing on the surface. So, for example, an expressivist about moral discourse might say that, while it may look like when we assert 'murder is wrong' we are describing the world by attributing the property of wrongness to murder, we are in fact expressing our own state of mind, for example, a revulsion towards, or disapproval of, murder.

A crucial first step is to understand this notion of 'expression'. What is *expressed*, in the relevant sense, is to be distinguished from what is *articulated* or *described*. Thus 'Ouch!' is an expression of being in a state of pain, whereas the utterance 'I am in pain' is a description of that state. Expressivists want to think of moral claims as expressions in a way somewhat analogous to the way that 'Ouch!' is an expression of pain. What a certain utterance (or indeed other piece of expressive behaviour) expresses is the mental state that it *reveals that you have*, not that it *describes you as having*.

Note that fact-stating assertions express things too, but, unlike 'Ouch!', they express in virtue of describing. 'The cat is black' is a description of the world, namely, that the cat is black, but, if sincerely asserted, it is an expression of my *belief* that the cat is black; stipulating sincerity on my part, it *reveals* that I have that belief. In this respect, it is a bit misleading to say that an expressivist thinks that the domain of discourse that is getting an expressivist treatment expresses a state of mind: even fact-stating, descriptive, discourse expresses a state of mind. The point is that it expresses a state of mind that is not a belief.

So, if it is not a belief that is expressed, what is? Many candidates have been advanced, including emotions, desires, pro-attitudes, etc. The precise details of these alternatives are not what interest us now, but rather this general move. Some domains of discourse look like they are describing the world, stating facts, but they are in fact doing something else. Expressivism about delusion attribution is the view that 'delusion' discourse is such a domain of discourse.

### 2.3 Why be an expressivist about delusion attribution?

Many of the considerations that motivate expressivism about moral discourse apply to delusion. These are:

1 Parsimony
2 Intrinsic motivation
3 Deep disagreement

Let's examine these in turn. I present them each by analogy with the moral case.

### 2.3.1 Parsimony

Some theorists are reluctant to posit a strange realm of moral properties or facts (Mackie 1977). Furthermore, the claim is that they don't need to. It is far more parsimonious to appreciate that it will be adaptive for social animals like ourselves to find ways of regulating behaviour within the group by expressing our approval or disapproval of certain kinds of behaviour.

In a similar manner, the argument would go, there are no *sui generis* delusion-pertaining (or indeed knowledge-pertaining) facts or properties. Social creatures like us who communicate and try to live in groups, will find it adaptive to give rough-and-ready signs of approval (thumbs up) to good epistemic states and practices, and give rough and ready signs of disapproval (thumbs down) to poor ones. The fact that the *words* 'knowledge' and 'delusion' emerged in English, and became roughly regimented, is just a distraction. We don't need to think of these as things or properties, but as constructs that we might read off our group practices.

### 2.3.2   Intrinsic motivation

Moral discourse, the argument goes, is intrinsically motivating (Stevenson 1937; Hare 1952; Blackburn 1998). There is a certain contradiction to sincerely claiming 'Murder is wrong but I do not thereby feel any reluctance to murder, nor do I wish discourage others from murdering etc.' Similarly, one could argue that delusion attribution is also intrinsically motivating. Calling someone delusional enjoins certain courses of action, certain responses, on the part of society. As with the moral case, there is a certain contradiction to saying 'This person is delusional, but I will take what they say seriously, engage with them rationally, etc.' Since beliefs do not intrinsically motivate: they only inform, and need to be coupled with a motivational state, what is expressed by these attributions (of moral disvalue or, by analogy, delusion) cannot simply be belief but must, at the very least, have a non-cognitive, motivational component.

### 2.3.3   Deep disagreement

In cases of 'deep disagreement', all of the facts pertaining to a particular case are agreed by two individuals, and yet there is still disagreement, e.g. in the moral case, about whether something is morally wrong. There is no further fact that can be learnt in order to bring the two disagreeing subjects in line with one another. Therefore, the argument goes, it is not a disagreement about facts, but about something else. For example, it might be a clash of emotions, or values, or similar (Stevenson 1937; Ayer 1952; Gibbard 1990).

Of course on many very serious moral infringements (murder), unanimity is not hard to find, but for more contentious culturally specific 'beliefs' (sex before marriage, homosexuality, abortion etc.) disagreements are rife. And bringing people in line with each other is not a matter of informing people of new facts, but of making them *feel* differently (of course, this can sometimes be done indirectly via the drawing attention of certain facts).

A similar thing could be said for delusion attribution. There are not only deep disagreements about what counts as good/bad, acceptable/unacceptable belief *contents*; there are also disagreements about what counts as good *methods and procedures* for forming beliefs, conversational standards for expressing those beliefs, and so on.

### 2.4   *The consequences of expressivism about delusion attribution*

The consequences of expressivism can be seen as further motivation for the view. In other words, since some of its consequences align with what we observe, we can adopt expressivism as an inference to the best explanation.

### 2.4.1   *Heterogeneity is to be expected, and attempts at definition are misguided*

If delusion attribution expresses (reveals) our folk epistemological evaluative attitudes, then we would certainly not expect these attitudes to track consistent properties and nor should we expect 'delusion' to be definable in terms of necessary and sufficient conditions. As we have seen, these definitions are highly vulnerable to counter-example, and rightly so. Indeed, we can ask ourselves, where does our intuitive sense of these *as counter-examples* come from? I'd say, our folk epistemological evaluative attitudes. The definitions themselves can't function to tell us what's delusional since we have a sense of that already. After all, it is that pre-existing intuitive sense of what counts as delusional that allows us to point to these examples *as counterexamples*.

### 2.4.2  Disjunctive norm pluralism

There are many different ways in which a belief (and related phenomena, like inquiry, reasoning, etc.) can be good or bad. As Lisa Bortolotti (2023) puts it, it 'explains why delusions are not always charged with the same epistemic sin' (p. 25). All that matters is that there is enough folk-detectable badness. It doesn't matter where it comes from. Take reverse Othello delusion. The belief that the subject's wife is not cheating on him is a perfectly plausible content taken in isolation. What makes it delusional is the subject's baffling blindness in the face of counter-argument. On the other end of the spectrum, it matters little what evidence a delusional patient might cite for the claim 'I am the left foot of God'. We just don't see how that could possibly be true. Arguably, something similar applies to delusional misidentification. No matter what private evidence you may have, we simply do not accept that people can be replaced by identical-looking doppelgangers. People just don't look, act and live exactly like someone and yet somehow fail to be them.

As we are about to see in more detail, there are likely many other folk-epistemic norms that we detect and they may all be involved in tipping the balance towards the (folk-epistemically) bad or good. Since it doesn't matter of what types of norms are broken as long as there is enough 'epistemic sin', we have what we might call *disjunctive norm pluralism*.

### 2.4.3  Intuitive folk norms are more important than theoretical norms

Observable things like 'understandability' or 'plausibility' rather than things like 'support from evidence', at least where evidence includes private experiential evidence (rather than public argument), are more likely to play a role in the expressivist delusion attribution mechanism. To call someone delusional is to react to them in a certain way, but it is also to flag them as suspect, as problematic for our folk epistemic, social epistemic, community. But these flags and warnings accommodate competing factors.

Recall Nozick's example of the mother who refuses to believe that her son is a murderer. According to the expressivist, we don't think that she's delusional because we can recognise her motivations, and we can recognise the influences that these can have on belief-formation and maintenance. This means that we find her epistemic irrationality unsurprising and *understandable*. This is just part and parcel of our *folk models* of other human beings. We might even recognise (implicitly or explicitly) that in similar circumstances, we would do similarly. We might even be repulsed by a mother who calmly and dispassionately evaluated evidence pertaining to her son's guilt. We model other human beings (and ourselves) as *understandably* biased, emotional creatures. Furthermore, since we and other members of our society do this too, we don't *need* to flag the mother in this case as suspect, as a threat to the social epistemic ecology: the context itself does that for us, and, in any case, we would be similarly biased in her position. In a related manner, maternal bias is not something that we as a society wish to discourage.

### 2.4.4   *The power of delusion attribution*

For the expressivist, when you inappropriately attribute delusion, namely, call something a delusion that shouldn't be, that is not an inaccuracy: it's an injustice. Just as calling something morally wrong that shouldn't be so called, it is not a description that lacks factual accuracy, but is a call to arms for an inappropriate course of action. In other words, it has a different direction-of-fit: it is not descriptive but projective/declarative/action-driving.

## 3.   A hybrid approach

We have seen descriptivist and expressivist approaches to delusion attribution. Very recently, there has been an approach that incorporate elements of both in ways that I am about to explain.

### 3.1   *Delusion attribution as not entirely non-descriptive*

While Bortolotti (2023) is sympathetic to the core insight of the expressivist approach ('Wilkinson's account of our practice of delusion attribution as evaluative is spot-on' [p. 26]) thinking of delusion as *entirely* non-descriptive is taking things too far. She puts it as follows.

> We can further unpack this sense of disapproval and identify the epistemic sins delusions are guilty of, without denying the heterogeneity of the phenomenon of delusions. We can think of delusions as having a core and a periphery. At the periphery variation occurs. But the core is shared, and it is epistemic in nature.
>
> *(Bortolotti 2023, p. 26)*

This retains a degree of descriptivism. In particular, Bortolotti insists that there is interesting theorising to be done about the criteria of delusion attribution. Having said this, it is very important to appreciate that Bortolotti's project, though criterial like the orthodox descriptivist project, is in fact fundamentally different. I'll explain why.

Descriptivism thinks of delusion as a thing in the world and tries to define it, via description, via criteria. This definition furnishes us with a descriptive concept of delusion, and the things that fall under that description are all and only those things that fit that description. An upshot of this is that the psychological act of judging someone to have a delusion is descriptive; it involves the formation of a factual belief. It is like attributing any other property to them. Saying: 'This person has a delusion' is like saying 'This person has brown hair'. And it expresses a belief with that content, and is true if and only if said person has a delusion or has brown hair.

Bortolotti disagrees with this. Instead, Bortolotti agrees with me that delusion attribution is irreducibly evaluative. However, she does want to theorise about criteria. Nevertheless, this need not mean that the attribution of delusion is, on the part of the attributer, an attribution of descriptive content either.

What Bortolotti is doing, as she herself writes, is trying to 'unpack this sense of disapproval' (p. 26). This could mean two things. The first is that delusion attribution is a partly descriptive, and partly evaluative/expressive, enterprise. The second claim is that delusion attribution is an evaluative/expressive enterprise, but that we can, as theorists, make sense of which phenomena trigger the (non-descriptive) delusion attribution response (in the attributors). We can, as it were, theorise about what things in the world tend to trigger the response, without the response itself being descriptive of what that theorising unearths. By analogy, disgust can be a primitive response, intrinsically speaking, but we can theorise in great detail about the things that trigger disgust. We can, for example, look at what those things have in common. We can also, for example, theorise about why, evolutionarily speaking, it is those things towards which we feel disgust. In this sense, there is a complex story behind the simplicity of the response, and the intelligence behind the response outstrips that of the responder.

I take Bortolotti to be doing the latter. In other words, she should be understood as endorsing and theoretically unpacking the expressivist view, rather than criticising it.

## 3.2  *The criteria that are tracked by delusion attribution*

So, what are the (relatively complex) criteria that are tracked by the (relatively simple) delusion attribution response? What is, to use a clunky metaphor, the epistemic pepper that triggers the sneeze of delusion attribution?

Bortolotti outlines three properties that the sorts of things that trigger delusion attribution tend to have. As I understand it, the relationship is one of causal tendency rather than hard conceptual necessity. Pointing to a delusion that doesn't have these properties is not a counterexample, because that's not the nature of the claim in the first place. The three properties are:

i Implausibility
ii Unshakeability
iii Centrality to identity

Let's examine these in turn.

### 3.2.1  *Implausibility*

A crucial first step in understanding the criterion of implausibility is that it must be distinguished from the sorts of definitional criteria that have tended to be put forward by orthodox descriptivist accounts, and, most prominently, (i) falsehood and (ii) bizarreness of content. Falsehood, in particular, is typically considered an objective, and individual, feature of belief. A belief either is or isn't false, and what makes it false is its content and the relationship of that content to how things stand in the world, regardless of what anyone else might think of the matter.

In contrast, an interesting and important feature of Bortolotti's criterion of plausibility is how social it is. A belief is *implausible* if it is unlikely to be true, given the existing beliefs of both the speaker (the person expressing their belief) and the interpreter (the person attributing that belief). This accommodates the well-rehearsed counter-examples about accidentally true delusions, but not through the lens of irrationality, but the far more social notion of implausibility. Something that is deeply implausible may turn out, by sheer fluke, to be true. The caricatural 'madman' prophesying the end of the world may be helped out by a freak asteroid, but that doesn't make their claim any more plausible. The implausible is sometimes true.

This also accommodates the observation that, while very bizarre beliefs tend to be delusional, not all delusions are bizarre. 'Bizarreness' can be given a more thorough gloss as having at least one of the following three properties (Cermolacce et al. 2010):

a  not merely false, but logically or physically impossible
b  incomprehensible within the speaker's culture
c  the situations talked about are not ordinary life situations.

So, bizarre beliefs, on this account, are delusional because the bizarre is implausible. But not everything that is sufficiently implausible as to be a delusion is bizarre. Indeed, some, like reverse Othello delusion, or erotomania (the delusional belief that someone, typically a celebrity, is in love with you), are mundane. It is perfectly possible that this person's partner is being faithful to them (indeed it is true of many people) it's just that, given that the partner has moved out and is now romantically involved with someone else, it's just deeply *implausible*. It is perfectly possible that this famous celebrity is in love with a normal member of the public, Notting Hill-style, but it's just deeply implausible since the celebrity in question has never met that member of the public and has no idea who they are.

Conversely, there are beliefs that are false, and resistant to evidence, but they are not delusional. These include racist beliefs, conspiracy theory beliefs, and so on. This is where the socially distributed force of the implausibility criterion really kicks in, because, while they may be implausible to the interpreter in the sense that the interpreter would never believe them, they are not implausible *tout court*: indeed, they are all-too-familiar and widespread, because, sadly, racist people do have racist beliefs, and conspiracy theories gain currency. Plausibility is about whether a belief is likely to be true, given the beliefs not just of the interpreter, but of the speaker, too.

### 3.2.2  Unshakeability

Just as implausibility distinguishes itself from the more traditional criteria of falsehood or bizarreness of content, so does 'unshakeability' distinguish itself from the traditional criteria of evidential support. A belief can be 'unshakeable' but still be heavily supported by evidence. What makes it 'unshakeable' is determined by our social epistemic practices of exchanges of reasons, and it is when a belief *stands firm in the face of external challenge*. (This is very much in keeping with Kengo Miyazono and Alessandro Salice's Social Epistemic Conception of Delusion, which grounds delusion in testimonial abnormalities [Salice and Miyazono 2021].)

Crucially, an unshakeable belief, in the relevant sense, is not one where the believer doesn't engage in that practice at all, but rather where they do not seem to acknowledge that they should give up their beliefs. Bortolotti (2023) uses the analogy of a five-year old child who plays snap, but does not contemplate the possibility of losing.

This fits particularly well with my expressivist account, insofar as the calling of someone delusional could function as a flag to disengage rationally, or, at least, to signal that such engagement is likely to be futile.[5] It effectively serves to say: 'By all means play "the game" with this person, but there will only be one outcome'. However, it is important to see that this is a folk, external, surface phenomenon. It doesn't matter what the mechanism underpinning the unshakeability is, and we should, as cognitive scientists, expect it to be heterogenous. At times, it may come from overwhelming experiential certainty, at other times, it may come from testimonial abnormalities, at other times, it may come from reasoning biases, and so on.

One more important thing to say about the 'unshakeability' criterion is that it does not imply that, if a belief is to count as a delusion, it could *never* be abandoned. Delusions are indeed sometimes abandoned. Delusional individuals cease to be delusional. However, the point is more to do with the *way* in which they are abandoned. They are, as Bortolotti points out, typically not abandoned as part of the normal receiving and accepting of reasons, but as part of a profound and transformative paradigm shift.

### 3.2.3 Centrality to identity

This criterion feels like an outlier from the other two, in that it doesn't seem epistemic (the others are at least folk-epistemic, in my view). As Bortolotti puts it:

> Another criterion for delusionality is that the belief reflects and shapes our identity. First, it emerges out of processes that are affected by our sense of self and group affiliation, reflecting those aspects of ourselves that make up our identity. Second, it moulds the interactions we have with the world, other people, and groups, contributing to how our identity evolves.
>
> *(Bortolotti 2023, p. 100)*

I'd like to make two observations here. First, it is not entirely clear that this constitutes an entirely separate criterion from the other two. It seems connected to both implausibility and unshakeability, with an especially strong link to the latter. Second, while the other two criteria (implausibility and unshakeability) are entirely compatible with my expressivist account, this third one is slightly at odds, in ways that I will explain.

One of the reasons why a belief may prove unshakeable is because it is central to someone's identity. This unpacks the idea that 'unshakeability' and 'centrality of identity' are closely related. People don't readily give up beliefs that are central to their identity, and these sorts of beliefs are often the sorts of beliefs that precisely aren't open to rational scrutiny. Furthermore, a longstanding tradition in the evolutionary psychology of belief would precisely claim that these beliefs serve in-grouping/out-grouping functions, and so, no *wonder* they aren't open to rational scrutiny, otherwise they would be too widely held to serve precisely the function that justifies their existence, namely that of marking group membership (for a recent development of these ideas see Williams 2020).

There is also a link between centrality to identity and 'implausibility', and it is as follows. Identity-central beliefs will tend to be epistemically isolating in that they don't take the interpreter along with them. *You* believe *that*, because it's central to *your* identity, but it's not central to *mine*. Even though implausibility is a distributed notion, a function of credibility on the part of both speaker and interpreter, an identity-central belief is very likely to score low on interpreter credibility (with the exception of another in-group member, who shares the relevant identity). But is this typically low enough to warrant delusion attribution?

This brings us onto the second observation. What is the potential incompatibility here between Bortolotti's third criterion ('centrality to identity') and the expressivist picture? First, a quick reminder of the compatibility of the first two criteria. The expressivist claims that delusion attribution is an expression of folk epistemic disapproval, an epistemic reactive attitude, if you like (Tollefsen 2017). One way of unpacking the properties tracked by that disapproval is to point out the sorts of things that those reactions may latch onto. So these will be surface and social phenomena, they will be folk phenomena, in the sense that they will not be theoretically fleshed out. Two such folk epistemic phenomena (which are to be distinguished from the more traditional and theoretically fleshed out epistemic notions like truth, evidence, epistemic rationality, etc.) could very probably be things like Bortolotti's notions of plausibility and unshakeability.

But what about centrality to identity? First of all, this is not epistemic. But there is a more pressing issue. The folk-epistemic reactive attitude appealed to in Wilkinson (2020) is not simply one of disapproval. It is also one of *bafflement*. This fits very nicely with unshakeability, since signalling such bafflement also serves to signal that rational engagement will be futile. It recommends rational disengagement. However, knowing that a belief is identity-central makes it *less* baffling to the interpreter, even to an out-group member, even to someone who is deeply opposed to it. Really implausible and unshakeable beliefs, like QAnon beliefs, the expressivist might argue, are *less likely*, not *more likely*, to attract delusion attribution if they are also identity central, because that's what these kinds of people (e.g. the American far-right) tend to believe. In other words, unshakeability (and implausibility for that matter) become less baffling, not more so, when coupled with centrality to identity.

One thing that both Bortolotti and I acknowledge (along with many others besides) is that social pressures can lead people to adopt epistemically bad beliefs. Where there is disagreement is about whether a subset of this social aetiology, namely, centrality to identity, makes it more (Bortolotti) or less (me) likely that it will attract the attribution 'delusion'.

How might this disagreement be resolved? Here are two interesting ways in which the two positions might be aligned. One strategy could be to distinguish clinical/serious attributions of 'delusion' from political/weaponised uses. In the former context, centrality to identity will lower your delusionality (i.e. the appropriateness of delusion attribution) in the eyes of clinicians. In contrast, in the latter context, it may make you a more prominent target of a weaponised use, a folk-epistemic denigration, on the part of your political opponents. After all, a moment's observation points to the fact that political opponents do call each other 'delusional' (even in the august context of the House of Commons).

The second strategy, which can be coupled with, or kept separate from, the first is to take the folk-epistemic bafflement as peripheral to delusion attribution, and to take rational disengagement to be the main function of it. This would explain why staunch political opponents call each other 'delusional': there's a pessimism about a meeting of minds. The political opponent, like the psychotic patient, is a rational lost cause. This would also explain why centrality to identity may causally contribute towards (although not *define*) delusionality: people do not give up their identities easily.

## 4.  Remaining issues and future directions

In this final section, I point towards some remaining issues and future directions.

### *4.1  Non-factualist and non-cognitivist alternatives to expressivism*

Non-cognitivism, non-factualism, and expressivism are closely related, although they do not strictly entail one another. The first move in expressivism about delusion attribution, as in meta-ethical expressivm, is a negative move that is then built upon with the positive expressivist proposal.

That first negative move, the claim that delusion attribution is not fact-stating (since there are no objective delusion-properties that make delusion-facts obtain) we could call *non-factualism*. Coupled with certain views about mind and world, about belief and fact, we might think that non-factualism relates quite closely to *non-cognitivism*, namely, the idea that the thoughts in that domain (e.g. delusion attributions) are not beliefs (i.e. not cognitive), since, firstly, there is no reality for those beliefs to latch onto, and, secondly, they are intrinsically motivating. It is then a small step from that negative position (thoughts pertaining to that domain are not beliefs, and the discourse is not fact-stating) to the more positive story about what *is* going on, rather than what isn't, namely, expressivism: linguistic assertions in that domain (e.g. delusion attributions) are expressions of something other than beliefs (e.g. folk-epistemic evaluative attitudes that are intrinsically motivating).

This has two limitations that can be met with positions that still hold onto the initial non-factualism and non-cognitivism. The two limitations are as follows:

Limitation 1: Expressivism places unrealistic constraints on the state of mind that the attributer needs to be in.

Limitation 2: Expressivism seems to suit primitive reactions that are clearly adaptive (e.g. moral revulsion) rather than more institutionally and theoretically scaffolded ones (e.g. epistemic disapproval).[6]

I will quickly sketch three paths to take from here.
Path 1: Clarifying that expressivism can be 'detached'
The first limitation only applies to a particularly primitive form of expressivism. The meaning of a word is derived from what the word *functions* to express, not what it actually expresses in every instance of utterance. So, on this view, it is not that 'delusion' means what it does only in contexts where it is actually used to express a negative epistemic evaluative mental state, but because that is what its function is. So 'delusion' can mean what it does, even when the asserter is not in the evaluative mental state. That is how it can be used in 'cold' theoretical contexts, in contexts with negations and conditionals.

You may notice that this applies quite naturally to all other uses of language. An assertion still means what it means, because it *functions* to express belief, and continues to mean what it does even if the asserter doesn't believe or otherwise endorse its content. Indeed lying works to mislead the hearer precisely because it exploits this belief-expressing function.

This addresses Limitation 1, but not Limitation 2. The latter presents us with the challenge of fleshing out in more detail how a non-factualist approach could work in more sophisticated contexts.

Path 2: Epistemic reactive attitudes

Another path (that can build on the first) is to retain a broadly expressivist framework, and to go into more detail about the precise state of mind expressed. We know it's not a factual belief, but, in Wilkinson (2020), I merely vaguely gestures towards folk-epistemic negative evaluation, disapproval, bafflement, and flagging as suspect. This is in need of more detail.

A promising avenue for this is to look at what Deborah Tollefsen (2017) calls 'epistemic reactive attitudes'. This framework builds on Peter Strawson's notion of 'reactive attitudes', like resentment, while reveal something deep about our moral commitments. Tollefsen's basic idea is that there is something similar, but across an epistemic dimension that reveal our epistemic commitments. As she puts it, '[o]ur practice of epistemic appraisal is steeped with emotions that are part and parcel of interpersonal exchange' (p. 357).

Thus, there are 'epistemic reactive attitudes' such as 'epistemic ridicule' or 'epistemic indignation', or 'epistemic disappointment'. Within this rich landscape of epistemic reactive attitudes, is there space for an attitude (or attitude cluster) that can be aligned with delusion attribution? Epistemic disappointment, for example, flags that you feel someone should have known better. Does delusion absolve the epistemic agent of that level of responsibility? Is it to flag, at least in part, that they *can't* have known better, because something is epistemically wrong with them? More generally, this avenue encourages interesting reflections about how delusion attribution interacts with interpersonal attribution (or absolution) of epistemic autonomy and responsibility.

Path 3: Epistemic inferentialism

Another quite different path might view the focus on emotion-laden interpersonal interaction as misguided. What matters instead, when thinking about a domain of discourse, is the role that it plays as a public linguistic item in society, not as something derived, even initially, from the mental state, emotional or otherwise, of the speaker. Developing this further, we might theorise about the inferential moves, both practical and theoretical, that are made by a particular attribution. What does calling something a 'delusion', or, indeed, calling something an instance of "knowledge", result in, theoretically and practically? This focus on the social function of epistemic claims has been explored by Matthew Chrisman (2010), especially with regard to knowledge attribution, and in particular as a way of addressing its context-sensitivity. This gives rise to what Chrisman calls 'epistemic inferentialism'. Perhaps something similar could be explored with regard to delusion attribution, and presumably this could integrate some of the institutional and theoretical richness surrounding delusion that motivates Limitation 2.


## 4.2   *The 'social turn' and our informational ecology*

While this entry is about delusion attribution, and has presented certain ways in which delusion attribution can be seen as a social phenomenon, it has said nothing about social ways of thinking about the formation of delusions themselves. Quite right, too, you might think, since it is a different topic (see Williams, Chapter 35). However, one might think that there is an interesting relationship, given the sorts of animals we are, between our public, intersubjective practices of epistemic evaluation, and the processes whereby we come to believe certain things. In particular, to think of these two things as separate would be to suggest that the way in which we form beliefs and evaluate them do not interact. But if we think along broadly expressivist lines, that, as a social species, our evaluations (whether moral or folk-epistemic) serve to (and exist because they) encourage and discourage certain behaviours, procedures and courses of action, then the evaluation of belief and its formation surely must interact. In other words, we could see belief-formation as deeply sensitive to social incentives, and one important feature of that landscape of social incentives is how one is epistemically evaluated. How questions about the formation of delusions and the evaluation of delusions relate to each other is explored in detail in Williams, Wilkinson, and Miyazono (forthcoming).

## Notes

1 There is then a challenge concerning what we mean by "harm" and to whom it should be harmful.
2 As Dominic Murphy very nicely puts it: "A delusion is a false belief, just as knowledge is true belief, but, as with knowledge, philosophers do not rest there. Knowledge is true belief plus something else. So too, philosophers try to find that extra property of the false belief that converts it from a mere false belief into a delusion" (Murphy, 2013, p. 115, emphasis added).
3 As Noordhof and Sullivan-Bissett (2023) convincingly point out, in "strong self-deception" we are confronted with cases that are more irrational than many instances of delusion.
4 See Sullivan-Bissett (2020) for a defence of a "one-factor account" grounded in the important distinction between pathological and non-pathological levels of irrationality.
5 This also fits well with the role of delusion attribution in psychiatry: you are unlikely to be able to talk this person out of their beliefs, so you will need to engage clinically (with either antipsychotics or CBT).
6 This second limitation may speak to one of the reasons why Bortolotti has misgivings about delusion attribution being purely devoid of descriptive content.

## References

American Psychiatric Association 2013: *Diagnostic Statistical Manual of Mental Disorders. DSM-5.* Washington, DC: American Psychiatric Association.
Ayer, A. J. 1952. *Language, Truth and Logic,* New York: Dover Publications, first Dover edition.
Bayne, T. and Pacherie, E. 2005. "In defence of the doxastic conception of delusion," *Mind & Language,* 20 (2): 163–188.
Blackburn, S. 1998. *Ruling Passions,* Oxford: Clarendon Press.
Bortolotti, L. 2009. *Delusions and Other Irrational Beliefs,* Oxford: Oxford University Press.
Bortolotti, L. 2022. "Are delusions pathological beliefs?" *Asian Journal of Philosophy,* 1 (1): 1–10.
Bortolotti, L. 2023. *Why Delusions Matter,* London: Bloomsbury Publishing.
Cermolacce, M., Sass, L., and Parnas, J. 2010. "What is bizarre in bizarre delusions? A critical review," *Schizophrenia Bulletin,* 36 (4): 667–679. https://doi.org/10.1093/schbul/sbq001
Chrisman, M. 2010. "From epistemic expressivism to epistemic inferentialism," in A. Haddock, A. Millar & D. Pritchard (eds.), *Social Epistemology,* Oxford: Oxford University Press, pp. 112–128.
Coltheart, M. 2007. "Cognitive neuropsychiatry and delusional belief" (The 33rd Sir Frederick Bartlett Lecture), *The Quarterly Journal of Experimental Psychology,* 60 (8): 1041–1062.
Currie, G. and Jureidini, J. 2001. "Delusions, rationality, empathy: Commentary on Davies et al.," *Philosophy, Psychiatry and Psychology,* 8 (2–3): 159–162.
David, A. S. 1999. "On the impossibility of defining delusions," *Philosophy, Psychiatry, and Psychology,* 6 (1): 17–20.
Gibbard, A. 1990. *Wise Choices, Apt Feelings,* Cambridge, MA: Harvard University Press.
Hare, R. M. 1952. *The Language of Morals,* Oxford: Clarendon.
Mackie, J. L. 1977. *Ethics: Inventing Right and Wrong,* Harmondsworth: Penguin.
Maher, B. A. 1974. "Delusional thinking and perceptual disorder," *Journal of Individual Psychology,* 30 (1): 98–113.
Miyazono, K. 2015. "Delusions as harmful malfunctioning beliefs," *Consciousness and Cognition,* 33: 561–573.

Miyazono, K. and Salice, A. 2021. "Social epistemological conception of delusion," *Synthese*, 199 (1–2): 1831–1851.

Murphy, D. 2012. "The folk epistemology of delusions," *Neuroethics*, 5 (1): 19–22.

Murphy, D. 2013. "Delusions, modernist epistemology and irrational belief," *Mind & Language*, 28 (1): 113–124.

Noordhof, P. and Sullivan-Bissett, E. 2023. "The everyday irrationality of monothematic delusion," in P. Henne & S. Murray (eds.), *Advances in Experimental Philosophy of Action*, London: Bloomsbury, pp. 87–111.

Nozick, R. 1993. *The Nature of Rationality*, Princeton, NJ: Princeton University Press.

Radden, J. 2010. *On Delusion*, Abingdon and New York: Routledge.

Samuels, R. 2009. "Delusions as a natural kind," in M. R. Broome & L. Bortolotti (eds.), *Psychiatry as Cognitive Neuroscience: Philosophical Perspectives*, Oxford: Oxford University Press, pp. 49–82.

Stevenson, C. 1937. "The emotive meaning of ethical terms," *Mind*, 46: 14–31.

Sullivan-Bissett, E. 2020. "Unimpaired abduction to alien abduction: Lessons on delusion formation," *Philosophical Psychology*, 33 (5): 679–704.

Tollefsen, D. P. 2017. "Epistemic reactive attitudes," *American Philosophical Quarterly*, 54 (4): 353–366.

Wakefield, J. C. 1992. "The concept of mental disorder: On the boundary between biological facts and social values," *American Psychologist*, 47 (3): 373–388. https://doi.org/10.1037/0003-066X.47.3.373

Wilkinson, S. 2020. "Expressivism about delusion attribution," *European Journal of Analytic Philosophy*, 16 (2): 59–77.

Williams, D. 2020. "Socially adaptive belief," *Mind and Language*, 36 (3): 333–354.

Williams, D., Wilkinson, S., and Miyazono, K. forthcoming. *The Social Roots of Delusions*, Oxford: Oxford University Press.

# 16

# DELUSION AND INTROSPECTION

*Chiara Caporuscio*

## 1.  Introduction

A widely studied symptom in the psychiatric population is the presence of delusions. Delusions are described in the *DSM-IV* as 'false beliefs based on incorrect inference about external reality that are firmly sustained despite […] what constitutes incontrovertible and obvious proof or evidence to the contrary' (American Psychiatric Association [APA] 1995), and in the *DSM-5* as 'fixed beliefs that are not amenable to change in light of conflicting evidence' (APA 2013). Delusions vary in content and origin: they can be caused by localized brain damage, typically resulting in monothematic, insulated beliefs ('my father is an impostor', 'mirrors are windows to another reality', 'I am dead'), or they can emerge as symptoms of an organic condition, like schizophrenia or bipolar disorder. Organic delusions are often polythematic, involving more than one belief and gradually spreading into an interconnected web of false convictions.

The *DSM-IV* definition seems to suggest that delusions can only be about external reality; however, this definition has been changed in the *DSM-5* (2013) because of controversial prima facie counter-examples. As Max Coltheart (2007) and Robyn Langdon (2011) point out, delusional agents can have beliefs about their own experiences (and not just about external reality) that appear odd at the very least: blind subjects that claim that they are seeing (Carvajal et al. 2012; Chen et al. 2015; Khalid et al. 2016; Martín Juan et al. 2018), schizophrenic subjects that believe they can hear other people's thoughts (Fernández 2010; Hoerl 2001; Pickard 2010; Sollberger 2014), people who have lost the sense of smell that claim they are able to feel the scent of coffee (Sacks 2012), and survivors of traumatic injuries that believe they can feel pain in limbs that are not any longer attached to their body (Halligan et al. 1993; Lotze et al. 2001). These cases lend themselves to two possible interpretations: (1) subjects could be having extremely peculiar experiences that go undetected by third-person perspective but are accessible to introspection, or (2) they could be wrong about their own experience. The first interpretation preserves the *DSM-IV*'s assumption that subjects jump to inaccurate conclusions about the external world, but they are not wrong about the internal world of their own experience. If the second interpretation

    DOI: 10.4324/9781003296386-20

is correct for at least some of these cases, instead, these should be treated as introspective delusions (henceforth ID): false pathological beliefs whose content includes one or more introspective mistakes.

In this chapter, I will review the debate concerning delusions and introspection. The possibility of IDs depends on how the relationship between hallucinatory experience and delusional belief is spelled out. In part 1, I will introduce the relevant debates concerning delusions and introspection and clarify the assumptions that make the concept of being deluded about experience possible. In part 2, I will discuss the entangled relationship between experience and delusion and focus on three case studies: Anton-Babinski syndrome, thought insertion and supernumerary limb delusion. I conclude that only endorsement models of delusional belief formations are incompatible with delusional beliefs that are not in line with experience, and it is unlikely that all delusions can be explained by a purely endorsement account. However, as our methods to access experience independently from introspective reports are still imperfect, it is still controversial whether specific delusions might come with introspective mistakes.

For the purposes of this chapter, I will assume throughout that delusions are pathological beliefs, meaning that they are still somewhat responsive to evidence, action-guidance and integration in one's belief system, although they might fail to respond appropriately more often or more drastically than the norm (for more on delusion and pathology see Petrolini, Chapter 1 for more on delusion and evidence see Flores, Chapter 12, and for more on delusion and action, see Tumulty, Chapter 18).

## 2.   Introspective mistakes

Introspection is our capacity to access our own conscious mental states and experiences from a first-person perspective (Schwitzgebel 2010). I refer to introspection as the process that starts with having an experience with a phenomenal quality and ends with the formation of a belief about that experience.

Introspection has been traditionally assigned a privileged epistemic status (Alston 1971; Chalmers 2003; Descartes 1641; Gertler 2012; Locke 1690; Smithies 2012). The extreme version of this claim goes as far as saying that introspection is infallible: no error can be possible in a genuine introspective judgement. On the other side, philosophers and psychologists like Eric Schwitzgebel (2008) and Emily Pronin (2009) have pointed out the shortcomings of introspection as an imprecise or inconsistent measure of conscious experience.

I have argued in a recent paper (Caporuscio 2021) that the disagreement here is based on different conceptions of what an introspective belief is and, consequently, what counts as an introspective error. According to some defenders of the incorrigibility thesis, pure introspective judgements are exclusively determined by their target mental state, therefore their truth does not depend on anything other than the experience itself. For example, the judgement 'I am feeling *this*' cannot be wrong when *this* is a demonstrative that directly refers to the phenomenal quality of my experience (Gertler 2012). It is hard to doubt that these kinds of judgements are somehow privileged.

However, even if we might have uniquely infallible access to the raw what-it-is-like of our experience, this does not mean we always have the capacity to correctly translate that experience into a full-fledged introspective belief. That requires us to encapsule our mental states into concepts, and relate them to each other and to the external world. Beliefs like

'I am feeling happy', 'I am having an experience of geometric visuals in my periphery', or 'I am feeling a throbbing pain' are examples of this kind of introspective beliefs.

For the possibility of ID to get off the ground, we need to assume that full-fledged introspective beliefs are not fundamentally different from our beliefs about the external world – both start with an experience, followed by a search for meaning and a selection of candidate hypothesis that culminates in a new belief (for a full discussion of this, see Connors & Halligan 2015, 2020; Caporuscio 2021). This means that the same failure conditions that cause mistakes and inaccuracies in our beliefs about the external world are threatening introspective beliefs as well: we can be mistaken when we choose the wrong concept to communicate or express our phenomenal experience, for example when we are led astray by our background beliefs or motivational factors. If I mistake hunger for anxiety, or furiously state that I am perfectly calm, I am committing an introspective error.

### 3.   What is an introspective delusion?

So far, we have established four assumptions:

Delusions are beliefs that fail more drastically than the norm at the test of rationality (responsiveness to evidence, action-guidance and integration).

Pathological deviations from the norm in the process of belief formation can give rise to delusions.

Introspection is our capacity to form beliefs about our conscious mental states from a first-person perspective.

At least some introspective judgements are susceptible to errors in a similar way to regular belief formation.

Note that all assumptions can be resisted or argued against – but if all these premises are accepted, it follows that there can be beliefs about our conscious mental states formed from a first-person perspective that contain introspective errors, and that fail more drastically than the norm at the test of rationality.

Pathological deviations from the norm in the process of introspective belief formation can give rise to IDs.

Even if this basic premise is accepted, the matter of IDs is still controversial. Delusions about the external world are easily spotted because psychiatrists can independently check the external world and notice inconsistencies with a subject's beliefs. To use a straightforward example, if a subject is convinced that the earth is in the middle of an alien invasion but there are no flying spaceships in sight, the psychiatrist can safely conclude that the subject is holding false beliefs about the external world. This type of access is more problematic when it comes to accessing subjects' private mental states and experiences – especially in the context of delusions – that often come together with bizarre hallucinations. When diagnosing delusions about one's own mental state, experience and belief seem irreversibly entangled: delusions often come together with bizarre experiences, and methods to access one's experience independently from the reported belief are lacking. In the following sections, I will review the literature on the relation between experience and belief (3) and argue, with the help of case studies (4) that most of these accounts allow for a dissociation between experience and belief that would make IDs possible. Finally, I will address the question of how to disentangle experience and belief on a case-by-case basis (5).

## 4.    From experience to belief and from belief to experience

Delusion and hallucination are as conceptually distinct as belief and perception: delusions are normally described in terms of pathologically irrational and false beliefs, while hallucinations are experiences that do not reflect reality. However, this conceptual distinction can become blurry in practice. Belief and perception can mutually influence each other: our beliefs about the world are often grounded in what we can perceive from our senses, and a long-standing debate in the philosophy of perception regards to what extent our percepts are cognitively penetrable, i.e. they can be influenced by beliefs and other higher-level mental states (Macpherson 2017; Marchi 2017; Newen & Vetter 2017).

There are good reasons to think that the link between delusions and experience might be even tighter than the one between belief and experience. It is easily observable in clinical cases that delusions often come together with hallucinatory experiences. Capgras delusion, with the paradigmatic content 'my loved one has been replaced by identical impostors', comes hand in hand with the experience of having an impaired affective reaction to a familiar stimulus (Coltheart & Davies 2022; Nuara et al. 2020). Subjects claiming that mirrors are windows to a different reality, or that their doppelganger is following them wherever there is a reflective surface, are usually diagnosed with mirror anosognosia, or the inability to recognize reflected images. The belief 'there are insects crawling under my skin' comes with the experience of tickling and itching, and subjects suffering from persecutory delusions typically experience paranoia and discomfort.

If strange experiences and irrational beliefs are observed together, two outstanding questions arise: which one came first and what is the causal relationship between them? This question is of particular importance in the regards to ID: if the content of the experience and the content of the delusion are always identical, or are completely shaped by one another, it is difficult to see how someone could be deluded about their own experience.

Two macro categories of answers have been given to these questions. Bottom-up or empiricist accounts ground the delusion in an abnormal experience (Bayne & Pacherie 2004b, for more on empiricist accounts see Bongiorno and Parrot, Chapter 26). According to top-down or rationalist accounts, abnormal experiences are grounded in deluded beliefs and not vice versa (Campbell 2001, for more on rationalist accounts see Ohlhorst, Chapter 27).

### 4.1   Bottom-up accounts

Bottom-up accounts of delusional belief-formation, instead, explain the link between delusion and hallucination by arguing that the abnormal experience has a prominent causal role in triggering the false belief and determining its content (Bayne & Pacherie 2004a). In other words, subjects are deluded by experience (Noordhof & Sullivan-Bissett 2021; Sullivan-Bissett 2020): the reason why they adopt and maintain such bizarre beliefs in spite of strong counterevidence and inconsistency with prior beliefs is their capacity to make sense of their bizarre, private internal reality. The hallucinatory experience comes first, and shapes belief. A similar intuition is shared by some versions of the predictive processing account of delusional belief-formation, according to which delusions are formed and maintained because the costs of leaving a salient experience unexplained are higher than the costs of making highly significant revisions to the rest of the belief system. In Andy Clark's words, the deluded brain forms 'increasingly bizarre hypotheses so as to accommodate the unrelenting waves of (apparently) reliable and salient yet persistently unexplained information' (Clark 2016, p. 206, see Corlett, Chapter 30 for more on prediction error accounts).

Bottom-up accounts are committed to the idea that subjects are deluded *because* of the anomalous experience, which prompts the bizarre hypothesis to be considered and determines its content. Experience might not be the only factor at play: while some empiricists argue that delusions are 'justified by the application of unimpaired procedural rationality to an anomalous experience' (Gerrans 2001: 162), others think that cognitive biases or deficits could still play a role in the maintenance of the delusional belief, for example by preventing it from being discarded when counterevidence is presented (Coltheart 2005). All empiricist accounts, however, agree that at the core of the delusional belief there is an anomalous experience that shapes and determines its content (Sullivan-Bissett 2018). This causes a prima facie reason to resist IDs: if subjects are deluded *by* experience, can they also be deluded *about* experience? If we concede that delusions emerge from powerful hallucinations, is there room for a dissociation not only between reality and experience, but between experience and belief as well? Can someone be deluded by experience and about experience at the same time?

The answer to this question will vary in different versions of the empiricist claim. Empiricist theories of delusion formation agree that the aetiology of delusions can be understood as bottom-up: irrational beliefs are caused by unusual experiences. However, there is one important respect where disagreement still stands, namely in how tight the link between experiential and doxastic content needs to be. Is the bizarre belief just formed by taking the experience at face value, or is there more to the delusional content?

According to endorsement theories of delusion formation, delusions are the result of the subject doxastically endorsing the content of their unusual experience. If delusions are simply an endorsement of experience, then the subjects' beliefs about their own experiences are always correct: their mistake resides only in the generalization from 'I experience the world as if P were true' to 'P is actually true'. This suggests that delusions arise from a dissociation between reality and experience, and not between experience and belief: a delusion is a hallucination so believable that it drives belief-formation astray. Endorsement theories are therefore committed to the claim that there can be no dissociation between experience and belief: delusional subjects believe what they experience.

Explanationist theorists, instead, believe that the link between experiential and doxastic content is much less tight than what is defended by endorsement models. According to these accounts, the delusional belief serves to provide an explanation for an unusual experience. The content of the delusional belief does not need to match the content of the unusual experience, because the experience only works as an initial precursor that triggers a search for meaning (often unconscious: see Bongiorno & Bortolotti 2019) and urges the subject to come up with an interpretation, which can be very far from the original content of the experience (Connors & Halligan 2015, 2020).

### 4.2 Top-down accounts

In top-down accounts, delusions are not caused by unusual experiences, but involve a 'top-down disturbance in some fundamental beliefs of the subject, which may consequently affect experiences and actions' (Campbell 2001: 89). Distorted belief comes first: because of motivational factors (Gunn & Bortolotti 2018), cognitive disturbances or organic malfunction, the subject comes to be convinced of something bizarre. It is only as a consequence of the delusional belief that hallucinations start to happen. This process is known as cognitive penetration, namely, the influence of higher-order cognitive states on perceptual experience (Macpherson 2012, 2017). For example, the belief of being followed can turn a perfectly normal experience of a day at the beach into a paranoid nightmare of shadows and creepy noises, and the phobia of insects can create the hallucinatory experience of itching.

This is not incompatible with IDs. Top-down disturbances affecting experience and belief do not necessitate that the two must always be aligned: while it is likely that some elements of the belief will trickle down to experience, this does not mean that the entirety of the subject's experience will be shaped by their beliefs (Macpherson 2017).

Summing up: ID are not compatible with endorsement models of delusional belief-formation, but they are compatible with explanationist and top-down models. Note that I am not arguing that adopting an explanationist or top-down account necessitates IDs, but merely that these account make it plausible that there might be delusions where agents come to endorse a false belief about their experience.

## 5.  Case studies

In this section, I will illustrate the point made in Section 4 by developing competing interpretations of specific delusions. Depending on which account is preferred (top-down, explanationist or endorsement), it is possible to interpret these cases both as an ID as as not an ID. The three candidate IDs are thought insertion, namely the false belief that one's thoughts belong to someone else, supernumerary limb delusion, namely the false belief of possessing and experiencing a limb that no longer exists, and Anton-Babinski syndrome, namely the false belief of having visual experiences after becoming blind.

### *5.1  Thought insertion*

> Thoughts are put into my mind like 'Kill God'. It is just like my mind working, but it isn't. They come from this chap, Chris. They are his thoughts.
>
> *(Frith 1992: 66)*

This is an example of thought insertion, a common delusion in schizophrenic subjects that involves experiencing one's thoughts as someone else's. Prima facie, thought insertion may look like a delusion about one's own experience: subjects think that they are hearing someone else's thoughts, while their true experience is one of thinking, or hearing voices. However, different accounts of thought insertion have something different to say about whether or not this delusion involves a belief that is mistaken about one's experience.

Michael Sollberger (2014) put forward an endorsement account of thought insertion. According to this model, subjects do not only believe that their thoughts belong to someone else but also experience them as if they belonged to someone else: the attribution of their thoughts to an external entity is not a doxastic stance on their experience, but it is part of their experience itself. Their mistake, then, is not introspective: their access to their own experience is flawless, but they incorrectly take the experience at face value and generalize it to the external world. They are right in believing that they are having an experience as of inserted thoughts, but they are wrong in believing that someone is actually inserting thoughts in their mind. In this account, thought insertion is not an ID: it's a false belief about the external world (someone else is thinking these thoughts), but not about their experience (thoughts without a sense of ownership).

According to the explanationist model put forward by Hanna Pickard (2010), instead, schizophrenics disown mental events if they are manifestations of mental states they do not endorse: the impulse of laughing without a background state of happiness, or intrusive thoughts that express beliefs they do not recognize as their own. Despite this, they are unable to suppress the mental states in question. In this account, the experience of thought insertion subjects is extremely minimal: all there is in the experiential state is a very salient mental event that they do not endorse or identify with. It is the (faulty) interpretation of this experience that leads them to form the delusional introspective belief that the disowned thoughts are not theirs, but are inserted from an external agent.

A possible top-down interpretation of thought insertion could hold that the thought insertion subject has severe paranoia, which causes them to believe that they can hear other people's thoughts (for example, negative things about the delusional person). Eventually, this belief causes auditory hallucinations and the experience of thought insertion. Paranoia is a known symptom of schizophrenia, that is, often associated with thought insertion.

In the last two interpretations of thought insertion, there is a dissociation between the delusional person's experience and their belief about the experience. Their belief is a mistaken interpretation of their phenomenal state (ID).


## 5.2   Anton-Babinski syndrome

Here, a doctor (G.G.) is asking a blind patient (H.S.) about her vision.

G.G.: What can you see of me?
H.S.: The head and… you are wearing a white coat
G.G. (covers his face with a black fan): Do you see my eyes?
H.S.: Yes.
G.G.: Do I wear glasses?
H.S.: I think not.

*(Goldenberg et al. 1995: 1378)*


This is an example of Anton-Babinski syndrome, namely the false belief[1] held by blind subjects that they are still able to see. Unlike Charles-Bonnet syndrome, a similar condition where blindness is caused by peripheral damages, leaving the visual cortex intact and free to conjure up dream-like hallucinations (Kazui et al. 2009), in Anton-Babinski syndrome, blindness is caused by severe damage to the visual cortex itself, making it doubtful whether visual experiences can be possible at all.

Endorsement models of ABS claim that subjects are undergoing experiences that are are phenomenally indistinguishable from perception: hallucinations (Allen-Hermanson 2017) or vivid imagination that is phenomenally indistinguishable from perception (Goldenberg 1995). The Anton-Babinski patient takes that experience at face value to endorse the belief that they are not blind. Thus, ABS is not an ID in this account.

Patricia Churchland (2002) and Fiona Macpherson (2010) disagree with this account, and defend the view that ABS subjects have an impaired access to their own experience. According to their accounts, ABS is an ID. The difference-maker between a regular person experiencing a vivid act of imagination and a delusional subject suffering from

Anton-Babinski syndrome is not to be found in the experience itself, but in motivational factors and biases that affect the subjects' belief but not (or to a lesser extent) the experience. This means either that ABS subjects have a special kind of experience that they interpret as vision (explanationist account), or that there is no kind of experience present, and the delusion is entirely caused by motivational factors and difficulty in accepting one's own loss of sight, leading to anosognosia, namely cognitive anawareness of one's condition.

### 5.3  *Supernumerary limb delusion*

Here, the participant (P) is talking to the experimenter (E) about his non-existent third hand.

> E. Does it get cold?
> P. Yes, it does get cold.
> E. Can you feel it?
> P. Yes, I do!
> E. So sometimes this third hand gets cold?
> P. Yes, it does.

*(Halligan et al. 1993: 162)*

This is a report from a case of supernumerary limb delusion. According to Peter Halligan and colleagues (1993), destruction of the sensory roots leads to the phenomenological experience of a supernumerary limb. Phantom pain has also been widely studied as a relatively common phenomenon following the loss of a limb (Di Pino et al. 2021; Lotze et al. 2001; Melzack 1990). If subjects can feel a limb that is not there, it would simply take an endorsement of that experience to come to believe that they possess such limb. Supernumerary limb delusion could only count as an ID if experience and belief were further apart: for example, if the experience of deluded subjects amounted to purely imagined pain or other sensations in the missing limb (explanationist account) or if their delusion were purely driven by motivational factors and refusal to accept one's illness, without any background experience in the missing limb (top-down account).

The cases I've discussed in this chapter show that the close relationship between experience and belief does not rule out the possibility of IDs – at least not unless we claim that accounts of delusional belief-formation should be exclusively limited to endorsement models. In the next section, I will argue that this is implausible: delusions are more likely to differ in whether and how much belief is dissociated from experience. Whether a specific delusion entails false introspective beliefs or not is better assessed on a case-by-case basis.

## 6.  How can we know?

The literature on delusional belief formation widely agrees that it is unlikely that all delusions might be explained in the same way. Robyn Langdon and Tim Bayne talk about a received-reflective spectrum (Langdon 2011; Langdon & Bayne 2010): on one end lie delusions that arise directly from experience, while on the other lie delusions whose content is elaborated and therefore distant from experience.

Consider the following reports:

'FE believed that his own reflection was another person who was following him around, not only in his home, but anywhere that there was a reflecting surface' (Breen et al. 2001: 240).

'As I walked along, I began to notice that the colors and shapes of everything around me were becoming very intense. And at some point, I began to realize that the houses I was passing were sending messages to me: Look closely. You are special. You are especially bad. Look closely and ye shall find. There are many things you must see. See. See. I didn't hear these words as literal sounds, as though the houses were talking and I were hearing them; instead, the words just came into my head – they were ideas I was having. Yet I instinctively knew they were not my ideas. They belonged to the houses, and the houses had put them in my head' (Saks 2007: 27).

'A woman [reports that she] is plagued by wireless phones, the blue is put upon her. She has under hypnosis had many children with 'astronomas'. Astronomas are different people, who are mutually identical… astronomas speak to her and can perform 'indications'. That is what one sees. If the doctor kills you, they can perform an indication' (Strømgren 1956).

The first report seems easily explainable with an endorsement-like model of delusion. FE had significant face processing deficits and deficits in his ability to interpret reflected space (Breen et al. 2001): his experience of looking at the mirror was plausibly the same experience as if he was looking through a window and seeing a face he could not recognize. The second report is harder to analyse in endorsement terms. While it is still plausible to imagine an experience with the content 'these thoughts are not mine', the report suggests otherwise: Saks talks about her experience as extremely similar to her regular experience of thinking ('the words just came into my head – they were ideas I was having') but with an added component that she describes in cognitive terms ('I instinctively knew they were not my ideas'). Furthermore, there are elements to her experience that do not seem to be mirrored in the delusion ('The colors and shapes around me were becoming very intense'). In the third report, an experience in line with the delusion seems downright impossible: the woman had a number of apparently unrelated beliefs (some about wireless phones, some about astromas, and some about the doctors), her delusions are extremely conceptual and difficult to imagine as experiences. The hypothesis that she formed these beliefs in an attempt to interpret a vague but persistent experience of discomfort and paranoia seems more plausible.

How to distinguish received from reflective delusions? I believe this is better assessed on a case-by-case basis. Delusions where the experience is understood as being highly specific and in line with the delusional belief are more likely situated at the received end of the spectrum. Delusions stemming from vague discomforting experiences are instead likely to be more elaborated. At the current state of research, our methlogies to access experience independently from introspective reports are far from perfect, both in terms of spatial and temporal resolution and in terms of our understanding of how brain processes map into experience. Thus, disentangling experience and belief will be easier for some delusions than for others.

There are good reasons to think that supernumerary limb delusion is at the received end of the spectrum. Research with fMRI and other neural imaging methods has identified neural correlates of phantom limb sensations and phantom limb pain (Lotze et al. 2001) and subjects' reports and behaviour offer ulterior support to the hypothesis that phantom pain is really being experienced, and not only imagined. The origin of these sensations has also been studied: according to a popular theory, phantom pain emerges from a mismatch between the lack of sensory signals from the amputated limb and its preserved representation and movement attempts by the neuromatrix, a widespread neural network representing the bodily self (Di Pino et al. 2021; Melzack 1990). This suggests that the precursor triggering the delusion is the phenomenological experience of pain and other sensations in a limb that does not exist. The hypothesis that is selected to explain the precursor ('I have a supernumerary limb') is excessively driven by experience, while previous knowledge and other sources of evidence are overruled. Motivational factors might play a role in accepting experience as correctly representing reality despite counterevidence. In this model, supernumerary limb delusion does not entail any introspective error, but only a false inference from experience to external reality.

The Anton-Babinski case seems different for a number of reasons. First, the extent of the damage to the visual cortex present in Anton-Babinski subjects raise doubts regarding whether these subjects can have visual experiences at all. Furthermore, the reported visual images seem to derive from confabulation, memory, and synesthetic imagination: subjects are likely to report that their doctor is wearing a white robe because they know they're in a hospital, or that they can see a match being lit when they hear the sound or feel the warmth (MacPherson 2010; Redlich & Bonvincini 1911). Subjects have strong motivational reasons not to want to believe they've gone blind: thus, they might mistake the experience of vividly imagining something for a visual experience. Neither of these elements is proof that the subjects' experience is not one of vision, and more investigation is needed as we shed light on the neural underpinnings of perception, hallucination and imagination. However, this is a case where there are at least have good prima facie grounds to doubt the subject's report of their introspected experience. The possibility that this is a delusion involving an introspective error should be taken seriously.

I will not address the question of whether thought insertion could involve introspective errors because the absence of a specific physical or neurological deficit makes it difficult to investigate the experience of thought insertion subjects. However, as the mechanism and origins of schizophrenic delusions become more clear, it might be possible to shed light on this case.

## 7. Concluding remarks and future directions

The possibility of IDs opens the door for rejecting introspective incorrigibility, namely the claim that in case of disagreements between the subjects' introspective access to their experience and any kind of external access, introspection will always be right. The example of Anton-Babinski syndrome suggests that, as our third-person methods of accessing conscious experience get refined, introspective reports might be corrected by external observations. This raises an important question for psychiatric practice: Is it ever ethically acceptable to question a subject's introspective report based on second or third-person evidence?

Further work is needed to explore the ethical dimension of rejecting introspective incorrigibility. However, it is crucial to point out that critically evaluating introspective reports should never mean overwriting the subject's perspective. On the contrary, psychiatrists should focus their interpretative efforts on understanding why subjects come to believe what they believe given what they are experiencing: when evaluating disputes, dialogue and empathy are necessary for successfully considering first, second, and third-person perspectives and come to a conclusion together with the patient.

In this chapter, I have reviewed the literature on the relationship between experience and belief in delusional belief formation from the perspective of ID, namely, false pathological beliefs about one's experience. I have argued that the current understanding of the relationship between experience and delusional belief leaves space for the possibility of ID:

only endorsement models of delusional belief formations are incompatible with delusional beliefs that are not in line with experience, and it is unlikely that all delusions can be explained by a purely endorsement account. However, as our methods to access experience independently from introspective reports are still imperfect, it is still controversial whether specific delusions like Anton-Babinski syndrome might be ID.

## Note

1 Anton-Babinski Syndrome is sometimes classified as confabulation. A detailed discussion on the distinction between confabulation and delusion goes beyond the scope of this chapter, but confabulatory explanations are often taken to have a lot in common with delusional beliefs. For a more detailed discussion on the difference between delusion and confabulation, see Langdon and Turner (2010).

## References

Allen-Hermanson, S. (2017). Introspection, Anton's syndrome, and human echolocation. *Pacific Philosophical Quarterly, 98*(2), 171–192.

Alston, W. (1971). Varieties of privileged access. *American Philosophical Quarterly, 8*(3), 223–241.

American Psychiatric Association (APA). (1995). *Diagnostic and statistical manual of mental disorders* (4th ed.). Arlington, VA: Author.

American Psychiatric Association (APA). (2013). *Diagnostic and statistical manual of mental disorders* (5th ed.). Arlington, VA: Author.

Bayne, T., & Pacherie, E. (2004a). Bottom-up or top-down: Campbell's rationalist account of monothematic delusions. Philosophy, *Psychiatry, & Psychology, 11*(1), 1–11. https://doi.org/10.1353/ppp.2004.0033

Bayne, T., & Pacherie, E. (2004b). Experience, belief, and the interpretive fold. *Philosophy, Psychiatry, & Psychology, 11*(1), 81–86. https://doi.org/10.1353/ppp.2004.0034

Bongiorno, F., & Bortolotti, L. (2019). The role of unconscious inference in models of delusion formation. In T. Chan & A. Nes (Eds.), *Inference and consciousness* (1st Ed., pp. 74–96). New York: Routledge. https://doi.org/10.4324/9781315150703

Breen, N., Caine, D., & Coltheart, M. (2002). The role of affect and reasoning in a patient with a delusion of misidentification. *Cognitive Neuropsychiatry, 7*(2), 113–137.

Campbell, J. (2001). Rationality, meaning, and the analysis of delusion. *Philosophy, Psychiatry, & Psychology, 8*(2–3), 89–100. https://doi.org/10.1353/ppp.2001.0004

Caporuscio, C. (2021). Introspection and belief: Failures of introspective belief formation. *Review of Philosophy and Psychology*, 1–20.

Carvajal, J. J. R., Cárdenas, A. A. A., Pazmiño, G. Z., & Herrera, P. A. (2012). Visual anosognosia (Anton-Babinski syndrome): Report of two cases associated with ischemic cerebrovascular disease. *Journal of Behavioral and Brain Science, 2*(3), 394–398.

Chalmers, D. (2003). The content and epistemology of phenomenal belief. *Consciousness: New Philosophical Perspectives, 220*, 271.

Chen, J. J., Chang, H.-F., Hsu, Y.-C., & Chen, D.-L. (2015). Anton-Babinski syndrome in an old patient: A case report and literature review: Anton-Babinski syndrome. *Psychogeriatrics, 15*(1), 58–61.

Churchland, P. S. (2002). *Brain-wise: Studies in neurophilosophy*. Cambridge: MIT Press.

Clark, A. (2016). *Surfing uncertainty: Prediction, action, and the embodied mind*. Oxford: Oxford University Press. https://doi.org/10.1093/acprof:oso/9780190217013.001.0001

Coltheart, M. (2005). Conscious experience and delusional belief. *Philosophy, Psychiatry & Psychology, 12*, 153–157.

Coltheart, M. (2007). Cognitive neuropsychiatry and delusional belief. *Quarterly Journal of Experimental Psychology, 60*(8), 1041–1062.

Coltheart, M., & Davies, M. (2022). What is Capgras delusion? *Cognitive Neuropsychiatry, 27*(1), 69–82.

Connors, M. H., & Halligan, P. W. (2015). A cognitive account of belief: a tentative road map. *Frontiers in Psychology, 5*, 123666.

Connors, M. H., & Halligan, P. W. (2020). Delusions and theories of belief. *Consciousness and Cognition, 81*, 102935. https://doi.org/10.1016/j.concog.2020.102935

Descartes, R. (1641/2016). Meditations on first philosophy. In *Seven masterpieces of philosophy* (pp. 63–108). New York: Routledge.

DI Pino, G., Piombino, V., Carassiti, M., & Ortiz-Catalan, M. (2021). Neurophysiological models of phantom limb pain: What can be learnt. *Minerva Anestesiologica, 87*(4), 481–487. https://doi.org/10.23736/S0375-9393.20.15067-3

Fernández, J. (2010). Thought insertion and self-knowledge. *Mind & Language, 25*(1), 66–88. https://doi.org/10.1111/j.1468-0017.2009.01381.x

Frith, C. (1992). *The cognitive psychology of schizophrenia*. Hillsdale, NJ: Erlbaum.

Gerrans, P. (2001). Delusions as performance failures. *Cognitive Neuropsychiatry, 6*, 161–173.

Gertler, B. (2012). Renewed acquaintance. In D. Smithies & D. Stoljar (A c. Di), *Introspection and consciousness* (pp. 89–123). Oxford: Oxford University Press.

Goldenberg, G., Muellbacher, W., & Nowak, A. (1995). Imagery without perception—A case study of anosognosia for cortical blindness. *Neuropsychologia, 33*, 1373–1382. https://doi.org/10.1016/0028-3932(95)00070-J

Gunn, R., & Bortolotti, L. (2018). Can delusions play a protective role? *Phenomenology and the Cognitive Sciences, 17*(4), 813–833.

Halligan, P. W., Marshall, J. C., & Wade, D. T. (1993). Three arms: A case study of supernumerary phantom limb after right hemisphere stroke. *Journal of Neurology, Neurosurgery & Psychiatry, 56*(2), 159–166. https://doi.org/10.1136/jnnp.56.2.159

Hoerl, C. (2001). On thought insertion. *Philosophy, Psychiatry, & Psychology, 8*(2), 189–200. https://doi.org/10.1353/ppp.2001.0011

Kazui, H., Ishii, R., Yoshida, T., Ikezawa, K., Takaya, M., Tokunaga, H., Tanaka, T., & Takeda, M. (2009). Neuroimaging studies in subjects with Charles Bonnet syndrome. *Psychogeriatrics, 9*(2), 77–84. https://doi.org/10.1111/j.1479-8301.2009.00288.x

Khalid, M., Hamdy, M., Singh, H., Kumar, K., & Basha, S. A. (2016). Anton Babinski syndrome—A rare complication of cortical blindness. *GMJ, 1*(1), 4.

Langdon, R. (2011). The cognitive neuropsychiatry of delusional belief. *WIREs Cognitive Science, 2*(5), 449–460. https://doi.org/10.1002/wcs.121

Langdon, R., & Bayne, T. (2010). Delusion and confabulation: Mistakes of perceiving, remembering and believing. *Cognitive Neuropsychiatry, 15*(1–3), 319–345. https://doi.org/10.1080/13546800903000229

Langdon, R., & Turner, M. (2010). Delusion and confabulation: Overlapping or distinct distortions of reality? *Cognitive Neuropsychiatry, 15*(1–3), 1–13.

Locke, J. (1690/1998). *An essay concerning human understanding*. London: Penguin Classics

Lotze, M., Flor, H., Grodd, W., Larbig, W., & Birbaumer, N. (2001). Phantom movements and pain. An fMRI study in upper limb amputees. *Brain: A Journal of Neurology, 124*(Pt 11), 2268–2277. https://doi.org/10.1093/brain/124.11.2268

Macpherson, F. (2010). A disjunctive theory of introspection: a reflection on zombies and Anton's syndrome. *Philosophical Issues, 20*, 226–265.

Macpherson, F. (2012). Cognitive penetration of colour experience: rethinking the issue in light of an indirect mechanism. *Philosophy and Phenomenological Research, 84*(1), 24–62.

Macpherson, F. (2017). The relationship between cognitive penetration and predictive coding. *Consciousness and Cognition, 47*, 6–16. https://doi.org/10.1016/j.concog.2016.04.001

Marchi, F. (2017). Attention and cognitive penetrability: The epistemic consequences of attention as a form of metacognitive regulation. *Consciousness and Cognition, 47*, 48–62. https://doi.org/10.1016/j.concog.2016.06.014

Martín Juan, A., Madrigal, R., Porta Etessam, J., Sáenz-Francés San Baldomero, F., & Santos Bueso, E. (2018). Anton–Babinski syndrome, case report. *Archivos de La Sociedad Española de Oftalmología* (English Edition), *93*(11), 555–557.

Melzack, R. (1990). Phantom limbs and the concept of a neuromatrix. *Trends in Neurosciences, 13*(3), 88–92. https://doi.org/10.1016/0166-2236(90)90179-e

Newen, A., & Vetter, P. (2017). Why cognitive penetration of our perceptual experience is still the most plausible account. *Consciousness and Cognition, 47*, 26–37. https://doi.org/10.1016/j.concog.2016.09.005

Noordhof, P., & Sullivan-Bissett, E. (2021). The clinical significance of anomalous experience in the explanation of monothematic delusions. *Synthese, 199*(3–4), 10277–10309.

Nuara, A., Nicolini, Y., D'Orio, P., Cardinale, F., Rizzolatti, G., Avanzini, P., Fabbri-Destro, M., & De Marco, D. (2020). Catching the imposter in the brain: The case of Capgras delusion. *Cortex, 131*, 295–304.

Pickard, H. (2010). Schizophrenia and the epistemology of self-knowledge. *European Journal of Analytic Philosophy, 6*(1), 55–74.

Pronin, E. (2009). Chapter 1: The introspection illusion. In *Advances in experimental social psychology* (pp. 1–67). https://doi.org/10.1016/S0065-2601(08)00401-2

Redlich, E., & Bonvincini, G. (1911). Weitere klinische und anatomische Mitteilungen fiber das Fehlen der Wahrnehmung der eigenen Blindheit bei Hirnkrankheiten. *Neurological Centralblatt, 30*, 227–235.

Sacks, O. (2012). *Hallucinations* (pp. xiv, 326). New York: Alfred A. Knopf.

Saks, E. R. (2007). *The center cannot hold: My journey through madness.* Paris: Hachette UK.

Schwitzgebel, E. (2008). The unreliability of naive introspection. *Philosophical Review, 117*(2), 245–273. https://doi.org/10.1215/00318108-2007-037

Schwitzgebel, E. (2010). *Introspection,* in the stanford encyclopedia of philosophy (winter 2019 edition), Edward N. Zalta (ed.). https://plato.stanford.edu/archives/win2019/entries/introspection/.

Smithies, D. (2012). A simple theory of introspection. In D. Smithies & D. Stoljar (A c. Di), *Introspection and consciousness* (pp. 259–294). Oxford: Oxford University Press.

Sollberger, M. (2014). Making sense of an endorsement model of thought-insertion. *Mind & Language, 29*(5), 590–612. https://doi.org/10.1111/mila.12067

Strømgren, E. (1956). *Psykiatri.* Copenhagen: Munskgaard.

Sullivan-Bissett, E. (2018). Monothematic delusion: A case of innocence from experience. *Philosophical Psychology, 31*(6), 920–947. https://doi.org/10.1080/09515089.2018.1468024

Sullivan-Bissett, E. (2020). Unimpaired abduction to alien abduction: Lessons on delusion formation. *Philosophical Psychology, 33*(5), 679–704. https://doi.org/10.1080/09515089.2020.1765324

# 17

# DELUSION AND EPISTEMIC INJUSTICE

*Eleanor Palafox-Harris*

This chapter explores how epistemic injustice might arise in interactions with people with delusions. I begin by introducing Miranda Fricker's (2007) classic account of epistemic injustice and briefly survey the current landscape of research into epistemic injustice and psychiatry. I then explore how epistemic injustices can arise in encounters with people with delusions. I present a significant objection to applying epistemic injustice frameworks to interactions with people with delusions, which I label the *challenge of irrationality*. The chapter ends by arguing that people with delusions are vulnerable to epistemic injustices because of inaccurate stereotypical attributions of irrationality.

## 1.  The background: epistemic injustice, identity prejudice, and psychiatry

The concept of *epistemic injustice* was first articulated by Fricker (2007) to capture a range of distinctly epistemic kinds of injustice, involving harms to a person in their capacity as a *knower* (Fricker 2007: 20). A person is harmed as a knower when they are wrongfully and harmfully prevented from engaging in epistemic practices such as imparting information to others and interpreting their own experiences. Fricker distinguishes between two separate but related kinds of epistemic injustice: *testimonial injustice* and *hermeneutical injustice*. In its most general formulation, testimonial injustice involves a speaker being dealt an *'identity-prejudicial credibility deficit'* (Fricker 2007: 28): we view them as less credible than they are due to prejudices relating to their social identity, and therefore treat their testimony with distrust or suspicion.

Hermeneutical injustices, broadly speaking, involve having 'some significant area of one's social experience obscured from collective understanding owing to a structural identity prejudice' (Fricker 2007: 155). In other words, hermeneutical injustice occurs when someone is prevented from understanding or articulating an important aspect of their social experience. This is due to defects or gaps in collective hermeneutical resources. Fricker maintains that hermeneutical injustice is *structural*, and thus not perpetrated by individuals (Fricker 2007: 159; 2016: 172). However, others have argued that hermeneutical injustice is (at least partly) *agential*, and therefore there is a role for individuals after all. Gaile Pohlhaus Jr has put forward the notion of 'wilful hermeneutical ignorance' to capture

DOI: 10.4324/9781003296386-21

258

instances where dominantly situated knowers refuse to give uptake to hermeneutical resources created by marginalised groups and wilfully 'continue to misunderstand and misinterpret the world' (Pohlhaus Jr. 2012: 716). In a similar vein, Rebecca Mason (2011) argues that Fricker's characterisation of hermeneutical injustice overlooks the way in which gaps in hermeneutical resources can be maintained by the ethically bad epistemic practices of dominant knowers (Mason 2011: 301).

Though distinct, testimonial injustice and hermeneutical injustice can compound each other (Fricker 2007: 159). When testimonial and hermeneutical injustices consistently co-occur, the result can be *epistemic oppression*, characterised by Kristie Dotson as 'persistent epistemic exclusion' (Dotson 2014: 115).

On Fricker's account, both testimonial and hermeneutical injustice are bound to *negative identity prejudice* (Fricker 2007: 28). Standard examples include negative identity prejudice related to a person's gender or race. For example, prejudicial attitudes about women can cause testimonial and hermeneutical injustice. The negative stereotype that women are less rational than men can distort a hearer's judgement about a woman speaker's[1] epistemic credibility; such distortions can lead to a speaker's credibility being *deflated*, *denied*, or made highly *conditional*, where a speaker is only trusted if certain conditions are met (such as corroborating evidence), or where they are only trusted in specific contexts or on specific topics. Consequently, the hearer might dismiss or distrust her testimony, as in testimonial injustice. Negative stereotyping can also generate hermeneutical injustices. For example, the prevalence of the stereotype that *women are less rational than men* may have prevented women from contributing equally to our shared interpretative resources, whilst – in the absence of a corresponding stereotype for men – men's perspectives dominate. This puts women at an 'unfair disadvantage' (Fricker 2007: 1) when making sense of their own experiences, because the concepts available to interpret and articulate their experiences have been created by the dominant group. Thus, in cases of testimonial and hermeneutical injustice towards women, the role of prejudice in undermining a speaker's epistemic position is clear.

Since Fricker's original 2007 account of epistemic injustice, the concept has been developed in a number of ways. These developments include refinements to Fricker's classic account, such as Jeremy Wanderer's (2017) addition of *structural testimonial injustice*, and Lucienne Spencer's (2023) expansion of testimonial injustice to include cases involving non-verbal communication (see n. 1). The notion of epistemic injustice has also been developed by the identification of other types of epistemic injustice, such as Kristie Dotson's (2011) account of *testimonial smothering*, and Christopher Hookway's (2010) identification of other pre-emptive epistemic injustices.

Recently, the epistemic injustice framework has been fruitfully applied to psychiatry, to illustrate how those with a psychiatric diagnosis are also vulnerable to testimonial and hermeneutical injustice. Most work so far has proceeded within the original Frickerian framework of epistemic injustice (Kidd, Spencer, and Carel 2022). Research on epistemic injustice and psychiatry has aimed to elucidate the *epistemic asymmetries* that exist within psychiatric healthcare in general (Scrutton 2017) and the heightened vulnerability of those with mental illness to epistemic injustice (Crichton, Carel, and Kidd 2017). Other research has been narrower in scope, focusing on a specific group within the psychiatric context, such as young people (Houlders, Bortolotti, and Broome 2021; also Harcourt 2021), or those with specific diagnoses (see Jackson 2017 for a discussion of depression). There are people who are critical of the applicability of epistemic injustice frameworks to psychiatry (such as Kious, Lewis, and Kim 2023, for a response see Kidd, Spencer, and Harris 2023), however everyone agrees about the vital importance of patients being able to communicate with their practitioner and receive appropriate care. Many patient testimonies and experiences sound like reports of epistemic injustice, such as complaints that they are *not listened to* or *not heard* by their practitioners (see Newbigging and Ridley 2018; see also Steslow 2010 for a perspective from lived experience). Epistemic injustice provides one way to theorise about the complaints of patients relating to their treatment as epistemic agents.

## 2.  The ethical and epistemic implications of epistemic injustice

Epistemic injustice carries significant ethical costs, particularly within the context of psychiatric care. Testimonial injustice can hinder communication between a patient and their practitioner, as dismissals of a patient's viewpoint can undermine their willingness to engage with treatment (Kurs and Grinshpoon 2018: 342). As positive engagement with mental health services can be a predictor of a good clinical outcome (Houlders, Bortolotti, and Broome 2021), testimonial injustice-driven disengagement with services puts the patient's clinical outcome at risk. Moreover, wrongfully distrusting a patient's claims can lead to misdiagnoses and incorrect treatment. One way this can occur is via *diagnostic overshadowing*, which is when a patient's physical symptoms are mistakenly attributed to a pre-existing mental illness because the patient's reports of physical symptoms are discredited and 'incorrectly interpreted as psychogenic' (Bueter 2021: 1139).

Epistemic injustice also carries considerable epistemic costs. Testimonial injustice is straightforwardly epistemically costly, as it potentially leads to discounting genuinely informative testimony. When a hearer dismisses the testimony of a speaker because of a prejudicial credibility deficit, the hearer misses out on 'knowledge and other rational input' (Fricker 2007: 59). This is particularly problematic for some contexts, including the clinical context, where gathering information about a patient's history and symptoms is vitally important for forming a diagnosis, creating a treatment plan, and evaluating a patient's progress. Epistemic injustice causes both epistemic losses to specific practices (such as the diagnosis of a particular patient) and wider epistemic losses to psychiatric practice more generally, such as losses to psychiatric classification (see Bueter 2019). Relatedly, hermeneutical injustice is epistemically costly because the gaps in hermeneutical resources hinder attempts for patients to pass on knowledge. As Fricker argues, 'that which remains insufficiently intelligible to the relevant social other cannot be passed on to them as knowledge' (Fricker 2016: 164). In other words, hermeneutical gaps act as *communicative roadblocks* between interlocuters, effectively preventing the flow of information. Within the context of psychiatric healthcare, this type of hermeneutical injustice creates obstacles to making the experiences of the patient intelligible to the clinician. This can give rise to feelings of frustration, isolation, or even despair for the patient, as they struggle to make their experiences understood. Other things can cause people with mental health conditions to experience hermeneutical estrangement aside from hermeneutical injustice, such as features of the illness itself, and as a result people with mental health conditions often *already* feel misunderstood. Hermeneutical injustice risks compounding these feelings of estrangement and misunderstanding.

Let us now turn to the more specific case of delusion. Mitigating the harmful effects of epistemic injustice in this context requires understanding how and when testimonial and hermeneutical injustice could occur in encounters with people with delusions. It is only by locating where the injustices occur and exploring how the epistemic positions of those with delusions come under threat that we can begin to put ameliorative strategies in place.

## 3.  Delusions and testimonial injustice

As we have seen, testimonial injustice occurs when a credibility deficit causes us to distrust or dismiss what a speaker is telling us. In such cases, the speaker's testimony is 'wrongfully mistrusted' (Fricker 2007: 46) due to the operation of prejudice. Are people with delusions vulnerable to being *wrongfully mistrusted*?

Fricker argues that negative stereotypes are the 'main point of entry' for prejudice (2007: 30). She suggests that negative stereotypes lead a hearer to make 'an unduly deflated judgement of the speaker's credibility' (2007: 17). Abdi Sanati and Michalis Kyratsous (2015) have argued that speakers with delusions are vulnerable to experiencing testimonial injustice due to the existence of a number of negative stereotypes. In particular, they argue that people with delusions are frequently stereotyped as being '*bizarre, incomprehensible,* and *irrational*' (Sanati and Kyratsous 2015: 484). Such negative stereotypes work to deflate perceptions of epistemic credibility, since irrationality, bizarreness and incomprehensibility are not markers of testimonial credibility or epistemic competence. If the stereotype is applied more generally to the cognition of people with delusions, it is plausible that we distrust the testimony of speakers with delusions even when they provide information on a topic that is unrelated to their delusion. Sanati and Kyratsous argue that this because we *generalise* epistemic irrationality from the speaker's delusional belief to other beliefs held by the speaker, such that irrationality is 'held as an attribute of the person's general psychic life' (Sanati and Kyratsous 2015: 484). In other words, the stereotype is not simply that a particular delusional belief is irrational (or bizarre or incomprehensible), but rather, that people with delusions are *generally* or *globally* irrational. So, we can see how the stereotype facilitates a generalisation from one site of irrationality (the delusional belief) to a presumed broader epistemic irrationality. It is important to note that this stereotype should not be understood as claiming that people with delusions are irrational in an unremarkable way (i.e., in the same way or to the same extent as the non-delusional population, for whom epistemic injustice does not occur as a result of perceptions of irrationality). Rather, there is an important difference in the *degree* or *kind* of irrationality taken to characterise subjects with delusions.

Moreover, once a person has been classified as globally irrational, they can suffer a 'lock-out' effect, whereby they then cannot engage in the epistemic practices that would ordinarily restore their epistemic status. Cynthia Townley (2011) likens having low epistemic credibility to 'Cassandra's Curse'. In Greek Mythology, Cassandra was cursed by Apollo so that no one would believe her true prophecies. Cassandra was unable to defend her claims because the curse of her low credibility completely excluded her from the epistemic community: no amount of truth-telling could restore her epistemic status (Townley 2011: 44–45). Like Cassandra, those who have been ascribed low epistemic credibility struggle to regain their epistemic status, because that low credibility precludes them from being able to successfully defend their claims to those who already perceive them to be untrustworthy epistemic agents. Similarly, Dotson (2014) suggests that epistemic exclusion is *persistent*: 'it is difficult to impossible to break out of this kind of epistemic exclusion when *one's own capacities to engage in a given epistemic community is compromised to this degree*' (Dotson 2014: 125, source emphasis). There is empirical support for the existence of a lock-out effect. A study by Toby Pilditch and colleagues found that 'sources accompanied by low trust cues not only have truthful communications rejected, but have their low trust penalized even further' (2020: 1). In other words, once a person has been assigned low epistemic credibility their subsequent truthful testimony is disbelieved and the fact that the testimony is true has no positive effect on repairing perceptions of their epistemic credibility (Pilditch, Madsen, and Custers 2020: 12). Applied to the case of delusions, we can see reason to think that a person who is classified as globally irrational (and therefore an untrustworthy epistemic agent) would struggle to regain their epistemic status, even when subsequent testimony is rational.

Sanati and Kyratsous describe two case studies of epistemic injustice involving individuals with a prior diagnosis of psychosis. In the first, J.N. is admitted to a psychiatric ward 'with an acute onset of psychotic phenomena' (including delusions). J.N. expresses concern that her partner is being unfaithful to her, which the psychiatric team takes to be a case of 'delusional jealousy'. In fact, J.N. was correct – her partner confirmed that he was being unfaithful (Sanati and Kyratsous 2015: 248).[2] In the second case study, M.G. is arrested and detained under the Mental Health Act after being evaluated as 'acutely psychotic' and resisting treatment. The reason for M.G.'s initial arrest was that he was threatening to attack another person who M.G. claimed had abused a close relative of his. Given M.G.'s other irrational and delusional beliefs, the psychiatric team assumed that M.G.'s claim about the abuse was also a delusion. However, it was later discovered that M.G. had been telling the truth about the abuse. In both cases, J.N. and M.G. are *wrongfully mistrusted*: their testimony is assumed to be unreliable or irrational because of their prior history of psychosis and delusional beliefs.

Moreover, both examples illustrate the epistemic and ethical ramifications of testimonial injustice. The credibility deficits sustained by J.N. and M.G. led to misdiagnoses, as both J.N's claim about her partner's infidelity and M.G.'s claim about abuse were attributed to their psychosis and mistakenly interpreted as delusions. Epistemically, this means that the psychiatric teams missed out on gaining important knowledge from the patients' testimonies. Ethically, the misdiagnosis could have led to incorrect treatment or caused damage to the relationship between the person with delusions and their practitioners – for example, J.N. felt 'betrayed' by the team – which could affect the quality of clinical outcomes.

## 4.   Delusions and hermeneutical injustice

In Fricker's original account, hermeneutical injustice occurs when 'a gap in collective interpretive resources puts someone at an unfair disadvantage when it comes to making sense of their social experiences' (Fricker 2007: 1). Hermeneutical injustices stem from hermeneutical *marginalisation*; that is, when a marginalised group is prevented from participating equally in the development of shared interpretive resources. This marginalisation causes important gaps in our hermeneutical resources, such that members of the marginalised group are rendered less able to understand their experience, or less able to articulate their experience to others. José Medina (2017) suggests that the *degree* to which hermeneutical injustice limits one's capacity for interpreting and articulating one's own experiences can differ:

> We can identify a continuum of cases: from skin-deep cases, in which subjects face unfair uptake in an isolated aspect of their life without leaving any mark in their interpretive power and hermeneutical agency [...] to marrow-of-the-bone cases, in which the hermeneutical harms become so pervasive that they compromise one's epistemic

life. [...] The most radical case would be the one in which one's voice is *killed* – what I have called *hermeneutical death*.

*(Medina 2017: 47)*

One key example Fricker uses to illustrate hermeneutical injustice is of women struggling to express the issue of sexual harassment or have a proper understanding of what was happening to them at a time when the concept and term for that experience did not yet exist (2007: 150–152). Fricker's example demonstrates how such gaps in our collective interpretive resources prevent a person from being able to understand and articulate 'a significant patch of her own experience' (2007: 151).

We can now see reasons to think that hermeneutical injustice affects people with delusions. People with delusions are hermeneutically marginalised due to power imbalances and epistemic asymmetries within psychiatric contexts. Havi Carel and Ian James Kidd argue that, in healthcare settings, healthcare professionals enjoy *epistemic privilege* as a result of their medical training and expertise (2014: 534–535). This epistemic privilege hermeneutically marginalises patients in a number of different ways. Firstly, healthcare professionals, rather than patients, are the people who set the language for medical discussions. Healthcare professionals define the concepts and terms for illness, the standards of intelligibility, the terms for symptoms, names for diagnostic categories, and so on (Carel and Kidd 2014: 535–536). All this can hermeneutically marginalise patients, as the interpretative resources available for a patient to make sense of their own experiences of ill-health are those created by clinicians and other healthcare professionals instead of those with similar experiences. In some cases, patients might feel that these medical terms and concepts do not adequately describe their experience. Kristen Steslow (2010), with lived experience of involuntary detention at two institutions, writes:

> Psychiatrists have developed a powerful vocabulary to render their patients' experiences medically intelligible and to carry out treatment, and its prevalence in psychiatric clinics is to be expected. But when those who speak this language assert its epistemic supremacy, much of its healing power is lost in a wake of alienation, disempowerment, and silencing. The patient loses her ability to speak with authority except to the extent that her language conforms to the standard medical discourse.

*(Steslow 2010: 30)*

Steslow suggests that in order to make herself heard and intelligible to the psychiatric team she had to adopt the medicalised language of her clinicians, thereby 'forsaking the uniqueness of [her] own perspective, understanding, and expression' (2010: 30). Steslow suggests that in so doing, the patient is alienated from her own experiences, thereby creating a 'fragmented' mind and impeding her recovery. This self-silencing could be understood as an example of *testimonial smothering* (Dotson 2011).

Alternatively, rather than adopt medical terms that do not fit their experience, the patient can create their own hermeneutical resources. Consider this example of a patient experiencing hip pain from Jaspers (1968):

> When asked whether what he felt was a 'twitching', he said: 'No, it isn't a twitching, it's a "plotching"'.

*(Jaspers 1968: 1319)*

Although patients can create new terms, like 'plotching', to describe experiences that medical language does not adequately capture, such terms will not be taken as seriously as the authoritative medical concepts and descriptions. Patients are therefore faced with two unsatisfactory options: to either adopt the medicalised language that cannot fully capture their experience, and in doing so silence their own expression, or create new hermeneutical resources which are not given uptake (an example of Pohlhaus Jr's *wilful hermeneutical ignorance* [2012]). In this way, the privileged position of healthcare professionals in creating our hermeneutical resources for medical conditions limits the ability of patients to express their experiences, resulting in hermeneutical injustice.

Secondly, healthcare professionals are accorded the epistemically privileged position of evaluating interpretations of a patient's experience. In other words, not only do healthcare professionals set the *language* for interpretations of patient experience, they also assess which interpretations are *ratified*. Rosa Ritunnano (2022) explores hermeneutical injustice in clinical encounters with people with psychosis. In such encounters, the clinician occupies the role of judging whether a patient's interpretation of their experience is delusional, and provides counter-interpretations. Ritunnano suggests that clinicians are likely to be assumed to be in the position of 'dominant knower' relative to the patient (Ritunnano 2022: 250). As such, Ritunnano argues that the clinician's counter-interpretations of a patient's experience can *distort* the patient's own 'interpretative attempts' (2022: 250). The epistemic asymmetry in the relation between the patient and the clinician means that greater weight is implicitly placed on the clinical counter-interpretation of the patient's experience than the patient's own interpretation. Consequently, the person with delusions is hermeneutically marginalised.

Moreover, Anastasia Scrutton argues that features of medical diagnosis can give rise to hermeneutical injustice for those with mental health conditions: in a diagnostic context, the experiences of a speaker can be 'forced into an existing mold' (2017: 349). In other words, the rich subjective experiences of the person being diagnosed can be reduced into fixed, pre-existing diagnostic criteria, often to the exclusion of other interpretations of those experiences (such as the patient's own non-medical, personal interpretation). According to Scrutton, clinical diagnosis *monopolises* how experiences are interpreted, as the clinical interpretation is considered authoritative. Consequently, patients are hermeneutically marginalised because their personal interpretations are overridden by clinical interpretations which fit the patient's experience into diagnostic classifications. We can apply this picture to delusion more precisely as follows: in diagnostic contexts, the various experiences of speakers with delusions are reduced into a discrete set of diagnostic categories, which overlooks the heterogeneity of delusional experience, and the subjective interpretations of delusional experiences which may be personally meaningful to the individual with the delusion (for more on delusion and meaning see Ritunnano and Littlemore, Chapter 2). People with delusions can therefore suffer hermeneutical injustice because of the diagnostic process.

In summary, people with delusions are vulnerable to hermeneutical injustice for at least three reasons: (i) healthcare professionals have epistemic privilege in creating the terms and concepts for distress and illness, (ii) clinicians enjoy an epistemically privileged position in evaluating patient interpretations and providing counter-interpretations to delusional experience, and (iii) the diagnostic process reduces subjective experiences of delusions into pre-existing moulds.

Having overviewed the ways in which two key types of epistemic injustice – testimonial and hermeneutical – can arise in encounters with people with delusion, we can now shift to a discussion of the main challenge facing applications of epistemic injustice to delusion.

## 5. The challenge of irrationality

There are a number of objections to applying epistemic injustice in the psychiatric context (Kious, Lewis, and Kim 2023), but the one most salient for the topic of delusions relates to irrationality. Fricker suggests that testimonial injustice is epistemically costly because 'knowledge or other rational input they [a speaker] have is missed out by others' (Fricker 2007: 59). Thus, for a dismissal of a person's testimony to count as epistemic injustice, the testimony needs to contain *rational input*. Arguably, this criterion is not met when a speaker is testifying about their delusion, as delusions are typically defined as irrational beliefs (for more on delusion and irrationality see Bradley and Gibson, Chapter 14). Now is not the time to give a precise characterisation of when beliefs are rational, but for our purposes we can presume that rational beliefs are those which are based upon and responsive to evidence. In contrast, delusions are commonly defined as those beliefs which are strongly held despite counter-evidence, for example on the *DSM-5* definition, they are 'not amenable to change in light of conflicting evidence' (American Psychiatric Association 2013: 87). If my previous quick characterisation of a rational belief is roughly right, delusions come out as irrational by definition.[3] It might seem then that dismissing delusional testimony would not count as testimonial injustice, because the testimony is not 'rational input'. Edward Harcourt (2021) raises this challenge. Harcourt argues that epistemic injustice frameworks are useful for theorising the wrongs experienced by *some* groups of healthcare service users. In particular, his argument focuses on the applicability of the notion of testimonial injustice to encounters with children and young people in healthcare. However, Harcourt objects that the concept of epistemic injustice has been applied 'too freely' to other cases such as people with delusions (2021: 731). Harcourt contends that because delusional testimony fails to meet standards for rationality, speakers with delusions do not meet the criteria for suffering epistemic injustice: 'the concept of epistemic (testimonial) injustice ... fits cases involving delusions badly' (Harcourt 2021: 734).

Moreover, the epistemic injustice framework arguably comes under tension even when speakers with delusions testify on non-delusional topics. In cases of testimonial injustice, a speaker is 'wrongfully mistrusted' (Fricker 2007: 46). That mistrust is *wrongful* implies that a speaker's epistemic credibility is called into question unduly. This is clear to see in the exemplar case of testimonial injustice affecting women. When a woman's testimony is dismissed because of negative stereotypes of lesser rationality, this constitutes testimonial injustice because the woman is mistrusted unduly. She is mistrusted unduly because the stereotype appealed to in our credibility judgement is *false*: it is not true that women are less rational agents than men. Thus, we are wrong to mistrust her. Hence, wrongful mistrust seems to require that a speaker's credibility is deflated to a level which is undue, as a result of false stereotypes distorting our credibility judgements.

However, it might be objected that the stereotypes at play in our credibility judgements about people with delusions are *true*. As noted earlier, Sanati and Kyratsous suggest that people with delusions are stereotyped as '*bizarre, incomprehensible,* and *irrational*' (Sanati and Kyratsous 2015: 484). Here I will focus on the stereotype of irrationality, because I take this stereotype to undermine perceptions of epistemic credibility most forcefully (and most directly), however parallel arguments could be made for bizarreness and incomprehensibility. We have seen reason to think, in line with Sanati and Kyratsous (2015), that stereotypical ascriptions of irrationality to those with delusions cause deflated perceptions of epistemic credibility, and consequently unjust dismissals of testimony. However, a critic might argue that people with delusions are stereotyped as irrational because they are *in fact* irrational. Thus, a critic of applying the epistemic injustice framework to cases involving people with delusions might argue that speakers with delusions are not dealt an undue credibility deficit: we view them as less credible epistemic agents because they are *in fact less credible*.

Arguably then, dismissing the testimony of speakers with delusions due to perceived irrationality is disanalagous to the example of dismissing women's testimony due to perceived irrationality; whereas women are mistrusted wrongfully because the stereotype of lesser rationality is false, the credibility of people with delusions is deflated in line with actual irrationality. If the credibility deficit sustained by speakers with delusions is not undue, then dismissing their testimony does not constitute testimonial injustice. In other words, whilst people with delusions are certainly mistrusted, they are not *wrongfully mistrusted*, even when they testify on topics which are unrelated to their delusion.

The challenge of irrationality for the applicability of epistemic injustice frameworks to delusion can therefore be summarised as the following two claims:

1 Dismissing the testimony of people with delusions when they are speaking about their delusion does not constitute testimonial injustice because delusions are not 'rational input'.
2 Dismissing the testimony of people with delusions when they are speaking about non-delusional topics does not constitute testimonial injustice because they are not dealt *undue* credibility deficits and are thus not mistrusted wrongfully.

In what remains of the chapter, I will respond to the second part of the challenge of irrationality. By narrowing my focus to the second challenge I do not mean to suggest that the first challenge is insurmountable. On the contrary, I think an argument could be made that even if delusional testimony does not constitute 'rational input' it nevertheless communicates subjective meaning or other information important to the person with delusions (such as cultural information). Therefore, it might still be wrong to dismiss delusional claims, as in so doing we miss out on other epistemic goods (such as meaning) even if we do not miss out on *knowledge* per se. However, making this argument would require a thickening of our conception of testimonial injustice. Thus, for the purposes of this chapter, I will concede the first challenge of irrational *beliefs* and focus instead on the second challenge of irrational *believers*.

The second challenge of irrationality has it that speakers with delusions are not *wrongfully mistrusted* because the negative stereotypes (namely, irrationality) which influence our credibility judgements are in fact true. I will respond to this objection by disputing the claim that the stereotypical ascription of irrationality to people with delusions is true.

## 6. Responding to the second challenge: disputing false stereotypes

The claim that delusions are irrational beliefs does not entail that people with delusions are ipso facto irrational agents, and therefore all their beliefs are irrational. All people have some irrational beliefs – beliefs which we lack evidence for or which we refuse to give up even in the face of counter-evidence. That we have irrational beliefs is not contentious, and there are whole industries in philosophy, social psychology, and cognitive science seeking to understand everyday irrational beliefs (see e.g. Bortolotti 2009). Over-optimistic appraisals are just one example of everyday irrational beliefs (other examples include paranormal beliefs and self-deception, explored by Noordhof and Sullivan-Bissett 2023). Often, people are over-optimistic about some aspect of their lives, such as their ability to control external events (the illusion of control), their perception of themselves and their skills (the better-than-average effect), or the likelihood of positive events occurring to them (unrealistic optimism) (Jefferson, Bortolotti, and Kuzmanovic 2017: 4). These over-optimistic appraisals are *epistemically irrational* when they are based on insufficient evidence or are insufficiently responsive to new evidence (Jefferson, Bortolotti, and Kuzmanovic 2017: 7). That a person holds an over-optimistic belief is not usually taken to be an indictment on the person's general epistemic rationality. Similarly, that a person holds a delusional belief does not mean that *all* their beliefs are irrational. This is particularly clear with monothematic delusions, which exist within a system of beliefs that is 'otherwise entirely unremarkable' (Coltheart, Langdon, and McKay 2007: 642). The fact that monothematic delusions co-exist with other 'unremarkable' beliefs negates the stereotype that people with delusions are *generally* epistemically irrational.

We can see the implausibility of this stereotype by turning to competing views on delusion formation, all of which would deliver the verdict that the stereotype that people with delusions are generally irrational is false. Consider the debate over the number of clinical abnormalities involved in the formation of monothematic delusions. On either one-factor or two-factor accounts of delusion formation, we can resist the conclusion that people with delusions are generally irrational and thus cannot be *wrongfully* mistrusted. Put briefly, *one-factor accounts* of delusion formation (most prominently Maher [1974 and elsewhere], see also Noordhof and Sullivan-Bissett [2021]) posit only one clinically abnormal factor to explain how a delusion comes about or is maintained; this factor is some anomalous experience (for more see Sullivan-Bissett, Chapter 28). In contrast, *two-factor accounts* stipulate that delusions are formed and/or maintained because of some anomalous experience *and* a second clinically significant factor, usually a cognitive bias, deficit, or performance error (for more see Davies and Coltheart, Chapter 29).

First, let us consider the one-factor theory, as, if true, this would offer the most straightforward rebuttal of the claim that people with delusions are generally epistemically irrational. The one-factor theory has it that although delusion formation might be the product of a number of causal influences (such as upbringing, trauma, socio-economic factors and so on), only one factor is *abnormal*. For one-factor theorists, this clinically anomalous factor is some anomalous experience that a delusion is formed in response to. For example, the Capgras delusion is characterised as the belief that *a loved one has been replaced by an imposter*. It has been hypothesised that the anomalous experience behind this delusion is a lack of affective response to a familiar face (Ellis and Young 1990; Ellis et al. 1997). One-factor theorists argue that the delusional belief is a *normal response* to the anomalous experience.

On one way of developing the one-factor account, Paul Noordhof and Ema Sullivan-Bissett appeal to the idea of a *normal range* and argue that speakers with delusions do not display irrationality beyond that which occurs within the normal range of individuals without delusions (2021: 10300). Thus, although the specific delusional belief is irrational, the person with the delusion need not be any less rational than any other person without delusions. The one-factor account clearly challenges the stereotypical claim that people with delusions are especially generally epistemically irrational and therefore all their testimony is irrational, as one-factor accounts deny that whatever irrationality is present in delusional subjects is clinically significant. Thus, the stereotype that speakers with delusions are particularly generally irrational is untrue on a one-factor account, since people with delusions display no irrationality beyond what everyone else does.[4] For one-factor theorists of delusion formation, speakers with delusions can be wrongfully mistrusted, because the stereotypes involved in our credibility judgements are false.

Secondly, I will now argue that even on a two-factor account of delusion formation, we can resist the claim that speakers with delusions are irrational in any generalised sense, such that irrationality spills over into their non-delusional beliefs. I will briefly consider the three main candidates for the second involved in delusion formation: *bias*, *deficit*, and *performance failure*.

On bias accounts, the person with the delusion is taken to have a *tendency* to process information in a biased way. There are various candidates for the reasoning bias at work in people with delusions. I will focus on the 'jumping to conclusions' (JTC) reasoning bias proposed by Philippa Garety and colleagues, though the argument could be applied to other biases (for research into JTC bias and delusion see Garety 1991; Garety, Hemsley and Wessely 1991; Dudley et al. 1997; Dudley et al. 2016). In brief, the thought is that people with delusions require less evidence to reach a conclusion than those without delusions. In the paradigmatic Beads Task, two jars are filled with beads of two colours in equal and opposite ratios: for example, Jar A contains 85 yellow and 15 black beads, whereas Jar B contains 15 yellow and 85 black beads (Garety, Hemsley, and Wessely 1991: 196). Participants are presented with beads pulled one at a time from one of the jars, for example, *yellow bead, black bead, yellow bead, yellow bead*. The participant is tasked with deciding which jar the beads are being pulled from. Results from the beads task demonstrate that participants with delusions require fewer beads before deciding which jar the beads are from than participants without delusions (Garety, Hemsley and Wessely 1991: 198; Dudley et al. 2016: 656). This suggests that people with delusions 'jump to conclusions' based on less evidence than those without delusions.[5] We can apply the JTC bias to the example case of the Capgras delusion. A two-factor bias explanation of the Capgras delusion could be that (Factor 1) a person has an anomalous experience (namely, lack of affective response to a familiar person), and (Factor 2) the person too quickly jumps to the conclusion that the familiar person has been replaced by an imposter (due to having a reasoning bias).

However, even if one accepts a two-factor account of delusion formation where the second factor is a reasoning bias such as the JTC bias, we can nevertheless resist the conclusion that the stereotype that people with delusions are generally irrational is true. With respect to the JTC bias in particular, findings suggest that the difference in the tendency to jump to conclusions of people with delusions and without delusions is found in *neutral* topics (such as the beads task). In cases involving *non-neutral* topics, such as personally meaningful content or emotive content, both participants with delusions and those without delusions show an increased tendency to jump to conclusions (Dudley et al. 1997: 580; Kemp et al. 1997: 402). Thus, if one argues that having a JTC bias demonstrates that the person with the bias is an irrational agent, then many people *without* delusions should also be labelled irrational.

A critic might point out that an important difference is that people with delusions exhibit the bias in both neutral and non-neutral cases, whereas people without delusions have been found to exhibit the bias in non-neutral cases *only*. Thus, they might argue that the JTC reasoning bias found in people without delusions is more circumscribed and context-specific, whereas the reasoning bias found in people with delusions appears more widespread, arguably pointing to a more generalised irrationality in people with delusions. One might argue that this difference lends credence to the stereotype that people with delusions are in fact generally epistemically irrational, and as a result, dismissing their testimony does not constitute wrongful mistrust.

However, the JTC reasoning bias is not tantamount to irrationality. Results from the beads task show that, for participants with delusions, the average number of beads needed to make a decision is more closely aligned with *Bayesian rationality*[6]:

> The deluded group appear better (more Bayesian) reasoners with respect to hypothesis formation.
>
> *(Garety, Hemsley, and Wessely 1991: 200)*

In contrast, participants without delusions were shown to be 'overcautious' with respect to Bayesian rationality (1991: 200). Therefore, if we accept Bayesian rationality as a good measure of rationality, then the presence of the JTC bias in people with delusions does not confirm the stereotype that those with delusions are generally epistemically irrational. Consequently, two-factor theorists who appeal to a JTC bias at the second clinically anomalous factor in delusion formation can resist that conclusion that the stereotype about people with delusions is true. As the JTC bias is not evidence of irrationality, speakers with delusions are wrongfully mistrusted when their testimony on nondelusional topics is dismissed.

On deficit accounts, the second factor involved in delusional belief is a reasoning deficit rather than a bias. For example, Max Coltheart and colleagues suggest that people with monothematic delusions suffer from damage to the right frontal lobe (Coltheart, Langdon, and McKay 2007: 644). They argue that damage to the right frontal cortex hinders the belief evaluation system, thereby preventing people with delusions from abandoning a delusional belief when presented with evidence against it. If we assume a two-factor deficit account of delusion, such as one which takes the second factor to be damage to the right frontal lobe, we can still resist the claim that people with delusions are generally epistemically irrational. This is because the reasoning deficit which constitutes the second factor is *localised*, rather than widespread. In other words, the putative reasoning deficit does not render *all* beliefs held by a person irrational. As such, two-factor theorists who posit a belief evaluation deficit as the second factor do not suggest that people with delusions are generally epistemically irrational. Rather, it is only in the context of some anomalous experience (the first factor) that the reasoning deficit causes a delusion (the irrational belief) to be maintained. Thus, in spite of damage to the right frontal cortex, the deficit in rationality is isolated to the delusional belief, rather than impacting the entire belief system of the person with delusions. Consequently, one can adopt a two-factor deficit account of delusion without entailing that the stereotype of generalised irrationality is true.

On performance failure accounts (such as Gerrans 2001), the person with a delusion does not lack *competence* for some exercise of rationality, but rather fails to *perform* this capacity for rationality. Gerrans illustrates performance failures with the example of a person losing and regaining the ability to speak after a stroke: the possibility of regaining speech suggests that the inability to speak is not a deficit in the person's linguistic *competence*, as this remains intact (Gerrans 2001: 166). Instead, the inability to speak following a stroke is a *performance failure*. In a similar way, a person having a delusion does not point to a lack of competence for some exercise of rationality, but simply a failure to perform in their capacity for rationality at that time. More precisely, on Gerrans' account, the second factor responsible for delusions is a performance failure of the capacity for *pragmatic rationality*, understood as 'the inability of delusional subjects to apply procedural rationality *in context*' (2001: 166, emphasis added). Thus, performance failure two-factor accounts of delusion formation, such as Gerrans (2001), do not ascribe generalised irrationality to people with delusions. On this account, we can reject the stereotypical portrayal of speakers with delusions as generally epistemically irrational.

In sum, neither one-factor nor two-factor accounts of delusion formation support the idea that people with delusions are generally epistemically irrational. On both one-factor and two-factor accounts, people with delusions can be mistrusted *wrongfully*, and are therefore vulnerable to epistemic injustices.

## 7.  Conclusion

I have explored the ways in which people with delusions are vulnerable to experiencing the two main types of epistemic injustice from Fricker's (2007) framework: testimonial and hermeneutical injustice. I considered a response to the *challenge of irrationality*, that is, the challenge that speakers with delusions are generally irrational and therefore cannot properly be said to have their epistemic authority undermined in ways which constitute epistemic injustice. I argued against the truth of the stereotypical attribution of irrationality to speakers with delusions. Thus, one can apply epistemic injustice frameworks to cases of interactions with people with delusions, and properly characterise them as *wrongfully mistrusted*.

Having concluded that those with delusions are vulnerable to experiencing epistemic injustice, the next step is to design ameliorative strategies. The literature on epistemic injustice and delusion is still in its infancy, so there has not yet been a great deal of research into ways to mitigate epistemic injustice in cases involving those with delusions specifically. Nevertheless, broader research into epistemic injustice in psychiatry more generally has suggested that tackling epistemic injustice will require ameliorative strategies at both an *individual* level and a *systemic* level (for a recent survey of ameliorative work see Kidd, Spencer, and Carel 2022). Individual-level strategies focus on changes individual clinicians can make to the way they interact with people with delusions, for example, it has been proposed that adopting a phenomenological approach to patient testimony would help us better understand and mitigate epistemic injustices (Carel and Kidd 2014; Ritunnano 2022). On the other hand, systemic-level strategies focus more broadly on structural and social changes in clinical practice, such as 'sustained engagement and interaction with service-user communities' (Miller Tate 2019: 99). Tackling epistemic injustice in relation to those with delusions will require a combination of individual and systemic changes, but most fundamentally all amelioration requires first an understanding of how the epistemic positions of those with delusions comes under threat, through both testimonial and hermeneutical injustice.

## Acknowledgements

I am grateful for funding from the Arts and Humanities Research Council Midlands4Cities Doctoral Training Partnership. Thanks to Ema Sullivan-Bissett, Ian James Kidd, and Lisa Bortolotti for their helpful feedback on earlier drafts of this chapter. I am grateful to audiences at the Association for the Advancement of Philosophy and Psychiatry (AAPP) Annual

Meeting (New Orleans), and the Mind, Mental Health, and Epistemic Injustice Workshop (Nottingham) for comments on material relating to the work in this chapter.

## Notes

1 Throughout, I use the terms 'speaker' and 'hearer' to describe the people involved in an instance of testimonial injustice, as per convention in the epistemic injustice literature. However, Lucienne Spencer (2023) has argued that our notion of testimonial injustice should be expanded to include *non-verbal* cases, such as testimonial injustices against people with late-stage dementia. Thus, though I use the term 'speaker' to denote the person whose testimonial agency is harmed in testimonial injustice, this should not be taken to exclude non-verbal testimonial injustices.

2 Of course, a belief merely being *not false* is not enough for it to be not delusional, as the latest DSM revision (DSM-5) replaces 'false belief' with 'fixed belief', and thus a delusion could be *accidentally true*. Sanati and Kyratsous (2015: 483) recognise this, but suggest that J.N's belief about her partner's unfaithfulness is not a case of an accidentally true delusion. I will also presume that M.G.'s case is not an instance of an accidentally true delusion either, though the authors do not speak to this.

3 This is not very controversial. Even those who take the irrationality of delusions to (a) exist along a continuum with other irrational beliefs (e.g. Bortolotti 2009) or to (b) not be clinically significant (e.g. Noordhof and Sullivan-Bissett 2023) nevertheless accept the claim that delusions are irrational (although see Noordhof and Sullivan-Bissett 2021, §5.1 for a way of resisting this).

4 It is open to the one-factor theorist to claim that speakers with delusions *are* actually generally irrational, as long as they are willing to ascribe generalised irrationality to *all humans*.

5 Although there is some evidence of the JTC bias in people with schizophrenia, there is little evidence of it in those with monothematic delusions (Noordhof and Sullivan-Bissett 2021: 10288).

6 Bayesian rationality is a probability-based measure of rationality which employs Bayes' Theorem, a formula for calculating conditional probabilities: $P(h/e) = P(e/h) \cdot P(h)/P(e)$.

## References

American Psychiatric Association (2013), *Diagnostic and Statistical Manual of Mental Disorders: DSM-5*, 5th edition. Washington, DC: American Psychiatric Publishing.

Bortolotti, L. (2009), *Delusions and Other Irrational Beliefs*. Oxford: Oxford University Press.

Bueter, A. (2019), 'Epistemic Injustice and Psychiatric Classification', *Philosophy of Science*, 86:5, 1064–1074.

Bueter, A. (2021), 'Diagnostic Overshadowing in Psychiatric-Somatic Comorbidity: A Case for Structural Testimonial Injustice', *Erkenntnis*, 88:3, 1135–1155.

Carel, H. and I.J. Kidd (2014), 'Epistemic Injustice in Healthcare: A Philosophical Analysis', *Medicine, Health Care and Philosophy*, 17, 529–540.

Coltheart, M., R. Langdon, and R. McKay (2007), 'Schizophrenia and Monothematic Delusions', *Schizophrenia Bulletin*, 33:3, 643–647.

Crichton, P., H. Carel, and I. Kidd (2017), 'Epistemic Injustice in Psychiatry', *BJPsych Bulletin*, 41:2, 65–70.

Dotson, K. (2011), 'Tracking Epistemic Violence, Tracking Practices of Silencing', *Hypatia*, 26:2, 236–257.

Dotson, K. (2014), 'Conceptualizing Epistemic Oppression', *Social Epistemology*, 28:2, 115–138.

Dudley, R., P. Taylor, S. Wickham, and P. Hutton (2016), 'Psychosis, Delusions and the "Jumping to Conclusions" Reasoning Bias: A Systematic Review and Meta-Analysis', *Schizophrenia Bulletin*, 42:3, 652–665.

Dudley, R.E.J., C.H. John, A.W. Young, and D.E. Over (1997), 'The Effect of Self-Referent Material on the Reasoning of People with Delusions', *British Journal of Clinical Psychology*, 36, 575–584.

Ellis, H.D. and A.W. Young (1990), 'Accounting for Delusional Misidentifications', *The British Journal of Psychiatry*, 157:2, 239–248.

Ellis, H.D., A.W. Young, A.H. Quayle, and K.W de Pauw (1997), 'Reduced Autonomic Responses to Faces in Capgras Delusion', *Proceedings of the Royal Society of London B: Biological Sciences*, B264, 1085–1092.

Fricker, M. (2007), *Epistemic Injustice: Power and the Ethics of Knowing*. Oxford: Oxford University Press.

Fricker, M. (2016), 'Epistemic Injustice and the Preservation of Ignorance', in Peels, R. and Blaauw, M. (eds.), *The Epistemic Dimensions of Ignorance*, pp. 160–177. Cambridge: Cambridge University Press.

Garety, P. (1991), 'Reasoning and Delusions', *British Journal of Psychiatry*, 159:14, 14–18.

Garety P.A., D.R. Hemsley, and S. Wessely (1991), 'Reasoning in Deluded Schizophrenic and Paranoid Patients: Biases in Performance on a Probabilistic Task', *The Journal of Nervous and Mental Disease*, 179:4, 194–201.

Gerrans, P. (2001), 'Delusions as Performance Failures', *Cognitive Neuropsychiatry*, 6:3, 161–173.

Harcourt, E. (2021), 'Epistemic Injustice, Children and Mental Illness', *Journal of Medical Ethics*, 47, 729–735.

Hookway, C. (2010), 'Some Varieties of Epistemic Injustice: Reflections on Fricker', *Episteme*, 7:2, 151-163.

Houlders, J., L. Bortolotti, and M. Broome (2021), 'Threats to Epistemic Agency in Young People with Unusual Experiences and Beliefs', *Synthese*, 199, 7689–7704.

Jackson, J. (2017), 'Patronizing Depression: Epistemic Injustice, Stigmatizing Attitudes, and the Need for Empathy', *Journal of Social Philosophy*, 48:3, 359–376.

Jaspers, K. (1968), 'The Phenomenological Approach in Psychopathology', *The British Journal of Psychiatry*, 114:516, 1313–1323.

Jefferson, A., L. Bortolotti, and B. Kuzmanovic (2017), 'What is Unrealistic Optimism?', *Consciousness and Cognition*, 50, 3–11.

Kemp, R., S. Chua, P. McKenna, and A. David (1997), 'Reasoning and Delusions', *British Journal of Psychiatry*, 170:5, 398–405.

Kidd, I.J., L. Spencer, and H. Carel (2022), 'Epistemic Injustice in Psychiatric Research and Practice', *Philosophical Psychology*, online ahead of print, https://doi.org/10.1080/09515089.2022.2156333.

Kidd, I.J., L. Spencer, and E. Harris (2023), 'Epistemic Injustice Should Matter to Psychiatrists', *Philosophy of Medicine*, 4:1, 1–4.

Kious, B.M., B.R. Lewis, and S.Y.H. Kim (2023), 'Epistemic Injustice and the Psychiatrist', *Psychological Medicine*, 53:1, 1–5.

Kurs, R. and A. Grinshpoon (2018), 'Vulnerability of Individuals with Mental Disorders to Epistemic Injustice in Both Clinical and Social Domains', *Ethics & Behaviour*, 28:4, 336–346.

Mason, R. (2011), 'Two Kinds of Unknowing', *Hypatia*, 26:2, 294–307.

Medina, J. (2017), 'Varieties of Hermeneutical Injustice', in I. Kidd, J. Medina, and G. Pohlhaus Jr. (eds.), *The Routledge Handbook of Epistemic Injustice*, pp. 41–52. Abingdon: Routledge.

Miller Tate, A.J. (2019), 'Contributory Injustice', *Journal of Medical Ethics*, 45, 97–100.

Newbigging, K. and J. Ridley (2018), 'Epistemic Struggles: The Role of Advocacy in Promoting Epistemic Justice and Rights in Mental Health', *Social Science & Medicine*, 219, 36–44.

Noordhof, P. and E. Sullivan-Bissett (2021), 'The Clinical Significance of Anomalous Experience in the Explanation of Monothematic Delusions', *Synthese*, 199, 10277–10309.

Noordhof, P. and E. Sullivan-Bissett (2023), 'The Everyday Irrationality of Monothematic Delusion', in P. Henne and S. Murray (eds.), *Advances in Experimental Philosophy of Action*. London: Bloomsbury, pp. 87–111.

Pilditch, T.D., J.K Madsen, and R. Custers (2020), 'False Prophets and Cassandra's Curse: The Role of Credibility in Belief Updating', *Acta Psychologica*, 202:102956, 1–12.

Pohlhaus, G. (2012), 'Relational Knowing and Epistemic Injustice: Toward a Theory of "Willful Hermeneutical Ignorance"', *Hypatia*, 27:4, 715–735.

Ritunnano, R. (2022), 'Overcoming Hermeneutical Injustice in Mental Health: A Role for Critical Phenomenology', *Journal of the British Society for Phenomenology*, 53:3, 243–260.

Sanati, A., and M. Kyratsous (2015), 'Epistemic Injustice in Assessment of Delusions', *Journal of Evaluation of Clinical Practice*, 21:3, 479–485.

Scrutton, A. (2017), 'Epistemic Injustice and Mental Illness', in I. Kidd, J. Medina, and G. Pohlhaus Jr. (eds.), *The Routledge Handbook of Epistemic Injustice*, pp. 347–355. Abingdon: Routledge.

Spencer, L. (2023), 'Epistemic Injustice in Late-Stage Dementia: A Case for Non-Verbal Testimonial Injustice', *Social Epistemology*, 37:1, 62–79.

Steslow, K. (2010), 'Metaphors in Our Mouths: The Silencing of the Psychiatric Patient', *Hastings Centre Report*, 40:4, 30–33.
Townley, C. (2011), *A Defense of Ignorance: Its Value for Knowers and Roles in Feminist and Social Epistemologies*. Plymouth: Lexington Books.
Wanderer, J. (2017), 'Varieties of Testimonial Injustice', in I. Kidd, J. Medina, and G. Pohlhaus Jr. (eds.), *The Routledge Handbook of Epistemic Injustice*, pp. 271–313. Abingdon: Routledge.

# PART 4

# Delusion's place in the mind

# 18
# DELUSION AND ACTION

*Maura Tumulty*

## Introduction

Attitudes and actions relate in complicated ways. Because attitudes like belief cause action in fairly reliable ways, we look to beliefs to help predict whether our partner will stop to pick up dinner on the way home from work—as well as whether someone's on-line radicalization indicates a drift toward violence. On the other hand, hypocrisy, weakness of will, ambivalence, and procrastination provide cases of tension between apparent beliefs and important tasks left undone. Some patterns of inaction make us wonder if people actually believe what they claim they do.

When we're interacting with other people, we are often quite confident about which actions they intended and performed. (I know you put the glass container in the cupboard, not the fridge.) We use that information to work out what they believed. (You must have believed the container was empty; you must not have noticed it held a hard-boiled egg.) Sometimes, instead, we have a better grip on what someone believes, and we use that to work out what she was doing. Working out what someone *did*, especially in any sense relevant to moral assessment, usually requires making some connection to her attitudes—because not just any change in the physical location of her limbs will count in the relevant sense as something she did.[1] Falling on you with sufficient force to grind all your clothes into the dirt might be one accurate description of something I did; whether it is the best one might turn on whether or not I believed you were in danger from an oncoming train (in which case 'push you to safety' is probably a better specification). Sometimes, neither starting from the attitude nor the action seems easier; we just have to repeat tentative interpretative steps all round. My friend might be destroying the eyes in the photo of her ex because she believes it will cause harm to befall him; or she might just be expressing her feelings (Hursthouse 1991). Both scenarios are possible, but the action/attitude pairs will be quite different in each case—and it might take some doing to figure out what is going on. Finally, in some cases, the circle between attitude-specification and action-specification feels anything but virtuous: we are equally unsure about both, and unsure about how to make progress. Any tentative interpretation we propose seems to undo itself almost immediately.



DOI: 10.4324/9781003296386-23

That kind of uncertainty can arise when we are interpreting people who come to clinical attention with delusional thinking. Resolving the uncertainty is pressing, because we want to identify when people with delusions might take actions that seriously harm themselves or others, or might engage in patterns of behavior that leave them vulnerable to harm (indirectly, because they stop eating enough, or directly, because others victimize them). There are also theoretical questions, of the kind that matter for this volume: How do delusions and action relate? What light would answering that question shine on the question of how attitudes and actions relate more generally?

Most of the questions about delusions and action will fall into one of two broad categories. (Initial answers we give to questions in one category are likely to affect how we frame and answer questions in the other, and vice versa.) The first category includes questions about the relevance of action to the nature of delusions—in particular, to the question of whether delusions ever count as beliefs. In debates about the doxastic status of delusions, decisions turn just as much on our (developing) views of the nature of belief as on our views about the nature of delusion.[2] The same is true in this particular, action-focused thread in that larger debate. That is, resolution of relevant questions will turn as much on which views of action we endorse as on which views about delusion we find compelling. In both domains, we can ask whether rationality is simply a term of praise for a belief, intention, or action, or whether rationality is ever relevant to the identity conditions of an attitude or action.[3]

The second category of question is more internally diverse. It includes all the practical, legal, and clinical questions about the interplay between delusion and action, both as those questions arise for subjects with delusions, their clinicians, their family and friends, and for legal, medical, and social institutions with which they interact. Questions about what marks a respectful, humane stance toward a person with delusions also fall in this category, when those questions connect to issues about his autonomy and his own sense of himself as an actor in the world.

Obviously, the two categories of question can't be completely separated, and the influence runs in both directions. How we answer questions about moral responsibility for actions connected to delusions might, for example, be affected by whether we take relevant delusional contents to have been *believed* by the person (for more on delusion and moral responsibility, see Scholten, Chapter 34). On the other hand, a better understanding of 'what it's like' to live with a persistent delusion, and a more nuanced understanding of the psychologically protective effects of some delusions, might lead us to frame new questions about what kind of actions could provide evidence for the character (doxastic or otherwise) of delusions. A significant reason, I contend, why questions in the two categories can't be addressed in isolation concerns the social character of reasoning, including practical reasoning. Getting at the truth of how *this* delusional content relates to *this* action will almost always require a wide-angle view that takes in how the subject is (or is not) able to position herself in future-directed social practices of self-explanation and self-justification.

In this chapter, I will present a number of questions in the first category before explaining why it is so difficult to use the relation between delusion and action in any effort to secure positive evidence for the claim that delusions have doxastic status (Sections 1–3). I will then look at a particular question in the second category: the relation of intention-specification to questions about moral responsibility, and urge epistemic caution (Sections 4 and 5). In conclusion, I'll suggest that some recent work on delusional disorders and social cognition might resonate with work in moral psychology on scaffolded responsibility—in ways that may recommend epistemic caution about ascriptions of determinate delusion-related intentions.

## 1.   What does (in)action imply about the doxastic character of delusion?

Because people with delusional thinking make what sound like assertions of the contents of their delusions, and sometimes act in ways that lead others to ascribe their delusion to them as believed, delusions are often categorized as beliefs (albeit unusual ones), both unofficially and officially.

Belief has implications for action, though exactly what those implications are depends on one's preferred account of belief. Belief is usually taken to be action-guiding in some distinctive way. That a state appears to play an action-guiding role may be taken as evidence that it is a belief (that framing may be especially appealing to some representationalists); action-guiding may, instead, be taken to partially constitute a state *as* a belief (that framing may be especially appealing to some dispositionalists). Right off the bat, two complications emerge. First, some states—like pretenses and intrusive thoughts—cause action, and may even appear to guide it, and yet are certainly not doxastic states.[4] So the fact that a delusion has a doxastic-like effect on action is not sufficient to establish the delusion is a belief. And second, some states commonly counted as beliefs fail to produce actions in the way we'd expect them to, if they were playing a distinctively doxastic action-guiding role (Bortolotti 2009: 172–175). If we let some of those states continue to pass as doxastic, oughtn't we do the same for delusions?

Consider the first complication. Because subjects with delusions often don't speak, act, or appear to have the emotional responses we'd expect if they believed the contents of their delusions, some theorists argue delusions are not genuinely doxastic states. Many of their arguments focus on the ways delusions, or deluded subjects, seem to be epistemically irrational. Someone in the grip of delusional thinking may seem to form her delusion on the basis of no, or insufficient evidence; or appear to maintain it in the face of serious counter-evidence (see Flores, Chapter 12 for more on delusion and evidence); or be unbothered when it contradicts her other beliefs. Other anti-doxasticist arguments, however, focus on practical irrationality. Delusions look oddly compartmentalized; subjects are apparently uninterested in actions that would be desirable, even urgent, if the content of their delusions were true. (This is especially striking in the case of monothematic delusions of misidentification: a supposedly kidnapped daughter may never be searched for, nor reported missing; an 'imposter' spouse gets into the marital bed at night, but the subject with delusions may placidly stay in place.) In many of these discussions of 'delusion and action', the actions being foregrounded are not merely verbal ones, such as the assertions or descriptions of the content of the delusion by which the person's delusion may first come to clinical attention.[5] Nor are they actions which aim to convince others (or even the speaker) that the content of the delusion is true (such as a young man with Cotard's displaying to his mother-in-law the absence of bleeding from his self-inflicted stab wound, as purported evidence that he was dead [Young & Leafhead 1996]). Rather, the focus is on actions that would be practically rational (on a belief-desire model) if the content of the delusion were true.

Actions in this category would be the protective actions taken by individuals with persecutory delusions, such as covering up house windows with cardboard to prevent spies from being able to see inside. Actions of this type are the ones that seem most promising for demonstrating that an action is being guided, not merely caused, by a delusion; and that it is being guided by the delusion in the way that beliefs are normatively expected to guide action. (Perhaps I *believe* spies threaten my *desired* safety and privacy; I *believe* the cardboard will thwart them, and secure it to the window.) In Section 3, we'll look more closely at options for handling cases where the delusion doesn't produce the action we might have expected. For now, the issue is this: even when a delusion seems to be guiding the production of action congruent with its content, that may not be sufficient to establish the doxastic character of the delusion.

That's because guidance of a quasi-doxastic type can be provided by attitudes that are clearly non-doxastic. (Some anti-doxasticists then claim that delusions in fact belong to one of the attitude categories [e.g. imagination] already familiar to us from folk-psychology [Currie & Jureidini 2001]; others hold that delusions belong to a distinct attitude category, but one they've devised, and recommend adding to our folk- and scientific-psychology repertoires [Doggett & Egan 2007; Egan 2008][6].) After all, pretending to be an elephant could lead to some of the same behaviors as believing oneself to be an elephant (Velleman 2000). One might announce 'I am an elephant'; one might rub dust on one's skin; one might seek out peanuts in the shell; etc. Perhaps when pretending one might take more actions designed to *show* others one's elephant status. One might be less concerned with these actions if one truly believed one were an elephant, but there would still be a good bit of overlap. So dust-bathing behavior alone wouldn't be evidence that an 'I am an elephant' delusional content was believed rather than imagined. If one wants to push a doxastic account of delusions generally, or use *this* action by *this* deluded subject as evidence in favor of such an account, you'd have to secure something additional.

Now consider the second complication. There are many beliefs that recommend nothing by way of actions in daily life at all; most banal biological generics like, 'Humans are bipeds' are of this sort (Bortolotti 2011). Then there are beliefs whose abstraction or complexity are such that, especially with a bit of imagination, an enormous variety of actions could be construed as recommended by them (e.g. 'Recession is looming'). So even when we know we've got not just some attitude-or-other, but a belief, confidence about what type of action we should be expecting—if any—isn't always obvious; and that's before we've added in obvious points about the holism of the mental and the importance of *ceteris paribus* clauses! (Obviously, my belief that *there is chocolate ice cream in the freezer* will lead me to walk toward the freezer to get some only if I *want* some, and only if a masked intruder hasn't suddenly burst in the room and commanded me not to get up from the couch, and so on.) So for a narrow slice of time, and especially absent much additional information, the fact that a state doesn't seem to be leading to this or that particular action need not be evidence against that state's being doxastic.

Most importantly, however, many beliefs that would demand particular types of action frequently appear not to produce anything of the sort—and yet everyone goes on comfortably ascribing (and even avowing) the belief. Many people sincerely assert a belief in the equal moral worth of every human person, but many fewer people act in anything like the ways one might expect if that content were guiding their actions in a doxastic way. Consider, too, weakness of will. While some hardline positions insist that apparent weakness of will is always really a change of mind about what ought to be done, many of us—for personal and theoretical reasons—think we can point to cases where we apparently believed that $\phi$ ought, all things considered, be done with some urgency right now—and yet we didn't $\phi$. We could respond to these cases by saying: these failures of action are analogous to the compartmentalization observed in delusion; these people aren't really in states of belief either (Schwitzgebel 2010; Tumulty 2014). A more common move has been to adopt some version of the continuity thesis (Bortolotti 2009): to say that we all have some beliefs that meet conditions for being *beliefs* while failing to meet conditions for being epistemically or practically *rational* beliefs; and that the forms of failure subjects with delusions display are not different in kind from everyone else's. Either way, it seems advisable to avoid double standards. Absent compelling reasons to do so, we should not hold someone with delusions to a higher standard for acceptable, genuinely doxastic-type relations to action than we hold someone without (present) delusions.

## 2.   Apparently doxastic states not producing much action?

Further exploration of the fact that many beliefs don't appear to recommend any very specific actions reveals additional complexity in the general relationship between attitudes and actions. Consider a context and a proposition for which we can identify a couple of actions (say, $\phi$ and $\phi^*$) such that a subject S's failure to perform (or sincerely attempt to perform) them in that context puts pressure on the claim that she has a doxastic-type attitude toward that proposition. If you'd been thinking of ascribing the belief that $p$ to S, but you notice S is failing to $\phi$ or $\phi^*$, you have options.

1   You could say that $p$ is imagined or desired rather than believed; or that S's determinate attitude toward $p$, whatever it is, isn't very belief-like; or that S has no determinate attitude toward $p$ at all.
2   You could ask whether $p$ was the best content-specification for S's attitude (doxastic or otherwise).
3   You could insist on the truth of a full-throated attribution to S of the belief that $p$, by arguing that the expectation re: $\phi$-ing or $\phi^*$-ing is *not* relevant to doxastic status here—but only to some other, additional claim we might want to make, about the belief that $p$, or about S as a believer that $p$ (e.g. that either is *rational*). (That is, you could adopt less strict standards for the proper attribution of beliefs.)
4   You could insist on the truth of a full-throated attribution to S of the belief that $p$, continue to see $\phi$ or $\phi^*$ as in some way relevant to that attribution's appropriateness, but seek to justify or excuse S's failure to $\phi$ or $\phi^*$. One could justify the failure by pointing out something previously unreported about S's beliefs and desires that, when revealed, makes sense of why S would not see either $\phi$ or $\phi^*$ as wise in the context. Or one could excuse the failure: acknowledge that given S's belief that $p$, it would be appropriate for S to either $\phi$ or $\phi^*$, but indicate something that prevents this *without* undermining the doxastic status of S's attitude toward p.[7] (That is, you could maintain strict standards, but find a justification or excuse for S's failure to meet them in this case.)

Strong doxasticists about delusion—who want to count all delusions as beliefs—almost always have to go down the 'excusing' branch of the fourth option at some point (Bayne & Pacherie 2005). There are many instances of delusional content rendering certain very specific actions quite urgent—looking for the kidnapped child, getting out of the marital bed after the imposter gets in. When such actions are not taken, there may not be anything inside the subject's perspective that looks like a justification. (Consider contents like, 'The kidnapper told me if I leave the house, they'll kill her' or 'If I let the imposter know I'm on to him, I'll be in trouble.' Such contents [in the relevant contexts] would not merely explain but would justify inaction.) In the absence of such justifications, excuses are needed. The difficulty, when formulating excusing conditions, is to identify factors that are strong enough to excuse the relevant failure to act—but aren't so strong that they undermine our confidence in the correctness of the content and attitude we ascribed to the deluded subject in the first place (Tumulty 2011).

This sets up an asymmetry. It can be fairly easy, in any particular case, to suggest that some factor—say, general apathy or anhedonia—might be sufficient to explain why S could both believe that $p$ and yet fail to $\phi$. This ensures that the failure to act as expected doesn't count as decisive evidence *against* the doxastic character of the delusional content that would, were it believed, represent that action as practically rational. It is harder to secure positive evidence that the relation between some delusional content and an agent's pattern of (in)action is doxastic, however. That's because most excuses strong enough to work should also make us question the accuracy and security of our ascriptions to this subject overall. If your anhedonia is severe enough to complicate not just your ability to hold onto (representations) of the goodness of your future professional projects but also of your family members' safety, that hugely complicates the task of identifying specific attitudes and determinate intentions to potentially ascribe to you. (Among other things, it makes it much harder to make assessments about how you rank your priorities, which affects how I specify your intentions.)

If we are faced with someone's lack of action to recover her supposedly missing daughter, we may be choosing between descriptions like 'She believes her daughter has been kidnapped, but has trouble holding on to the idea of urgency associated with this' and 'Her relation to the idea of her daughter's kidnapping isn't quite doxastic'. The kind of excuse strong enough to interfere with the action-guidance normally provided by such a distressing, urgent belief will be strong enough to raise concerns about the distance between how we are specifying the content of the delusion (her daughter is *in danger*) and how the deluded subject experiences that content. It will also raise concerns about how confident we should be in any decision to go with the supported-by-excuse, doxastic interpretation of the subject's attitude toward her delusion, rather than another interpretation of her attitude. Taking subjects' attitudes toward their delusions to be beliefs might seem the best way to continue to engage them as conversational or epistemic peers, but as this example shows, that won't always be the case. Attributing to someone the type of excusing conditions required to explain why she didn't act on a 'my daughter has been kidnapped' belief itself pushes her quite far away from the status of our clear epistemic peer. It isn't obvious that by doing this we push her any farther away than we do by attributing her delusion to her as the content of a non-doxastic attitude. To the extent that pragmatic or ethical considerations should shape attribution decisions in such cases, they may not always tilt in the doxastic direction.

## 3. Apparently non-doxastic states guiding action in quasi-doxastic way?

Recall the first complication: the fact that states that are clearly not beliefs sometimes guide action, and sometimes do so in belief-ish ways. When wondering if a delusion's relation to action is evidence for doxastic status, then, how should we distinguish merely belief-ish from fully doxastic guidance? We certainly don't want to count only the fully explicitly deliberative considerations of reasons for and against $\phi$-ing, followed by an explicit judgment that $\phi$-ing is what one has all-things-considered reason to do, followed by an explicitly articulated intention to φ, followed by a self-aware and complete φ-ing as 'doxastic guidance'! (Among other things, that holds us hostage to a form of practical decision making we almost never go in for, and rides roughshod over continuing debates about the nature of practical deliberation, the relation between judgment and intention, etc.; it can't be that our most general idea of belief-style action guidance lines up only with one very particular theory of practical decision-making!) On the other hand, we do need to be holding on to the idea of *guidance*, and some connection to the idea of a belief speaking in favor of an action. That's because many things reliably cause specific actions without being beliefs; and many psychological factors other than attitudes can be appealed to in explanations that indicate causes of people's actions, and render them more intelligible. Explanations that appeal to personality traits like extroversion, or moods like despair, bring actions and agents within the fold of mutual intelligibility, but they don't advert to factors agents would themselves put forward to explain why it seemed right to them to act as they did (Alvarez 2017). My extroversion may explain why a lively party appeals to me this gloomy Friday evening; but it is the likely liveliness of the party, not my extroversion, that *I* would cite in explaining why I want to go. Aspects of my current psychology and mental lay-out may cause—and hence explain—my action, in a variety of ways; some of that causation may be fine-grained enough to warrant some talk of 'guiding'. But the kind of guiding that would be positive evidence for the claim that I am guided by a *belief* must be connected in some way with my own view of the situation within which I (plan to) act.

There are ongoing debates—whole cottage industries in metaethics—about what it is to act for or on a reason, or what it is to view something as a consideration in favor of acting, etc. We can abstract from those for now (but engaging with them more fully is unlikely to make the questions about delusions and action easier to settle). The main point is that there is a way our beliefs—our takes on ways the world is—shape our action that is different from the way our moods, traits, and energy levels shape our action. We might appeal to a mood, trait, or degree of apathy in order to explain away someone's failing to do what a belief should make it very pressing for them to want to do.[8] And we might appeal to such non-attitude factors to explain why someone acts. But in neither case will we have made a connection with how the world appears to a subject, as favoring certain actions over others—the connection that would suggest she *believes* the world is this way, and that is (part of) why she acted.

Even when we do appeal to an attitude—and not just to a trait or mood—we still might not be cleanly getting at the kind of connection that would show the attitude-action relation to be of the doxastic-guidance type. That's because beliefs (and other attitudes) can have both global and local effects on our actions. The belief that I've done hard things before, combined with a belief that a record of overcoming past challenges is predictive of future success, may together induce an optimistic mood and sense of myself as efficacious in the world. That optimistic self-efficacy may make it easier for me to carry out *any* of my intentions, and easier for me to stick with complex deliberations long enough to form clear intentions in the first place. But now suppose we were uncertain what my attitude was toward the content 'I have done hard things in the past'. Noticing this global effect on action after I entertained this content would not suffice to prove my attitude toward it was doxastic.

It surely matters—clinically, and in familial relationships—that a delusion might have (for a time at least) a general action-supporting effect. If delusions implying I have been singled out for a special mission boost my mood, self-esteem, and sense of competence, it could be counter-productive for anyone to try and disrupt the hold of the delusion on me without some plan for what might replace its supportive work (Gunn & Bortolotti 2018; Ritunnano et al. 2022; for more on delusion and adaptiveness, see Bortolotti and Murri, Chapter 3).[9] But such purely global effects won't necessarily mean that the content of the delusion figures in any of the considerations in light of which I take any action I do. (And of course, the state need not be doxastic at all to have whatever global effects it does. For example, perhaps periodically *visualizing* myself as singled out for a special mission might nudge me to look more kindly at myself, elevate my mood and self-esteem, etc., in ways that increase my efficacy as an agent.)

The kind of 'local' connection relevant to evidence of truly doxastic-style action guidance from delusional content does sometimes occur. It happens tragically, as when someone harms themselves or someone else and the content of the delusion was (from the subject's perspective) a consideration favoring her action (e.g. a delusion that this person is not a person but an evil robot who must be disassembled [Sullivan-Bissett et al. 2016]). It can happen with the protective actions that are taken by those with persecutory delusions (covering windows with cardboard, unplugging phones, avoiding certain forms of transit); such actions may not directly harm anyone, but their obvious oddness can accelerate social isolation. And it can happen helpfully, as when a delusion that God has chosen you for a special mission but can't reveal it to you yet leads someone who previously planned to kill themselves to delay their plans—and this allows time for treatment to help (Gunn & Bortolotti 2018). In each of these cases, there is a way in which the content of the delusion would, if true, rationalize the action/decision in question, by displaying it as worth doing (from the agent's perspective): either directly, or as a means to some end. In these cases, we are closer to having not just belief-ish action-guidance, but positive evidence that the subject's attitude toward the content in question is doxastic.

Because the metaphysics of belief are still in dispute, and because on some accounts of belief, failures to act in ways a belief would render practically rational are fairly easy to excuse, it is risky to defend on action-related grounds a full-blown anti-doxastic view about all delusions. At the very least, some of the complexity in how delusion relates to action can be explained as no different in kind from how non-pathologized beliefs relate to action; and some of the relevant complexity can perhaps be excused as compatible with a doxastic character for delusion. But it is also risky to defend, on action-related grounds, a view ascribing doxastic status to all or most delusions. The amount of information required to move from 'we can disarm what looks like negative evidence against doxastic status in this case' to 'we have positive evidence for doxastic-style, content-driven action-guidance in this case' is significant, and we may not have it as often as doxasticists would hope.

## 4.  Intention-specification and higher-stakes attributions

In addition to wondering whether people believe their delusions, and how this connects to their likelihood of acting on them, we may wonder how delusional disorders affect responsibility generally. We might wonder whether a delusion diminishes responsibility for all and only those actions it somewhat directly provokes, or whether someone prone to delusional thinking might be confused enough in certain key ways that it wasn't fair to hold her responsible for any of her actions, whether they seemed connected to the themes of her most prominent delusions or not. These questions matter in institutional and legal contexts, but also in ordinary ethical ones. Consider, for example, a person who developed a Capgras-like duplicative delusion as a result of dementia with Lewy bodies (von Siebenthal et al. 2021) but has now passed into such a late phase of the disease that for large stretches of time it isn't clear she is aware of what is going on around her at all. If she shoves a caregiver hard enough to cause a fall and subsequent injury, the question of blame might never come up—because everyone had already stopped treating her as morally responsible, in the sense of morally assessable, at all. Earlier in the disease progression, that action might have been attributed to her but understood as excused. Perhaps we took her to have a false belief that she was being attacked, and agreed that shoving would have been an appropriate response if the attack had been real. Assuming someone is otherwise apt for moral assessment, the mere fact that they have a delusion will rarely suffice to render some relevant action not blameworthy (Sullivan-Bissett et al. 2016).[10] That's because many such actions would be blameworthy even if the content of the delusion were true. Consider, for example, a persecutory delusion about a supposedly loud-music-playing neighbor. Suppose both parts of your delusion are false: your neighbor isn't playing loud music, and he has no aim to annoy you. However, even if both were *true*, that would not justify your killing him (Sullivan-Bissett et al. 2016). So you would still be blameworthy. Similarly, some patterns of action that reveal vices of character don't seem to do so any less when accompanied by delusions. If you are a tyrannical personality dripping with disdain for the 'little people', you really may have the relevant vices, whether or not you also take yourself to be the reincarnation of Cleopatra.[11]

However, recall how inaction puts pressure on the claim that a deluded subject genuinely believed the content of her delusion (and, perhaps, on our confidence that we have accurately specified the content of her delusion). Similar pressures play out with respect to intentions. That's because the very cases in which delusions appear to lead people to act in ways that violate social and ethical norms are also cases where we might just as well wonder whether we had accurately specified their intentions—what it was they were aiming to do. Precisely because 'killing someone for playing loud music' is so very ethically wrong, we should wonder: are we sure *that's* the correct specification of the agent's intention? (Is there any chance, for example, that part of the delusion of persecution included a fear that the loud music would eventually cause him irreparable harm?) If we can't be confident we are specifying intentions clearly, we can't be confident we are applying justifying, excusing, and blaming conditions properly—because we aren't confident about *what* we are justifying, excusing, or blaming. General worries about transparent ascriptions to deluded subjects of attitudes and intentions come up again here, with special force. Sometimes people with delusional disorders do make assertions that look like rationalizations of some of their behavior. Sometimes, however, others assume that several behaviors are connected to the same rationalization—without it being clear that the person in question would share *that* understanding of what they were doing. The distinction between those attributions that merely allow third parties to capture a subject's persecuted mood or style and those that express a content providing doxastic-style guidance for her actions matters a good deal—especially when assessments of responsibility are at stake.


## 5.   Meaning, conversation, and scaffolding

That the formation of a delusion could be associated with, or even cause, a sense of calm; that it could help create a sense of overall life-meaning and in some cases directly reduce the likelihood of self-harm—these facts emerge from careful attention to the descriptions people with delusional thinking give of the role of delusions in their lives, during and sometimes after a stretch of delusional thinking (Isham et al. 2022; Ritunnano & Bortolotti 2022; Ritunnano et al. 2022; see also Ritunnano & Littlemore, Chapter 2). That such attention and conversational effort could be not just a kindness but also clinically effective and generative for academic research hasn't always been sufficiently appreciated. It's been important for researchers to trace the ways delusional thoughts could, despite being caused by disorders and having harmful effects over long time-horizons, provide people with senses of purpose and resolution, and so provide medium-term supports for both a subjective sense of agency and an ability to carry out objectively useful plans.

Of course, as defenders of the continuity thesis point out, deluded subjects are hardly the only ones who frequently violate standards for practical rationality. Few of us who claim that every human life deserves equal moral consideration spend even ten minutes each day acting in any of the ways made practically rational by that belief. And those of us now capable of reading this essay were all once too young to have the stable attitudes required for full-blown moral responsibility; some of us will lose capacities required for full-blown moral responsibility as we age. At any given moment, therefore, there are more folks being ascribed folk-psychological attitudes like 'wanting a cookie' and 'believing the cookies are in the jar' then are in fact living up to the standards that (in part) individuate those attitudes. To the extent that our ascriptive practices help nudge us into compliance by attributing to us attitudes and underlying capacities we don't quite (or quite consistently) have (McGeer 2007; Zawidzki 2013), this might be a feature rather than a bug. Both very young children and adults with various cognitive deficits rely on others to provide conversational scaffolding and other environmental cues to help support appropriate action. A young child may be helped to become reliable at following through on her stated intentions by being proleptically treated as if she already were; an older man in the early stages of dementia may be supported in maintaining his capacities for independent action by being ascribed desires and wishes that are a bit more determinate than the ones he could easily report.

Interviews with populist election deniers in the United States and Brazil provide examples of individuals who are only too happy to offer justifications for their actions, explanations of why they deserve praise rather than blame, and confident assertions of belief. There are complicated empirical questions about how conspiracy theories, cultish articles of faith, and delusions differ (Bortolotti, Ichino, and Mameli 2021; for more on delusion and conspiracy theories, see Pierre, Chapter 37). There are also complicated theoretical choices to be made about which thought-patterns should be labeled pathological (Bardon 2019; Sakakibara 2022; for more on delusion and pathology, see Petrolini, Chapter 1). But at a basic, folk-psychological level, one difference between the conspiricist or cult figure and many deluded subjects is obvious. The former have *some* conversational community within which they work out with peers—if only by confabulating elaborate, socially acceptable excuses—explanations and justifications for their failures to act in ways their supposed beliefs make practical rational. Because of the social isolation that delusional disorders may precipitate and be exacerbated by, subjects with delusions may not participate in many of those conversations—even if they retain some capacity to do so.

A woman with persecutory delusions who shies away from questions about why she keeps unplugging the phone of her elderly, shut-in mother is quite different from a regular churchgoer who squirms under probing questions about how much she donates to charity. The latter may offer some defense of her choices; dispute your implication that her actions were insufficient; turn to the 'no one is perfect' cliché; or own her hypocrisy and confess how much it troubles her. In contrast, the former may avoid clarificatory conversation to such an extent that it is legitimate to wonder: How confident should we be that 'someone is spying on my mother, and wishes her harm' is a belief of hers, or 'protecting my mother from the spies' is an intention with which she acts? The social contexts and interactions that support greater determinacy of attitude and intention, and clarify both for interpreters, are often missing for subjects with delusions—at least during key stretches of their delusional thinking (Bell et al. 2021). Perhaps, quite generally, a capacity to participate in ongoing clarificatory conversation is needed for agency and attribution. People need such conversation to help relieve their confusion about what someone's intentions are, but individuals may need such conversations to help fix their intentions in the first place.[12] If so, the social isolation that both exacerbates delusional thinking (and accelerates during it) may affect what determinate intentional actions can confidently be ascribed to a deluded subject.[13]

## 6. Conclusion

In the case of subjects with delusions, their attitudes and actions, there are going to be hitches; things that don't quite fit. In navigating those hitches, we need to avoid dismissive attitudes toward people with delusions, and avoid flattening the complexity of their lives and the agency they do preserve. But the best way to avoid these pitfalls, in our theorizing and our practical interactions, may not always be to grant doxastic status to as many delusional contents as possible. Nor will theoretical nuance or respectful practical engagement always be best served by the confident attribution of highly determinate intentions and actions to individuals with active delusions.

In a welcome development, more researchers are listening to subjects describe their delusional thinking, and listening to descriptions of how delusions function in their lives. This has led some researchers to wonder if an over-emphasis on the doxastic aspects of delusional consciousness could produce its own kind of flattening. For example, if delusions prompt more focus on the way an experience of the world is *your experience* rather than a means of access to *the world*, subjects might be less inclined toward goal-directed action during stretches of delusional experience (Feyaerts et al. 2021). A subject who feels the personal significance of delusional experiences may be drawn to reflect on them and not take those experiences to be disclosing suggested actions in the world she shares with others (Feyaerts et al. 2020); this could further reduce her access to social scaffolds for developing determinate intentions, and complicate others' efforts to assess her attitudes. Such possibilities prompt new questions about the implications of inaction for attitude attribution. Careful attention to the variety of ways delusion could affect action is not dismissiveness. Acknowledging the gap between our ability to predict what actions a deluded subject might take, and our ability to grasp what speaks to her in favor of her acting, is not itself a lack of respect. Delusions may sometimes guide action in belief-typical ways. But attention to the times they *don't* will help us better understand delusions, and perhaps illuminate broad questions about how actions and attitudes interact.

## Acknowledgments

I am grateful to conversations with Carolina Flores, which helped shape the approach I took to this chapter. Ema Sullivan-Bissett provided deft guidance and insightful feedback on an earlier draft.

# Notes

1 There are contentious questions about how to specify important differences among categories like these: what someone does (recognize her mother at 20 paces); an intentional action she performs (light the candles on her mother's birthday cake); an activity she can voluntarily modulate but can't voluntarily initiate (weep, after getting bad news about her mother); a bodily motion that may or may not *also* have a description that marks it out as an intentional action (air moves out from her lungs, mouth, and lips). For the purposes of most questions about delusion and action, people are interested in the category of intentional action where that implies something more than mere behavior (e.g. an arm flinging out) or something done by a person without being an action (tasting the milk in the coffee). But there is no agreed-on way of cashing out that 'more'; see Piñeros Glasscock and Tennenbaum (2023) for a helpful overview.

2 Many authors (e.g. Kengo Miyazono 2019) note how hard it is to say anything significant about the nature of delusion while remaining neutral on key metaphysical questions about belief. Eric Schwitzgebel (2022) is especially clear on just how many metaphysical questions there are (e.g. are beliefs token representations, or sets of dispositions?). He notes that settling those question still wouldn't fully settle questions about the cognitive architecture that implements beliefs. Admittedly, 'belief' is often used in clinical definitions of delusion; the American Psychiatric Association's *Diagnostic and Statistical Manual* defines delusion in part as a "belief…that is firmly held despite what almost everyone else believes…The belief is not ordinarily accepted by other members of the person's culture" (DSM-5, 2013, p. 819). Participants in the debates about the doxastic status of delusions don't take such definitions to settle the relevant empirical or conceptual issues.

3 Lisa Bortolotti (2005, 2009) argues that irrationality need not undermine an attitude's doxastic status; Donald Davidson's reliance on rationality to individuate belief was the main target of her 2005 (see, for example, Davidson 1974).

4 That non-doxastic attitudes *cause* behavior is not in dispute. What is disputed is the exact shape of each attitude's causal-functional profile, with reference to behavior; and what distinctive role beliefs (or other attitudes) play in rationalizing, as opposed to merely causing, behavior. David Velleman (2000) argues that imagination and belief have the same motivational role (he argues that, therefore, no purely functional account will suffice to individuate belief from other attitudes of taking-true). Lucy O'Brien (2005) and Neil van Leeuwen (2009) contend (on different grounds) that Velleman has missed features of belief's motivating role that *do* distinguish it from imagination. Anna Ichino (2019) argues that imagination and belief *share* a functional profile with respect to the motivation of behavior. Ichino argues that in many cases where imagination appears not to motivate action, a belief would not have done so either, other things being equal—because the subject in question had meta-cognitive attitudes sufficient to block motivation to act. The result is a picture that has, ironically, some similarity to van Leeuwen's. Both authors acknowledge the distinctive role of belief in linking agents to first-order representations—including representations of their contexts for action—needed for effective action. Van Leeuwen takes this 'grounding' to give belief a distinctive motivational role. Ichino argues that if we focus on the role played by the meta-cognitions that keep track of (and sometimes misrepresent) first-order mental states, we'll appreciate that the motivational roles of belief and imagination are identical. (She does hold that belief has a distinctive functional profile with respect to evidence and inference.) As we'll see, as long as such general questions about the individuation conditions of belief's motivational role remain this unsettled, appealing to any particular account of a belief-action link to help settle questions about action and delusion will be fraught.

5 Verbalizations need not be what brings someone to clinical attention, but something must (for those who *do* come to clinical attention). As Bortolotti argues, '[t]here is a sense in which all clinical delusions are manifested in behaviour: minimally, they are reported and are diagnosed *as delusions* partially for the negative consequences that follow from the subject's conviction that the content of the delusion is true' (2009: 163).

6 Amy Kind (in press) argues that the case of delusion doesn't require us to add novel attitudes to our mental state taxonomies (or, at least, that the arguments presented in Doggett and Egan [2007] and Egan [2008] don't succeed in making that case). In the conclusion of that paper, Kind suggests that when various phenomena appear to put pressure on standard taxonomical categories, we may instead wish to amend those categories (perhaps by allowing them a kind

of 'smudginess'). Attention to the different uses we make of such categories is another way of relieving such pressures; see Tumulty (2014).

7   You might also say the person is φ-ing or φ*-ing (and that this supports your claim that she believes that *p*), but in a novel way. It might require some imagination to recognize her particular action as an instance of φ-ing or φ*-ing. Some of the protective behaviors undertaken by people with persecutory delusions might merit this sort of response.

8   The presence of such moods or states might sometimes be related to the underlying disorder (dementia with Lewy bodies, or schizophrenia) that made the formation of delusions more likely. But in appealing to the trait or tendency—apathy, for example—we would be appealing to an action-suppressing effect of the delusional disorder, but not to an action-suppressing effect of any specific delusion's *content*.

9   Similarly, the general lessening of anxiety that seems to accompany and be caused by the exit from the prodromal phase of a delusional disorder—perhaps because the formation of the delusion brings about a 'now everything makes sense' feeling—could have general agency-supporting effects. It can be hard to take any kind of decisive action when in the fog of anxiety. But such improvement wouldn't have any semantic tie to the particular content of the delusion that formed; anything that reduced anxiety would work as well. Such general agency-supporting effects will again provide only low-quality evidence that the relevant delusions have a distinctively doxastic character.

10  Philosophers are often interested in monothematic delusions like Capgras precisely because of their interesting implications for moral responsibility. Those discussions rarely note the fact that the majority of the Capgras cases that come to clinical attention are linked to neurodegenerative disorders such as Alzheimer's or dementia with Lewy bodies (for example, 38 of the 47 patients in ten years in the Mayo Clinic records; Joseph 2007). Every patient with such a disorder will fail to meet global conditions on moral responsibility at *some* point along that disease trajectory. Even in the middle phases of disease progression, while the *topic* of the delusion may be encapsulated, so that the delusion can be picked out as distinctive against all the rest of the person's cognition, it is unlikely that all the person's cognition and capacity for reasoning and conversational engagement is typical. See Section 5 for why this might matter to assessments of responsibility.

11  This framing is meant to be neutral between 'answerability' and 'attributability' understandings of responsibility (Shoemaker 2011).

12  Some of the research based on detailed conversations with people who have experienced delusions is retrospective—that is, the conversations are taking place after, not during, the time when the person was fully in the grip of her delusion (e.g. Dickson et al. 2016). This can make it hard to separate questions about whether a person had trouble having conversations with others because others were unwilling to engage with the unusual or off-putting *content* of the delusion, or whether she had general difficulties maintaining conversational back-and-forth, responding to requests for clarification, accepting mild challenges to her statements, etc. Either way, there was likely to be a reduction in the kind of conversation that helps in the formation of determinate intentions (let alone in the conversations that provide evidence to others of such intentions' content).

13  I am bringing, all the way down to the capacity for intention formation, Victoria McGeer's account of how social scaffolding helps in the development and on-going maintenance of our capacity for responsible agency (McGeer 2019). McGeer is especially interested in how our abilities to participate in *forward*-looking practices of explanation, justification, and self-improvement can impact which backward-looking responsibility attributions it is appropriate to make to us.


# References

American Psychiatric Association (2013) *Diagnostic and statistical manual of mental disorders (DSM-5)*. Washington, DC: American Psychiatric Association.

Alvarez, M. (2017) "Reasons for Action: Justification, Motivation, Explanation," in *The Stanford Encyclopedia of Philosophy (Winter 2017 Edition)*, Edward N. Zalta (ed.). https://plato.stanford.edu/archives/win2017/entries/reasons-just-vs-expl/.

Bardon, A. (2019) *The Truth about Denial: Bias and Self-Deception in Science, Politics, and Religion*. Oxford: Oxford University Press.

Bayne, T., and Pacherie, E. (2005) "In Defence of the Doxastic Conception of Delusions," *Mind and Language* 20(2): 163–188.

Bell, V., Raihani, N. and Wilkinson, S. (2021) "Derationalizing Delusions," *Clinical Psychological Science* 9(1): 24–37.

Bortolotti, L. (2005) "Delusions and the Background of Rationality," *Mind & Language* 20(2): 189–208.

Bortolotti, L. (2009) *Delusions and Other Irrational Beliefs*. Oxford: Oxford University Press.

Bortolotti, L. (2011) "Double Bookkeeping in Delusions: Explaining the Gap between Saying and Doing," in J.H. Aguilar, A.A. Buckareff, and K. Frankish (eds.), *New Waves in Philosophy of Action*. London: Palgrave Macmillan, 237–256.

Bortolotti, L., Ichino, A., and Mameli, M. (2021) "Conspiracy Theories and Delusions," *Reti, Saperi e Linguaggi: Italian Journal of Cognitive Sciences* VIII(2): 183–200.

Currie, G. and Jureidini, J. (2001) "Delusion, Rationality, Empathy: Commentary on Martin Davies et al.," *Philosophy, Psychiatry, & Psychology* 8(2): 159–162.

Davidson, D. (1974) "On the Very Idea of a Conceptual Scheme," *Inquiries into Truth and Interpretation*. Oxford: Clarendon Press.

Dickson, J.M., Barsky, J., Kinderman, P., King, D. and Taylor, P.J. (2016) "Early Relationships and Paranoia: Qualitative Investigation of Childhood Experiences Associated with the Development of Persecutory Delusions," *Psychiatry Research* 238: 40–45.

Doggett, T. and Egan, A. (2007) "Wanting Things You Don't Want," *Philosophers' Imprint* 7(9): 1–17.

Egan, A. (2008) "Imagination, Delusion, and Self-Deception," in T. Bayne and J. Fernández (eds.), *Delusion and Self-Deception: Affective and Motivational Influences on Belief Formation*, Hove: Psychology Press, 263–280.

Feyaerts, J., Henriksen, M.G., Vanheule, S., Myin-Germeys, I. and Sass, L.A. (2021) "Delusions Beyond Beliefs: A Critical Overview of Diagnostic, Aetiological, and Therapeutic Schizophrenia Research from a Clinical-Phenomenological Perspective," *The Lancet Psychiatry* 8(3): 237–249.

Gunn, R. and Bortolotti, L. (2018) "Can Delusions Play a Protective Role?," *Phenomenology and the Cognitive Sciences* 17(4): 813–833.

Hursthouse, R. (1991) "Arational Actions," *Journal of Philosophy* 88: 57–68.

Ichino, A. (2019) "Imagination and Belief in Action," *Philosophia* 47: 1517–1534.

Isham, L., Loe, B.S., Hicks, A., Wilson, N., Bird, J.C., Bentall, R.P. and Freeman, D. (2022) "The Meaning in Grandiose Delusions: Measure Development and Cohort Studies in Clinical Psychosis and Non-Clinical General Population Groups in the UK and Ireland," *The Lancet Psychiatry* 9(10): 792–803.

Josephs, K.A. (2007) "Capgras Syndrome and its Relationship to Neurodegenerative Disease," *Archives of Neurology* 64(12): 1762–1766.

Kind, A. (2024) "Contrast or Continuum? The Case of Belief and Imagination," in E. Sullivan-Bissett (ed.), *Belief, Imagination, and Delusion*. Oxford: Oxford University Press. pp. 42–59.

McGeer, V. (2007) "The Regulative Dimension of Folk Psychology," in D.D. Hutto and M. Ratcliffe (eds.), *Folk Psychology Re-Assessed*. Dordrecht: Springer, 137–156.

McGeer, V. (2019) "Scaffolding Agency: A Proleptic Account of the Reactive Attitudes," *European Journal of Philosophy* 27(2): 301–323.

Miyazono, K. (2019) *Delusions and Beliefs: A Philosophical Inquiry*. New York: Routledge.

O'Brien, L. (2005) "Imagination and the Motivational View of Belief," *Analysis* 65(1): 55–62.

Piñeros Glasscock, J.S. and Tenenbaum, S. (2023) "Action," *The Stanford Encyclopedia of Philosophy* (Spring 2023 Edition), Edward N. Zalta & Uri Nodelman (eds.). https://plato.stanford.edu/archives/spr2023/entries/action/.

Ritunnano, R., and Bortolotti, L. (2022) "Do Delusions Have and Give Meaning?," *Philosophy and the Cognitive Sciences* 21: 949–968.

Ritunnano, R., Kleinman, J., Oshodi, D.W., Michail, M., Nelson, B., Humpston, C.S. and Broome, M.R. (2022) "Subjective Experience and Meaning of Delusions in Psychosis: A Systematic Review and Qualitative Evidence Synthesis," *The Lancet Psychiatry* 9(6): 458–476.

Sakakibara, E. (2022) "Delusions and Beliefs as a Symptom of Illness," in J. Musolino, J. Sommer, and P. Hemmer (eds.), *The Cognitive Science of Belief*. Cambridge: Cambridge University Press, 440–461.

Schwitzgebel, E. (2010) "Acting Contrary to Our Professed Beliefs or the Gulf between Occurrent Judgment and Dispositional Belief," *Pacific Philosophical Quarterly* 91(4): 531–553.

Schwitzgebel, E. (2022) "The Nature of Belief from a Philosophical Perspective, With Theoretical and Methodological Implications for Psychology and Cognitive Science," *Frontiers in Psychology* 13: 947664.

Shoemaker, D. (2011) "Attributability, Answerability, and Accountability: Toward a Wider Theory of Moral Responsibility," *Ethics* 121: 603–632.

Sullivan-Bissett, E., Bortolotti, L., Broome, M. and Mameli, M. (2016) "Moral and Legal Implications of the Continuity between Delusional and Non-Delusional Beliefs," in G. Keil, L. Keuck, and R. Hauswald (eds.), *Vagueness in Psychiatry, International Perspectives in Philosophy and Psychiatry*. Oxford: Oxford Academic, 191–210.

Tumulty, M. (2011) "Delusions and Dispositionalism about Belief," *Mind and Language* 26(5): 596–628.

Tumulty, M. (2014) "Managing Mismatch between Belief and Behavior," *Pacific Philosophical Quarterly* 95(3): 261–292.

Van Leeuwen, D.N. (2009) "The Motivational Role of Belief," *Philosophical Papers* 38(2): 219–246.

Velleman, D. (2000) *The Possibility of Practical Reason*. Oxford: Oxford University Press.

von Siebenthal, A., Descloux, V., Borgognon, C., Massardi, T. and Zumbach, S. (2021) "Evolution of Capgras Syndrome in Neurodegenerative Disease: The Multiplication Phenomenon," *Neurocase* 27(2): 160–164.

Young, A.W. and Leafhead, K.M. (1996) "Betwixt Life and Death: Case Studies of the Cotard Delusion," in P.W. Halligan and J.C. Marshall (eds.), *Method in Madness: Case Studies in Cognitive Neuropsychiatry*. Hove: Psychology Press, 147–171.

Zawidzki, T.W. (2013) *Mindshaping: A New Framework for Understanding Human Social Cognition*. Cambridge: MIT Press.

# 19
# DELUSION AND DOXASTICISM

*Paul Noordhof*

People with delusions claim to believe very strange things and we can't see why they do, or reason them out of it. Some argue that when subjects with delusions say that their loved one has been replaced by an imposter or that they themselves are dead, these aren't really their beliefs but rather something else. The prevailing terminology is that *doxasticists* hold that delusions essentially involve beliefs that have a content characteristic of the delusion in question (hereafter, 'delusion-characterising content') and *non-doxasticists* (or *anti-doxasticists*) hold that delusions essentially involve other kinds of cognitive states with that content. However, many non-doxasticists allow that some delusions may involve beliefs and commensurately some doxasticists allow that delusions may involve other kinds of cognitive states with delusion-characterising content in virtue of which subjects with these states have a delusion (e.g. Bayne & Pacherie 2005: 179). Let's call positions that allow for these possibilities: *weak non-doxasticism* and *weak doxasticism* respectively.

Successful defence of doxasticism depends upon a proper characterisation of belief, and the relation of this characterisation to other competitor states for the delusion-characterising content; the arguments that identify features of delusion that beliefs allegedly fail to have; and the success of the competitor states in explaining these features. The latter issue will be evaluated further in the chapter on delusion and non-doxasticism (Noordhof, Chapter 20). I will set one issue aside. For some, the peculiarity of the ostensible delusion-characterising content implies that subjects with delusions don't have states with that content at all. They believe different 'framework propositions' to us which we cannot interpret or just mouth the words that putatively express the content (Campbell 2001: 96–98, for further critical discussion see Thornton (2008) and Ohlhorst, Chapter 27, this volume). At least in the monothematic case, these claims are implausible because subjects with such delusions show an appreciation of how other people use the words and, outside of the delusional context, seem to appreciate their meaning (Bayne & Pacherie 2004: 8–9, Hamilton 2006: 228). The issue of doxasticism versus non-doxasticism does not resolve the question of how delusions are to be fully explained but just focuses upon one aspect of their characterisation.

The discussion will have the following structure. First, we will consider the nature of belief. The conclusion of this section is that a particular type of functional theory is to be preferred (independently of a commitment to physicalism or functionalism generally).

DOI: 10.4324/9781003296386-24

In the second section, we will outline the arguments that have been offered against delusions involving beliefs and explain how the functional theory may deal with them without any substantial adjustment. In Chapter 20, we will consider the nature of non-doxastic alternatives and how they hope to explain, better, the features of delusions that suggest that delusions don't involve belief. Generally, the non-doxastic alternatives will be found wanting. The conclusion will be that the general arguments against delusions involving beliefs don't work although there may be cases in which there are no grounds for attributing to a subject a belief with delusion-characterising content.

## 1.  The nature of belief

Part of the reason why doxasticism continues to be contested is that there is no generally agreed approach to the nature of belief. Different approaches yield different verdicts. Discussion of eliminativist approaches would take us too far afield. It is an assumption of the debate that they are false. Dual level approaches, which break down our common understanding of beliefs into two types of states that work in different ways to capture our full understanding of beliefs, will be discussed towards the end of Chapter 20, drawing upon discussion of single state approaches, and non-doxastic states, that taken together make up the two types of states that they envisage.

Single state accounts of belief may be distinguished between those which appeal to a feature that is potentially independent of the present potential for the belief to stand in relations to other beliefs, mental states more generally, and behaviour, and those which aren't. On the former side, there are phenomenological, biological-functional, and representationalist accounts of belief, on the latter dispositional or functional theories and normative interpretive theories. I will explain how the former don't help to decide the issue between doxasticists and non-doxasticists before turning to the latter where the issue is more pressing.

### 1.1  *Phenomenological approaches to belief*

Phenomenological approaches to belief take belief to involve the entertaining of a proposition in consciousness in a certain way, typically assenting to or feeling convinced that it is the case (Bagehot talks of the emotion of conviction, Bagehot 1871: 32–34). Such approaches are largely recognised to be untenable unless integrated into one of the other approaches identified below. We attribute beliefs to a subject in the absence of any phenomenological properties relating to them when the subject is asleep or their consciousness is occupied with something else (Armstrong 1973: 7–8). The approach faces two related issues. The first concerns whether the characteristic feeling is compatible with a subject having no inclination to the cognitive responses and behaviour typical of the belief identified by the characteristic feeling. Feeling convinced that the bridge across which you are walking is going to collapse should, at the least, make you anxious and hasten your pace. The second is that it is natural to suppose that the feeling of conviction may be either, at least partly, a functional property of a certain kind or part of the characterisation of the functional role of belief. If the former, then it does not avoid the puzzles to which cases of delusion give rise. The functional role of feeling convinced *that p* is likely to involve acting as if *p* is true and integrating *p* in one's mental life. As an example of the latter option, a recent defence of doxasticism holds that a subject S believes that *p* if and only if S is disposed immediately to judge that *p* (understood to be an intentional occurrent state with a phenomenal character of judging that *p*) when p-entertaining triggers obtain (Clutton 2018: 201, Kriegel 2015: 123). Apart from the problem of justifying a narrowly focused functional role in terms of phenomenological dispositions, the analysis doesn't get past the difficulty of divorcing the phenomenal character of judging completely from its natural articulation in acting as if *p* and integrating the content of the judgement with the rest of a subject's mental life. We will discuss functional theories more generally below.

## 1.2   Representationalist approaches to belief

Representationalists hold that the belief that *p* is partly constituted from a representation that *p*. The approach can give the impression that inquiring whether there is a representation that *p* in the belief box in a subject's psychology may yield a fact of the matter over whether a subject believes that *p*, independent of the belief's relationship to other mental states, or responsiveness to evidence. Such an approach would provide a quick way with the arguments for non-doxasticism. However, just as with phenomenological accounts of belief, the issues that non-doxasticists use to motivate their position affect the present approach at crucial points. Talk of a belief box is a metaphorical way of describing representations that have a particular functional role with respect to other mental states and behaviour. Likewise, giving an account of what makes a representation a representation of *p* involves relations to other mental states and also the environment. So, even if representational accounts of belief can deal with the various problems that have been raised concerning them, for example, tacit beliefs, what access a subject must have to a representation for that to be the content of a belief, and so on, there is no reason to expect that this will bear on the question of whether doxasticism or non-doxasticism holds in the case of delusions (for discussion of some of these issues, see Field 1978: 36–37 fn. 9, Lycan 1988: 58, Quilty-Dunn & Mandelbaum 2018: 2359–2360, Schwitzgebel 2001: 76–78).

## 1.3   Biological-functional approaches

Biological-functional approaches hold that an essential feature of beliefs is that they have a biological function derived from the biological function of the cognitive mechanisms that give rise to them. Biological function is the result of a history of evolutionary selection in which creatures with that type of mechanism were favoured because of the survival advantage it conferred. Some have argued that delusions involve malfunctioning beliefs that may lack the features that the arguments against doxasticism take to be essential to beliefs (Miyazono 2019: 35–37).

While this approach provides the possibility of a defence of doxasticism, it faces the following issues that make its successful development difficult. First, the approach has to explain why the malfunctioning of the cognitive apparatus is producing malfunctioning *beliefs* rather than producing something else. Second, the selection history behind the cognitive apparatus producing the delusion-characterising content state has to be shown to be that behind belief production rather than behind the production of non-doxastic states which, in itself, either may be correctly functioning or malfunctioning in certain ways to produce non-doxastic states with some belief-like features. We can sidestep these issues if the grounds for supposing that delusion-characterising states are non-doxastic are inadequate. We shall find this to be the case with respect to the two approaches outlined below, those most directly challenged by non-doxasticism. There is no need to understand the nature of beliefs in terms of biological function but rather as possessors of biological function which their character enables us to assess as successfully or unsuccessfully carried out (just as a heart is a pump which, in virtue of its selection history, has the function of being a pump).

## *1.4 Normative-interpretive approaches*

According to the normative-interpretivist approach, the nature of belief is given in terms of its role in a normatively characterised interpretative framework involving the attribution of beliefs and desires to a subject to make sense of their behaviour. The nature of belief is generally given in terms of the circumstances in which an ideally rational subject would have particular beliefs, how they would reason, and, how the beliefs should interact with desires to give rise to the subject's behaviour (Dennett 1981a: 18–22). In applying the framework to human subjects, we should seek to minimise a subject's departure from how an ideally rational subject concerned with the truth would be. Beyond a certain point, an envisaged departure is too great and the interpretative framework becomes inapplicable. However, all that there is to learn about beliefs can be learnt by a fully informed interpreter applying the interpretive framework (Child 1994: 1, Davidson 1973: 144, 1974: 236–239, 1983: 148).

Actual subjects approximate to the idealisations of the interpretative framework. Daniel Dennett has suggested that we should see the approximation as similar to the existence of a pattern in a noisy system (Dennett 1991: 42–51). But what happens when the departure gets too much, the pattern lost, and yet it is plausible the subject has beliefs? Broadly speaking there are two not necessarily exclusive approaches: partitioning and adopting a more minimal appeal to rationality.

According to the first approach, when the departure gets too great at the level of subjects, it is restored by fragmentation into elements in which the pattern is restored. In the case of self-deceived subjects, when they seem to believe *p* and believe that *not-p*, Donald Davidson puts the belief that *p* on one side of the partition and the belief that *not-p* on the other side, along with the requirement of total evidence: give credence to the hypothesis most highly supported by all available relevant evidence (Davidson 1985: 140). The partition reflects a lack of rational connection between parts of the subject together with rational connections between the elements in the partition (for further discussion see Davidson 1985: 211, Noordhof 2003: 90–91, Pears 1984, 1986: 97–98). It is possible for the agent to come to believe that *p* as a result of their desire to believe that *p* because the unacceptable belief that not *p*, that generated the self-deception, is on the other side of the partition (Davidson 1985: 205–212). In general, the idea is that partitions are recognised when, as a result, the partitioned systems more closely approximate the ideal pattern than the whole system does in the absence of the partition (Davidson 1982: 181).

Some cases of delusion have the same character as self-deception and so can be treated in the same way. One illustration is a form of anosognosia involving the denial of a hemiplegia (paralysis or weakness) in the left side due to a stroke in which a subject's desire to believe that there is nothing wrong with them is uninhibited by reality-checking mechanisms standardly occurring in the affected right hemisphere (Noordhof & Sullivan-Bissett 2023: 104–106, Ramachandran 1996, Fernández, Chapter 22).

Many delusion-characterising contents are distressing, for instance, believing that you are dead or a loved one has been replaced by an imposter. These cases are not naturally assimilated to self-deception or other ways in which a mind may be fragmented, for example, failure to imply information in long term memory (Cherniak 1986: 57–59, 62–67). For this reason, it is tempting for proponents of normative-interpretive approaches to adopt a more minimal account of rationality to characterise it (e.g. Dennett 1981b: 94–97, drawing from Cherniak's work amongst others, Bortolotti 2010, 2012, Cherniak 1986).

> If a subject has a particular belief-desire set, the subject would undertake some, but not necessarily all, of those actions that are apparently appropriate.
>
> *(Cherniak 1986: 9)*

The difficulty is that the interpretive framework becomes under characterised and its conditions of application unclear. For example, in further articulation of it, Lisa Bortolotti suggests that all we should say is that beliefs are integrated into a system with some inferential relations with other intentional states, that they should display a sensitivity to evidence (without this necessarily corresponding to epistemic rationality and how a subject should respond to evidence) and have some manifestation in behaviour, and that these beliefs can be self-ascribed, self-reported, and defended with reasons to some extent (Bortolotti 2010: 261–265). It is far from clear that an interpretive approach of this character provides a complete characterisation of when it is legitimate to ascribe a belief to a particular subject, when it is not, and what the implications of such an ascription should be for the mental life of a subject. All of this has no prospect of being further specified if the normative framework is taken to exhaust the nature of belief.

One response is to take the more moderate rationality condition to characterise what must hold for somebody to count as a believer and yet argue that there is a further story to characterise what belief is like for different kinds of believer (humans, other higher mammals, robots). There would be a normative generality to belief but the beliefs of particular kinds of believers would constitute natural kinds discovered by further kind-specific psychological investigation.

A hybrid approach to belief of this type is hard to motivate when there is an alternative way of capturing the same idea that does not involve this normative-descriptive split between belief in general and kind-specific belief. The alternative is to develop a functional or dispositional approach to belief and recast the moderate rationality condition as a requirement on the functional role having certain features. The general objection that John McDowell makes against a functionalist understanding of the interpretative approach – namely that *ideal* rationality is uncodifiable – doesn't work against a position that appeals to a moderate rationality requirement to place a constraint upon the features that a belief's functional role should have (McDowell 1985). The success of the normative-interpretive framework is further qualified when it is appreciated that the epistemic norms that characterise the framework are given different weight in conscious attention than outside conscious attention (Noordhof 2001, 2003, 2024).

## 1.5 *Functional or dispositional approaches*

The standard distinction between functional and dispositional accounts of belief turns upon whether the nature of belief is understood in terms of a causal role that focuses upon the characteristic links of beliefs to behaviour (in the case of dispositional accounts) or to include, in addition, reference to the non-mental antecedents of beliefs such as the input to the senses, and the relations of beliefs to other mental states (in the case of functional accounts). More recently, some proponents of dispositional accounts of belief have also talked about dispositions to give rise to other mental states (e.g. Schwitzgebel 2002: 2513, 2013: 87–88). Equally, early proponents of dispositional accounts of beliefs antedating functional accounts partly characterised beliefs in terms of what we dwell upon in imagination and feeling (e.g. Ryle 1949: 129, leading later proponents to identify themselves as producing a Rylean account, Schwitzgebel 2002: 249, 259–260). So the picture is confused, probably due to the attempt to characterise the shift from behaviourism to functionalism as a decisive shift involving an overlooked element (Putnam 1967: 420–424). I'm going to suppress the issue of whether there's an element of context sensitivity in the ascription of belief, on the basis of a subject's satisfaction of its stereotypical dispositions, because the aim of the present discussion is that it is appropriate to attribute delusion-characterising beliefs in both clinical contexts and a wide range of everyday contexts (Schwitzgebel 2002: 256–257). Both functional and dispositional accounts of belief can be developed independently of, or inclusive of, the results of psychology in the characterisation of the causal role of belief. Recent dispositionalists such as Eric Schwitzgebel who emphasise that they are providing a superficial theory of belief – rejecting a deep nature of belief to be discovered by empirical investigation – are best thought of as taking on an additional commitment to which we need not adhere here.

Functionalism as a general theory of mind claims that every kind of mental state can be characterised in terms of input conditions, output conditions, and mental states where the latter are also functional states. Functionalists have recognised the possibility of a weaker position in which a particular kind of mental state is characterised functionally but some of the mental states mentioned in the characterisation need not be functional states (Shoemaker 1981b: 310–311). It is the weak functionalist position that we are going to consider in the case of belief (of which Schwitzgebel's phenomenal dispositional account is an instance, Schwitzgebel 2002: 257–259).

Proponents of functionalism draw a distinction between the core realisation of a mental state and its total realisation (Shoemaker 1981a: 264–265). The core realisation is what is required for the presence of a state characterised in terms of a causal role. The total realisation are the conditions that must hold, along with the core realisation, for the functional state to be a kind of mental state, namely the minimal conditions for there to be a mind of which it is a state. Precisely the same issue afflicts dispositional accounts of belief developed in terms of a cluster of stereotypical causal relations. These relations don't have to be present for the disposition to be realised, just their potential (Schwitzgebel 2002: 252–257). If beliefs cannot be instantiated out of minds, then they are not simply functional states but rather a complex state involving a functional state in a certain context.

If the total realisation conditions are those that are required for any mental state to be present, then there is no reason to assume that, when these hold, the functional state that partly constitutes a belief should stand in the expected causal relations to other mental states. This represents a clear difference between functional theories of belief and normative-interpretative theories. Nevertheless, functionalist accounts of belief can introduce further conditions which, they may claim, should hold if a functional state is going to count as a belief. We may call these supplementary total realisation conditions, *belief realisation conditions*. Brian Loar calls them *L constraints* (Loar 1981: 72). An illustration of a L constraint is if S were to believe that *p*, then it is not the case that S would believe that *not-p*. However, as Loar makes clear, the L constraints are meant to hold *in general* and allow for exceptions. The functional role characterises the expected potential for causal relations in standard circumstances, where this records a tendency rather than an invariable occurrence of these relations, and in non-standard (excusing) circumstances the subject will not respond as expected (Bayne & Pacherie 2005: 181).

This point gives rise to an important distinction when dealing with the way in which subjects with delusions don't seem to behave, and emotionally respond to, the delusion-characterising cognitive states in the way that we would expect if they were beliefs. There is a difference between being in excluding conditions in which the expected causal role of state fails to be manifested and being in a state that only has some of the expected causal role of belief in standard circumstances. When Eric Schwitzgebel writes,

> it is not sufficient for believing that p that one be in a state, or possess an entity, that typically, for members of your population plays a certain functional role. That state has to actually play that functional role, for you
>
> *(Schwitzgebel 2012: 14)*

he overlooks the distinction. If you are a subject with delusions, the belief need never play the expected functional role, if you are always in excluding circumstances.

Although a defence of doxasticism is clearly available within a functional approach to belief, the success of such defence of doxasticism turns upon whether a plausible account of the functional role of belief can be provided that still allows for the accommodation of cases of delusion. The features upon which I focus are of particular importance for the contrast with non-doxastic states.

A central aspect of the functional role of belief is its *motivational role*, the role it plays in combination with desire, to produce action. When we act, we often rely upon means-end beliefs. To illustrate, if I desire that $p$ is the case now (over everything else) and I believe that if I make it the case that $q$, then $p$ will be the case (and no other option presents itself), then I will act to make $q$ the case (given I can). Merely thinking or imagining that this is so won't play the same role. Similarly, if I believe that $p$ is the case, then I won't act on my desire that $p$, indeed my desire may even be extinguished once I have the belief, but merely thinking or imagining that p is the case may sharpen my desire and make me act. Beliefs can give rise to emotions which then play out in bodily responses and actions. Motivational role, in the most general sense, should be understood as the potential for impact on behaviour in all of these ways.

David Velleman has argued that motivational role is insufficient to characterise belief because our imaginings may play the same role as belief in cases of play. Children pretending to be elephants can imagine that they have put their trunk (arm touching their nose) in a pail of water, inhaled, and that if they blow through it, then they will be able to spray another child with water. As a result of this imagining, they act accordingly because they desire to spray another child (Velleman 2000: 255–263). Even if imagining plays the role of belief in these circumstances, outside the context of play, imaginings do not play the motivational role of beliefs, whereas beliefs continue with their motivational role. Even in contexts of play, many beliefs retain their motivational role and only those that are explicitly set aside by play (e.g. the belief that one is not an elephant) fail to play the role. When children make-believe that a piece of playdough is a pie, they still act surprised if somebody actually tries to eat the playdough suggesting they monitor the reality that the playdough is a prop and don't let their imagining give rise to the belief that the playdough is good to eat

(Golomb & Kuersten 1996, Van Leeuwen 2014: 701). It is plausible that beliefs have the following functional role: they are the most context-insensitive state that has the motivational role in question (Noordhof 2001: 253, 2024, Section 2). They may sometimes fail to play the role because the subject forgets, or does not focus on this belief, or because of situations of play, but generally, they play the motivational role in question. The times when they do not play the role will often be covered by excusing conditions. If you sought to characterise beliefs and imaginings in terms of the same motivational role, the latter would require a larger number of different types of excusing conditions. The failure of imagining that $p$ generally to result in a meta-cognitive belief that you believe that $p$ doesn't provide an excusing condition that restores parity between belief and imagination (contrary to what Anna Ichino suggests, Ichino 2019: 1524–1531). There are cases where we don't believe that we believe that $p$ but find that we do as a result of how we are disposed to act. I don't believe that I believe my partner is unfaithful to me and yet I find myself anxious and checking her movements. This is not so in the case of imagining.

The context insensitivity of the motivational role in question is relative to the stakes involved given the truth of a particular content. Consider a familiar case in which I believe that a gun is unloaded and am offered £5 to point it at my head and pull the trigger. This may give me pause since £5 is not a lot of money and the risks are huge. That doesn't mean I don't believe that the gun is unloaded but imagine it. If we compare believing that the gun is unloaded, with imagining that the gun is unloaded, then the motivational role characterising the belief that the gun is unloaded will be present in more contexts than any of these other states.

Relative context-insensitivity of motivational role is one kind of stability that characterises the functional role of beliefs. The point I have just made relates to a second form of stability that some have attributed to beliefs, namely that our beliefs should, at the least, persist unless a subject becomes aware of *epistemic* reasons that make the holding of the belief theoretically irrational (Ross & Schroeder 2012: 277–280). The loaded gun case can be taken to show that I did not believe that the gun was unloaded because it did not display stability in the sense just identified. An alternative is that I believed that the gun was unloaded but the high stakes circumstances of the gun being pointed at my head is an excusing condition. According to this view, beliefs are the default basis for a subject's motivation unless the stakes are high. In those circumstances, a subject is aware that their credence in the content of the belief may not be enough to make an action made on the basis of the content of the belief have a better expected value than that based upon the negation of the content.

We needn't resolve the question of whether to understand the functional role of belief partly in terms of persistence in the face of non-epistemic reason or in terms of excusing conditions that allow the attribution of belief even though it does not lead to relevant action in the case of high stakes situations. Either way, it is unclear why the evidence-resistance of delusion-characterising contents should throw into question the attribution of belief. Delusion-characterising states would display greater stability rather than less.

Perhaps it will be argued that failure to be evidence-responsive stops a state from having the distinctive motivational role of belief because the subject could not take the content of their belief to be true if unsupported by evidence. There are familiar circumstances in which a belief may have its distinctive motivational role in the absence of evidence in support of its content. First, the belief may strike us as independently plausible. Many propositions seem to recommend themselves to reason and, in those circumstances, evidence against the propositions is often dismissed. Second, we make take ourselves to experience the truth of the proposition and this often outweighs evidence against it from other sources. Third, we may see how a proposition is supported by other propositions but lack the attention, ability, or motivation, to see how those propositions rely upon the truth of other propositions that are presented to us as false. Fourth, we may remember that we established that $p$ but forget the details. Nevertheless, this memory still supports the proposition in the sense of making us believe that we, previously, had a reason for taking $p$ to be true. Fifth, it may seem unacceptable for us to believe that a proposition is false – some politically contested propositions are like this – and so we retain the proposition in the absence of overwhelming evidence against a particular proposition (Noordhof 2003, 2024, Section 2).

In the absence of such a link between evidence-responsiveness and motivational role, the existence of delusion-characterising states with the latter character supports doxasticism. With this in mind, we will review the arguments in favour of non-doxasticism.

## 2.   Arguments against delusions involving beliefs

Arguments against weak doxasticism usually involve noting the way that the delusion-characterising states are inappropriately epistemically based, lack integration, or fail to guide action in the way that one would expect of belief.

### 2.1   *Argument from inappropriate epistemic basis*

The first argument is that states with delusion-characterising content are not appropriately related to epistemic reasons, specifically evidence concerning their content, to be beliefs. There is either not sufficient evidence for the content in the first place or the states are not revised appropriately when evidence comes along which conflicts with their content (Dub 2017: 29–30, Egan 2009: 265, Hamilton 2006: 221, 225–226, for more on this issue, see Flores, Chapter 12). It is not claimed that subjects with monothematic delusions fail to respond to evidence at all. Most are *sensitive* to evidence (Bortolotti 2010: 117, 262–264, who claims this is enough for belief). Many subjects show a recognition of the fact that there is strong evidence against the content of the delusion-characterising state (e.g. Alexander, Stuss, & Benson 1979: 335). It is the failure to be *appropriately* responsive to evidence that makes the attitude to the delusion-characterising content something other than a belief.

One influential response to this objection, due to Bortolotti, is that many of our beliefs in other areas are also merely sensitive to, rather than appropriately responsive to, evidence. Religious and superstitious beliefs involve contents that are similarly poorly supported by evidence and improbable as an explanation of what evidence there is. Determined non-doxasticists respond that the states characterised by religious and superstitious contents should not be taken to be beliefs either (e.g. Dub 2017: 34–35, Ichino 2020: 212–215, 2024: 82–84, Van Leeuwen 2014).

We can break out of the impasse by making three moves. First, the characterisation of belief, in terms of motivational role given above, does not require an appropriate response to evidence. We could add appropriate evidence-responsiveness to a belief's functional role but we would be left with the question of how to classify states without this evidence-responsiveness but which played the distinctive motivational role. They look very much like things it is plausible that the subject believes however misguidedly.

There is some evidence that subjects with delusions, in general, show a relative bias against disconfirming evidence to the delusion-characterising content of their states (Woodward et al. 2006: 611–613). The question is whether such differences provide grounds for restricting our talk of belief to a sub-category of states with the motivational role of belief, those without the bias. The implied exclusion of some subjects (those with the bias against disconfirming evidence), and limitation to certain kinds of states, excluding those with religious and superstitious contents, represents a loss of generality that needs to be justified given that our talk of belief seems focused on attributing the most general kind of state about the world upon which we act.

Second, even if the delusion-characterising states are less responsive to evidence than non-delusory beliefs generally, subjects with delusions treat the contents of these states in a way that is more in line with them being beliefs than some other kind of mental state. They recognise the conflict between these contents and the evidence that they have. For example, LU, who believed that she was dead, slowly abandoned this belief when it was pointed out that other dead people she had come across did not move and talk whereas she did (McKay & Cipolotti 2007: 253). Similarly, MF corrected his belief that his wife was an imposter when it was pointed out to him that the ring he had bought his wife that she wore had his initials engraved (Coltheart 2007: 1054). Subjects with delusions respond to cognitive behavioural therapy (Brakoulias et al. 2008: 162 –163, Chadwick & Lowe 1990). All of this shows that they *display* a capacity to respond to evidence against the delusion-characterising content, even if they are resistant to, and avoid, disconfirmatory evidence. In addition, their delusion-characterising states resemble more unproblematic cases of belief by showing themselves to be move evidence-responsive across contexts than non-doxastic states. During play, imaginings may be corrected to the same degree as beliefs. A child's imagining that daddy has magical powers may be as responsive to features of the game (one cannot imagine that daddy has magical powers if he is not holding the wooden stick [the magic wand]) as their belief that daddy is approaching is sensitive to the presence of daddy coming towards them. These conditions of play do not make such imaginings evidence-responsive outside this context. Beliefs are a different matter.

Such features are explained by non-doxasticists as either because subjects with delusion-characterising states mistakenly take themselves to have beliefs, when they don't, and respond accordingly or because they are in some half-way house state between belief and a non-doxastic state. In Chapter 20, I explain why the first alternative is problematic. The second alternative fails to appreciate the significance of the presence of excusing conditions in the functional role of belief.

The two points just made are independent of the question of whether delusions are based on a subject's, typically anomalous, experiences (as Empiricists about delusion claim, for more on Empiricism, see Bongiorno and Parrott, Chapter 26) and whether subjects with delusory beliefs are rational to persist in having the beliefs (Noordhof and Sullivan-Bissett 2023). If part of the functional role of beliefs included a greater responsiveness to evidence than I have acknowledged, the anomalous experiences to which subjects with delusions are responding are a very plausible candidate for excusing conditions. Regardless of whether a subject is rational to adopt a delusory hypothesis, it is certainly the case that our experiences have a strong influence on the beliefs we form in everyday life and are often responsible for our own strongly held beliefs. To the extent that the subject's response is rational, anomalous experiences won't be excusing conditions but proper displays of evidence-responsiveness (Tumulty 2011: 606). Where the response departs from rationality, anomalous experiences excuse the failures to respond appropriately (a possibility Tumulty seems to overlook, Tumulty 2011: 606).

It is an open question whether all delusions have a basis in, or support from, experience in the sense just specified. Even if there are no *anomalous* experiences to explain some delusions, this does not mean that subjects' apparent failure to respond to evidence appropriately can't be partly explained in terms of a whole complex of experiences they have over time as a result of which they have a certain world view and set of emotional responses.

## 2.2   *The argument from lack of integration*

The second argument is that the content of delusion-characterising states is not well-integrated with a subject's beliefs, and other aspects of their mental life, in the way that one would expect if the state were a belief (Dub 2017: 31, Egan 2009: 266, calls this 'theoretical circumscription'). Subjects with Capgras delusion don't seem to think through the consequences of their loved one being replaced by an imposter and alter their world view accordingly (Davies and Coltheart 2000: 10–27, Young 1999: 581–583). Relatedly, emotional responses one might expect if the delusion-characterising content was the content of a belief seem to be absent. Those who take their loved ones to be replaced by imposters often aren't too concerned about what happened to them or try to see their loved ones rather than accepting the imposters (Alexander, Stuss, & Benson 1979: 335–336, Young 2000: 53). Louis Sass writes of flatness of affect in schizophrenic cases (Sass 1994: 23–24, 43–45). Where subjects with delusions appear to believe contradictory things, it is more plausible to suppose that one of the contradictory contents characterises an imaginary state than to attribute contradictory beliefs (Currie & Ravenscroft 2002: 15–18).

The impact of the argument is limited. It is rare that subjects with delusions have beliefs that are directly contradicted by their delusion-characterising states. They have beliefs that *we* judge should be seen as in conflict with their delusion-characterising states. To take the most extreme example, in Cotard's delusion, subjects believe that they are dead and yet, acknowledge they can feel their heart beating and that, for people generally, they wouldn't feel this unless they were alive. Nevertheless, they count themselves an *exception* (Young & Leafhead 1996: 157–158). Counting oneself as an exception to generalisations we otherwise accept is a familiar phenomenon from everyday life.

The more general point is there are some very plausible excusing conditions to account for why a belief with the delusion-characterising content sometimes fails to be integrated. First, the content of the belief is often radically at odds with, and so disruptive of, their previously held beliefs and a subject's daily existence. Subjects are motivated not dwell on all the consequences but try to isolate the belief (Davies & Coltheart 2000: 29–30). Second, subjects often face a situation in which there is competition between two bases of belief. The first is that they are trying to make sense of highly anomalous experiences. In the case of Cotard delusion, the subject was suffering from depression and her experiences of eating and her body felt unreal. The second is that other experiences, including testimony from those around them, present counterevidence to the delusion-characterising content. In the case of Capgras delusion, the basis of the imposter belief is visual experience but auditory experience is unaffected and so the subject can hear the imposter as their loved one (Young 1999: 576, drawing on Hirstein & Ramachandran 1997). Other people will claim that the loved one is not an imposter and medical professionals will challenge the delusion-characterising content (Young 1999: 583). Even though the subject has rejected this counterevidence it is still plausible that it has an effect. One aspect will be an increased suspiciousness of other people who challenge the belief but another aspect will be an inhibition of integration. The experiences and testimony of others may serve to distract the subject with Capgras delusion from dwelling on the danger their loved one may be in.

The failure of integration is often overstated and its significance open to question. Although there are typically connections between a subject's beliefs and their emotional responses, these aren't invariable. Let me give some illustrations of these points. In a variant case of Capgras, in which a subject believed his wife to be a disliked ex-colleague, although he was prepared to leave hospital and be looked after by her, which might seem rather puzzling, he reacted angrily when she tried to kiss him, brandished his walking stick, and later said to his doctor that part of his concern was that his wife would not have been happy with him being kissed by another woman (Breen et al. 2002: 119). A subject with Capgras delusion addressed the 'imposter' in a very gentle way and seemed pleased to see her. Nevertheless, had an inquiring manner when talking of their past, or her characteristics, left the house on one occasion to go looking for his real wife, and urged the imposter to come with him to the police station to report the disappearance of his wife (Lucchelli & Spinnler 2007: 189–190). A mother who became convinced her daughter an imposter became depressed and refused food from concern they might poison her (Christodoulou 1977: 557). Many subjects with a syndrome of doubles (Capgras, Fregoli, Intermetamorphosis, and Subjective Doubles) were suspicious of, observed intently the appearance and behaviour of, and inquired into past events and acquaintances of, the person whom they misidentified in one of the distinctive ways. This suggests that they had a good sense of the implications of the delusory hypothesis. They displayed this behaviour again when they were in the process of making a recovery from the delusion (Christodoulou 1978a: 69–70). It is also worth noting that the avowals of delusion-characterising content have significant costs for the subject with delusions which is both indicative of the conviction with which the content must be held and also the integration between having the belief, having an occurrent expression of the belief, and believing that they have the belief.

These observations support weak doxasticism. Recognition of circumstances in which it is plausible that subjects have a delusion-characterising belief supports seeking to understand their mental life in other circumstances in terms of excusing conditions or the fact that while a delusion-characterising belief typically has certain mental consequences, these aren't invariable. There will be situations in which subjects no longer have the delusion-characterising beliefs due to non-epistemic changes that remove enough of the motivational role identified but identifying these is not straightforward. Subjects with delusions should be understood as instantiating mental processes which have believing the delusion-characterising content as a likely, albeit perhaps intermittent, outcome.

### 2.3   *The argument from failure to guide action*

The third argument is that beliefs tend to guide action, whereas the delusion-characterising states do not to the same extent (Currie & Ravenscroft 2002: 177, Dub 2017: 32, Egan 2009: 266, Hamilton 2006: 221–226, Sass 1994, 3, Tumulty, Chapter 18). A typical illustration is the subject with Capgras delusion who does not act in the way that one might expect if they believed their loved one had been replaced by an imposter.

As before, one influential response is to note that subjects often don't behave was we would expect concerning their moral and religious beliefs either (e.g. Bortolotti 2010, Young 1999: 583). As already noted, determined non-doxasticists can extend their non-doxasticism to cover these cases.

The extension is facilitated by overly strict interpretations of what the motivational role of belief involves. Earlier I suggested that beliefs were the most context-insensitive state that played the motivational role distinctive of them. Talk of the *most* context-insensitive state, rather than context-independent state, captured the fact that even when we have a certain belief, our mind may be distracted or otherwise disturbed, so that the belief does not manifest itself in action as expected. The connection is what typically holds and is subject to excusing conditions. In his version of the argument from failure to guide action, Neil Van Leeuwen appeals to full 'practical setting independence' (Van Leeuwen 2014: 702). Although Van Leeuwen ostensibly draws this idea from Michael Bratman's work, it is much stronger than Bratman's notion. For Bratman, beliefs are the default cognitive background for an agent's deliberations. It is not the case that, *without changing their mind*, in one context of deliberation, an agent takes $p$ to be true, in another context of deliberation, the agent does not, where $p$ is the content of a belief (Bratman 1992: 18). When a belief fails to be operative in a context, it may still be part of the *default cognitive background* for the agent's deliberations. It is just that, for one reason or another, the agent has failed to take $p$ into account, for example, by being distracted or bracketing the belief (Bratman 1992: 27–30). For example, I believe Isabel is untrustworthy and will betray all my secrets. I don't want my secrets betrayed. Yet, in the charm of the moment, I find myself confiding in her, not attending to my belief and my want. These are not circumstances in which I fail to have the belief or desire. Assimilating failure to be operative with not being part of the default cognitive background makes it all too easy to find other cognitive attitudes than beliefs at work in a host of contexts and, indeed, may make one conclude that there are no beliefs. Taking beliefs to be the most context-insensitive state with a certain motivational role, where failures to be operative are covered by excusing conditions, removes much of the support for weak non-doxasticism to be derived from the failure to guide action.

Apart from a subject's apparently sincere avowals of the content of the delusory state, there is a range of non-verbal behaviour that attest to the fact that the delusion-characterising content is the content of a belief. A subject with perceptual delusional bicephaly shot at what he took to be his second head (which was of his wife's suspected lover) (Ames 1984). Subjects with Capgras delusion have attacked or killed the suspected imposters, and in one case searched for batteries and micro-film in the head of his 'imposter' stepfather (Blount 1986: 207, de Pauw & Szulecka 1988: 92, Silva, Leong, & Weinstock 1992: 80). Subjects with Fregoli delusion have attacked individuals who they take to be familiar individuals in disguise and those who believe that someone else is becoming them (subjective doubles) have attacked the people who they take to be becoming them (Christodoulou 1978b: 250, de Pauw & Szulecka 1988: 91–92). Nearly one-fifth of those with delusional misidentification of some kind or another showed violent behaviour as a result (de Pauw and Szulecka 1988, Förstl et al. 1991). Even those with Cotard delusion, who believe that they are dead, which is one of the most puzzling delusory beliefs to attribute, may stop eating, retain their urine and faeces, stop bathing, become mute, and fail to respond to noxious stimuli (Weinstein 1996: 20–21, Young & Leafhead 1996: 152).

## 3. Conclusion

The case against weak doxasticism is weak. The most plausible account of belief allows for the possibility of attributing beliefs to subjects with delusions. The arguments against this claim are ineffective. The success of the defence of doxasticism also turns on whether non-doxastic states can provide a more plausible explanation of some of the phenomena that have been taken to threaten doxasticism. If non-doxasticism faces similar problems, then the argument in support of weak doxasticism provides support for strong doxasticism.

## Acknowledgements

I acknowledge the support of the Arts and Humanities Research Council (*Deluded by Experience*, grant no. AH/T013486/10) for the research underpinning this chapter, and thank Ema Sullivan-Bissett for her very helpful comments on a previous draft.

## References

M. P. Alexander, D. T. Stuss & D. F. Benson (1979), 'Capgras Syndrome: A Reduplicative Phenomenon', *Neurology*, 29, pp. 334–339.

David Ames (1984), 'Self Shooting of a Phantom Head', *British Journal of Psychiatry*, 145, pp. 193–194.

D. M. Armstrong (1973), *Belief, Truth and Knowledge* (Cambridge, Cambride University Press).

J. Arturo Silva, Gregory B. Leong and Robert Weinstock (1992), 'The Dangerousness of Persons with Misidentification Syndromes', *Bulletin of the American Academy of Psychiatry and the Law*, 20, 1, pp. 77–86.

Walter Bagehot (1871), 'On the Emotion of Conviction', *The Contemporary Review*, 17, April, pp. 32–40.

Tim Bayne and Elizabeth Pacherie (2004), 'Bottom-Up or Top-Down: Campbell's Rationalist Account of Monothematic Delusions', *Philosophy, Psychiatry and Psychology*, 11, 1, pp. 1–11.

Tim Bayne and Elisabeth Pacherie (2005), 'In Defence of the Doxastic Conception of Delusions', *Mind and Language*, 20, 2, pp. 163–188.

Gary Blount (1986), 'Letter to the Editor', *Nebraska Medical Journal*, 71, p. 207.

Lisa Bortolotti (2010), *Delusions and Other Irrational Beliefs* (Oxford, Oxford University Press).

Lisa Bortolotti (2012), 'In Defence of Modest Doxasticism about Delusions', *Neuroethics*, 5, pp. 39–53.

Vlasios Brakoulias, Robyn Langdon, Gordon Sloss, Max Coltheart, Russell Meares and Anthony Harris (2008), 'Delusions and Reasoning: A Study Involving Cognitive Behavioural Therapy', *Cognitive Neuropsychiatry*, 13, 2, pp. 148–165.

Michael Bratman (1992), 'Practical Reasoning and Acceptance in a Context', *Mind*, and in his (1999), *Faces of Intention* (Cambridge, Cambridge University Press), pp. 15–34.

Nora Breen, Diana Caine and Max Coltheart (2002), 'The Role of Affect and Reasoning in a Patient with Delusion of Misidentification', *Cognitive Neuropsychiatry*, 7, 2, pp. 113–137.

John Campbell (2001), 'Rationality, Meaning, and the Analysis of Delusion', *Philosophy, Psychiatry and Psychology*, 8, 2/3, pp. 89–100.

P. D. J. Chadwick and C. F. Lowe (1990), 'Measurement and Modification of Delusional Beliefs', *Journal of Consulting and Clinical Psychology*, 58, 2, pp. 225–232.

Christopher Cherniak (1986), *Minimal Rationality* (Cambridge, The MIT Press).

William Child (1994), *Causality, Interpretation and the Mind* (Oxford, Oxford University Press).

G. N. Christodoulou (1977), 'The Syndrome of Capgras', *British Journal of Psychiatry*, 130, pp. 556–564.

G. N. Christodoulou (1978a), 'Course and Prognosis of the Syndrome of Doubles', *The Journal of Nervous and Mental Diseases*, 166, 1, pp. 68–72.

G. N. Christodoulou (1978b), 'Syndrome of Subjective Doubles', *American Journal of Psychiatry*, 135, pp. 249–251.

Peter Clutton (2018), 'A New Defence of Doxasticism about Delusions: The Cognitive Phenomenological Defence', *Mind and Language*, 33, 2, pp. 198–217.

Max Coltheart (2007), 'Cognitive Neuropsychology and Delusional Belief', *The Quarterly Journal of Experimental Psychology*, 60, 8, pp. 1041–1062.

Gregory Currie and Ian Ravenscroft (2002), *Recreative Minds* (Oxford, Oxford University Press).

Donald Davidson (1973), 'Belief and the Basis of Meaning', reprinted in his (1984), *Inquiries into Truth and Interpretation* (Oxford, Oxford University Press), pp. 141–154.

Donald Davidson (1974), 'Psychology as Philosophy', reprinted in his (1980), *Essays on Actions and Events* (Oxford, Oxford University Press), pp. 229–239.

Donald Davidson (1982), 'Paradoxes of Irrationality', reprinted in his (2004), *Problems of Rationality* (Oxford, Oxford University Press), pp. 169–187.

Donald Davidson (1983), 'A Coherence Theory of Truth and Knowledge', reprinted in his (2001), *Subjective, Intersubjective, Objective* (Oxford, Oxford University Press), pp. 137–153.

Donald Davidson (1985), 'Deception and Division', in Ernest LePore and Brian McLaughlin (eds.), Actions and Events (Oxford, Blackwell), pp. 138–147, reprinted in his (2004), *Problems of Rationality* (Oxford, Oxford University Press), pp. 199–212 [page references in text to latter].

Martin Davies and Max Coltheart (2000), 'Pathologies of Belief', *Mind and Language*, 15, 1, pp. 1–46.

J. David Velleman (2000), 'On the Aim of Belief', in his (2000), *The Possibility of Practical Reason* (Oxford, Oxford University Press), pp. 244–281.

K. W. de Pauw and T. K. Szulecka (1988), 'Dangerous Delusions: Violence and the Misidentification Syndromes', *British Journal of Psychiatry*, 152, pp. 91–97.

Daniel C. Dennett (1981a), 'True Believers', reprinted in his (1987), *The Intentional Stance* (Cambridge, The MIT Press), pp. 13–35.

Daniel C. Dennett (1981b), 'Making Sense of Ourselves', reprinted in his (1987), *The Intentional Stance* (Cambridge, The MIT Press), pp. 83–101.

Daniel C. Dennett (1991), 'Real Patterns', *The Journal of Philosophy*, 88, 1, pp. 27–51.

Richard Dub (2017), 'Delusions, Acceptances, and Cognitive Feelings', *Philosophy and Phenomenological Research*, 94, 1, pp. 27–60.

Andy Egan (2009), 'Imagination, Delusion and Self-Deception', in Tim Bayne and Jordi Fernández (eds.), *Delusion and Self-Deception* (New York and London, Taylor and Francis Group), pp. 263–280.

Hartry Field (1978), 'Mental Representation', *Erkenntnis*, 13, pp. 9–61, reprinted in his (2001), *Truth and Absence of Fact* (Oxford, Oxford University Press), pp. 30–82 [page references in text to latter].

Hans Förstl, Osvaldo P. Almeida, Adrian M. Owen, Alistair Burns and Robert Howard (1991), 'Psychiatric, Neurological and Medical Aspects of Misidentification Syndromes: A Review of 260 Cases', *Psychological Medicine*, 21, pp. 905–910.

C. Golomb and R. Kuersten (1996), 'On the Transition from Pretense Play to Reality: What Are the Rules of the Game?', *British Journal of Developmental Psychology*, 14, pp. 203–217.

Andy Hamilton (2006), 'Against the Belief Model of Delusion', in Man Cheung Chung, Bill Fulford and George Graham (eds.), *Reconceiving Schizophrenia* (Oxford, Oxford University Press), pp. 217–234.

William Hirstein and V. S. Ramachandran (1997), 'Capgras Syndrome: A Novel Probe for Understanding the Identity and Familiarity of Persons', *Proceedings of the Royal Society: Biological Sciences*, 264, 1380, pp. 437–444.

Anna Ichino (2019), 'Imagination and Belief in Action', *Philosophia*, 47, pp. 1517–1534.

Anna Ichino (2020), 'Superstitious Confabulations', *Topoi*, 39, pp. 203–217.

Anna Ichino (2024), 'Religious Imaginings', in Ema Sullivan-Bissett (ed.), *Belief, Imagination and Delusion* (Oxford, Oxford University Press), pp. 81–106.

Uriah Kriegel (2015), *The Varieties of Consciousness* (Oxford, Oxford University Press).

Brian Loar (1981), *Mind and Meaning* (Cambridge, Cambridge University Press).

F. Lucchelli and H. Spinnler (2007), 'The Case of Lost Wilma: A Clinical Report of Capgras Delusion', *Neurological Science*, 28, pp. 188–195.

William Lycan (1988), *Judgement and Justification* (Cambridge, Cambridge University Press).

John McDowell (1985), 'Functionalism and Anomalous Monism', in Ernest LePore and Brian McLaughlin (eds.), *Actions and Events: Perspective on the Philosophy of Donald Davidson* (Oxford, Basil Blackwell), pp. 387–398.

Ryan McKay and Lisa Cipolotti (2007), 'Attributional Style in a Case of Cotard Delusion', *Consciousness and Cognition*, 16, pp. 349–359.

Kengo Miyazono (2019), *Delusions and Beliefs* (London, Routledge).

Paul Noordhof (2001), 'Believe What You Want', *Proceedings of the Aristotelian Society*, 101, 3, pp. 247–265.

Paul Noordhof (2003), 'Self-Deception, Interpretation and Consciousness', *Philosophy and Phenomenological Research*, 57, 1, July, pp. 75–100.

Paul Noordhof (2024), 'Irrationality and the Failures of Consciousness', in Ema Sullivan-Bissett (ed.), *Belief, Imagination and Delusion* (Oxford, Oxford University Press), pp. 266–304.

Paul Noordhof and Ema Sullivan-Bissett (2023), 'The Everyday Irrationality of Monothematic Delusion', in Paul Henne and Sam Murray (eds.), *Advances in Experimental Philosophy of Action* (London, Bloomsbury), pp. 87–111.

David Pears (1984, 1986), *Motivated Irrationality* (Oxford, Oxford University Press).

Hilary Putnam (1967), 'The Mental Life of Some Machines', H. Castaneda (ed.), *Intentionality, Minds and Perception* (Detroit, Wayne State University Press), reprinted in his (1975), *Mind, Language and Reality* (Cambridge, Cambridge University Press), pp. 408–428 [page references in text to latter].

Jake Quilty-Dunn and Eric Mandelbaum (2018), 'Against Dispositionalism: Belief in Cognitive Science', *Philosophical Studies*, 175, pp. 2353–2372.

V. S. Ramachandran (1996), 'The Evolutionary Biology of Self-Deception, Laughter, Dreaming and Depression: Some Clues from Anosognosia', *Medical Hypotheses*, 47, pp. 347–362.

Jacob Ross and Mark Schroeder (2012), 'Belief, Credence, and Pragmatic Encroachment', *Philosophy and Phenomenological Research*, 88, 2, pp. 259–288.

Gilbert Ryle (1949), *The Concept of Mind* (Harmondsworth, Penguin).

Louis A. Sass (1994), *The Paradoxes of Delusion* (Ithaca, IL and London, Cornell University Press).

Eric Schwitzgebel (2001), 'In-Between Believing', *The Philosophical Quarterly*, 51, 202, pp. 76–82.

Eric Schwitzgebel (2002), 'A Phenomenal, Dispositional Account of Belief', *Noûs*, 36, 2, pp. 249–275.

Eric Schwitzgebel (2012), 'Mad Belief?', *Neuroethics*, 5, pp. 13–17.

Eric Schwitzgebel (2013), 'A Dispositional Approach to Attitudes: Thinking Outside of the Belief Box', in Nikolaj Nottelmann (ed.), *New Essays on Belief* (Houndmills, Basingstoke, Palgrave Macmillan), pp. 75–99.

Sydney Shoemaker (1981a), 'Some Varieties of Functionalism', *Philosophical Topics*, 12, 1, pp. 83–118, reprinted in his (2003), *Identity, Cause and Mind* (expanded edition) (Oxford, Oxford University Press), pp. 261–286.

Sydney Shoemaker (1981b), 'Absent Qualia Are Impossible' *The Philosophical Review*, 90, 4, pp. 581–599, reprinted in his (2003), *Identity, Cause and Mind* (expanded edition) (Oxford, Oxford University Press), pp. 309–326 [page references in text to latter].

Tim Thornton (2008), 'Why the Idea of Framework Propositions Cannot Contribute to an Understanding of Delusions', *Phenomenology and the Cognitive Sciences*, 7, pp. 159–175.

Maura Tumulty (2011), 'Delusions and Dispositionalism about Belief', *Mind and Language*, 26, 4, pp. 596–628.

Neil Van Leeuwen (2014), 'Religious Credence Is Not Factual Belief', *Cognition*, 133, pp. 698–715.

Edwin A. Weinstein (1996), 'Reduplicative Misidentification Syndromes', in Peter K. Halligan and John C. Marshall (eds.), *Method in Madness* (Hove and New York, Psychology Press), pp. 13–36.

Todd S. Woodward, Steffen Moritz, Carrie Cuttler, Jennifer C. Whitman (2006), 'The Contribution of a Cognitive Bias Against Disconfirmatory Evidence (BADE) to Delusions in Schizophrenia', *Journal of Clinical and Experimental Neuropsychology*, 28, 4, pp. 605–617.

A. W. Young (1999), 'Delusions', *The Monist*, 82, 4, pp. 571–589.

Andrew W. Young (2000), 'Wondrous Strange: The Neuropsychology of Abnormal Beliefs', *Mind and Language*, 15, 1, pp. 47–73.

Andrew W. Young and Kate M. Leafhead (1996), 'Betwixt Life and Death: Case Studies of the Cotard Delusion', in P. Halligan and J. Marshall (eds.), *Method in Madness: Case Studies in Cognitive Neuropsychiatry* (Hove, Psychology Press), pp. 147–171.

# 20

# DELUSION AND NON-DOXASTICISM

## Paul Noordhof

Non-doxasticists about delusion are united by the idea that at least some kinds of delusion involve subjects in which the state whose content characterises the delusion (hereafter the delusion-characterising state) is not a belief. Non-doxasticism can come in different strengths depending upon whether a delusion-characterising non-doxastic state is an essential feature of delusion (Strong Non-Doxasticism) or a feature of some cases of delusion (Weak Non-Doxasticism). A key question for non-doxasticists is the kind of non-doxastic state that is delusion-characterising because there are variety of such states and some differences of view as to their proper characterisation. In the first section of the chapter, I shall make some preliminary clarifications about the nature of these states and their relationship to empirical work on belief. In the second section, I will discuss grounds that have led non-doxasticists to espouse their approach, revisiting the arguments against doxasticism discussed in the chapter on Delusion and Doxasticism (Chapter 19). In Section 3, I will consider the particular versions of non-doxasticism that have been offered and the challenges they face, dividing the territory into those which add an appeal to meta-cognitive states, those that postulate a hybrid state, and those that are developed within a two-level account of cognition.

My conclusion will be that none of the non-doxastic approaches so far are successful. They suffer from a number of failings that, taken together, point the way to a more successful non-doxasticist approach. The approach must avoid a dilemma. When non-doxasticists appeal to standard non-doxastic states to understand subjects with delusions, these introduce puzzles of the same order as doxasticism. When non-doxasticists appeal to hybrid states which capture subjects overall state of mind better, then their explanatory implications are quite unclear. The difficulty is to strike a balance between fitting and informing. At the close, I shall make some suggestions about how this can be done.

## 1.  Non-doxastic states

Relevant non-doxastic cognitive states include cognitive imaginings, acceptances, and suppositions.

In contrast to imaginings involving sensory imagery, *cognitive imaginings* have a content of the same type as belief. Cognitive imaginings are often under our control although

DOI: 10.4324/9781003296386-25

they can be brought about spontaneously or guided by a particular purpose. We shouldn't assume that spontaneous cognitive imaginings are passive. I might spontaneously imagine a lurking man when coming home late at night. I didn't seek to do so and yet my imagining was not something that happened to me but something that, in a highly general sense, I did to myself. When our imaginings are guided by a particular purpose, then what we imagine is subject to constraint. For example, we may seek to imagine what beliefs and desires another person has on the way to predicting what they will do. The key point is that, by being under our control, our cognitive imaginings don't have to display the sensitivity to evidence that some urge is distinctive of beliefs. This is one source of their attraction as a delusion-characterising state. On the other hand, it also makes the delusion-characterising state something over which the subject with delusions has potential control and is something they are doing to themselves. These elements should be born in mind.

Cognitive imaginings are sometimes contrasted with supposings. The former are more closely linked with affective consequences than the latter. When we *imagine* that a friend has had a serious accident, we are emotionally engaged. When we suppose that they have, this need not have the same emotional consequences (Arcangeli 2019: 31). The distinction does not require that suppositions always fail to give rise to an emotional response or, indeed, that cognitive imaginings produce them. The contrast is that, where a particular content may engender an emotional response in the case of a cognitive imagining, the subject could have supposed that content without the same level of emotional response. Supposition is more divorced from the affective system in this sense. Equally, although our emotions can give rise to suppositions – for example, the anxious father supposing that his son might be ill to consider whether there is anything he should do – our emotions engage with the development of our cognitive imaginings in a more pervasive fashion whereas, in the case of suppositions, the subsequent development is broadly inferential (Arcangeli 2019: 40–46, for one way to develop these points). On the other hand, cognitive imaginings are relatively insulated from the guiding of action otherwise our cognitive imaginings in response to fiction might involve more fight and flight (Weinberg & Meskin 2006b: 222–226).

Suppositions can involve contradictions, whereas cognitive imaginings are typically taken not to. There is no problem with supposing that a contradiction holds and considering what follows from that (Weinberg & Meskin 2006a: 193). Imagining that a contradiction holds is a different matter. One way of drawing the contrast is to note that, when we suppose that *p*, we entertain a content, that *p*, for a particular purpose. By contrast, when we imagine that *p*, we consider how *p* is true (cf. Kind 2013: 149–151). This might involve fleshing out our understanding of the circumstances in which p holds. For example, David Chalmers takes cognitive imagination to have the content that *p* mediated by an object, a situation, in which *p* is true (Chalmers 2002: 151). A more committed version of this position takes the object to be an experience in which *p* is presented as so (Peacocke 1985: 20 –21). The latter reduces the distinction drawn between sensory and cognitive imaginings.

Other philosophers adopt an account of cognitive imaginings that does not differentiate them from suppositions. Both of them are taken to be a re-creation of belief in imagination (Currie 2002: 215–220). Imagination is process of re-creation of mental states independent of the standard ways in which they are produced, and their standard connections to action. The apparent difference between cognitive imaginings and suppositions stems from the fact that some imaginative projects are more richly developed involving a subject's disposition to have imaginary desires. The latter are a re-creation of desire in imagination without the standard ways in which they are produced and their standard connections to action. We can remain neutral on this except to note that subjects with delusions should typically be taken to have a richer project if a non-doxasticist theory draws upon cognitive imaginings.

Acceptances are usually understood in terms of taking a proposition as true in a certain context for a certain purpose (e.g. Bratman 1992: 20, Stalnaker 1984: 79–81). They are naturally distinguished from simply entertaining a certain proposition. There is no commitment to taking a proposition as true in simply entertaining it. It is conceivable that acceptances could be assimilated to imagined beliefs. However, acceptances are propositions taken as true in an actual context and not taken as true in an imaginary context. Acceptances are acted upon, whereas the connection between an imagined belief and action is typically suspended. To that extent, it is plausible that acceptance is distinct from supposition and cognitive imagining.

A necessary condition for a successful non-doxastic position is that, when subjects are in the relevant non-doxastic state, it does not follow that they believe the contents of these states. This makes non-doxasticism potentially in conflict with Spinozan theories of belief formation. According to such theories, when a subject entertains, supposes, or cognitively imagines a proposition, the subject immediately believes it (e.g. Gilbert 1991: 108–109, Mandelbaum 2014: 61–62). Rejecting the proposition requires mental effort governed by a distinct process. The proposition's endorsement or unacceptance occurs at a later stage. In which case, any non-doxastic cognitive state with a delusion-characterising content implies that the subject in that state believes the delusion-characterising content (Bongiorno 2022: 728–729).

There is only a conflict if the states Spinozans classify as beliefs are plausibly contrasted with the states in terms of which non-doxasticists offer a distinct account of delusion. Otherwise, the difference is terminological. Suppose that when a subject understands an utterance, they accept the content. The question is whether this acceptance is belief in the sense that non-doxasticists deny that subjects with delusions have beliefs. Spinozans recognise that the state their theory concerns may be thought of as 'thin' belief as opposed to the thick belief of epistemologists (Levy & Mandelbaum 2014: 27, Mandelbaum 2016: 236). They also do not differentiate between beliefs and credences that p where the measure of the credence is enough to have behaviour consequences but need not be as high as 0.9 (Mandelbaum 2014: 58, fn. 11). It is not obvious that this is sufficient to distinguish their notion of belief from guesses and or run of the mill acceptances. Non-doxasticists can argue that they deny delusions are believed in the thick sense.

A second challenge from Spinozan theories of beliefs derives from their idea that, after a subject has contemplated and believed a content, they may (unless cognitively loaded with competing activities) go through a process of endorsement or rejection. Subjects with delusions have attention-grabbing anomalous experiences which place them under a cognitive load so that they are unable to go through the process of rejection or endorsement with regard to the content of the delusion-characterising state (Bongiorno 2022: 733–735).

The experimental support for the effect of load on subjects' capacities to evaluate their beliefs comes from the following kind of set up. Subjects are asked to give sentences to offenders for crime incidents. They look at a video screen with a top scrolling line of text and a bottom one. The top contains true (in black) and false (in red) statements which are either extenuating or exacerbating concerning the personality of the perpetrator. The bottom is a string of numbers. Loaded subjects are those who have to identify when a 5 occurs, unloaded subjects don't. It was found that loaded subjects were more likely to take the information flagged as false (i.e. occurring in red) into account in determining the sentences, than unloaded subjects (unloaded, extenuating, 6 years, unloaded, exacerbating 7 years; loaded, extenuating, 5 years, loaded, exacerbating 11 years) (Mandelbaum 2014: 83–84, from experimental work by Gilbert, Tafarodi, & Malone 1993). This is not because the subjects were prepared to use *false* information as the basis of the judgements because they were also found to misremember the false-flagged information as true. The influence upon sentencing judgements is taken to illustrate the inferential promiscuity of the contents making them contents of beliefs. The inferential promiscuity identified is thin. It involves an influence on sentencing judgement exercised in an experimental rather than real-life situation and the influence in question is independent of any beliefs about which features are relevant for taking into account in a sentencing judgement.

Setting aside the question of whether this thin notion of inferential promiscuity is enough for a thick understanding of belief, it is questionable whether subjects with anomalous experiences are under cognitive load in a way analogous to the notion of cognitive load to which the experimenters appeal. A subject with Capgras delusion only has anomalous experiences when they have visual experience of the loved one they claim to be replaced by an imposter. They are not under load for large parts of the day or, for that matter, when interviewed by psychiatrists.

## 2. Arguments in favour of non-doxasticism

### 2.1 *Argument from lack of evidence responsiveness*

Those who argue that weak non-doxasticism is true tend to emphasise the importance of a delusion-characterising state's failure to be rationally responsive to evidence. The emphasis is natural bearing in mind the single most striking feature of subjects with delusions is the bizarre contents they assert in the face of any evidence offered against them. They will argue that doxasticists underplay this feature.

There have been two recent challenges to the argument from lack of evidence responsiveness. First, it has been argued that research into the character of belief shows that beliefs generally are not formed in response to evidence and they may not be revised in the light of evidence unless the circumstances are right. Second, it has been argued that the correct notion of evidence-responsiveness is much weaker than non-doxasticists suppose it to be. I will consider these in turn.

Spinozan theories of belief hold that, standardly, there are no evidential constraints on the formation of beliefs. The experiment concerning sentencing judgements described above is taken to be one illustration of this point. In spite of the fact some statements about a man to be sentenced are flagged as false, the subject still forms beliefs with those statements as contents.

As things stands, the experiment is open to another interpretation. Subjects are forming their beliefs on the basis of written testimony. Written testimony is a perfectly appropriate and familiar basis for beliefs. When placed under load, their ability to differentiate between true and false testimony is affected. The difficulty is to distinguish between the hypothesis that we believe anything presented to us (or even entertained by us) and the hypothesis that we prima facie trust what is delivered to our senses and testimony unless we recognise it to be false.

Two considerations have been offered in favour of the former hypothesis. First, when subjects, and observers of their performance, are pre-briefed without being cognitively loaded, that the feedback relating to whether the subjects have successfully distinguished genuine from fake suicide notes is bogus, the judgements, of both subjects and observers, was still affected by the feedback. Where the feedback had been positive, the judgement concerning how many suicide notes were, in fact, correctly identified, and the subjects' ability, were both inflated and, conversely, if the feedback had been negative (Wegner, Coulton, & Wenzlaff 1985: 343). If a subject were just taking testimony to be prima facie trustworthy, one would expect that the pre-briefing would set this aside (Mandelbaum 2014: 70–71).

It is plausible that what is going on here is an anchoring effect. The subjects are meant to generate a guess as to how good they are at the task where the feedback, although bogus, isn't necessarily false. Subjects make an adjustment using the initial feedback value as an anchor against which they make their judgement. If this is the correct diagnosis, then the significance of the experiment turns on whether the Spinozan has a plausible account of anchoring effects.

When a subject is asked to guess the answer to a question, for example, the population of Chicago, the final answer they give is influenced by the answer that is immediately suggested to them, or by them (an anchor). I will arrive at different answers regarding the population of Chicago if I start by thinking 'Is the answer 200,000?' or if I start by thinking 'Is the answer 5,000,000?' The effect is present even when the subject has generated the initial answer for themselves and takes it to be fatuous (Mandelbaum 2014: 71, fn. 40). Mandelbaum takes this as evidence that subjects believe whatever they entertain. The details of the phenomenon do not support this.

First, if a subject *believed* the initial answer, they should not be inclined to adjust their answer as opposed to stick with it. The initial answer seems to be used as a stimulus for accessing information that either might support it or, if it does not, inclines a subject to make an adjustment to the nearest answer that seems plausible in the light of the information accessed.

Second, subjects respond differently when they are the source of the initial answer rather than somebody else, such as the experimenter. This is shown in the experiments on manipulation of the adjustment. When a subject is the source of the initial answer, the extent to which they adjust from the initial answer differs depending upon whether they shake their head or nod their head. They adjust more if they shake their head, less if they nod their head (Epley & Gilovich 2001: 392–395). This does not occur if somebody else has proposed the initial answer. A natural way to interpret the difference is that the subjects have different attitudes to the original answer depending upon the source. Otherwise the nodding and shaking behaviour would apply to both. Even if we were to take the anchoring effect to be explained by a subject believing the anchoring proposition suggested by others, it would be a mistake to take a subject's own entertaining of a certain anchor to result in belief. The difference is to be expected if the prima facie trust in testimony hypothesis is correct.

The second challenge stemmed from a weaker notion of evidence-responsiveness. The suggestion is that the key connection between belief and evidence is that if a subject believes that $p$, then they should have the *capacity* to respond rationally to evidence for and against $p$ (Flores 2021: 6305). The capacity to respond rationally to evidence is specifically related to a particular proposition $p$, the characteristic content of a delusion, rather than the subject having a general capacity to respond to evidence concerning the propositions they believe and the response should be in rationally permitted ways (Flores 2021: 6306). That does not mean that a subject usually responds rationally to evidence concerning $p$ because the capacity may be masked by various factors: the anomalous experiences supporting the delusion; motivational states which favour the delusory belief; and a subject's biases for example, a liberal acceptance bias that allows for a greater range of explanatory hypotheses that can be used to set aside counter-evidence (Flores 2021: 6305–6311).

It is questionable whether this doxasticist response is successful. One issue is whether the three masking conditions mentioned above are masking conditions for the exercise of the general capacity to respond rationally to evidence or, more specifically, as Carolina Flores argues, masking conditions for the particular capacity to respond rationally to evidence relating to the delusory content.

Suppose that somebody suffers a sports injury as a result of which, if they try, they have to stop because of the pain before completing a two mile run. It is plausible that while they have the capacity to run they, *currently, do not* have the capacity to run two miles. Flores seems to think otherwise because she claims injury is a mask of a capacity to run 10 miles in under 40 minutes (Flores 2021: 6306). It is implausible that the sports injury sufferer is currently capable of running 10 miles in under 40 minutes. Some things that get in the way of the manifestation of a capacity strike at the grounds for attributing it in the first place. The question is whether what are alleged to be masks of the particular capacity to respond to evidence relating to *p* in fact strike at the grounds for attributing the capacity in the first place, for example, by implying that a subject cannot apply their general capacity to respond to evidence rationally.

Flores suggests that one reason for thinking they have the particular capacity is that subjects try to explain evidence against their delusory belief away and seek to avoid further evidence of that type. They seem aware of what the rationally permissible response to counter-evidence is even if they are not able to make it. Avoiding the evidence against one's belief suggests that the subject is concerned that they might rationally respond to it (Flores 2021: 6308–6309).

The behaviour does not indicate that the subject has the particular capacity to respond *rationally* to the evidence against *p*. It is plausibly explained by attributing the general capacity to respond rationally to evidence and a particular capacity to respond to evidence relating to p, although not necessarily rationally. In a more every day case, when we find a subject unwilling to accept strong evidence against a proposition they believe and we consider it due to some motivational state – for example, that one's son is innocent of some terrible crime – it is plausible to say that the subject is not capable of responding rationally to the evidence against their son's innocence.

Flores claims that when subjects *actually* give up their delusions and rationally respond to the evidence against p (as they often do in cognitive behaviour therapy), then it follows (trivially) that they have had the capacity to respond rationally to the evidence against p (Flores 2021: 6312, 6314). However, this is a mistake. We don't have a capacity trivially if we actually do what the capacity is defined in terms of. Suppose I throw a dart and hit a bullseye. This is a fluke. It doesn't follow that I have the capacity to hit the bullseye. To have the capacity to do A, I have to be able to do it reliably in the circumstances. The reliability requirement implies that Flores hasn't successfully identified a substantially weaker plausible constraint on evidence-responsiveness.

Flores suggests that it would be architecturally too disruptive to suppose that subjects with delusions failed to have the capacity to respond rationally to evidence with respect to *p* but that when they undergo cognitive behaviour therapy, they develop the capacity (Flores 2021: 6014). This overlooks a natural way of describing the situation. The subject with delusions has the general capacity to respond rationally to evidence. The general capacity is masked with regard to propositions falling within the delusionary theme although they do have the particular capacity to respond to evidence. Cognitive behaviour theory assists them in having the capacity to respond *rationally* to evidence against their delusionary belief. No great architectural disruption is attributed to occur during cognitive behaviour therapy.

The concerns I have raised don't presuppose that, if a subject has the capacity to do A, they should invariably do A in favourable conditions when appropriate. Instead, the point is that if there are some persistent features of the subject that make it the case they are not reliably able to do A in favourable circumstances, then those features count against it being the case that the subject has the capacity rather than just being classified as masking conditions. That's a plausible explanation for why subjects with monothematic delusions should not be attributed the capacity to respond rationally to evidence against their delusory belief.

Lack of rational evidence-responsiveness remains a significant basis for a successful defence of the non-doxasticist position (For more on delusion and evidence, see Flores, Chapter 12).

## 2.2  *Argument from lack of integration and failure to guide action*

In Chapter 20, we saw how a functional theory of belief was able to defend itself against the claim that the lack of integration of the delusion-characterising state, and its failure to guide action, showed that the state was not a belief. On the one hand, integration and action guidance did take place and, when it did not, there were plausible excusing conditions which were always a distinctive part of a plausible functional theory.

Proponents of weak non-doxasticism more effectively defend their position when they argue that they offer an alternative account of these features that might plausibly fit some cases. Such a defence will have two features. First, the way in which the non-doxastic state explains the occasions when there is lack of integration and guidance of action more naturally follows from the way in which we may take the non-doxastic state to play its mental role, than the excusing conditions that would have to be attributed to the delusion-characterising state if it were a belief. Second, it is plausible that a subject with such a non-doxastic state would, intuitively, count as a subject with a delusion.

The proposals below should be assessed with these features in mind.

## 3.  Types of non-doxastic theory

There are broadly three strands of theoretical development in the non-doxastic position. There are those which take delusions to involve a non-doxastic delusion-characterising state but add a meta-cognitive element. There are those whose appeal is to a hybrid first-order state. There are those that draw on a two-level conception of cognition.

## 3.1  *Non-doxastic delusion-characterising states with meta-cognitive states*

An appeal to cognitive imagining, rather than belief, recognises that cognitive imaginings may interact inferentially with a subject's beliefs. The inferences drawn are to assist the imaginative project further. This is most typically the case in when cognitive imaginings are in the service of our understanding of fiction. The important difference between the

314

inferential promiscuity of belief and cognitive imagining is that when a subject cognitively imagines that $p$, when $p$ is in conflict with some of the subject's beliefs, these are backgrounded but available for use when the imagining is ended. Cognitively imagining that $p$ is not a challenge to a subject's belief that not-p nor does the subject's belief vitiate the imagining in question (Currie & Ravenscroft 2002: 15–17, 178–179). This approach to delusion has a meta-cognitive element because subjects with delusions generally take themselves to believe what the theorist says they merely imagine (Currie 2000: 176). More specifically, it holds that a subject with delusions 'fails to monitor the self-generatedness of her imagining that p' (Currie 2000: 177, Currie & Jureidini 2001: 160). As a result, the imagining that $p$ presents itself as something generated by the world beyond itself. In typical cases, it is taken to be a response to precipitating, and validating, experiences.

One problem with this position concerns the appeal to a failure of source-monitoring. On the one hand, the delusion-characterising cognitive imaginings are a response to experiences, and more easily generated by experiences than beliefs (Currie & Jureidini 2001: 159). On the other hand, when we arrive at judgements on the basis of experience, we take ourselves to be judging. Otherwise, the contents would not be taken to be our judgements but rather have an external origin inserting them into our minds. The difference to which Gregory Currie and Jon Jureidini seem to be appealing is that subjects fail to recognise *the way* in which the imaginary state is an exercise of mental agency. Experience is insufficient to support a belief (otherwise experience would be the basis of a self-ascription of belief) but subjects are unaware that the experience is insufficient. Lack of awareness of the nature of their own contribution makes them think that the imagining is a belief. The problem is that it is unclear why this kind of monitoring failure only gives rise to a meta-cognitive belief (about the imagining) that it is a belief as opposed to generating a first-order belief that is ill-grounded in experience. The move from believing that one believes that $p$ to believing that $p$ seems almost immediate when a subject does not appreciate that they are responsible for the content of the state but take it to be based in experience.

A second problem concerns the explanatory benefits of appeal to imaginings together with a meta-cognitive belief. The suggestion is that, whereas beliefs have a functional role that results, when we have a new belief, in adjusting our other beliefs in conflict with it, imaginings do not have this functional role. Imaginings may be adopted while putting beliefs that clash with the content of the imaginings in the background. Appeal to imaginings explain why subjects with delusions fail to respond to contradictions between the content of their delusion and their other beliefs.

The problem is with the meta-cognitive element. Contradictions in our beliefs are most difficult to understand when subjects are aware of the contradiction. In this situation, subjects will believe that they believe that $p$ and that they believe that they believe that not-$p$. If subjects with delusions have a state of imagining that $p$ that they take to be a belief that $p$, then they both believe that they believe that p and believe that they believe that not-p, in cases where they have beliefs that contradict their delusory belief. Why don't they seek to resolve the contradiction that they believe is present? The explanation of this cannot be that the belief contradicting the delusion-characterising state is in the background because, as far as the subject is concerned, it is conflicting with the delusion-characterising state taken as a belief (Currie & Jureidini 2001: 160). Any other explanation of their puzzling state of mind is one to which the doxasticist could easily appeal to explain why subjects with delusions fail to resolve contradictory beliefs. For example, if they are distracted from resolving the contradiction that their meta-cognitive states claim is present in their beliefs, then appeal to this distraction can explain why a subject persists in having contradictory beliefs in the first place. It seems that the distinctive meta-cognitive element has been set aside when identifying the explanatory advantages of imaginings over beliefs with regard to contradictory beliefs.

This is not the only difficulty deriving from the meta-cognitive element. Currie himself notes that a subject who believes that they believe that $p$ is likely to end up believing that $p$ because a subject would, if they believed that they believe that $p$, assume that $p$ was true, and so, as a causal consequence, believe that $p$ (Currie 2000: 177–178). However the connection is tighter than this. If a subject believes that they believe that $p$, the functional role of the higher order belief will include much of that of the belief that $p$. If a subject has this higher order belief, then they will be disposed to act upon the truth of $p$ and make sure it is integrated with their other beliefs. For example, if I believe that I believe that my wife has been replaced by an imposter, don't we expect that I should be concerned by what has happened to her and whether the imposter is out to do me harm and puzzled if I am not? Perhaps it will be suggested that the meta-cognitive belief need not be a conscious one. But in that case, we have no explanation of why subjects with delusions report themselves as believing what the non-doxasticist says that they merely imagine.

A final problem with the metacognitive approach is that it fails to explain why a subject only mistakes *some* of their imaginings in response to their experiences for beliefs. If subjects with delusions mistake cognitive imaginings for beliefs, one might expect this failure to distinguish them to show up more generally (Bayne & Pacherie 2005: 177).

Other proponents of the meta-cognitive approach broaden the first order states from cognitive imaginings to include beliefs, emotions, hunches, forebodings, premonitions, opinions, and even empty speech acts which they take to be the object of a complex higher-order attitude, characterised as a delusional stance, to interpret the lower order attitude in various ways (Stephens & Graham 2004: 239). They characterise the delusional stance as follows:

> S is deluded that p just in case p is the representational content of a lower order state or attitude of S: (a) with which S personally identifies, (b) to which S clings in the face of strong contrary considerations and (c) about which S lacks insight into the nature and imprudent costs of maintaining.
>
> *(Stephens & Graham 2004: 240)*

S identifying with the content means that they don't take the content as intrusive.

Suppose that the subject has the non-doxastic delusion characterising state that their bones are being consumed by worms. The contrary considerations to this referred to in (b) are taken to be prudential ones relating to the impact upon the quality of their life and reputation as a thinker. It is hard to understand how they can be characterised as clinging onto $p$ in the face of contrary considerations in (b) but, at the same time, having no insight into the nature of these pragmatic considerations in (c). How can both (b) and (c) be true and how can the subject with delusions lack insight into the costs of maintaining that the delusory content is the case. Equally, it is unclear why there should be a problem with persistently imagining that one's bones are being consumed by worms in itself.

The situation is changed if the content of this imagining is taken to be true by the subject. It would be a disturbing thought, something that a subject would wish to communicate whatever the cost, and explain why the subject persisted in being in a state with this content even though there were strong prudential considerations against it. The puzzle is to explain the nature of the subject's distress and the reason for their lack of insight in a way that does not appeal to their belief in the delusion-characterising content. This puzzle is comparable with the puzzle that motivates going non-doxastic in the first place, namely that a subject may claim to believe that their bones are being consumed by worms and yet not seek medical attention.

Doxasticists can agree with non-doxasticists that the delusion-characterising state does not explain the delusion. An important element is the surrounding mental context or mental stance they take to these contents. Current characterisations of the meta-cognitive element involved either seem to undermine the explanatory utility of non-doxastic states or work better if they are directed to doxastic states (for more on delusion and imagination, see Kind, Chapter 21).

### 3.2  Hybrid first-order states

One version of this strategy holds that delusions do not involve either beliefs or imaginings but rather an intermediary state with a functional role involving elements of each but is, in fact, of neither. Andy Egan calls them bimaginings (Egan 2009: 263). The ways in which subjects with delusions seem to depart in their behaviour from that we would expect if they believed, or imagined, the typical delusory content provides reason to recognise these intermediate states between belief and imagining.

A general problem with all identifications of hybrid states of this kind is that their motivation derives from the fact that some delusion-characterising content states fail to behave in the way that we would expect if they were beliefs. The hybrid state is tailor-made to fit this kind of case (Egan 2009: 265–269). However, apart from fitting the case, the functional role of these states more generally is unclear. If you bimagine something, what are the circumstances in which it interacts with our beliefs, what is the impact of bimagining on our emotions, and so on. It does not look as if we identify a functional role that has wider articulation to justify postulating these states within scientific psychology (Matthews 2013: 107–109). By contrast, we can seek to explain the case of delusion by appealing to a standard case of belief in which there are excusing conditions with predictable results. Imagining ourselves in those circumstances, we can see how we might display similar behaviour to subjects with delusions.

Part of the appeal of bimagining is that it draws on the fact that we can envisage a continuum of states from those with most of the expected functional role of belief being manifested to those with most of the expected functional role of imagining being manifested. Aspects of the role don't come as a package. Yet, it is unclear whether the envisaged variation is due to exceptional circumstances holding in which the role is not manifested or due to the state being a different state which don't have certain expected manifestations as part of its role. As Amy Kind points out, disruptive beliefs (like the true belief that one's partner has just died) may fail to be properly integrated with one's other beliefs (Kind 2024: 55). For example, one might hear noises in the next room and take it to be her for a moment, forgetting that she's dead. We wouldn't conclude that this is evidence that one doesn't believe it. It's just that the belief hasn't sunk in. Deciding which is appropriate is a matter of the explanatory potential of the recognition of the states in question. The tailor-made character of bimagining which looked to be its strength is currently its major weakness.

Another hybrid position suggested by delusions and other phenomena is to take the subject to in-between or half-believe the delusion-characterising content. We might call this a semi-doxasticist position, rather than a non-doxasticist position, but I discuss it here because it denies the appropriateness of saying that a subject believes the delusion-characterising content.

Eric Schwitzgebel illustrates the attractiveness of attributions of half-belief by the following kind of case. Juliet is politically liberal, claims that all races are equally beautiful, will remark upon and favour (if asked) the beauty of non-white ethnic groups while nevertheless being more emotionally engaged by, and more spontaneously aware of, beauty in white people. In her most reflective moments, she is aware of this in herself. Schwitzgebel resists the claim that there might be a psychological reality such as the representation of 'white people are more attractive' in her belief box. Rather, the thought is that she half-believes this and half-believes the opposite reflecting the way that her dispositions don't accord with the stereotype of one belief or another (Schwitzgebel 2013: 85–88).

Understanding the attribution of half belief as a kind of summary judgement about the whole network of dispositions present in the subject has some plausibility. As before, the question is whether this also gives us an explanatory purchase on subjects in the state of half-belief or whether we get more insight by the attribution of belief and the recognition of excusing conditions. How would you expect someone who half believes that p to behave and to what extent is this distinct from them bimagining that *p*?

Consider the case of Juliet. If she is negotiating a social context in which all her friends are politically liberal and she wants their good opinion, then one might suppose that she secretly believes that white people are more beautiful but the rest can be explained by the social context. On the other hand, if the excusing condition for this belief isn't there and she displays these dispositions, then we might say that, although she believes that the races are equally beautiful, she might find the physical characteristics of white people more emotionally engaging. It is plausible that in characterising Juliet in these ways we get more explanatory grip on her behaviour even if either or both of them count as ways of half believing a particular proposition taking her whole state of mind into account.

While it is true that according to the functional account of belief, once information about the dispositions are fixed, there is no further matter to investigate for the attribution of belief (e.g. whether there is a sentence in the language of thought with a particular content in the belief box), the correct attribution of the dispositions is not a straightforward matter (contrary to what Schwitzgebel seems to assume, for example, Schwitzgebel 2002: 261–262). There is significant play off between the attribution of different beliefs with different excusing conditions, the role of social context in evaluating them, and attributing more complex states of emotional engagement (as Schwitzgebel acknowledges in principle, Schwitzgebel 2010: 534–535). The capacity of a dispositional account to avoid questions of whether there is deep fact about whether a subject believes that *p* or not is overrated. Schwitzgebel suggests that dispositions may not distinguish between affective, evaluative, and belief states – or, at the least, stereotypical dispositions may not – however this seems implausible (Schwitzgebel 2013: 90). We are well aware, in everyday life, of verbal and other behaviour that distinguishes between these states and discuss these differences between ourselves when attributing to somebody one state or another. Affective states don't always correspond to what it is quite plausible that we believe, as one development of the Juliet case would display.

In the case of delusions, there are good reasons for thinking that subjects are in excusing conditions for delusion-characterising beliefs. Subjects with delusions receive counter-evidence concerning their delusion-characterising beliefs, both from other people and their own experience, and they may be anxious about thinking through the implications of their beliefs given their nature. The explanatory worth of the attribution of half-belief, in contrast to its accuracy as a summary judgement, is yet to be made out.

### 3.3 Two level accounts of cognition: delusions as acceptances

Those who take the delusion-characterising state to be an acceptance that $p$ develop the proposal within a two-level framework for cognition. Level 1 involves credences measured in terms of probabilities from 0 to 1, and desires measured by degrees of valuing (to be distinguished from level 2 desires). On this level, even if a subject has a credence of 1 in a particular proposition $p$, it doesn't follow in itself that you have a flat out belief that $p$. Flat-out belief relates to facts that hold on level 2. On level 2, you have acceptances and goal adoptions (level 2 desires). A sub-category of acceptances are those that count as flat-out beliefs. They involve the policy of taking their content as an unrestricted premise in deliberation subject to exceptions such as when one fails to remember the content, or doesn't take it to be relevant, or because one has another pragmatically based restricted policy of taking a countervailing content as a premise in practical deliberation. Illustrations of the latter would be when a lawyer professionally takes their client to be innocent or games of pretence (Frankish 2004: 130–132, this is drawn from Cohen's account of acceptance, see Cohen 1992: 4–5). These policies of taking the content of the acceptance as a premise in practical deliberation are caused by (Frankish says realised in) level one credences and desires. The framework is neutral between doxastic and non-doxastic positions. Non-doxastic positions focus on level two acceptances that fail to be unrestricted policies for premises in practical deliberation.

In Keith Frankish's development of a non-doxastic version (at times he remains neutral about the truth of non-doxasticism), he suggests that the desire behind the policy of using the delusion-characterising content as a premise is outweighed by other desires concerning the ways in which, if the delusion-characterising content were true, life would be unacceptable, for example, the desiring to continue to live in your home, avoid estrangement from your wider family, and consequent upheaval (Frankish 2009a: 279–280). The policy of using the delusion-characterising content as a premise in practical deliberation is restricted as a result.

A non-doxastic version of Frankish's proposal might be plausible for cases of delusion that seem to be cases of self-deception. One illustration is a form of anosognosia involving the denial of a hemiplegia (paralysis or weakness) in the left side due to a stroke in which a subject's desire to believe that there is nothing wrong with them is unchecked by reality-checking mechanisms standardly occurring in the affected right hemisphere (Ramachandran 1996, for more discussion see Noordhof and Sullivan-Bissett 2023: 104–106, Fernández, Chapter 22, this volume). However, many delusion-characterising contents are distressing. Why is a subject adopting the policy of accepting that they are dead or that their loved one has been replaced by an imposter? Frankish's suggestion is that we should look into the subject's motivation to find out the answer, but it is natural to think that one reason why the subject adopts such a relatively unrestricted premising policy is because they take the content to be true (Frankish 2009a: 281). At best, gesturing towards some sort of motivation operating at level one is a promissory note that struggles with those monothematic delusions for which a motivational element has seemed harder to identify, for example, Capgras and Cotard.

A second issue concerns the explanation of the typical behaviour of subjects with delusions. Frankish explains the role that delusion-characterising acceptances play in terms of a subject with delusions high confidence in the desirability of acting upon the outcome of practical deliberation in which the content of the acceptance is taken as a premise (Frankish 2009a: 277–279, 2009b: 88–90). Consider what the proposal says about the action of the subject with delusions if the non-doxasticist picture is correct. In this case, the subject's failure to respond in the expected ways in other circumstances means that the premising policy they have is not considered a belief and, thus, is not accurately thought of as indicative of what they take to be true (as opposed to what they accept to be true as part of a policy). When the subject expresses their belief that their partner has been replaced by an imposter and calls the police, this is not because they take it to be true that their partner has been replaced by an imposter but rather because they are (usually unconsciously) confident that the premising policy involving the content that their partner has been replaced by an imposter will, as part of their practical deliberation, result in an outcome that is desirable, namely that they contact the police. As far as what is before their conscious mind, they have an acceptance which, in itself, is not different structurally from professionally accepting your client is innocent if you are a lawyer although the acceptance may be more persistent. The issue is whether we can understand what a subject is up to better than if we were to attribute a belief. It is hard to see the proposal as an improvement in comprehensibility unless we appeal to the extent to which a subject with delusions takes the delusion-characterising content as a premise for practical deliberation as the basis for an illusion that they believe the content in question (Dub 2017: 36–40, gives examples of how this may lead to meta-cognitive mistakes). Otherwise, the delusion is something that they are doing to themselves for obscure motivation that makes little sense even to themselves.

Perhaps, in part, to answer this challenge, Richard Dub supplements the picture. He appeals to cognitive feelings to explain why a subject accepts that *p* and persists in accepting that *p* in various contexts. These cognitive feelings are experienced as internal evidence (Dub 2017: 50). Dub suggests that the subject with Capgras delusion has a cognitive feeling of unfamiliarity with respect to what seems like a loved one and the persistent acceptance that they are an imposter is a consequence of this (Dub 2017: 47–48, 51). Dub suggests that these feelings exist to produce a 'temporary simulated belief' that motivates us to engage in the relevant reasoning. Temporary simulated beliefs enable us to respond quickly to an alarm while not setting in train the process of updating all our beliefs (which, if the cognitive feeling gave rise to a belief, we would otherwise go through) (Dub 2017: 52).

The position raises a number of issues. First, it requires a sharp distinction between a cognitive feeling supported acceptance and a belief. Even in a case where the content of a subject's acceptance is part of an unrestricted policy of using it as a premise in practical deliberation, this will still be, by Dub's lights, acceptance rather than belief. By extending cognitive feeling supported acceptances to explain phobias (such as arachnophobia), Dub also allows that they might have significant impact upon behaviour otherwise suggestive of belief (Dub 2017: 52–53). The motivation for doing so is unclear.

For one thing, there seems no advantage over the idea that belief formation may be relatively swift – generated by prima facie trust in our senses, testimony and cognitive feelings – with the process of belief evaluation and integration with other beliefs being a more lengthy process. So long as there is some check between these two stages there is little reason for separating off the first as involving acceptances which are not beliefs. The earlier discussion of Spinozan theories of belief involved the recognition that there might be adjustment to other judgements that we might be inclined to make as a result of what we accept. So it is not the case that our acceptances are relatively isolated from the rest of our cognitive system. Equally, monothematic delusions undergo elaboration which is harder to understand if acceptances backed by cognitive feelings are simulated beliefs avoiding wider updating of beliefs. By connecting the occurrence of cognitive feeling backed acceptances with phobias, Dub also undermines the motivation for denying that delusion-characterising states are beliefs derived from their relative failure to be action-guiding.

My point is not that theories cannot be developed relating to cognitive feeling backed acceptances to answer these questions. It is rather that, since these questions arise, the theoretical motivation for distinguishing cognitive feeling backed acceptances from belief is undermined and the kind of answers that will be given would naturally support understanding how delusion-characterising states may be beliefs operating in particular conditions.

It is unclear how cognitive feeling backed acceptances are supposed to explain the utterances of subjects with delusions. Why does the cognitive feeling of unfamiliarity relating to the loved one make the subject with Capgras delusion assert that their loved one is an imposter in a relatively unrestricted manner as opposed to their loved one about whom they have a funny sense of unfamiliarity? It is hard not think that the missing ingredient is that the feeling of familiarity makes the subject take the content of the acceptance to be true. But that would make it plausible that the subject is actually in a delusion-characterising state of belief some of whose typical consequences may be suppressed because of excusing conditions.

Although it is not an essential part of Dub's position, he also commits himself to strong non-doxasticism. If a subject with delusions does end up believing the content of their cognitive feeling backed delusion-characterising acceptances, then Dub claims they are no longer deluded (Dub 2017: 55). This seems to take the puzzle of understanding some subjects with delusions as the basis for isolating them from subjects which we might otherwise conceive of having fallen deeper into delusion.

A more plausible way to develop Dub's position would be to insist that a cognitive feeling backed acceptance may be a delusion-characterising state in circumstances in when a subject feels the conflict of their delusory state with other sources of beliefs that they typically trust – perception and testimony – and yet the content of the delusion is something that they find unavoidable to exclude as part of their perspective on the world. They don't take the content to be true due to the conflict, but, because of the cognitive feeling, they find themselves unable to abandon the content in question.


## 4.  Concluding remarks

It is plausible that there are two motivations for non-doxasticism. The first there are circumstances in which it is plausible that a subject has a delusion but the attribution of belief is not secure. They are engaged in an imaginative project that they take really seriously or have a cognitive feeling backed acceptance in the context described earlier. Non-doxasticism is at is strongest emphasising the potential diversity of delusion-characterising states rather than insisting that subjects with delusions can't be characterised as having beliefs because of the arguments identified earlier. The second motivation derives from the non-doxasticists attempt to identify a distinct attitude that the subject with a delusion bears towards the content taken in the round. Where the doxasticist attribute a belief which does not play an expected functional role because of excusing conditions related to the subject's circumstances, the non-doxasticist takes the combination of the state with the delusion-characterising content, together with the context in which the state occurs, as making it plausible to take the state in question to involve a different attitude to the content as a kind of summary judgement about their state of mind. A problem with this idea is moving from descriptive adequacy – which is a potential strength of the non-doxastic approach – to explanatory interest. Does the identification of a distinctive delusory attitude play a useful role the further explanation of the subject's behaviour? It is clear that non-doxasticists are motivated by thoughts that it does (e.g. Dub 2017: 35). Or is better explanatory purchase obtained by focusing on belief, and how the excusing conditions may operate to give rise to behaviour not typical of the belief? For the moment, matters seem to favour the doxasticist. Yet, delusion provides an interesting case study for the potential development of an understanding of other attitudes than the ones that we generally tend to attribute. For that reason, its further study is of immense value for the more general assessment of non-doxasticist positions.

## Acknowledgements

I acknowledge the support of the Arts and Humanities Research Council (*Deluded by Experience*, grant no. AH/T013486/10) for the research underpinning this chapter, and thank Ema Sullivan-Bissett for her very helpful comments on a previous draft.

## References

Margherita Arcangeli (2019), *Supposition and the Imaginative Realm* (London and New York, Routledge).

Tim Bayne and Elisabeth Pacherie (2005), 'In Defence of the Doxastic Conception of Delusions', *Mind and Language*, 20, 2, pp. 163–188.

Federico Bongiorno (2022), 'Spinozan Doxasticism about Delusions', *Pacific Philosophical Quarterly*, 103, 4, pp. 720–752.

Michael Bratman (1992), 'Practical Reasoning and Acceptance in a Context', Mind, and in his (1999), *Faces of Intention* (Cambridge, Cambridge University Press), pp. 15–34.

David Chalmers (2002), 'Does Conceivability Entail Possibility', in Tamar Szabó Gendler and John Hawthorne (eds.), *Conceivability and Possibility* (Oxford, Oxford University Press), pp. 145–200.

Gregory Currie (2000), 'Imagination, Delusion and Hallucinations', *Mind and Language*, 15, 1, pp. 168–183.

Gregory Currie (2002), 'Desire in Imagination', in Tamar Szabó Gendler and John Hawthorne (eds.), *Conceivability and Possibility* (Oxford, Oxford University Press), pp. 201–221.

Gregory Currie and Jon Jureidini (2001), 'Delusion, Rationality, Empathy: Commentary on Martin Davies et al', *Philosophy, Psychiatry and Psychology*, 8, 2/3, pp. 159–162.

Gregory Currie and Ian Ravenscroft (2002), *Recreative Minds* (Oxford, Oxford University Press).

Richard Dub (2017), 'Delusions, Acceptances, and Cognitive Feelings', *Philosophy and Phenomenological Research*, 94, 1, pp. 27–60.

Andy Egan (2009), 'Imagination, Delusion and Self-Deception', in Tim Bayne and Jordi Fernández (eds.), *Delusion and Self-Deception* (New York and London, Taylor and Francis Group), pp. 263–280.

Nicholas Epley and Thomas Gilovich (2001), 'Putting Adjustment Back In The Anchoring and Adjustment Heuristic: Differential Processing of Self-Generated and Experiment-Provided Anchors', *Psychological Science*, 12, 5, pp. 391–396.

Carolina Flores (2021), 'Delusional Evidence-Responsiveness', *Synthese*, 100, pp. 6299–6330.

Keith Frankish (2004), *Mind and Supermind* (Cambridge, Cambridge University Press).

Keith Frankish (2009a), 'Delusions: A Two Level Framework', in Matthew R. Broome and Lisa Bortolotti (eds.), *Psychiatry as Cognitive Neuroscience* (Oxford, Oxford University Press), pp. 269–284.

Keith Frankish (2009b), 'Partial Belief and Flat-out Belief', in F. Huber and C. Schmidt-Petri (eds.), *Degrees of Belief* (Springer), pp. 75–93.

Daniel T. Gilbert (1991), 'How Mental Systems Believe', *American Psychologist*, 46, 2, pp. 107–119.

Daniel Gilbert, Romin W. Tafarodi and Patrick S. Malone (1993), 'You Can't Not Believe Everything You Read', *Journal of Personality and Social Psychology*, 65, 2, pp. 221–233.

L. Jonathan Cohen (1992), *Belief and Acceptance* (Oxford, Oxford University Press).

Amy Kind (2013), 'Heterogeneity of Imagination', *Erkenntnis*, 78, pp. 141–159

Amy Kind (2024), 'Contrast or Continuum?', in Ema Sullivan-Bissett (ed.), *Belief, Imagination, and Delusion* (Oxford, Oxford University Press), pp. 42–59.

Neil Levy and Eric Mandelbaum (2014), 'The Powers that Bind: Doxastic Voluntarism and Epistemic Obligation', in Jonathan Matheson and Rico Vitz (eds.), *The Ethics of Belief* (Oxford, Oxford University Press), pp. 15–32.

Eric Mandelbaum (2014), 'Thinking Is Believing', *Inquiry*, 57, 1, pp. 55–96.

Eric Mandelbaum (2016), 'Attitude, Inference, Association: On the Propositional Structure of Implicit Bias', *Nôus*, 50, 3, pp. 629–658.

Robert J. Matthews (2013), 'Belief and Belief's Penumbra', in Nikolaj Nottelmann (ed.), *New Essays on Belief* (Houndmills, Basingstoke, Palgrave Macmillan), pp. 100–123.

Paul Noordhof and Ema Sullivan-Bissett (2023), 'The Everyday Irrationality of Monothematic Delusion', in Paul Henne and Sam Murray (eds.), *Advances in Experimental Philosophy of Action* (London, Bloomsbury), pp. 87–111.

Christopher Peacocke (1985), 'Imagination, Experience and Possibility', in John Foster and Howard Robinson (eds.), *Essays on Berkeley* (Oxford, Oxford University Press), pp. 19–35.

V. S. Ramachandran (1996), 'The Evolutionary Biology of Self-Deception, Laughter, Dreaming and Depression: Some Clues from Anosognosia', *Medical Hypotheses*, 47, pp. 347–362.

Eric Schwitzgebel (2002), 'A Phenomenal, Dispositional Account of Belief', Noûs, 36, 2, pp. 249–275.

Eric Schwitzgebel (2010), 'Acting Contrary to Our Professed Beliefs or the Gulf Between Occurrent Judgment and Dispositional Belief', *Pacific Philosophical Quarterly*, 91, pp. 531–553.

Eric Schwitzgebel (2013), 'A Dispositional Approach to Attitudes: Thinking Outside of the Belief Box', in Nikolaj Nottelmann (ed.), *New Essays on Belief* (Houndmills, Basingstoke, Palgrave Macmillan), pp. 75–99.

Robert Stalnaker (1984), *Inquiry* (Cambridge, The MIT Press).

G. Lynn Stephens and George Graham (2004), 'Reconceiving Delusion', *International Review of Psychiatry*, 16, 3, pp. 236–241.

Daniel M. Wegner, Gary F. Coulton and Richard Wenzlaff (1985), 'The Transparency of Denial: Briefing in the Debriefing Paradigm', *Journal of Personality and Social Psychology*, 49, 2, pp. 338–346.

Jonathan M. Weinberg and Aaron Meskin (2006a), 'Puzzling over the Imagination: Philosophical Problems, Architectural Solutions', in Shaun Nichols (ed.), *The Architecture of the Imagination* (Oxford, Oxford University Press), pp. 175–202.

Jonathan M. Weinberg and Aaron Meskin (2006b), 'Imagine That!', in Matthew Kieran (ed.), *Aesthetics and the Philosophy of Art* (Malden, MA, Blackwell Publishing), pp. 222–237.

# 21
# DELUSION AND IMAGINATION

*Amy Kind*

## 1. Introduction

Psychiatric case studies of subjects undergoing delusions contain a host of examples of rather bizarre reports that have been made by such subjects. These reports often share similar themes: that the subject's spouse or loved ones have been replaced by impostors; that people known to the subject are following them around, but in disguise, so that the subject can't tell who they are; or that someone else is causing the subject's limbs to move without their intending to bring about the movement.

Each of these three themes is associated with a specific form of clinical delusion. The first corresponds to Capgras syndrome, the second to Fregoli syndrome, and the third to alien control syndrome (often connected with schizophrenia). And other common themes abound. In Cotard syndrome, individuals typically report that they are dead or that they have ceased existing, while in mirrored-self misidentification syndrome, individuals typically report that they are unable to recognize or identify themselves when looking in a mirror; rather, the image reflected seems to them to be of a stranger.

Bizarre as these reports by subjects with delusions may be, they appear to be made sincerely. The individuals do not appear to be lying or otherwise confabulating but rather to be reporting on their beliefs. Indeed, delusions are typically characterized as false beliefs that are sincerely and persistently held despite an absence of real evidence. Consider, for example, the characterization of delusion in the *DSM-5*:

> A false belief based on incorrect inference about external reality that is firmly held despite what almost everyone else believes and despite what constitutes incontrovertible and obvious proof or evidence to the contrary.
>
> *(American Psychiatric Association [APA] 2013: 819)*[1]

Given this clinical definition of delusion, it's not at all surprising that much of the philosophical work on delusion aims to defend a doxastic conception of delusion that treats delusion fundamentally as a species of false belief.[2] In what follows, I will refer to this doxastic view as the *belief model*. Various versions of this model have been developed, and though they differ in the explanations offered for the etiology of the relevant beliefs and how such beliefs manage to be sustained, they all share the basic assumption that delusions behave like typical beliefs in giving rise to action and sincere report (for more on delusion and doxasticism see Noordhof, Chapter 19).

Despite the prevalence of the belief model, it has not been immune from criticism.[3] Why, we might wonder, must delusions be *beliefs*? As succinctly put by cognitive scientist Max Coltheart in the context of raising problems for the *DSM*'s characterization of delusion, perhaps these mental states might 'instead be imaginings that are mistaken for beliefs by the imaginer' (Coltheart 2007: 1043).[4] This line of thought underlines one prominent alternative to the belief model. According to what I will call the *imagination model*, it's not belief but imagination that should be assigned the central role in the explanation of these delusional syndromes. In what follows, I will explore the imagination model and assess its viability in accounting for delusion.

In order to understand the imagination model, it will be helpful to have before us a clear characterization of imagination – what it is and how it differs from other mental states like belief. Such a characterization will be instructive for seeing how the imagination model differs from the belief model and how the former model can avoid problems that have been raised for the latter. Providing such a characterization of imagination will thus be the task of Section 2.

In Section 3, I turn to the imagination model itself. In addition to clarifying the core commitments of the theory, I also consider two prominent versions of it, one that has been developed primarily by Gregory Currie (2000) and one that has been developed primarily by Shaun Gallagher (2009). With these two versions of the imagination model before us, we are also well positioned to see the advantages this model has over the belief model.

In the last section of the chapter, Section 4, I explore some common criticisms directed at the imagination model. At the heart of these criticisms is the charge that proponents of the imagination model have misconstrued the nature of belief and the way that it differs from imagination. As we will see, philosophers offering these criticisms are not all driven by the same theoretical motivations. Some are motivated to defend the belief theory, but others are motivated to defend a wholly different account of delusion, one that is in many ways a hybrid of the belief model and the imagination model. In my view, however, none of these criticisms is wholly successful.

## 2.  What is imagination?

In a famous passage from his *Confessions*, St. Augustine notes the surprising difficulty he has in explicating the nature of time: 'For what is time? Who can readily and briefly explain this? If no one asks me, I know: if I wish to explain it to one that ask[s], I know not'.[5]

A similar puzzlement arises when trying to provide an adequate characterization of imagination. As familiar an activity as it is in ordinary life – employed in a wide variety of contexts from games of pretend to daydreaming to planning for the future – philosophers have found it surprisingly difficult to 'readily and briefly' explain what it is.[6] That said, we can take as a useful starting point the characterization provided by Shen-yi Liao and Tamar Gendler in their entry on imagination in the *Stanford Encyclopedia of Philosophy*: 'To *imagine* is to represent without aiming at things as they actually, presently, and subjectively are' (Liao and Gendler 2020).

But what is the nature of the representation employed in imagination? What is the relation between imagination and mental imagery? And how does imagination differ from other similar kinds of mental representations like supposition and conception? Philosophers have given a variety of answers to these questions (for just a few illustrative examples, see, e.g., Kind 2001; Balcerak Jackson 2016; Arcangeli 2018; Langland-Hassan 2020). Fortunately, we can largely bypass these issues here. For our purposes, what's most important is a distinction often made in discussions of imagination between two structural forms that imagination often takes: objectual imagining and propositional imagining.

Sometimes when we engage in acts of imagination, we aim to represent a person or thing or event, as when I imagine Snow White or a strawberry milkshake or a massive earthquake along the San Andreas fault. The content of these imaginings can be said to be objectual in nature. In contrast, sometimes when we engage in acts of imagination, we aim to attribute some property to these objects. I might imagine that Snow White is dancing on the moon, that a strawberry milkshake has just magically appeared on the kitchen counter, or that a massive earthquake along the San Andreas fault results in a collapse of the 210 freeway. The content of these imaginings can thus be said to be propositional in nature.

One way to bring out the structural difference between these two kinds of imagining it to compare them to belief. Imagining a massive earthquake along the San Andreas fault isn't something that is structurally analogous to belief; it doesn't make any sense to talk of believing a massive earthquake along the San Andreas fault. Objectual imagining doesn't take a form appropriate to serve as the content of a belief. But imagining that a massive earthquake along the San Andreas fault results in the collapse of the 210 freeway is something that is structurally analogous to belief. The content of this imagining takes a form that is perfectly appropriate to serve as the content of a belief. Like belief, propositional imagining can be seen as a propositional attitude, i.e., an attitude that we take towards a particular content.

Of the two kinds of imagining just distinguished, it's propositional imagining that plays the primary role in the imagination model of delusion, and so that's what we'll focus on here. Perhaps unsurprisingly, what makes this kind of imagining a potential candidate for explaining delusion is precisely that it is like belief in being a propositional attitude; it has the right kind of structural form to capture the examples of delusional contents mentioned above. But, as we will see, it's the differences between propositional imagining and belief that give the imagination model some important advantages over the belief model.

Perhaps the most fundamental distinction between the attitude of belief and the attitude of imagination concerns their relationship to truth. If I *imagine* that the 210 freeway has collapsed, I need not have any commitment to the truth of that claim. But matters are different if I *believe* that the 210 freeway has collapsed. When someone believes a given content, they take that content to be true. Imagining does not have the same connection to truth that belief has. In the philosophical literature on belief and imagination, there are various different ways of characterizing the contrasting connection that these two attitudes have to truth. Sometimes it's put by saying that beliefs, but not imaginings, ought to be true. Sometimes it's put by saying that beliefs, but not imaginings, aim at the truth (for discussion, see Sinhababu 2016).

Importantly, this does not rule out the existence of beliefs with false contents, nor does it rule out the existence of imaginings with true contents. Sometimes when my sons polish off last night's leftovers without telling me, I might believe that there's enough casserole for dinner even though there's not. My belief has a false content. But now, sticking with that same scenario, suppose I were to imagine that there aren't any leftovers, perhaps as a prelude towards imagining dinner at my favorite restaurant. In that case, my imagining would happen to have a true content though I wouldn't realize that it does.[7]

A second fundamental contrast between belief and imagination concerns their functional profiles. With respect both to formation and revision, belief seems to be dependent on and responsive to evidence in a way that imagination is not. When dinner ends and I see that the casserole dish is still half full, that evidence undergirds my belief that there will be leftovers for dinner tomorrow night, but it need not have any effect on my imaginings. The next evening, my discovery of the empty casserole dish on the kitchen counter leads me to adjust my belief that there are leftovers in the fridge, but once again, it need not cause any adjustments to my imaginings. The discovery will, however, have effects on my other beliefs: my belief about what the family will be having for dinner, about how soon I need to go grocery shopping, and so on. All of these will be appropriately revised in light of my new evidence. Beliefs are integrated with one another, so a change to one belief will usually lead to change to other beliefs. Imaginings in contrast, are not integrated with one's beliefs. Instead, they are usually quarantined from them.

Belief and imagination also have different functional profiles when it comes to their relationship to action, emotion, and so on. Generally speaking, belief is thought to have a more expansive role with respect to guiding behaviour and generating affective responses, while imagining is thought to have a much more circumscribed role in these regards. My belief that my sons finished off the casserole without telling me is likely to result in irritation and annoyance. I might also slam the fridge door and sigh in frustration. The corresponding imagining is much less likely to have any such effects on my emotions and actions.

Though there's more that could be said about what imagination is, and about the differences between imagination and belief, the discussion of this section should provide us with a sufficient picture for our purposes here. In particular, it lays the groundwork that I need in order to explicate both the imagination model of delusion and the considerations offered in its favor. I'll turn to those tasks in Section 3.

## 3.   The imagination model

Hints of the imagination model appear as far back as the 17th century in John Locke's characterization of madness in terms of the 'violence' of imagination. On his view, those suffering from madness have mistakenly taken 'their fancies', that is, their imaginings, for realities (Locke 1689/1997: 157). Just as Locke seems to characterize delusions in terms of imagining and not belief, so too do proponents of the imagination model.

In introducing the imagination model in Section 1, I noted that accounts of this sort assign imagination a central role in explaining delusions. Importantly, however, the way that I am defining the model construes this role to be of a very specific sort, namely, a constitutive one. The imagination model sees imagination as playing a role analogous to the role that belief plays in the belief model. Just as the belief model sees a delusion as being constituted by a belief, the imagination model sees a delusion as being constituted by an imagining. Exactly what conditions imaginings have to meet to count as delusions varies across different versions of the imagination model, but what's key to the model is that the delusional content is imagined, not believed.

Defining the model this way has the advantage of treating the belief model and the imagination model as parallel to one another. But it's worth noting an important consequence of this way of proceeding. As I am defining things, not every way of invoking imagination in accounting for delusions will count as a version of the imagination model. Consider, for example, the account offered by Colin McGinn according to which delusion is seen as imagination-driven belief: 'Normally, our beliefs are detached from the imagination, and linked to perception; in [delusion], our beliefs become shaped by the imagination, and perception loses its hold on them' (McGinn 2004: 114). On McGinn's view, imagination certainly plays a central role in accounting for delusion. But this role is etiological rather than constitutive in nature. It thus doesn't count as a version of the imagination model, at least not in the sense in which I am using the notion. Despite his invocation of imagination and the fact that he refers to his account as 'the imagination theory', to my mind McGinn's account is actually best seen as a version of the belief model. In his view, though delusions are brought about by imagination, they are still classified as beliefs.[8]

One particularly influential development and defense of the imagination model comes from Gregory Currie, both in his solo-authored work (2000) and in co-authored work (Currie and Jureidini 2001; Currie and Ravenscroft 2002). According to Currie, an individual with delusions suffers from an inability to properly identify their own mental attitudes and, more specifically, from an inability to distinguish imaginings from beliefs. Consider someone with schizophrenia who is under the delusion that Martians have infiltrated the city. On Currie's analysis, the best explanation of the delusion is that the individual has imagined that there are Martians in the city but then mistakenly takes themselves to believe that there are Martians in the city (Currie 2000: 174). Likewise for other delusions. As a general matter, subjects with delusions misidentify something that they imagine as something they believe. In describing their situation, we might put things in metarepresentational terms, that is, in terms of beliefs about beliefs: Though subjects with delusions do not believe the contents of their delusions, they believe that they believe the contents of their delusions. For this reason, Currie's view is often referred to as the *metarepresentational account of delusions* (see, e.g., Bortolotti 2010: 73), though he himself refers to it as the *disorder of imagination theory* (Currie and Ravenscroft 2002: 170).

Of course, typically we can tell our imaginings from our beliefs. Thus, in offering this treatment of delusion, Currie owes an explanation as to how and why delusional imaginings come to be misidentified as beliefs. In doing so, he relies upon considerations about the relationship between imagination and the will. Typically, imaginings are thought to be subject to the will in a way that beliefs are not. Whether I *believe* that there's a coyote running around the neighborhood is not really in my control; rather, we might say, it's in the control of how the world is. But whether I *imagine* that there's a coyote running around the neighborhood is under my control. It seems plausible that these facts about will-dependence typically play a role in how we distinguish our imaginings from belief. Thus, insofar as delusions seem to have become decoupled from the individual's will – that is, the individual takes himself not to have any control over them – we could make sense of how the misidentification happens.[9]

A second version of the imagination model has been offered by Shaun Gallagher (2009). Gallagher's account relies crucially on the notion of multiple realities. On the one hand, all of us live in a reality of 'shared everyday life' – a reality in which we work, interact with friends and family, clean the house, walk the dogs, and so on. But consider what happens when we read a novel, watch a movie, play a video game, or daydream. In such cases, says Gallagher, we end up 'escaping into a different sort of reality' that takes us away from our everyday reality. Normally, we can keep track of the different realities in which we're entering. Even when I am engrossed in the world of Middle Earth, I know that from the perspective of everyday reality I am on ordinary Earth. Sometimes, however, my engagement becomes so deep that I no longer have the same attitude of distance from the alternate reality. In such a case:

> I may enter into it *body and soul*, so to speak ... I am *in-the-world* of the play, the film, the game, etc.; I can get excited and emotional, or remain cool under pressure; I may adopt a certain physical posture, I may act virtually ... Sometimes as I come back out of such realities, everyday reality can seem oddly unreal in relation to what I have been doing.
>
> *(Gallagher 2009: 255)*

For Gallagher, what happens in the case of delusion is very similar to this. An individual can enter delusional realities just as they enter the realities of novels, films, and games. This gives rise to Gallagher's *multiple realities hypothesis*: When a subject enters into a delusional state, they enter an alternative reality, one that may be firmly sustained and not accepted by others (Gallagher 2009: 256). Unlike in other cases when we enter alternative realities, however, someone who is deluded suffers from a 'failure to suspend belief in the ontological actuality of the delusional reality' – that is, they mistake the delusional reality for everyday reality (Gallagher 2009: 257).

In developing this account, Gallagher is clear in his rejection of the belief model – he expressly rejects the *DSM* definition and notes that delusions are not false beliefs. But, that said, he does not explicitly invoke imagination in laying out his account. We thus might naturally wonder what makes the multiple realities hypothesis a version of the imagination model. The answer lies in the fact that philosophers typically understand our engagement with works of fiction and film in terms of imagination (see, e.g., Walton 1990). When we're reading (or watching) *Lord of the Rings*, and we form a representation with the content, 'The ring Frodo carries is the one ring to rule them all', this isn't a false belief about everyday reality. We're not believing this content but imagining it. Likewise, when someone with Capgras syndrome forms a representation with the content, 'That's not really my wife', Gallagher claims that this isn't something that they falsely believe about everyday reality but rather something that they imagine to be true in virtue of their having entered a delusional reality. As put by Neralie Wise when developing an account of Capgras syndrome that is heavily influenced by Gallagher's multiple realities hypothesis, 'the subject enters an imaginative world which can accommodate the impostor existing in what otherwise appears to be the normal everyday world' (Wise 2016: 203).

Though there are important differences between the two versions of the imagination model that we have considered, they both treat delusional content as imagined content rather than believed content. This kind of account has several important advantages over the belief model. Recall some of the aspects of belief's functional role that we noted in the previous section: Beliefs tend to cause action and effect in line with their contents, and beliefs also tend to be integrated with one another. Often, however, delusions do not seem to have this functional profile, as there is a mismatch between the content of the delusion and the relevant behavioural and emotional responses. Many people with Capgras syndrome who claim that their loved ones are impostors are strangely complacent about the situation. They are not overcome with grief, they do not search for their missing loved ones, they do not try to leave the house but instead continue to cohabitate peacefully with the supposed impostor, and so on.[10] We see a similar mismatch in cases of other common types of delusions. For example, people with Cotard syndrome eat and drink despite professing themselves to be dead. But while this discrepant behaviour poses a deep threat to the belief model, it poses essentially no threat at all to the imagination model. Since imaginings tend to be much more circumscribed than belief in terms of causing action and effect, the issue of behavioural mismatch does not really arise. When engaging with this chapter, for example, a (non-delusional) reader might become intrigued by Capgras syndrome and start imaginatively exploring the idea that their loved ones are impostors. The fact that they stay seated at their desk, calmly reading on, while they undertake this imagining is not at all puzzling or even surprising.

A second advantage that the imagination model has over the belief model arises from the fact that delusions show remarkable persistence, even when the deluded subject is faced with strong evidence to the contrary. Normally, beliefs exhibit sensitivity to evidence. Consider someone who stopped watching the 2023 Superbowl at halftime with the Philadelphia Eagles leading the Kansas City Chiefs 24-14. They head to bed with the belief that the Eagles won the game. When they awake the next morning to headlines proclaiming Kansas City the champions, they revise their belief. More generally, when we are confronted with evidence that conflicts with one of our beliefs, we revise our belief so as to bring it into conformity with the evidence. This kind of revision does not happen with delusions. As indicated by the *DSM* definition quoted earlier, delusions tend to persist 'despite what constitutes incontrovertible and obvious proof or evidence to the contrary'. This relationship to evidence marks a second way in which delusions do not fit well with the functional profile of beliefs (for more on delusion and evidence see Flores, Chapter 12). But just as the behavioural mismatch poses no threat to the imagination, the evidential mismatch also poses no threat to it. As noted by Currie and Ravenscroft, when we imagine something 'we do not cease to believe things that are inconsistent with what we imagine, and we do not regard clashes between what we believe and what we imagine as in need of resolution' (2002: 178). When a depressed Eagles fan imagines that his team was the 2023 Superbowl champs, for example, they do not stop believing that Kansas City won the game. As Currie and Ravenscroft also note, imaginings 'are not apt to be revised in the light of evidence; the whole point of imagining is to enable us to engage with scenarios we know to be non-actual' (2002: 178–179). We might say something similar for our engagement with the alternate realities of fiction or film. In this way, by treating delusions as imaginings, proponents of the imagination model have an easy explanation for why delusions do not exhibit a sensitivity to evidence.

Before closing this section, it's worth noting that these problems facing the belief model do not force one to adopt the imagination model. There are other accounts on offer. For example, some theorists have suggestion that delusions should be treated as instances of empty speech. Having argued that delusions are structurally so unlike normal beliefs that it makes little sense to view them as beliefs at all, German Berrios puts forth a proposal of this sort:

> Properly described, delusions are empty speech that disguise themselves as beliefs. To use Austin's felicitous term, they are but 'masqueraders'. So, although delusions purport to be real statements, and hence convey information, they may turn out to be epistemically *manqué* [that is, epistemic failures].
>
> *(Berrios 2009: 114–115)*

But while this proposal avoids the mismatch problems facing the belief model that we have just discussed, it faces problems of its own. Perhaps most importantly for our purposes here, it does not explain why the deluded subject would be making these empty assertions, and why they would do so as persistently as they do. In this respect, it seems to have considerably less explanatory power than the imagination model.[11]

## 4. Criticisms of the imagination model

Though the imagination model seems to have some important advantages over the belief model, it has nonetheless been subject to criticism. Often, these criticisms come from proponents of the belief model as part of an attempt to defend their model (see, for example, Bayne and Pacherie 2005; Bortolotti 2010). As such, these criticisms are usually less of the form: 'Delusions can't be imaginings' and more of the form: 'The reasons offered for thinking that delusions can't be beliefs are inadequate'. But some of the points raised are explicitly meant to cast doubt on the claim that delusions can be appropriately understand as imaginings. I will here consider two such points.[12]

First, one might worry that proponents of the imagination model have been insufficiently attentive to evidence that delusional subjects are often aware that their delusional beliefs are in tension with their other beliefs. Tim Bayne and Elizabeth Pacherie raise a criticism of this sort. Among their examples is an individual with Cotard syndrome referred to in the literature as JK. During the period in which she claimed she was dead, she was asked by psychiatrists whether she had various bodily sensations, specifically, whether she could feel her heart beat, whether she could feel hot or cold, and whether she could feel whether her bladder was full. The patient said that she could. It was then explicitly suggested to her that these feelings should count as evidence that she was not dead. According to the case study:

> JK said that since she had such feelings even though she was dead, they clearly did not represent evidence that she was alive. ... We then asked JK whether she thought we would be able to feel our hearts beat, to feel hunger, and so on if we were dead. JK said that we wouldn't ... However, she eventually agreed that 'it might be possible.' Hence, JK recognized the logical inconsistency between someone's being dead and yet remaining able to feel and think, but thought that she was none the less in this state. JK found this conversation very unsettling, possibly because it had presented a challenge to her delusional belief system.
>
> *(Young and Leafhead 1996: 158)*

Bayne and Pacherie note that JK is not unique in recognizing this kind of tension and being unsettled by it: 'Other deluded patients exhibit discomfort and attempt to change the topic of conversation when confronted with inconsistencies between their background beliefs and their delusion' (Bayne and Pacherie 2005: 173). Since normally one isn't bothered or unsettled when the contents of one's imaginings are in tension with one's beliefs, Bayne and Pacherie take this evidence to suggest that delusions can't be imaginings.

But here proponents of the imagination model seem to have an obvious response. Recall that on Currie's version of this model, it's not just the case that delusions are imaginings but also that deluded subjects misidentify these imaginings as beliefs. Thus, even if JK is imagining and not believing that she is dead, the fact she takes this imagining to be a belief can explain why she feels uncomfortable when inconsistencies are pointed out to her.

Turning to a second line of criticism of the imagination model, some have charged that it cannot always adequately account for the behaviour of deluded subjects. For example, even though the majority of those with delusions do not engage in violent behaviour, there are still some who do (see n. 10). In order to account for the lack of violence and otherwise complacent behaviour exhibited by so many of the subjects with delusions, proponents of the imagination model note that imagination tends to play a more circumscribed role than belief with respect to motivating action and affect. But if imagination really does play this circumscribed role, then the imagination model cannot account for those cases in which delusions do seem to bring about considerable action and affect.

In raising this worry, Bayne and Pacherie make an interesting point. Though proponents of the belief model might be said to face a problem of *in*activity, proponents of the imagination model face a converse problem of *over*activity (Bayne and Pacherie 2005: 173). The upshot of this worry seems to be less an indictment of the imagination model as a cancellation of the behaviour mismatch problem raised for the belief model. This worry thus ends up being something of a wash. Given the vast range of behaviour (and lack of behaviour) exhibited by subjects with delusions, neither model has offered an explanation that seems applicable across all cases. Is it more problematic for the imagination model that it can't handle the cases where there is considerable delusion-concordant behaviour (overactivity) or for the belief model that it can't handle the cases where is considerable delusion-discordant lack of behaviour (inactivity)? Perhaps the proponent of the imagination model can point to the fact that inactivity occurs more often than overactivity, and thus that the problem here is more significant for the belief model. But as that response still leaves us without an explanation for the overactivity, it fails to be wholly satisfactory. It seems clear that more needs to be said to settle the issue.

Interestingly, one might draw a different moral from these considerations about action and affect, namely, that we need to revise our conceptions of belief and imagination. Though philosophical orthodoxy treats them as distinct cognitive attitudes, Andy Egan (2008) has suggestion that in order to account adequately for delusion, we should instead view them as lying on a continuum. Other philosophers have made a similar suggestion in connection with the phenomenon of over-coherence (Currie and Jureidini 2004) and in connection with pretense and immersion (Schellenberg 2013). In brief, the continuum hypothesis suggests that there is a continuum of mental states between imaginings analogous to the way in which there is a continuum of colors between yellow and red (Schellenberg 2013: 509). As Egan puts the point, there is reason to accept the existence of 'a spectrum of cases, from clear totally non-belief-like imaginings to clear, full-blooded paradigmatic beliefs, with intermediate, hard-to-classify states in the middle' (Egan 2008: 274).

Acceptance of the continuum hypothesis gives rise to a third way of accounting for delusion. In line with Egan's suggestion that we refer to the states intermediate between belief and imagination as *bimagination*, we can refer to this account of delusion as *the bimagination model*. To motivate this model, Egan suggests that delusion does not perfectly match the functional profile of either imagination or belief but instead partly matches one and partly matches another. Our earlier discussion of the belief model suggested various ways in which delusions do not exhibit the normal functional role of belief: they are formed without connection to any evidence, they persist in the face of contrary evidence, they are not well-integrated with one's overall belief system, and they often do not give rise to the kind of behaviour and affect that would be expected. But, says, Egan, they also do not exhibit the normal functional role of imagination. As we saw earlier in this section, there at least some cases in which delusions give rise to considerably more behaviour and affect than in typical cases of imaginings. A further problem comes from the fact that when individuals report their delusions, they appear to do so sincerely. As Egan notes, though imaginings do sometimes give rise to report about what's being imagined, as when a child playing a game of pretend with friends reports, 'I'm a pirate captain', such reports do not typically arise in contexts where one is making sincere assertions. Generally speaking, sincere reports are guided by beliefs rather than imaginings. In Egan's view, if delusions really were beliefs, they wouldn't display as much circumscription and evidence independence as they do, whereas if delusions really were imaginings, they would display more circumscription and evidence independence than they do (Egan 2008: 268). If we instead see delusions as states that are midway between belief and imagination, then we can understand why they would have some of the typical aspects of belief and some of the typical aspects of imagination.

In responding to the introduction of a state like bimagination, philosophers have raised various worries about its coherence and explanatory usefulness (see, e.g., Liao and Doggett 2014; Kind 2024). For our purposes here, however, the main target of scrutiny is not the notion of bimagination itself but the bimagination model of delusion. To my mind, there are some good reasons to think that it's insufficiently motivated. In particular, we might worry that it's based on an overly strict conception of the functional profiles of imagination and belief. As I've argued elsewhere, the functional roles of both imagination and belief are a good deal 'smudgier' than Egan's discussion suggests (Kind 2024). When we look at the wide range of mental states that are typically classified as imaginings, we see quite a range of circumscription, for example. Compare an imagining about an armed intruder in the house – one that comes to you, unwelcome, when you're home alone late at night – with an imagining about what kind of sofa would look good in your living room – one that you explore while shopping at the furniture store. The first gives rise to considerably more affect than the second. Sometimes when we imagine that the person sitting across from us is our mortal enemy, it gives rise to action – as is the case when this is imagined by an actor in the course of performing a role on stage. But sometimes this same imagining gives rise to no action at all – as is the case when this is imagined by a bored professor daydreaming during an interminable faculty meeting. By employing considerations such as these, the proponent of the imagination model can undercut the rationale for the bimagination model.[13]

## 5.  Concluding remarks

Ultimately, then, it seems that the proponent of the imagination model has various plausible options to respond to the criticisms that have been levied against it. As our discussion has shown, the typical criticisms raised seem to arise from a mischaracterization of the resources available to someone who wants to defend the model. Once we attend more carefully to how the imagination model treats delusions as imaginings, and what the functional role of imagining really is, the criticisms lose much of their force.

Granted, the considerations discussed here by no means provide a decisive case in favor of the imagination model of delusion. It's clear that there are more details to be worked out. On the whole, however, our discussion has shown that the imagination model should be given very serious consideration when it comes to providing an account of delusion. In light of the kinds of the persistent criticisms that arise for the belief model, it seems well worth further exploring the alternative that the imagination model provides.

## Notes

1 Compare the definition (dating back to the mid-16th century) provided by the *Oxford English Dictionary*: 'a fixed false opinion or belief with regard to objective things, *esp*. as a form of mental derangement'. www.oed.com/view/Entry/49546

2 For just a few notable defenses of the doxastic account, see Bayne and Pacherie (2005), Bortolotti (2010), and Miyazono (2015). Note that the doxastic view is also dominant among psychologists and psychiatrists; for discussion, see Bortolotti (2022).

3 Some of these criticisms come from proponents of the imagination model of delusion to be discussed in detail in this chapter. See, e.g., Currie (2000) and Gallagher (2009). But there are other criticisms as well. See, e.g., Berrios (1996), Campbell (2001), and Tumulty (2011).

4 Coltheart summarizes a number of other common criticisms as well. For example, we might think that the DSM is mistaken in limiting delusions to false beliefs, since it seems like a true belief might be delusional if the believer had no good reason for taking it to be true. See Coltheart (2007: 1043).

5 Full text available via Project Gutenberg at https://www.gutenberg.org/files/3296/3296-h/3296-h.htm.

6 No doubt this is at least partly due to the fact that the term "imagine" and its cognates are used in a multiplicity of different ways both in ordinary life and in philosophy. See Stevenson (2003) and Kind (2013) for discussion.

7 Although it won't matter for our subsequent discussion of delusion, it's worth noting that someone can even engage in imaginings with true content that they fully recognize as being true. Suppose it's a day on which my sons didn't finish off the leftovers. There are indeed leftovers in the fridge, and I know that they're there. Still, I might imagine this true content as part of a larger imaginative project: Perhaps I imagine taking out those leftovers and feeding them all to the dogs so that we'll have an excuse to go out to dinner.

8 In fact, McGinn intends his imagination theory to contrast not with the belief model but with what he calls *the hallucination theory*. On his theory, delusional belief results from malfunctioning imagination; on the hallucination theory, delusional belief results from malfunctioning perception, namely, hallucination. For criticism of McGinn's view, see Currie and Jones (2006).

9 In support of this hypothesis, Currie notes that schizophrenia is often associated with a loss of agency (Currie 2000: 177), and thus it might be natural to think that schizophrenic delusions might be decoupled from the will.

10 A recent meta-review that examined over 225 cases of Capgras syndrome did find a 'moderate association' with violence and aggression. When the syndrome occurred in the context of functional psychiatric disorder (such as schizophrenia or psychotic depression), there was aggression in about 38 per cent of cases, and when the syndrome occurred in the context of organic psychiatric disorder (such as dementia), there was aggression in the context of 23 per cent of cases. But as the researchers noted, this means that the majority of subjects with Capgras syndrome are non-violent, and they took this to raise 'puzzling philosophical questions' about why there is such 'frequent failure to act on the delusional content' (Pandis et al. 2019: 166). For more on delusion and action see Tumulty, Chapter 18.

11 See Campbell (2001: 91) for related criticisms.

12 Bayne and Pacherie make two other arguments that are specific to Currie's version of the imagination model: First, that he equivocates between different senses of imagining, and second, that he does not offer an adequate explanation for how imaginings can come to be misidentified as beliefs.

13 See Kind (2024) for additional ways that this model can be criticized.

## References

American Psychiatric Association (APA) (2013) *Diagnostic and Statistical Manual of Mental Disorders* (5th ed.). Available at https://dsm.psychiatryonline.org/doi/book/10.1176/appi.books.9780890425596

Arcangeli, M. (2018) *Supposition and the Imaginative Realm. A Philosophical Inquiry*, New York: Routledge.

Balcerak Jackson, M. (2016) "On the Epistemic Value of Imagining, Supposing, and Conceiving." In A. Kind and P. Kung, eds., *Knowledge through Imagination*, 41–60, Oxford: Oxford University Press.

Bayne, T. and Pacherie, E. (2005) "In Defence of the Doxastic Conception of Delusions." *Mind and Language* 20(2): 163–188.

Berrios, G.E. (1996) *The History of Mental Symptoms: Descriptive Psychopathology Since the Nineteenth Century*, Cambridge: Cambridge University Press.

Bortolotti, L. (2022) "Delusion." In E.N. Zalta, ed., *The Stanford Encyclopedia of Philosophy* (Summer 2022 Edition). Available at https://plato.stanford.edu/archives/sum2022/entries/delusion/

Bortolotti, L. (2010) *Delusions and Other Irrational Beliefs*, Oxford: Oxford University Press.

Campbell, J. (2001) "Rationality, Meaning, and the Analysis of Delusion." *Philosophy, Psychiatry, and Psychology* 8(2/3): 89–100.

Coltheart, M. (2007) "Cognitive Neuropsychiatry and Delusional Belief." (The 33rd Sir Frederick Bartlett Lecture). *The Quarterly Journal of Experimental Psychology*, 60(8): 1041–1062.

Currie, G. (2000) "Imagination, Delusion and Hallucinations." In M. Coltheart and M. Davies (eds.) *Pathologies of Belief*, 167–182, Oxford: Blackwell.

Currie, G. and Jones, N. (2006) "McGinn on Delusion and Imagination." *Philosophical Books* 47(4): 306–313.

Currie, G. and Jureidini, J. (2004) "Narrative and Coherence." *Mind and Language* 19(4): 409–427.

Currie, G. and Jureidini, J. (2001) "Delusions, Rationality, Empathy: Commentary on Davies et al." *Philosophy, Psychiatry and Psychology*, 8(2–3): 159–162.

Currie, G. and Ravenscroft, I. (2002) *Recreative Minds: Imagination in Philosophy and Psychology*, Oxford: Oxford University Press.

Egan, A. (2008) "Imagination, Delusion, and Self-Deception." In T. Bayne and J. Fernandez, eds., *Delusion and Self-Deception: Affective and Motivational Influences on Belief Formation*, New York: Psychology Press, pages 263–280.

Gallagher, S. (2009) "Delusional Realities." In L. Bortolotti and M. Broome, eds., *Psychiatry and Cognitive Neuroscience*, 245–266, Oxford: Oxford University Press, pages 245–266.

Kind, A. (2024). "Contrast or Continuum: The Case of Belief and Imagination." In Ema Sullivan-Bissett, ed., *Belief, Imagination, and Delusion*. Oxford: Oxford University Press, pages 42–59.

Kind, A. (2013). "The Heterogeneity of the Imagination." *Erkenntnis* 78: 141–159.

Kind, A. (2001). "Putting the Image Back in Imagination." *Philosophy and Phenomenological Research* 62: 85–109.

Langland-Hassan, P. (2020) *Explaining Imagination*, Oxford: Oxford University Press. http://doi.org/10.1093/oso/9780198815068.001.0001

Liao, S. and Doggett, T. (2014) "The Imagination Box." *The Journal of Philosophy* 111(5): 259–275.

Liao, S. and Gendler, T. (2020) "Imagination." In E.N. Zalta, ed., *The Stanford Encyclopedia of Philosophy* (Summer 2020 Edition). Available at https://plato.stanford.edu/archives/sum2020/entries/imagination/

Locke, J. (1689/1997) *An Essay Concerning Human Understanding*, edited by Roger Woolhouse, London: Penguin Books.

McGinn, C. (2004) *Mindsight: Image, Dream, Meaning*, Cambridge, MA: Harvard University Press.

Miyazono, K. (2015) "Delusions as Harmful Malfunctioning Beliefs." *Consciousness and Cognition* 33: 561–573.

Pandis, C., Agrawal, N. and Poole, N. (2019) "Capgras' Delusion: A Systematic Review of 255 Published Cases." *Psychopathology* 52: 161–173.

Schellenberg, S. (2013) "Belief and Desire in Imagination and Immersion." *Journal of Philosophy* 110(9): 497–517.

Sinhababu, N. (2016) "Imagination and Belief." In A. Kind, ed., *The Routledge Handbook of Philosophy of Imagination*, 111–123. New York: Routledge.

Stevenson, L. (2003) "Twelve Conceptions of Imagination." *British Journal of Aesthetics* 43: 238–259.

Tumulty, M. (2011) "Delusions and Dispositionalism about Belief." *Mind and Language* 26(5): 596–628.

Walton, K. (1990) *Mimesis as Make-Believe*, Cambridge, MA: Harvard University Press.

Wise, N. (2016). "The Capgras Delusion: An Integrated Approach." *Phenomenology and the Cognitive Sciences* 15(2): 183–205.

Young, A.W. and Leafhead, K.M. (1996) "Betwixt Life and Death: Case Studies of the Cotard Delusion." In P.W. Halligan and J.C. Marshall, eds., *Method in Madness: Case Studies in Cognitive Neuropsychiatry*, 147–172. Hove: Psychology Press.

22

# DELUSION AND SELF-DECEPTION

*Jordi Fernández*

## 1. Introduction

Delusion and self-deception are similar, but different, conditions. Delusions are mostly discussed in the literature from psychiatry and cognitive science, whereas self-deception is mostly discussed in the philosophical literature. My aim in this chapter is to highlight some important similarities, and some important differences, between delusion and self-deception. As we will see, there are enough similarities between the two conditions to consider them both, in some sense, a form of irrationality. The relevant form has to do with our belief-attribution practices, and how those practices do not seem to be well-suited to attribute beliefs to a subject who finds themselves in either of the two conditions. Given this similarity between delusion and self-deception, it is tempting to consider that one of the two conditions might be subsumed under the other one. Perhaps, one might think, self-deception is a specific type of delusion, or maybe being deluded is a particular way of being self-deceived. It turns out, however, that there are a number of important features that the two conditions do not share. These features concern the aetiology of delusion and self-deception, their social impact and their impact on the subject's well-being, the normative aspects of the two conditions and their connections to psychopathology. Given those features, the outcome of our discussion will be that, on the whole, there are more grounds for distinguishing delusion from self-deception than there are for assimilating either of the two conditions to the other one.

## 2. How to characterise delusion and self-deception?

It is remarkably difficult to define what it is to be deluded, and what is to be self-deceived. Theories of delusion and self-deception disagree on how to characterise the two conditions and, as a result, it is hard to offer a definition of either condition which does not beg the question against some account of the condition in the literature. The characterisations of delusion and self-deception offered below are not meant to propose necessary and sufficient conditions that a subject must meet in order to be deluded, or in order to be self-deceived. Instead, these characterisations are simply meant to provide a useful grasp on what the

DOI: 10.4324/9781003296386-27                    336

conditions of delusion and self-deception are; a grasp which is sufficiently useful for the purposes of determining to what extent delusion and self-deception are similar, and to what extent they are not.

In the *Diagnostic and Statistical Manual of Mental Disorders – Fifth edition* (*DSM-5*), delusions are characterised as follows (American Psychiatric Association [APA] 2013: 87):

> Delusions are fixed beliefs that are not amenable to change in light of conflicting evidence. Their content may include a variety of themes (e.g., persecutory, referential, somatic, religious, grandiose). Persecutory delusions (i.e., belief that one is going to be harmed, harassed, and so forth by an individual, organization, or other group) are most common. Referential delusions (i.e., belief that certain gestures, comments, environmental cues, and so forth are directed at oneself) are also common. Grandiose delusions (i.e., when an individual believes that he or she has exceptional abilities, wealth, or fame) and érotomanie delusions (i.e., when an individual believes falsely that another person is in love with him or her) are also seen. Nihilistic delusions involve the conviction that a major catastrophe will occur, and somatic delusions focus on preoccupations regarding health and organ function [...]. The distinction between a delusion and a strongly held idea is sometimes difficult to make and depends in part on the degree of conviction with which the belief is held despite clear or reasonable contradictory evidence regarding its veracity.

The *DSM-5* characterisation of a delusion is by no means uncontroversial, but it does highlight five features which are typically associated with delusions: The first of those features concerns the type of mental state under which delusions fall. A delusion appears to be, at least on the face of it, a belief. The second of those features concerns the epistemic status of the beliefs which qualify as delusions. A delusion is held in light of conflicting evidence (for more on the relationship between delusion and evidence, see Flores, Chapter 12). A third important feature concerns the manner in which those beliefs are held. A delusion is held strongly. It is, in that sense, 'fixed'. A fourth feature of delusions is that they are not circumscribed to a particular topic. Delusions concern many different subject matters. Sometimes, they are about the subject themselves. Sometimes, they are about the world. And, finally, a fifth characteristic feature of delusions is that, in most cases, the content of those beliefs which qualify as delusions is highly implausible.[1]

There is no characterisation of self-deception in the philosophical literature which plays an equivalent role to that of the *DSM-5* characterisation of delusion in the psychiatric literature. Instead, philosophers illustrate the condition to which they refer as 'self-deception' by means of particular examples, or vignettes. Here is, for instance, a particular case of self-deception:

> Tom has been smoking for years. Recently, he has repeatedly found himself out of breath and dizzy when he performs a task which involves minimum physical effort. He has been having some pain in his chest, and he has been having a persistent cough as well. Occasionally, he has found some specks of blood in his handkerchief when he coughs. At the same time, Tom has missed, several times, his regular appointment with his doctor. He insists on changing the channel if the program on tv contains any medical information. And he quickly changes the topic of the conversation if people around him begin to talk about medical issues. However, if, noticing Tom's cough or

acute shortness of breath, a friend asks Tom whether he is sick, Tom will honestly reply that he is not. He will sincerely say that he is healthy.

This example illustrates a number of features which are taken to be characteristic of self-deception. Firstly, self-deception is a condition in which, on the one hand, one sincerely makes a claim but, on the other hand, one behaves as if one thought that the claim that one is making was not true. Tom, for example, claims that he is not sick, but he does not behave as if he thought that he was healthy. Secondly, self-deception is a condition of the subject's own making. It is up to the subject to bring their behaviour and their speech into alignment but, for some reason, the self-deceived subject fails to do that. Tom, for instance, is free to either drop his claim that he is not sick, or to change his avoidance behaviour. The fact that he does neither is something for which Tom himself seems to be responsible. And, finally, self-deception is an objectionable condition; a condition for which we are inclined to criticise the subject. When we notice that Tom's claim that he is not sick is in tension with, for example, his avoiding seeing his doctor, we do not simply conclude that he is, somehow, in a disrupted state. We conclude, more strongly, that he is in a disrupted state for which he is blameworthy.[2]

There seems to be, then, some sense in which delusion and self-deception are alike. Consider, for example, the delusional subject who believes that another person is in love with them despite having evidence that this is not the case (Jordan and Howe 1980). They seem to be, in some sense, similar to the self-deceived subject who claims that they are healthy despite having evidence that this is not the case. The important question, though, is: In what precise sense are the two subjects and, more generally, the two conditions, alike? And in what sense are they different? Let us turn to those two issues now.

## 3. Similarities between delusion and self-deception

There are two main similarities between delusion and self-deception. One concerns the notion of belief, whereas the other one concerns the notion of evidence. Let us consider, first, the similarity which concerns belief. In both delusion and self-deception, there are prima facie reasons for attributing a certain belief to the subject. But, on reflection, there are also reasons why attributing the belief to the subject seems to be problematic. In other words, in both delusion and self-deception, our common practices for attributing psychological states, and in particular beliefs, to people appear to fail us. In both conditions, subjects seem, on the face of it, to have certain beliefs but, all things considered, it is ultimately unclear whether they can be credited with having those beliefs or not.

Take the case of delusions first. Consider, for example, the Capgras delusion, in which the subject claims that their spouse has been replaced by an impostor (Young 2008). What reasons are there for thinking that the subject with Capgras believes that their spouse has been replaced by an impostor? The main reason is that the subject *says* that their spouse has been replaced by an impostor. They are making a certain claim. If we assume that sincere claims express beliefs that the subject has, then, the fact that the subject with Capgras claims that their spouse has been replaced by an impostor constitutes prima facie grounds for attributing, to them, the belief that their spouse has been replaced by an impostor. And yet, there are also reasons for doubting that the subject really has this belief. One reason is that, sometimes, the claim that the delusional subject is making does not seem to have an impact on some of the other beliefs that the subject appears to have. A subject with

Capgras, for example, does not always seem concerned about where their spouse has gone, whether they are alive or dead, or how the process of replacement has taken place (Young 2000: 49, for more on double bookkeeping in delusion, see Porcher, Chapter 13).

Another reason is that, sometimes, the subject does not behave as if the claim that they are making was true. The subject with Capgras, for instance, does not always behave with antipathy towards the person who, they allege, has replaced their spouse. They may even seem quite pleased to cohabitate with the 'impostor' (Lucchelli and Spinnler 2007: 189, for more on delusion and action, see Tumulty, Chapter 18). Taking all these facts into consideration, it does not seem surprising that a debate has arisen on whether delusions are actually beliefs or not.[3] After all, there seem to be considerations which point in opposite directions on this issue.

In the case of self-deception too, we seem to have reasons for and against attributing some key beliefs to a subject. What reasons are there for thinking that Tom, for example, believes that he is healthy? The main reason is that Tom *says* that he is. Assuming that Tom is sincere, this constitutes grounds for attributing, to Tom, the belief that he is healthy. But, analogously to the case of delusions, there are also reasons for not attributing this belief to him. The main reason is that Tom does not behave as if he thought that he was healthy. By avoiding the sources of information that could confirm whether the troubling changes in his body are symptoms of a disease, Tom is behaving, in fact, as if he believed that he is sick. Thus, in the case of self-deception too, we seem to have grounds for attributing a belief to a subject, but we also have reasons for not attributing the belief to them. It is no wonder that, in the literature on self-deception, there is also a debate on what kinds of beliefs we should attribute to a subject who is self-deceived.[4]

A second similarity between delusion and self-deception concerns the notion of evidence. In the case of delusion, it seems clear that, whether the claim that the subject makes expresses a belief or not, that claim is held with firm conviction despite the fact that the subject has no evidence for the truth of the claim. The subject with Capgras, for example, will insist that their spouse has been replaced by an impostor even if they are not capable of explaining how that replacement could have happened. The tension between the claim that the delusional subject makes and the evidence that the subject has in support of that claim is, in fact, an essential characteristic of a delusion in the *DSM-5* characterisation of delusions mentioned above. The strength of the conviction with which the subject holds on to that claim despite the available evidence is also an essential characteristic of delusions on the *DSM-5* characterisation.

There is a similar conflict between the evidence which is available to the subject and the claims that the subject is prepared to make despite that evidence in the case of self-deception. Tom, for example, will insist that he is healthy even if there seems to be evidence that he is sick; evidence which is clearly available to Tom. As in the case of delusion, the self-deceived subject will continue to hold on to their claims despite the conflicting evidence available to them. In the literature on self-deception, the most common explanation for the strength of the conviction with which the subject will hold on to their claims appeals to motivational factors. We will return to the role of motivational factors in self-deception below.

There are two thoughts that one might pursue in order to explain these similarities between delusion and self-deception. Perhaps, one might think, the reason why it is hard to attribute beliefs to both the delusional and the self-deceived subject, and the reason why there is a conflict between their claims and their behaviour, is that delusion is not an on/off condition, but a spectrum, and self-deception is a low-intensity type of delusion, typically of the non-bizarre kind. Alternatively, one might think that the reason why we have trouble attributing beliefs to both the delusional and the self-deceived subject, and the reason why we perceive a tension between their claims and their behaviour, is that self-deception can be more or less extreme and, in extreme cases, we call that kind of self-deception, 'delusion'. The two possibilities are thought-provoking but, compelling as the similarities between delusion and self-deception are, there seem to be more reasons for distinguishing delusion and self-deception as two separate conditions than there are for assimilating either of the two conditions to the other one. Let us turn to the reasons for separating the two conditions from each other now.

## 4.   Differences between delusion and self-deception

Delusion and self-deception are different conditions in several respects. They have different aetiologies, they have a different impact on the subject's well-being and on their capacity for social interactions, they are different from a normative point of view, and they are different from a medical point of view.

With regard to the aetiology of both conditions, one might say that, for the most part, self-deception is explained by appealing to motivational factors, whereas delusions are explained by appealing to neurobiological factors. There are two main explanations of self-deception in the literature; intentionalism and motivationalism. Intentionalists believe that, in cases of self-deception, a subject intentionally causes themselves to believe something that they themselves think to be false (Bermúdez 2000). The idea would be that Tom, for example, has gotten himself to believe that he is healthy; something that he himself believes to be false. Motivationalists, by contrast, conceive self-deception by analogy to wishful thinking. According to motivationalists, in self-deception, a subject forms a belief due to the influence of some of their motivational states, such as desires and emotions (Mele 2001). The idea, in this case, would be that Tom, for example, does not want to face the fact that he is sick. That truth is too difficult to face and, for that reason, he does not pay attention to the evidence suggesting that he is sick. Notice, however, that this is a controversy about whether self-deception is an intentional act or not. It is not a controversy about whether motivational factors play a role in self-deception or not. Proponents of both intentionalism and motivationalism will need to agree that the source of self-deception is to be found in motivational factors. Otherwise, intentionalists will have no explanation for why a subject who believes something is getting themselves to form the opposite belief. Even intentionalists will accept that the subject's reason for performing this act is to avoid what they regard as the painful truth on some issue.

Delusions, by contrast, are normally explained by neurobiological causes such as odd perceptual experiences, biases in reasoning, or disrupted prediction-error signals. Three types of theories appeal to causes of this kind; one-factor theories, two-factor theories, and prediction error theories. One-factor theories of delusions, for example, explain the claims that delusional subjects make as expressions of certain beliefs which constitute hypotheses. These are hypotheses that the subject formulates in order to explain some unusual perceptual experiences that they are having. Now, the relevant hypotheses may or may not be plausible but, even when they are implausible, one-factor theorists believe that the fact that the subject formulates the hypotheses can be explained without appealing to any abnormal cognitive failing on the part of the subject. The unusual perceptual experiences that the subject is trying to explain by formulating those hypotheses, by contrast, are considered clinical anomalies by one-factor theorists of delusions. It is for this reason that one-factor theorists believe that we only need to appeal to a single factor in order to explain delusions. That single factor is the subject's unusual perceptual experience. In the Capgras case, for example, the thought is that the subject does not have the type of perceptual experience that one would normally have while looking at the face of one's spouse. Specifically, the thought is that the subject with Capgras has lower autonomic responses to familiar faces compared to subjects who lack the delusion (Ellis et al. 1997). And, in order to explain why there is something odd about the perceptual experience that they are having when they look at their spouse, the subject with Capgras forms the hypothesis that their spouse has been replaced by an impostor (Maher 1974; Sullivan-Bissett 2020; Noordhof and Sullivan-Bissett 2021, see also Sullivan-Bissett, Chapter 28). Two-factor theories, by contrast, explain delusions not only as the result of an unusual perceptual experience that the delusional subject needs to make sense of, but also as the result of a reasoning deficit, bias, or performance error, which accounts for why the subject would formulate or endorse a highly implausible hypothesis in the first place, and/or why they would subsequently fail to abandon it despite the available evidence against it (Coltheart et al. 2010, see also Davies and Coltheart, Chapter 29). According to prediction error theories, we have expectations about what the world is like based on a model that we have formed of the world and, when our experience does not meet those expectations, a prediction-error is coded so that our model of the world can be updated. What happens in a delusion is that, due to the type of abnormal experience to which one-factor theories appeal, a prediction error is coded incorrectly, and the subject updates their model of the world as a reaction to that signal, by forming a delusional belief. The subject with Capgras, for example, finds themselves being part of an unexpected event when they encounter their spouse, which generates a prediction error signal. The subject's reaction to this prediction error is to formulate the delusion that their spouse has been replaced in order to respond to the unexpected event and update their model of the world (Corlett et al. 2007, see also Corlett, Chapter 30).

What is common to all three accounts of delusions is that, in all three accounts, the explanation of delusions is not psychodynamic. If motivational factors are invoked in the explanation of delusions, it is always in a hybrid format, where a role for motivational factors needs to be found in conjunction with the types of neurobiological factors mentioned above (McKay et al. 2007).

Delusions and self-deception are also different with regard to their impact on the subject's well-being. Delusions, on the one hand, appear to have a negative effect on the subject's capacity for social interaction, leading to social withdrawal and isolation (Freeman et al. 2014). Self-deception, however, can have a positive effect on the subject's well-being. The reason is that the self-serving biases which are provided by self-deception can play a role in making us optimistic and happy (Von Hippel & Trivers 2011). At the very least, self-deception has the value of protecting us from the emotional impact of facing some fact which is difficult for us to face. Naturally, this is not to say that delusions are bad and self-deception is good. Things are more nuanced than that. Delusions may cause social withdrawal and isolation, but they also seem to have some pragmatic and epistemic benefits. For example, the formation of delusions arguably provides relief from anxiety to those subjects who, in the prodromal stage of psychosis, are in a state of heightened awareness and, as a result, are bombarded with hypersalient stimuli (Kapur 2003). Furthermore, it could be argued that delusions are adaptive in a different sense. They constitute a conceptual framework which provides a sense of order, stability and meaning to the anomalous experience that the subject is having (Roberts 1991, 1992). And, through those pragmatic benefits, delusions might indirectly contribute to improving the subject's epistemic functionality, by enhancing, for example, concentration, attention and, more generally, an active engagement with the environment which allows for the acquisition of new information (Bortolotti 2020). Self-deception, on the other hand, may generate optimism through self-serving biases, but a similar claim could be made, in some instances at least, about delusions as well. One might argue that delusions of grandeur, for example, can protect the subject from the low self-esteem effects of having a negative conception of themselves (McKay et al. 2005). And, similarly, the Reverse Othello syndrome (the delusion that one's romantic partner is faithful when they are not) can protect the subject from the sense of loss associated with a fractured relationship (Butler 2000). On the whole, however, it does seem that delusions have a disruptive effect in the life of the subject, whereas self-deception does not.

Delusions and self-deception are different in another important respect too. This is the extent to which we hold the subject responsible for their condition and, therefore, we are inclined to criticise the subject for it. Consider self-deception first. It seems that, no matter how we try to explain self-deception, this is a condition for which we will hold the subject responsible, and for which we will criticise them. If we explain self-deception in intentionalist terms, for example, then, clearly, we should hold the self-deceived subject responsible for their self-deception. For their self-deception is the result of an intentional action of theirs. It is the result of their getting themselves to have a belief which is contrary to another belief that they also have. And that complex state is a state which, from an epistemic point of view, they should not occupy, since it involves having two contradictory beliefs. Thus, self-deception seems to be, when construed in intentionalist terms, something for which the subject is blameworthy; blameworthy from an epistemic standpoint. Things are not different if we try to explain self-deception in motivationalist terms. In that case, self-deception is not the result of an intentional action of the subject. Nevertheless, the self-deceived subject is doing something which, epistemically speaking, they should not do. They are forming beliefs, not in accordance with the available evidence, but under the influence of their motivational states. Furthermore, this kind of bias is something which is within the subject's power to change. For that reason, self-deception seems to be, when construed in motivationalist terms, something for which the subject is blameworthy too.

Interestingly, we do not seem to have the same intuitions about responsibility and blame when it comes to delusions. Notice that, whether we explain delusions through one-factor accounts, two-factor accounts, or prediction-error accounts, one feature which is common to all of these accounts of delusions is that, on all of them, a delusion is not something that the subject does (or the result of something that the subject does). It is, instead, something which happens to the subject (or the result of something which happens to the subject). Having an unusual perceptual experience when one looks at a familiar person, for example, is not something which is under the subject's control. Neither is having a reasoning deficit, or reacting to a prediction error signal. On all of these accounts of delusions, then, delusions are not the kind of thing which is up to the subject to have, or not to have. And, for that reason, it does not seem surprising that we do not hold the delusional subject responsible for their delusions, and we do not take the delusional subject to be blameworthy for them.[5]

The final respect in which delusions and self-deception are different is that we take different positions on the issue of whether delusion or self-deception are pathological or not. That is, we take different positions on the issue of whether delusion or self-deception are a form of mental illness. The generally accepted position, when it comes to self-deception, is that it is not pathological.[6] By contrast, it seems plausible to consider delusions pathological beliefs. One reason for considering them pathological is that, as we have seen, they have a dysfunctional, or defective, aetiology. Another reason is that, as we have also seen, they have a harmful effect on the subject's well-being.[7] For these reasons alone, it seems natural to place the phenomenon of delusion under the scope of, not only philosophy or cognitive science more broadly, but also under the scope of psychiatry. (For more on delusion and pathology, see Petrolini, Chapter 1.) This is a feature that delusions do not share with the phenomenon of self-deception.

## 5. Conclusion

We have seen that self-deception and delusion have sufficiently different features as to consider them separate conditions. However, it is possible that they both constitute instances of irrationality, depending on how 'irrationality' is understood.

In a broad sense of 'irrational', a subject can be seen as being irrational if we cannot explain, and predict, their behaviour by attributing a set of beliefs and desires to them (Davidson 1982). One thing that the delusional subject and the self-deceived subject have in common is that, at least at first glance, they both seem to have this property. Our belief attribution practices do not work very well when we encounter a subject in either of the two conditions. And, for that reason, we have trouble explaining their verbal and non-verbal behaviour. They are, in that broad sense, irrational.

In a narrower sense of 'irrational', a subject can be seen as being rational if they have formed a belief through a process which is inappropriate in some epistemic sense. The inappropriateness at issue can be 'motivated', when desires, emotions, and other motivational states influence the way in which evidence is gathered and evaluated, or 'cognitive', when the way in which the evidence is gathered and evaluated is the result of some cognitive failure or deficit. Do self-deception and delusion share either of the two varieties of narrow irrationality?

Two-factor theorists of delusions appeal to the narrow type of irrationality, in its cognitive variety, in order to explain how delusions are formed and/or sustained.[8] To be clear, the exact clinical status of the relevant cognitive deficits in delusions is a controversial issue. In two-factor theories of delusions, the cognitive deficits which are responsible for the formation of delusions in response to unusual experiences are assumed to be clinical abnormalities, but this has been a contested point (Noordhof and Sullivan-Bissett 2021). It seems, then, that perhaps an argument could be made that narrow irrationality of the cognitive type is involved in delusions, but it would be a less straightforward argument than it might seem at first glance. However, there is, as far as I can see, no need to invoke this type of irrationality in an explanation of self-deception, whether one is an intentionalist or a motivationalist about self-deception. Thus, it seems that the narrow type of irrationality, in its cognitive variety, is not a property that delusion and self-deception are likely to share, whether two-factor theorists of delusions are correct in appealing to it or not.

What about the motivated variety of narrow irrationality? The issue of whether either delusion or self-deception is irrational, in that sense, is particularly unclear. Motivationalist accounts of self-deception do involve the narrow type of irrationality, in its motivated variety (Mele 2001). And some accounts of delusions appeal to motivational factors in order to explain the formation and/or the maintenance of delusions in response to unusual experiences.[9] One might think, then, that this type of irrationality is involved in both delusion and self-deception. But I think that claim needs to be approached with caution. For one thing, it is not certain that the motivated variety of narrow irrationality is involved in self-deception. Intentionalist accounts of self-deception must ultimately appeal to motivational factors in order to explain the reasons that the self-deceived subject has for forming a belief which they themselves think to be false. But that role for motivational factors in self-deception is consistent with a lack of narrow irrationality of the motivated variety. (Motivational states, such as desires, may give the self-deceived subject a reason for carrying out the act of forming a certain belief without causing a motivational bias in the formation of such a belief.) For another thing, motivational factors may play a role in some delusions but, even if they do, it is not clear that delusions involve more motivational factors than those involved in everyday instances of motivated irrationality, such as wishful thinking (Noordhof and Sullivan-Bissett 2023). If that is correct, it is not clear how clinically significant this type of irrationality would be in the case of delusions.

What can be granted about the similarity between delusion and self-deception, I believe, is that they are both irrational in the broad sense. They are both forms of broad, Davidson-type, irrationality. But they are importantly different, and any attempt to assimilate one of the two conditions to the other one will miss, in my view, the significant differences between the two conditions.

## Notes

1 'In most cases' because the *DSM-5* distinguishes between so-called bizarre and non-bizarre delusions, depending on whether the relevant delusions are 'clearly implausible and not understandable to same-culture peers and do not derive from ordinary life experiences' (APA 2013: 87). Thus, the delusion that one's thoughts have been removed by an outside force is considered to be a bizarre delusion whereas the belief that one is under surveillance by the police, if it is strongly held despite any evidence in support of it, is considered to be a non-bizarre delusion. As the examples in the *DSM-5* characterisation illustrate, most delusions tend to be highly implausible, which seems to render them bizarre according to the just-mentioned criterion.

2 What exactly do we find objectionable in self-deception? Why do we blame a self-deceived subject like Tom? One will take a different position on this issue depending on the types of mental states that one is inclined to attribute to Tom. If, for example, one takes Tom's claim that he is not sick at face value, and attribute to Tom the belief that he is not sick, then it seems reasonable to think that Tom is blameworthy because he is not forming that belief in accordance with the available evidence (Mele 1987). As we will shortly see, however, theorists of self-deception disagree on the types of mental states that one should attribute to a self-deceived subject like Tom.

3 See, for example, Bayne and Pacherie (2005) and Bortolotti (2009) in favour of the doxastic conception of delusions, and Currie (2000) and Dub (2017) against it. (For more on delusion and doxasticism and non-doxasticism, see Noordhof, Chapters 19 and 20.)

4 There are those who believe that a subject like Tom both believes and disbelieves that he is sick (or, for that matter, that he is healthy). See, for example, Sartre (1957: 47–67). There are also those who believe that Tom's case needs to be understood by attributing to him a belief and a desire, rather than two beliefs (Mele 1987). In Tom's case, for instance, the belief at issue would be the belief that he is healthy and the desire in question would be the desire to be healthy. And there are those who believe that Tom's case needs to be construed, instead, by attributing two beliefs to Tom, but two beliefs which are not contradictory; a belief about his health and a belief about his own beliefs (Fernández 2013). In Tom's case, for instance, the first-order belief would be the belief that he is sick and the higher-order belief would be the belief that he believes that he is healthy.

5 Notice that this is a different issue from the issue of whether a delusional subject is responsible for, not their delusions, but the behaviour caused by their delusions. On delusions and moral responsibility, see Bortolotti et al. (2014), see also Scholten, Chapter 34.

6 An exception can be found, perhaps, in Levy (2007), in which Neil Levy discusses what he assumes to be pathological instances of self-deception. Levy, however, offers cases of delusions as such instances of self-deception (Levy 2007: 262). Levy is taking, then, the starting position that delusions and self-deception are not different conditions.

7 On the different senses in which delusions might be considered pathological beliefs, see Miyazono (2015), and Bortolotti (2022).

8 The relevant cognitive deficit varies across different two-factor explanations of delusions. It has been argued, for example, that subjects with delusions jump to conclusions (Garety and Freeman 1999), that they have a tendency to prioritise observational data over adjustments to their beliefs (Stone and Young 1997), and that they fail to inhibit a pre-potent doxastic response to experience (Davies et al. 2001).

9 Psychodynamic accounts of the Capgras delusion, for example, have appealed to the fact that the subject feels suspicious towards the person they judge to be an impostor (Vogel 1974). That sense of suspicion is acknowledged outside of the psychodynamic approach to the Capgras delusion as well (Ellis and Young 1990: 241).

# References


American Psychiatric Association (APA) (2013) *Diagnostic and Statistical Manual of Mental Disorders*, Fifth Edition, Arlington, VA: American Psychiatric Publishing.

Bayne, T. and Pacherie, E. (2005) "In defence of the doxastic conception of delusions," *Mind & Language* 20: 163–188.

Bermúdez, J. (2000) "Self-deception, intentions, and contradictory beliefs," *Analysis* 60: 309–319.

Bortolotti, L. (2022) "Are delusions pathological beliefs?," *Asian Journal of Philosophy* 1: 31.

Bortolotti, L. (2020) *The Epistemic Innocence of Irrational Beliefs*, Oxford: Oxford University Press.

Bortolotti, L. (2009) *Delusions and Other Irrational Beliefs*, Oxford: Oxford University Press.

Bortolotti, L., Broome, M.R. and Mameli, M. (2014) "Delusions and responsibility for action: Insights from the Breivik case," *Neuroethics* 7: 377–382.

Butler, P. (2000) "Reverse Othello syndrome subsequent to traumatic brain injury," *Psychiatry: Interpersonal and Biological Processes* 63: 85–92.

Coltheart, M., Menzies, P. and Sutton, J. (2010) "Abductive inference and delusional belief," *Cognitive Neuropsychiatry* 15: 261–287.

Corlett, P., Murray, G.K., Honey, G.D., Aitken, M.R.F., Shanks, D.R., Robbins, T.W., Bullmore, E.T., Dickinson, A. and Fletcher, P.C. (2007) "Disrupted prediction error signal in psychosis: Evidence for an associative account of delusions," *Brain* 130: 2387–2400.

Currie, G. (2000) "Imagination, delusion and hallucinations," *Mind & Language* 15: 168–183.

Davidson, D. (1982) "Two paradoxes of irrationality," in R. Wollheim and J. Hopkins (eds.), *Philosophical Essays on Freud*, Cambridge: Cambridge University Press, pp. 289–305.

Davies, M., Coltheart, M., Langdon, R. and Breen, N. (2001) "Monothematic delusions: Towards a two-factor account," *Philosophy, Psychiatry, & Psychology* 8: 133–158.

Dub, R. (2017) "Delusions, acceptances and cognitive feelings," *Philosophy and Phenomenological Research* 94: 27–60.

Ellis, H.D. and Young, A.W. (1990) "Accounting for delusional misidentification," *British Journal of Psychiatry* 157: 239–248.

Ellis, H.D., Young, A.W., Quayle, A.H. and De Pauw, K.W. (1997) "Reduced autonomic responses to faces in Capgras delusion," *Proceedings of the Royal Society of London. Series B, Biological Sciences* 264: 1085–1092.

Fernández, J. (2013) "Self-deception and self-knowledge," *Philosophical Studies* 162: 379-400.

Freeman, D., Startup, H., Dunn, G., Wingham, G., Černis, E., Evans, N., Lister, R., Pugh, K. Cordwell, J. and Kingdon, D. (2014) "Persecutory delusions and psychological well-being," *Social Psychiatry and Psychiatric Epidemiology* 49: 1045–1050.

Garety, P.A. and Freeman, D. (1999) "Cognitive approaches to delusions: A critical review of theories and evidence," *British Journal of Clinical Psychology* 38: 113–154.

Jordan, H.W. and Howe, G. (1980) "De Clérambault syndrome (erotomania): A review and case presentation," *Journal of the National Medical Association* 72: 979–985.

Kapur, S. (2003) "Psychosis as a state of aberrant salience: A framework linking biology, phenomenology and pharmacology in schizophrenia," *American Journal of Psychiatry* 160: 13–23.

Levy, N. (2007) *Neuroethics: Challenges for the 21st Century*, Cambridge: Cambridge University Press.

Lucchelli, F. and Spinnler, H. (2007) "The case of lost Wilma: A clinical report of Capgras delusion," *Neurological Science* 28: 188–195.

Maher, B. (1974) "Delusional thinking and perceptual disorder," *Journal of Individual Psychology* 30: 98–113.

McKay, R., Langdon, R. and Coltheart, M. (2007) "Models of misbelief: Integrating motivational and deficit theories of delusions," *Consciousness and Cognition* 16: 932–941.

McKay, R., Langdon, R. and Coltheart, M. (2005) "'Sleights of mind': Delusions, defences and self-deception," *Cognitive Neuropsychiatry* 10: 305–326.

Mele, A. (2001) *Self-Deception Unmasked*, Princeton, NJ: Princeton University Press.

Mele, A. (1987) "Recent work on self-deception," *American Philosophical Quarterly* 24: 1–17.

Miyazono, K. (2015) "Delusions as harmful malfunctioning beliefs," *Consciousness and Cognition* 33: 561–573.

Noordhof, P. and Sullivan-Bissett, E. (2023) "The everyday irrationality of monothematic delusion," in P. Henne and S. Murray (eds.), *Advances in Experimental Philosophy of Action*, London: Bloomsbury, pp. 87–111.

Noordhof, P. and Sullivan-Bissett, E. (2021) "The clinical significance of anomalous experience in the explanation of monothematic delusions," *Synthese* 199: 10277–10309.

Roberts, G. (1992) "The origins of delusion," *The British Journal of Psychiatry* 161: 298–308.

Roberts, G. (1991) "Delusional belief systems and meaning in life: A preferred reality?" *The British Journal of Psychiatry* 159: 19–28.

Sartre, J.P. (1957) *Being and Nothingness: An Essay on Phenomenological Ontology*, London: Methuen.

Stone, T. and Young, A. (1997) "Delusions and brain injury: The philosophy and psychology of belief," *Mind & Language* 12: 327–364.

Sullivan-Bissett, E. (2020) "Unimpaired abduction to alien abduction: Lessons on delusion formation," *Philosophical Psychology* 33: 679–704.

Vogel, F. (1974) "The Capgras syndrome and its psychopathology," *American Journal of Psychiatry* 131: 922–924.

Von Hippel, W. and Trivers, R. (2011) "Reflections on self-deception," *Behavioural and Brain Sciences* 34: 41–56.

Young, A.W. (2000) "Wondrous strange: The neuropsychology of abnormal beliefs," in M. Coltheart and M. Davies (eds.), *Pathologies of Belief*, Oxford: Blackwell, pp. 47–73.

Young, G. (2008) "Capgras delusion: An interactionist model," *Consciousness and Cognition* 17: 863–876.

23

# DELUSION AND MEMORY

Sarah Robins and Si-Won Song

## 1. Introduction

Most research on the intersection between memory and delusion has focused on *confabulation* – a term initially used to characterize false memories in dementia patients, which has since expanded to include a broader range of errors in clinical and everyday settings. Confabulation has received a good deal of sustained treatment from philosophers of memory in recent years (Michaelian 2016, 2020; Bernecker 2017; Robins 2019, 2020). In the current chapter, our aim is to explore the intersection of memory and delusion beyond confabulation: Does memory play a role in other delusions?

Capgras delusion has been a delusion of interest for many philosophers and cognitive scientists. Amongst clinicians, and some philosophers, Capgras is viewed as an affective disorder, according to which the connection between familiarity and its response has been somehow severed (Ellis and Young 1990; Ramachandran 1999). Philosophers have, however, become increasingly interested in pointing out the inadequacies of the affective account, and have offered alternative proposals for understanding Capgras (e.g., Hirstein 2010; Bongiorno 2020; Coltheart and Davies 2021).

While these views are commendable for the increased attention and nuance they bring to the explanation of Capgras, they all continue to face challenges accounting for the full range and nature of the delusional phenomena in Capgras. In this chapter, we propose an alternative characterization according to which the Capgras delusion is a result of a malfunction in the way memories are updated. A version of this *memory updating view* was first proposed by Dennis Staton and colleagues in 1982, but received very little attention and uptake. We update and revive the view here, arguing that it has myriad advantages that warrant its serious consideration.

## 2. Capgras delusion

The Capgras delusion occurs when a person claims that someone familiar to them has been replaced by an imposter. Documented cases are rare. A recent metaanalysis (Pandis et al. 2019) includes 255 documented cases in the century since Joseph Capgras' initial

347

DOI: 10.4324/9781003296386-28

identification. Capgras (Capgras & Reboul-Lachaux 1923/1994) identified the delusion in a 52-year-old Parisian woman who insisted that her husband had been replaced by an imposter who bore a great resemblance to him. Subsequent cases have tended to follow this pattern: a person is brought in by a loved one for their insistence that they or another loved one has been replaced by an imposter. Often, these reports are made after repeated reassurances and attempts to provide evidence to the contrary by the alleged imposter and other friends and family. Despite all of this, persons experiencing Capgras delusion continue to insist that the loved one has been replaced with a duplicate.

The delusion has captured the attention of philosophers, as well as other scientists and clinicians, not because of its pervasiveness but because of its peculiarity. The delusion is alarming. It involves a person seeming to simultaneously recognize and fail to recognize someone they know well. After all, persons experiencing this delusion do, in some sense, recognize the familiar person. They are able to accurately identify their physical features, claiming them to be an imposter rather than a stranger. V.S. Ramachandran (1999), for example, reports a person experiencing the Capgras delusion to have said, 'That guy isn't my father. He just looks like him' (159). Occasionally, persons experiencing the delusion will offer justifications for their claims, which are based on alleged discrepancies between the imposter and the original. Persons experiencing Capgras delusion have, for example, suggested that the imposter's nose is a different size (O'Reilly and Malholtra 1987) or that their hand is softer (Rojo et al. 1991). However, many of these discrepancies are minor and would not be cause for concern, much less the basis for a claim that the person is an imposter, in standard circumstances.

The Capgras delusion is often directed toward a person who is emotionally significant; a spouse, parent, or child is often the one labeled an imposter. Pandis and colleagues' (2019) meta-analysis suggests that the determination of which of these emotionally significant relationships is affected by the delusion is influenced by the person's life stage. When the delusion onset is at a younger age, the imposter tends to be a parent, while those who first experience the delusion when they are older tend to claim either their spouse or child is the imposter. Most persons experiencing Capgras delusion focus their claim of duplicitous duplication on one or two persons. In a few cases, persons experiencing the delusion identify a handful of imposters. Regardless of who is selected, subjects experiencing Capgras delusion limit their claims about an imposter to only a select few. This is not a disorder that involves indiscriminate misidentification.

There is no standard demographic profile for a person experiencing Capgras delusion, as the delusion can result from different underlying causes. Often, Capgras delusion is a symptom of schizophrenia, but can also be caused by neurodegenerative diseases such as Alzheimer's (Edelstyn and Oyebode 1999, for more on delusions in the disorders of old age see Hughes, Chapter 11). Thus, generally, those affected tend to either be in their early twenties, the standard age of onset for schizophrenia, or in late adulthood, when neurodegenerative diseases are most common. Capgras delusion can also occur as a result of brain trauma – for example, a car accident – in which case the age of onset is more variable. Regardless of its underlying cause, Capgras delusion is persistent. A person experiencing it will continue to claim that the previously familiar person is an imposter for an extended period of time, typically corresponding to the duration of the underlying condition. Those who experience Capgras delusion as a result of the onset of schizophrenia, for example, will generally continue to experience the delusion until their schizophrenia is well-managed. When the delusion occurs as a result of brain trauma or neurodegeneration, the delusion can persist indefinitely.

## 3.  Affective responsiveness hypothesis

Clinicians have long favored an affective explanation of the Capgras delusion. William Hirstein (2010) dubs it the 'affective responsiveness hypothesis', according to which Capgras delusion is the result of a deficit in the autonomic response involved in facial recognition.

The affective responsiveness hypothesis is standardly credited to Hadyn D. Ellis and Andrew W. Young (1990), who developed the view. The general idea that the affective features of recognition are thwarted in cases of this delusion has, however, long been discussed. As Ellis and Young refer in their paper, Capgras (1923) discussed it in his original paper, and similar remarks can be found in Derombies (1935), Lewis (1987), Bauer (1986), Anderson (1988), Brochado (1936) and Weinstein and Burnham (1991). Ellis and Young were, however, the first to develop the claim into a full-fledged view, with neuroanatomical support for the explanation. Ellis and Young were inspired by work on *prosopagnosia*, a disorder where a person is unable to recognize faces. Prosopagnosia patients, peculiarly, show an autonomic response to familiar faces, but not to unfamiliar ones, even when they are unable to recognize the familiar faces (Bauer 1984; Tranel et al. 1985, 1988). Facial recognition, in standard cases, involves two distinct kinds of recognition: (1) reidentifying the facial features as belonging to a particular person and (2) an autonomic/physiological response (Bauer 1984). These two forms of recognition normally occur together when we recognize a person, but they are neurologically dissociable. So, for example, when I see a friend of mine, two types of recognition occur: one where I am able to recognize my friend by their physical features and can identify who the features belong to and another that involves a kind of 'glow of arousal'[1] where I have a physical response to the perception of familiar facial features. In many cases, the response may be so faint as to remain below the level of awareness, but can nevertheless be detected in experimental contexts.

The first kind of recognition is referred to as *overt recognition* in the literature, while the latter is referred to as *covert recognition*. Despite prosopagnosia patients' inability to overtly recognize familiar faces, they seemed to nonetheless have some covert recognition when looking at familiar faces, as detected by increases in their skin conductance response (SCR). SCR is a measure of the electrical conductivity of a person's skin, which increases when exposed to physically arousing stimuli. It is considered to be an empirical measure of a person's affective response to stimuli. The tendency for prosopagnosia patients to show heightened SCR to familiar faces suggests the persistence of covert recognition of familiar persons they are unable to overtly recognize.

The affective responsiveness hypothesis proposes that Capgras is the inverse phenomenon: overt recognition without a covert recognition response. In Capgras, familiar people are still registered as familiar, but the standard autonomic response to such familiar faces does not come along. Ellis and Young propose that while the subject can correctly recognize that the physical features they see belong to a familiar person, they do not experience the glow of arousal that normally also occurs during recognition. Because these two types of recognition usually occur together, lacking one type of recognition creates an anomalous perceptual experience that is thought to be the cause of the delusion.

## 4.  The etiological problem

Philosophers have explored the affective response proposal in more detail, asking questions about how precisely the recognition should be understood and how it accounts for the

Capgras delusion. A distinction is then made between *explanationist* and *endorsement* accounts, which focuses on how the anomalous experience and delusion are related. From this perspective, Ellis and Young's (1990) account is characterized as an *explanationist* account. The affective response itself has relatively minimal content – i.e., it registers only that the person is unfamiliar. The delusion then arises out of the attempt to explain this anomalous experience.

Alternatively, others have proposed an *endorsement* account (Bayne and Pacherie 2004; Pacherie 2008). On this view, the content of the affective response is understood to be much richer such that the delusion needs only to provide an endorsement of this state rather than an explanation. Such accounts have been viewed as particularly useful amongst philosophers trying to parse the relationship between abnormal perceptual experience and delusional testimony. Tim Bayne and Elisabeth Pacherie (2004), for example, assert that the statements delusional subjects make should be understood as a reflection of what their abnormal experience is like. If a subject asserts that they think that their father has been replaced by an imposter, an endorsement account would say that this assertion is more or less what the imposter is experiencing. To the subject, the supposed 'imposter' does appear to genuinely be a different person.

Both views face what Federico Bongiorno (2020) calls the *etiology problem*, which high-lights the distance between the affective disruption and the delusional content. Consider first the explanationist approach. A thinly characterized affective response could serve as the root of the delusion, but it is unclear how such a response could explain *why* the person goes on to claim that the person who fails to generate an affective response in them is an imposter. That is, the disconnect explains the anomalous experience, but not the subsequent interpretation of the anomalous experience. The challenge is especially striking considering how varied persons experiencing Capgras delusion are, in terms of personality, age, back-ground, and underlying medical condition.

The etiology problem presses on the endorsement account from the other side. While there are benefits to understanding anomalous experiences in the enriched way they favor, it is unclear that the mechanism involved is capable of doing so. The affective mechanisms supporting familiarity responses are not generally thought to be such that they could sup-port elaborate, nuanced contents of the sort that would directly invoke the idea of an imposter.

Ultimately, the etiological problem demonstrates that affective response cannot account for the Capgras delusion. There are competing accounts of the affective content involved in this endorsement (Bongiorno 2020; see also the expressivist proposal from Bradley and Gibson 2023). It remains unclear which way of thinking about the content is most apt – and more generally, there are no clear guidelines in place regarding how competing content attributions should be adjudicated.

Many philosophers have thus been motivated to look for ways that the affective response could be supplemented by patterns or forms of reasoning. This then leads to debates between one- and two-factor accounts over what these additional reasoning features are and whether they should be understood as abnormal or not.[2] The ensuing discussion often focuses on the additional reasoning factors, moving attention further away from the initial abnormality. We are setting this debate aside, proposing a return of focus to how the basic disruption to recognition and familiarity in the Capgras delusion should be understood. For this reason, we focus our discussion below on accounts that offer an alternative to the affective response hypothesis.

Hirstein (2010) and Sam Wilkinson (2016) both suggest abandoning the affective view of the Capgras delusion and replacing it with something else entirely. They differ over what they propose as a suitable replacement.

Hirstein (2010) suggests that Capgras is the result of damage to the representations featured in the person's theory of mind.[3] Mindreading is the ability to predict and explain the behavior of oneself and others in terms of mental states, most particularly beliefs and desires. Philosophers debate about how to best characterize this capacity as well as its scope in human development and in other organisms, but there is nonetheless consensus about the existence of such a capacity (Andrews, Spaulding, and Westra 2020). To explain how the Capgras delusion is related to this overall capacity, Hirstein emphasizes the role of perspective-taking in mindreading. Specifically, Hirstein characterizes perspective-taking in mindreading in terms of the ability to create egocentric representations of the minds of others. Not all mindreading involves such intense perspective-taking. But, Hirstein argues, in cases where we know a person well, it becomes possible to employ not just generic viewpoints, but person-specific perspectives on the world.

Suppose you are set to meet someone at the movie theater, and you arrive a few minutes late to find that they are not at the agreed-upon location. Given the context, where use of cell phones is prohibited, you cannot contact them. Instead, you have to reason about what they might have done. If the person is a casual acquaintance, you may engage in mindreading by taking a generic perspective: what would make a person do this? If, however, it is someone you know well, then you can deploy your own egocentric representation of their perspective, asking more specifically what *that person* is likely to do in such a situation. The ability to incorporate specific features presumably provides richer information that can yield more accurate predictions.

Damage to this ability for egocentric mindreading is, Hirstein (2010) claims, at the basis of the Capgras delusion. As he argues, it can be understood as 'caused by damage to the mind-representing part of this large egocentric representation system' (2010: 243). How does the loss of an egocentric representation of another person lead to the belief that the person is an imposter? Hirstein claims that the deficit occurs only to the egocentric representations of the person, leaving other information about the person intact. That is, a Capgras subject can still represent what their loved one looks like, but can no longer generate any sense of what the world is like from their perspective. It is this dissonance that leads to the conviction that the person is an imposter.

Wilkinson (2016) offers a different proposal for the primary deficit in the Capgras delusion, which he characterizes in terms of mental files. In developing this account, Wilkinson appeals to Recanati's (2012) approach to informational semantics, which explains the ability to have thoughts about individuals in terms of mental files that refer to those individuals. Mental files explain how thought about individuals is possible. As a disordered way of thinking about familiar individuals, Wilkinson reasons, Capgras delusion is best understood in terms of damage to this system – as the 'mismanagement of files' (2016: 396). The *mental file* is the referring concept that identifies a particular individual as the one we are thinking about, offering a metaphorical way of thinking about mental information storage. When we encounter an individual for the first time, a file is opened and filled with pertinent information about that individual. Subsequent thoughts about and interactions with that person reopen the file, allowing for information to be added and updated.[4] Appeal to mental files has been used in the literature on reference to explain errors in identifying individuals – e.g., cases when a new file is opened for a person that has been encountered previously. Capgras delusion is, then, a particular way of mismanaging files, where a completely new file is created for a well-known person rather than merging the new open demonstrative file with the file of the familiar person. What happens in the case of Capgras is that the subject notices the resemblance between the newly opened file and a previously built one, and concludes that the latter individual is an impersonator of the former rather than the same person. As Wilkinson sees it, the mental files approach offers a helpful way of distinguishing between identifying individuals and predicating over them, which can be used to explain the distinct elements of what goes wrong and right in Capgras, respectively.

## 5.   The selectivity problem

Each of the accounts of the Capgras delusion reviewed in the previous section offers a plausible way to address the etiological challenge. For the purposes of this chapter, we are not interested in adjudicating between them further on this point. Instead, we claim that even if the etiology challenge can be met, existing accounts of the Capgras delusion all face an additional and largely-overlooked challenge: *the selectivity problem*. As discussed above in Section 2, persons experiencing Capgras delusion experience it toward very few people. In most cases, the Capgras delusion is focused on a single person. In some cases, two or three familiar persons are claimed to be imposters. Why is the delusion selective? Any successful account of the Capgras delusion will have to explain how the anomalous experience arises in one or only a handful cases. This is the selectivity problem.[5]

Ellis and Young's (1990) original affective responsiveness hypothesis attempted to address selectivity via familiarity. If it is the reduced affective response that triggers the delusion, then the reduced response would be most prominent and most likely to do so, in the case of the person who is most familiar to the subject. This helps to explain why it is standardly a person who is emotionally significant to the subject who is claimed to be an imposter – e.g., a spouse, parent, or child. But familiarity is not selective enough. Nearly everyone is familiar with many people. Coltheart, Langdon, and McKay (2011) thus propose a slightly more nuanced approach to Capgras' selectivity, suggesting that it is only in cases where the familiarity reaction should have been so strong that the recognition discrepancy is large enough to produce the delusion. Familiarity admits of degree so there may be some such threshold. Even so, it seems strange that the delusion would be set such that it picks whatever level corresponds to one or possible two to three persons across all those who experience the delusion. There are also cases that directly challenge these proposals - for example, Nuara and colleagues (2020) discuss a patient who developed the delusion toward his son, but not his daughter, when all reports indicate equal familiarity with and fondness toward both children.

The selectivity problem is not only a challenge for explanationists. Endorsement accounts of the Capgras delusion are also not well-equipped to address the selectivity problem. Such accounts are focused on the delusion's content, not its origin. That is, endorsement accounts take hold at the point of the abnormal perceptual experience. They do not offer any account of how the abnormal perceptual experience was generated. This could mean that an account that answers the selectivity problem could be supplemented with an endorsement view of the delusion's content, but on its own endorsement cannot explain why Capgras is selective.

Replacement accounts like Hirstein (2010) and Wilkinson's (2016) show tacit sensitivity to the selectivity problem. In rejecting the affective approach, they both offer attempts to replace it with a mental process that includes discrete representations of individual people. Hirstein locates these representations within the mindreading system; Wilkinson locates them within mental files. Each architectural proposal makes it possible to lose or disrupt some representations but not others.

No account of the Capgras delusion is complete without an explanation of its selectivity. It must offer a way to make sense of the delusion's focus on only a select few individuals. Accounts based in the affective responsive hypothesis appear to lack the resources to account for Capgras' selectivity. Replacement accounts, in contrast, show promise. The question thus turns to evaluating the various replacement proposals: do either of the proposed capacities offer the right kind of individualized representations of persons? If not, what other candidates are available. We turn to these questions in the next section.

## 6. Selectivity and cognitive architecture

Replacement views of the Capgras delusion show potential for addressing the selectivity problem because they locate the delusion in a system that, in standard conditions, stores representations of individual persons. The delusion then represents a disruption to that system such that one or more representations are damaged. This makes it possible to have a delusion focused on a single person, leaving the majority of person representations intact and preventing the claim of imposter from spreading more widely. Both Hirstein (2010) and Wilkinson's (2016) replacement accounts are well-structured to address selectivity, but it remains to be determined whether the systems in which they locate this selectivity can provide such representations of individual persons and do so in a way that makes sense of the delusion.

### 6.1 *Mindreading*

Hirstein (2010) situates individual person representations within the mindreading system. According to Hirstein, Capgras delusion is the result of an egocentric representation of a familiar person becoming damaged and inaccessible. There are, however, at least three issues that arise for his account.

First, while there are many accounts of mindreading that include representations of individual persons, it is unclear that the kind of representations they use could accommodate the distinctively egocentric perspective that Hirstein proposes. According to 'model' views of mindreading (e.g., Godfrey-Smith 2005; Maibom 2009a,b; Spaulding 2018), mindreading happens in much the same way as much of scientific reasoning: it relies on the creation and systematic manipulation of a model of the world. Model views of mindreading incorporate many features, including representations of individual persons for individuals that the particular mindreader knows well. This, at least, is well-aligned with Hirstein. It is unclear, however, how these representations could account for a deficit in egocentric ways of representing those individuals. Model-based accounts include systematized information about individuals – what they believe, what they're prone to do, etc. They do not include information about what the world is like from that person's perspective. Such information would be not only burdensome to store, and of limited use for predicting and explaining behavior, which may require reasoning about situations where the mindreader was not present and situations that haven't happened yet.

Second, it is not clear that subjects with Capgras delusion have a mindreading deficit. Clinical reports of Capgras patients provide evidence of retained mindreading ability toward the person they now claim is an imposter. Staton and colleagues (1982) describe a patient who justified his claim that his father had been replaced by an imposter by detailing how his father's behavior contradicted his expectations. The patient expressed certainty that it was an imposter because, 'my father would never have expanded the milk business' (Staton et al 1982). Similarly, Frazer and Roberts (1994) describe a patient who claimed, 'my son would never kiss me', as the reason as to why she believed her son had been replaced with a stranger. There has not been, to our knowledge, any systematic testing of mindreading abilities in Capgras patients, but offhand remarks like these are suggestive of retained capacity for mindreading about the same persons toward whom the delusion is targeted.

Finally, there may be cases of Capgras delusion that target non-human or even non-minded individuals. A small but still notable proportion of Capgras cases involve the misidentification of animals and inanimate objects. According to the meta-analysis by Pandis and colleagues (2019), inanimate objects are the third most common target of Capgras delusion, behind spouse and parent. Islam and colleagues (2015) describe a patient who claimed that both her pet dog and the paintings in her home had been replaced with duplicates. Others claimed that their cutlery, book, or even favorite songs have been replaced with duplicates (Ghatak et al. 2023). In most accounts of mindreading, the capacity is focused on fellow humans. Even if it is taken to extend to include pets and other familiar animals, this would not explain cases where the delusion targets inanimate objects. Locating the individual representations inside of mindreading thus seems poorly fit to the full scope of individuals at which the delusion can aim.

### 6.2  *Mental files*

Wilkinson's appeal to mental files is intuitive. Mental files were proposed to account for our ability to have thoughts that refer to individuals (Recanati 2012). Wilkinson straightforwardly applies this framework to cases of Capgras, arguing that the delusion occurs when the files are 'mismanaged' such that multiple files are mistakenly created for the same individual.

First, Wilkinson's appeal to mental files inherits challenges raised to the overall framework. Much of the work on mental files operates at a metaphorical level – discussing cognitive processes in terms of office workflows. Many find the metaphor quite useful, and this has likely helped promote attention to and support for this view. It remains unclear, however, whether the notion of a mental file has any psychological or neural plausibility. Is there more to the view than metaphor?[6] This matters for the application to Capgras delusion because the implementation of this framework is critical to solving the selectivity problem. If mental files are just a loose way of speaking about the mind's organization that does not actually impose any such structure in the neurocognitive architecture, then there would be no way for this framework to account for damage to a particular component of that architecture.

Second, while the mental files approach is focused on thoughts about individuals, the concerns around which it is built are quite different from those at the heart of the Capgras delusion. Mental files were developed from broader concerns in the philosophy of language about the nature of singular thought and reference. The focus is largely on explaining how thoughts about and inferences over individuals are possible. There is a lot of work on how mental files can be used to make determinations of identity or distinctness. In cases of

Capgras delusion, however, what needs to be answered is why retrieval of the correct file failed. And why the file cannot be mended and updated, as happens in all cases other than the imposter.

Here the metaphorical nature of mental files compounds the confusion. What does it mean to 'mismanage' files and how might we make progress on understanding that in terms of plausible cognitive processes? In thinking through this question, we find a discussion in Ramachandran's (1999) helpful. Ramachandran describes his patient as a young man who developed Capgras delusion toward his parents as the result of a car accident. The patient had no prior history of psychiatric conditions, or other signs of psychiatric illness. Much like other Capgras patients, his delusion was selective. He took his parents to be imposters, but his ability to recognize other people remained intact. Ramachandran and colleagues ran many tests to investigate the nature and scope of the patient's facial recognition deficit. They engaged the patient in a task to test his ability to track gaze direction, showing the patient a series of pictures featuring strangers and asking him to judge which direction the person was looking and whether the direction of gaze changed across photos. The patient performed well across photos where there were slight changes in the subject's direction of gaze. When there were significant changes in the person's direction of gaze, however, the patient reported that it was a new model in the picture. The patient would offer some explanation for their judgment, claiming the person in the photo looked older, etc.

This intriguing result suggests that the Capgras deficit may involve some sort of failure of updating information about individuals over time. A failure to update is, in a sense, a form of mismanagement – but it is a more specific form, and one more closely tied to cognitive processing. Rather than attempt to expand the mental files approach to make sense of this, we think it is potentially more promising to develop an alternative replacement account centered on memory updating.

## 7.  Memory updating account

In this final section, we explore the idea that the Capgras delusion should be explained in terms of a deficit in memory updating. This idea has been around for a while. Staton and colleagues (1982) proposed it in a case report four decades ago. With its focus on a single study in the era just before Ellis and Young's (1990) affective responsiveness hypothesis took off, it was largely dismissed. Given how the literature on the nature of delusions and memory have both changed in the decades since, we think the view warrants a second look. We return to it here, elaborating and expanding on the initial proposal. Ultimately, we think the memory deficit theory is a plausible and promising account of the Capgras delusion, which is well-positioned to address both the etiological and selectivity problems discussed above.

In a short case report of a patient experiencing Capgras delusion, Staton and colleagues (1982) propose that the delusion derives from a memory deficit. More specifically, they argue that it is the patient's failure to update their memory of a familiar person that leads to the belief that the familiar person is an imposter. They describe a patient, RK with the Capgras delusion. RK was a 31-year-old male with no prior psychiatric or neurological impairment, who developed the Capgras delusion following brain damage from a car accident when he was 23. At the time of referral, he held the Capgras delusion about his parents, relatives, and friends. In defending his delusional states, RK repeatedly appealed to his memory as evidence that the current instantiations being imposters. For example, when

RK claimed that familiar people had been replaced, he cited differences between his recollections and their current appearance and behavior.

In describing his experience, RK is quoted as saying, 'The issue is that my memory is just too good' (Staton et al. 1982). We agree with the patient, and the assessment of Staton and colleagues, that the deficit appears to be memory-related. We also think it is worth probing further how a cognitive capacity performing too well could be the source of a deficit or delusion. In describing his memory as working too well, RK appears to be appealing to a common assumption about memory – namely, that the purpose of memory is to retain information. On such an 'archival view' of memory (Robins 2016), RK's would be exceptionally good, keeping track of so many details about familiar persons that even the smallest changes trigger a mismatch. This way of thinking about memory was more prominent several decades ago, at the time Staton and colleagues (1982) were evaluating RK's case. The archival view of memory helps to make sense of RK's remark, but it does not help to make sense of his deficit. How could memory performing its function too well be a malfunction?

In the decades since, an alternative way of thinking about the function of memory has become increasingly influential. According to the 'constructive view' of memory, memory is better understood as a fluid system, where information is retained, but in a way that permits dynamic changes and alterations over time (e.g. Schacter and Addis 2007). On such a constructive view, RK's deficit is more easily understood. A well-functioning memory retains information in a more loose and labile way so that representations of individuals can absorb a range of changes. On such a view, a memory that retains too many details in too fixed of a format would be malfunctioning. Thinking of Capgras in these terms thus fits well with current theorizing about the nature of memory.

Additionally, there are advantages to thinking of the Capgras delusion in terms of a memory deficit. The delusion clearly involves a deficit of recognition. Attempts to capture this deficit as part of the perceptual process and the accompanying affective response have not fared well, as was discussed above. Thinking of the recognition process in terms of memory may fare better. Failure to update a memory could lead to the mismatches that produce the kind of partial recognition experienced in Capgras, where the person is registered as familiar but suspicious. This would provide a straightforward response to the etiological problem. Further, it could situate Capgras within a broader set of strange phenomenal experiences that occur in cases of recognitional mishaps in memory. Much like deja vu is the false recognition of a new event as familiar; Capgras delusion could be the failed recognition of a familiar person.

The memory updating view also appears better equipped to account for phenomena that posed challenges to Hirstein (2010) and Wilkinson's (2016) accounts above. Consider again Ramachandran's (1999) patient who had difficulty tracking a single, novel individual across photos where there were significant changes in the person's direction of gaze, expression, etc. The case does not fit well with Hirstein's explanation in terms of psychological representations of well-known persons. Similarly, Wilkinson (2016) could characterize what's happening as the mismanagement of mental files, but this does not in any way explain the case. It merely describes the phenomenon. If we think about the case in terms of memory updating, a richer explanation is possible. A memory of the individual depicted is being formed, but the features included are represented in a rigid or inflexible way, such that a significant change in how the same person is depicted registers as the kind of break indicative of a new individual. Expanding this kind of explanation further, we can see how the memory updating view fares better than other available accounts in explaining how the Capgras delusion can, in some cases, be directed toward mere acquaintances rather than close friends or family.

Memory updating may also better explain cases where the Capgras delusion is directed toward pets, inanimate objects, and environmental contexts like one's house or city. Views like Hirstein's (2010) which situate the deficit within the mindreading capacity, struggle to explain cases of this kind. Wilkinson's (2016) mental files approach may have slightly wider scope but is still limited to individuals. Memory for particular people, places, and things need not be similarly restricted. There can be memory related to any item that is tracked over time and across events - and the same general issue of updating can explain the selective loss or disruption of particular memories over time. In this way, the memory updating view has the advantage of making clearer the connection between Capgras delusion and other delusional misidentification syndromes, such as reduplicative paramnesia where the failure to recognize previously familiar items is extended to locations. In fact, the patient RK (from Staton et al. 1982) had reduplicative paramnesia in addition to Capgras delusion. He not only reported his family members as imposters, but also thought that his city and pet had been replaced. Staton and colleagues describe him as claiming that Fargo (the city he was hospitalized in) could not be the real Fargo,[7] because 'they didn't have this kind of hospital in Fargo' (1982: 24), and his cat was a fake because of a new scar on its ear.

Framing the Capgras delusion in terms of memory updating also allows for a straightforward response to the selectivity problem. It makes sense for memory to be organized in a way that allows for discrete retention of familiar people, places, and things that are repeatedly encountered across time in different contexts. This kind of organization in memory makes it possible to explain how memory for some items could be degraded or lost while other memories are left intact.

To fully explore and develop this view requires a richer understanding of how memory for individuals is organized and updated. To do this would require a significant shift in the focus of current theorizing about memory. Theorizing about memory is currently guided by what James Openshaw (2022) refers to as *eventism* – our understanding of how memories are encoded, stored, and retrieved is guided by events. The standard way of thinking about declarative memory involves separating it into two distinct forms: episodic memory, which is memory for particular past experiences, and semantic memory, which is memory for general facts and information. This way of thinking about memory's organization only allows for memory of individuals as it is situated within events or tied to general pieces of information. Openshaw's focus is on the need to account for memory of objects. Here our aim is to echo this need, and encourage the expansion of this category to include persons.

In sketching a proposal for object memory, Openshaw (2022) proposes that object memory be understood as a collection of information about an individual. This initial proposal is promising, but does not yet have the fluidity or flexibility to explore how the memory of an individual, whether it's an object or a person, could be updated to allow for changes over time without loss of unity. Even for inanimate objects, there will be changes over time – in the perspective from which they are viewed, the available lighting, as well as surrounding items and noise, and so on. For pets and persons there will be all of these features and more as the individuals grow, age, and move around.

In thinking about the complexity of such cases, we are struck by the poignancy of an example from Mark Rowlands (2017), where he describes a childhood memory including his father. In reflecting on this memory, Rowlands comes to realize that, in his memory, his father's face is depicted as it looks now, rather than how it looked in his childhood. This kind of case is suggestive and compelling for thinking about how memory of persons in particular may exert an influence on episodic memory and its content rather than the other way around. There is much more to be explored here. We contend that the appeal of using such a framework to account for Capgras delusion provides key motivation for its development.

## 8. Conclusion

In this chapter, we have explored standard accounts of the Capgras delusion, highlighting an explanatory limitation that they all share: the selectivity problem. The Capgras delusion often targets a single person, or at most a handful of persons and other animals or objects. It is a constraint on any adequate account of this delusion to explain how such a selective disruption of recognition processes is possible. We argue that, at a minimum, this requires an account to include representations of individuals. Views based in an affective response cannot do this, and so accounts that seek to replace the affective responsiveness hypothesis have an advantage over views that seek instead to supplement the affective view. We argue that a view of the Capgras delusion in terms of memory updating offers the best such replacement account. Building off of a long-neglected proposal from Staton and colleagues (1982), we explain how such a view aligns with contemporary theorizing about memory and well accounts for the selectivity of Capgras.

## Notes

1 Term borrowed from Pacherie (2008).
2 Philosophical accounts of delusions can generally be divided into one- and two-factor accounts. One-factor accounts (Maher 1974; Gerrans 2002; Sullivan-Bissett and Noordhof 2021; Sullivan-Bissett, Chapter 28) locate the abnormality entirely within sensory or perceptual systems, arguing that all additional reasoning elements fall within the normal range. Two-factor accounts (Freeman and Garety 1999; Langdon and Coltheart 2000; Garety et al. 2001; McKay 2012; Davies and Coltheart, Chapter 29) couple the phenomenal abnormality with an additional cognitive, interpretive, or reasoning abnormality.
3 Hirstein's (2010) mindreading account is meant to explain not only Capgras delusion, but also other misidentification syndromes like asomatognosia.
4 As Wilkinson explains it, the information in the file includes things like "what they have done, when the subject has encountered them in the past, character traits etc., as well as what they look like" (397).
5 Note that the selectivity problem as posed is not a question about who was selected. We do not take the issue to be *Why did the subject claim their mother was an imposter rather than their father?* We suspect answers about which individual is selected are likely to be determined by the particular details of a subject's life. The selectivity question is thus not *Why X and not Y* but instead *why 1 not 100 (or all)?*
6 See Goodman and Gray (2022) for an extended and compelling argument that there is not.
7 This delusion is called Reduplicative Paramnesia, which is a monothematic misidentification delusion involving location.

## References

Anderson, D.N. (1988) "The Delusion of Inanimate Doubles," *British Journal of Psychiatry*, 153(5), pp. 694–699.
Andrews, K., Spaulding, S. and Westra, E. (2020) "Introduction to Folk Psychology: Pluralistic Approaches," *Synthese*, 199(1–2), pp. 1685–1700.

Bauer, R.M. (1984) "Autonomic Recognition of Names and Faces in Prosopagnosia: A Neuropsychological Application of the Guilty Knowledge Test," *Neuropsychologia*, 22(4), pp. 457–469.

Bauer, R.M. (1986) "The Cognitive Psychophysiology of Prosopagnosia," *Springer eBooks*, pp. 253–267.

Bayne, T. and Pacherie, E. (2004) "Bottom-Up or Top-Down: Campbell's Rationalist Account of Monothematic Delusions," *Philosophy, Psychiatry, & Psychology*, 11(1), pp. 1–11.

Bernecker, S. (2017) A Causal Theory of Mnemonic Confabulation. *Frontiers in Psychology*, 8, pp. 1–14.

Bongiorno, F. (2020) "Is the Capgras Delusion an Endorsement of Experience?," *Mind & Language*, 35(3), pp. 293–312.

Bradley, A. and Gibson, Q. H. (2023) "Monothematic Delusions and the Limits of Rationality," *British Journal for the Philosophy of Science*, 74(3), pp. 811–835.

Brochado, A. (1936) "Le syndrome de Capgras," *Annales M´edico-Psychologiques*, 15, pp. 706–717

Capgras, J.-B. and Reboul-Lachaux, J. (1923/1994) "L'Illusion des 'sosies' dans un délire systématisé chronique," *History of Psychiatry*, 5(17), pp. 119–133.

Coltheart, M. and Davies, M. (2021) "What Is Capgras Delusion?," *Cognitive Neuropsychiatry*, 27(1), pp. 69–82.

Coltheart, M., Langdon, R. and McKay, R. (2011) "Delusional Belief," *Annual Review of Psychology*, 62(1), pp. 271–298.

Davies, M. *et al.* (2001) "Monothematic Delusions: Towards a Two-Factor Account," *Philosophy, Psychiatry, & Psychology*, 8(2), pp. 133–158.

Derombies, M. (1935) "L'illusion de sosie, forme particuliers de la reconnaissance systematique," *Annales Medico-Psychologiques*, 94, pp. 706–717

Edelstyn, N.M.J. and Oyebode, F. (1999) "A Review of the Phenomenology and Cognitive Neuropsychological Origins of the Capgras Syndrome," *International Journal of Geriatric Psychiatry*, 14(1), pp. 48–59.

Ellis, H.D. and Young, A.J. (1990) "Accounting for Delusional Misidentifications," *British Journal of Psychiatry*, 157(2), pp. 239–248.

Frazer, S.J., and Roberts, J.M. (1994). "Three Cases of Capgras' Syndrome,"*British Journal of Psychiatry*, 164(4), pp. 557–559.

Freeman, D. and Garety, P.A. (1999) "Worry, Worry Processes and Dimensions of Delusions: An Exploratory Investigation of a Role for Anxiety Processes in the Maintenance of Delusional Distress," *Behavioural and Cognitive Psychotherapy*, 27(1), pp. 47–62.

Garety, P.A., Kuipers, E., Fowler, D., Freeman, D. and Bebbington, P. E. (2001) "A Cognitive Model of the Positive Symptoms of Psychosis," *Psychological Medicine*, 31(2), pp. 189–195. https://doi.org/10.1017/s0033291701003312

Gerrans, P. (2002) "Multiple Paths to Delusion," *Philosophy, Psychiatry, and Psychology*, 9(1), pp. 65–72.

Ghatak, M. et al. (2023) "The Capgras Delusion of Inanimate Objects: A Duplicate World," *Psychiatry Research*, 2(1), p. 100106.

Godfrey-Smith, P. (2005) "Folk Psychology as a Model," *Philosophers' Imprint*, 5, pp. 1–16.

Goodman, R. and Gray, A. (2022) "Mental Filing," *Noûs*, 56(1), pp. 204–226.

Hirstein, W. (2010) "The Misidentification Syndromes as Mindreading Disorders," *Cognitive Neuropsychiatry*, 15(1–3), pp. 233–260.

Islam, L., Piacentini, S., Soliveri, P., Scarone, S. and Gambini, O. (2015) "Capgras Delusion for Animals and Inanimate Objects in Parkinson's Disease: A Case Report," *BMC Psychiatry*, 15, p. 73. https://doi.org/10.1186/s12888-015-0460-7

Lewis, S. (1987) "Brain Imaging in a Case of Capgras' Syndrome," *British Journal of Psychiatry*, 150, pp. 117–121.

Maher, B.A. (1974) "Delusional Thinking and Perceptual Disorder," *Journal of Individual Psychology*, 30(1), pp. 98–113.

Maibom, H.L. (2009a) "In Defence of (Model) Theory Theory," *Journal of Consciousness Studies*, 16(6–8), pp. 6–8.

Maibom, H.L. (2009b) "Feeling for Others: Empathy, Sympathy, and Morality," *Inquiry: An Interdisciplinary Journal of Philosophy*, 52(5), pp. 483–499.

McKay, R. (2012) "Delusional Inference," *Mind & Language*, 27, pp. 330–355.

Michaelian, K. (2016) *Mental Time Travel: Episodic Memory and Our Knowledge of the Personal Past*. Cambridge, MA: MIT Press.

Michaelian, K. (2020) "Confabulating as Unreliable Imagining: In Defence of the Simulationist Account of Unsuccessful Remembering," *Topoi*, 39(1), pp. 133–148.

Nuara, A. et al. (2020) "Catching the Imposter in the Brain: The Case of Capgras Delusion," *Cortex*, 131, pp. 295–304.

O'Reilly, R.J. and Malhotra, L. (1987) "Capgras Syndrome – An Unusual Case and Discussion of Psychodynamic Factors," *British Journal of Psychiatry*, 151, pp. 263–265.

Openshaw, J. (2022) "Remembering Objects," *Philosophers' Imprint*, 22, pp. 1–20.

Pacherie, E. (2008) "Perception, Emotions and Delusions: The Case of the Capgras Delusion," in Tim Bayne and Jordi Fernàndez (eds.), *Delusion and Self-Deception: Affective and Motivational Influences on Belief Formation*. New York: Psychology Press. pp. 107–125.

Pandis, C., Agrawal, N. and Poole, N. (2019) "Capgras' Delusion: A Systematic Review of 255 Published Cases," *Psychopathology*, 52(3), pp. 161–173.

Ramachandran, V.S. (1999) *Phantoms in the Brain: Probing the Mysteries of the Human Mind*. New York: Harper Collins.

Recanati, F. (2012) *Mental Files*. Oxford: Oxford University Press.

Robins, S. K. (2016). "Misremembering," *Philosophical Psychology*, 29, pp. 432–447.

Robins, S. (2019) "Confabulation and Constructive Memory," *Synthese*, 196(6), pp. 2135–2151.

Robins, S. (2020) "Mnemonic Confabulation," *Topoi*, 39(1), pp. 121–132.

Rojo, V.I. *et al.* (1991) "Capgras' Syndrome in a Blind Patient," *American Journal of Psychiatry*, 148(9), pp. 1271–1272.

Rowlands, M. (2017) *Memory and the Self: Phenomenology, Science and Autobiography*. Oxford University Press.

Schacter, D.L. and Addis, D.R. (2007) "The Cognitive Neuroscience of Constructive Memory: Remembering the Past and Imagining the Future," *Philosophical Transactions of the Royal Society of London. Series B, Biological Sciences*, 362(1481), pp. 773–786.

Spaulding, S. (2018) "Mindreading Beyond Belief: A More Comprehensive Conception of How We Understand Others," *Philosophy Compass*, 13, p. e12526.

Staton, R.D., Brumback, R.A. and Wilson, H.R. (1982) "Reduplicative Paramnesia: A Disconnection Syndrome of Memory," *Cortex*, 18(1), pp. 23–35.

Tranel, D et al. (1985) "Electrodermal Discrimination of Familiar and Unfamiliar Faces: A Methodology," *Psychophysiology*, 22, p. 4.

Tranel, D et al. (1988) "Intact Recognition of Facial Expression, Gender, and Age in Patients with Impaired Recognition of Face Identity," *Neurology*, 38(5), pp. 690–696.

Weinstein, E.A. and Burnham, D.L. (1991) "Reduplication and the Syndrome of Capgras," *Psychiatry*, 54(1), pp. 78–88.

Wilkinson, S. (2016) "A Mental Files Approach to Delusional Misidentification," *Review of Philosophy and Psychology*, 7(2), pp. 389–404.

# 24

# DELUSION AND DREAMING

*Philip Gerrans*

*P:* I think I'm dead (…) it started during the night, *like it was some kind of a dream*, but this remains until now.

(…)

*E:* Do you rationally think you are dead?

*P:* I do. It may not make much sense since I realize I have blood pressure when they measure it but I rationally think I am dead (Gonçalves and Tosoni 2016: 35).

## 1.  Introduction: taking out the cognitive trash

It is a cliché that delusions *resemble* dreams. John Nash for example said of his delusions 'it's kind of like a dream. In a dream it's typical not to be rational'. In his deeply delusional state, he *accepted* the delusion.

'Acceptance' here is a term of art. I do not use it to indicate that the subject takes the content to be true, justified, or an accurate representation of the external world. Nor do I propose it as a distinctive type of non-doxastic attitude to experience (this formulation has been developed in detail for the case of delusion by Keith Frankish [2012]). Rather by acceptance I mean something very minimal: experience is accepted when it is incorporated in the subject's stream of consciousness without being registered as inconsistent or problematic. To register something is for it to attract attention and cognitive and behavioural resources because it is salient to the subject in a way that requires a metacognitive response. Registration can be epistemic, when the veracity or doxastic status of an experience is its salient feature, but novelty and goal relevance are the primary dimensions of salience (for more on delusion and salience see McKenna, Chapter 31). In the reports above the subjects register the epistemic incongruity of their delusion in retrospect, but typically during the depth of psychosis, its epistemic status is not salient. This is why subjects invoke dreams as an analogy for the delusional state. In dreams bizarre and impossible experiences are accepted.

Similarities and differences between delusions and dreams have been explained in different ways, most of which rely on epistemic notions. For example, delusions have been explained in terms of failure of 'reality testing', 'metacognition', or 'belief-evaluation'

                    DOI: 10.4324/9781003296386-29

whose neural substrates are also deactivated in dreams (Hobson 1999, Hobson et al. 2000, Kirberg 2022). I will argue that while these characterisations are not wrong (delusional subjects are irrational measured against procedural norms because they don't adjust their beliefs to conform to reality (Gerrans 2001), they are not pitched at the right level to explain the phenomena. Folk psychology interprets systemic behaviour under an assumption of minimal rationality, abstracting away from neurocognitive mechanisms. Consequently folk psychological definitions are unhelpful for multilevel integrative explanation. The assumption of minimal rationality creates a normative epistemic constraint on explanation that does not apply at lower levels of causal explanation. I prefer the neurocognitive approach to a description of the target phenomenon that is neutral between conceptual frameworks as in this definition of delusion.

> Delusions arise when *default cognitive processing, unsupervised* by *central executive processing,* is *monopolized* by *hypersalient information.*
>
> *(Gerrans 2014a, 2014b)*

This definition can be used without loss of information by a theorist whose focus is mechanistic, cognitive or phenomenological. Indeed the nature of mechanisms is illuminated when we consider for example what 'salience' means in terms of cognition and neuro-computational resource allocation. Similarly, at the level of phenomenology, properties of the stream of consciousness are illuminated when we understand the neurocognitive mechanisms of salience. My aim here is not to defend this explanation of delusion but to use the approach to explain the relationship between delusions and dreams. In particular to explain the difference between delusions and dreams in terms of the associative properties of the default mode network (DMN) in different contexts: sleep, wake, mindwandering, and dreaming (Windt 2010, 2015).

The key idea is that

> DMN activity immerses the subject in a simulated world. These simulations are constructed by processes that are *essentially associative,* not governed by rules of inference.

Association has never been better defined than by David Hume as the linking of representations according to relations of causation, contiguity, and resemblance. In modern-day parlance (see the discussion of Deep Dream below), we could put this as the idea that the outputs of a neural network are a product of its weight structure installed by training (experience). Thus, patterns of association are idiosyncratic reflecting individual differences in architecture and history.

The concept of active inference provides a framework for understanding this conceptualisation of DMN activity. Active inference treats cognition as a form of action whose goal is the stabilisation of an adaptive model (representation) of the internal and external world. That model predicts the consequences of iterative activity and is confirmed or modified by sensory evidence acquired though action (Barrett et al. 2016, Kirchhoff et al. 2018, Corcoran et al. 2020, Parr et al. 2022). Active inference requires the modelling (representation) of the self as the source and target of regulatory activity and the world as the source of sensory signals. Activity here is very broadly construed to include bodily regulation, overt behaviour, *and* cognition. The mind builds models at progressively higher levels of abstraction and generality in order to optimise organismic function through action. On this view cognition is a process of hierarchical model building.

Active inference is essentially cognitive foraging, construction, and exploration of an informational possibility space in order to confirm a model. A scientific experiment, for example, obtains evidence for theoretical hypotheses. Someone exploring a city is consolidating a model that maps the city. Someone trying alternative translations of a poem is building a semantic model. So the cognitive context for a form of active inference is set by the model that structures the possibility space for that activity. In perception, those models are quite rigid and specific. For example, visual saccades glean information about edges and contours that support perceptual models of the concrete structure of the world. Abstract and conceptual models such as theories and stories place fewer restrictions on active inference. There is in principle no restriction on what evidence is relevant to a confirmation of a scientific hypothesis for example so abductive inference is notoriously unconstrained. A narrative model is limited only by the imagination of its author. The level and nature of active inference determines the type of modelling. Planning, decision, autobiographical recollection, imaginative rehearsal, empathy, and social cognition all involve simulating actions and experiences by constructing complex representations that interleave the actual and the possible. Thus, we can imagine what it would be like to live as a different sex to help decide whether reconstructive surgery is a good match for our lifestyle. These are forms of active inference

immerse the self in a simulated world decoupled from the subject's actual situation. (Gerrans 2014a, 2014b). These types of simulation deploy narrative models that represents episodes of a life (the relation between episodes can be causal, temporal, intentional, or rational according to the model). The notion of narrative applies to these simulations because constraints on narrative are different to constraints of empirical adequacy and rationality that apply to belief fixation (Currie and Jureidini 2004, Menary 2008, Goldie 2011).

In the case of delusion, the simulation system that underwrites these types of cognition is activated in response to a salient experience. The result is a model that makes the experience ineligible as part of a narrative.

This is why the imaginative hypothesis of delusion is attractive. Imagination is not essentially constrained by doxastic norms which would explain explains why delusions are not true or revised to fit rational norms. However, once again the folk psychology of imagination is an obstacle here because delusions do not obey *all* the folk psychological constraints on the concept of imagination. They are not under actual or counterfactual voluntary control for example. It is possible to deal with arguments against the imaginative theory of delusion in different ways. One can to reinforce doxastic theories against objections (see Paul Noordhof, Chapters 19 and 20, and Amy Kind, Chapter 21) or construct hybrid accounts that try and reconcile the doxastic and imaginative accounts (Gendler 2008, Bayne 2010). However a better solution is to look at the cognitive properties of the processing system that generates the phenomenon. And when we examine those cognitive properties of the DMN, we find a system that generates (more or less) immersive simulations.

If we see both delusions and dreams as forms of immersive simulation differently embedded in the overall cognitive economy according to context, then a debate over whether delusions are imaginative, doxastic, dreamlike, or *sui generis* psychotic states *according to folk psychological categories* becomes irrelevant (for more on delusion and folk psychology see Dominic Murphy, Chapter 25).

The active inference framework provides a neutral way to conceptualise these different contexts. In alert waking, cognition simulations are constructed to verify models that support the subject's ability to act in the world in episodes of 'mental time travel' (Suddendorf and Corballis 2007, Suddendorf et al. 2009, Michaelian 2016). For example, when imagining emigrating and living in a different country knowledge about the destination helps construct the simulated experience of a life abroad. In these cases, background knowledge about the world constrains the process. In dreaming, there is no goal to constrain the simulation and hence dreams in general do not build models, although they rehearse model building machinery. The dreamscape reflects patterns of association produced by endogenous activation of the DMN 'from below'. That is to say by neurochemical activation of DMN and the suite of affective and motivational systems that innervate it (relatively) disconnected from metacognitive and early stimulus driven perceptual processing that provide a goal structure for waking cognition. In delusion, DMN activity produces a narrative or narrative fragment in response to salient experience but that model then rigidifies foreclosing further active inference.

## 2.  Cognitive trash?

It is this interpretation of the role of the DMN that rescues neurochemical theories of dreaming such as the AIM Model (Activation, Information, Mode) and delusion from criticisms that argue that they eliminate the intentional content of dreams and psychotic states. Versions of this idea can be found in the 'broken brain' hypothesis of psychosis and the 'cognitive trash' interpretation of dreams and psychosis proposed by Allan Hobson (Hobson et al. 2000). The idea behind eliminative theories is that the experience of psychosis and dreams is a by-product of activity in neural systems rather than a product. Another way to put this is to say that dreams and psychotic states are 'cognitive trash' as Hobson put it. On Hobson's view describing the neural differences between delusional and non-delusional subjects or dreaming and waking subjects exhausts the explanation of those differences. The content of psychosis or dreams does not matter to their explanation.

Hobson's target was psychodynamic or evolutionary theories of dreaming that treat dreams as cognitive processes whose states have intentional content. On these views, dream experiences have intentional content related to their purpose (Revonsuo 2000). Another way to put this is to say that psychodynamic (or evolutionary psychology) theories of dreams treat them as forms of active inference constrained by a model. Hobson's view can be put as the idea that there *is no model* constraining the activity of the DMN in dreams. Does this mean that dreams are 'cognitive trash' or that their content is epiphenomenal to their explanation? That kind of eliminativism is too extreme, as two examples from visual processing make clear.

Visual processing is a form of active inference that constructs models of the world that explain the distal cause of retinal input. In so doing, those models mirror the 'natural compositional structure of the world' building images from elements such as edges and contours drawing on templates that model naturally occurring features such as shading and motion. Normally that model building process is initiated by perceptual engagement with the world as the organism tries to confirm a model that enables adaptive behaviour. However, the visual system can also be activated endogenously in which case we do not perceive the world but we nonetheless experience imagery of colours, shapes and objects. The imagery we experience in the absence of perceptual input is a consequence of the architecture of visual processing. The difference between hallucination and perception is explained by the way the model building properties of the visual system give rise to different experiences under different conditions. The patterns of activity produced by endogenous activation are non-accidental precisely because they are produced by an architecture evolved to represent the structure of the world. Thus, the difference in experience between the two cases is not that in one case we have 'visual trash' and in the perceptual case vision. We cannot explain the experience produced by activation in the visual system without reference to the cognitive properties of the system it implements.

Another example is provided by 'Deep Dream' style neural networks. These networks have a weight structure that maps visual inputs to outputs to produce artificial visual imagery. In the standard case, weights are adjusted dynamically in response to changing input and the system learns to map inputs to correct outputs or predict the cause of a pattern of activity across an input array. In effect the weight structure tacitly represents a model of the stochastic structure of the training data. In the case of the Deep Dream network the process is reversed (Keshavan and Sudarshan 2017). Weights are held constant as input changes. So now all input is processed in terms of a static model. The result is analogous to hallucinogenic or psychedelic imagery or the phenomenon of pareidolia in which the mind imposes patterns on ambiguous or noisy input (seeing faces in clouds for example). A Deep Dream network trained on animals and then exposed to portraits will produce imagery of humans with oddly animal faces. Are these images 'visual trash'? Or another way to put the question is to ask whether the animalesque imagery is irrelevant to the explanation of the difference between a network trained on animals and portraits. We could focus on the weight and activation structure of two networks but in doing so we would lose information about what the system is doing (superimposing images of animals and people). The fact that a system represents animals or human faces is invisible at the unit level of statistical processing in the same way as the fact that activity in a visual system represents contours or colours is invisible when we focus at the neural level. But all this tells us is that the system needs to be understood as a multilevel model builder. When we understand it that way, its cognitive properties and phenomenological properties explain its mechanistic properties and vice versa.

In fact when we take this approach, the only level of analysis that seems to add nothing to understanding is folk psychological/epistemic. What neurobiological eliminativism gets right about dreams is that the folk psychological interpretation of dreams is a dead end. In dreams, simulation processes are active but the simulations that result are not part of a process of model building and consolidation driven by a cognitive goal. In dreams, the DMN is in screensaver mode, active but not constructing simulations to support action that verifies a model.

I now apply these ideas to the explanation of dreams and delusions. I first discuss the properties of the DMN as a simulation system that operates in different contexts. Two of those contexts, planning and decision, and mind wandering, are forms of active inference more or less tightly constrained by goals. Dreams reflect the operation of the simulation system in the absence of a goal to structure its activity.

> dreams can be seen as a unique and more fully developed form of mind wandering, and therefore as the quintessential cognitive simulation. They are the quintessential cognitive simulation not only because they have elaborate story lines that are often enacted with exquisite sensory, motor, and cognitive involvement, with some dreams

unfolding over a period of several minutes to half an hour or more. There is also the striking fact that they are usually experienced as real while they are happening.

*(Domhoff 2011)*

I then show how the AIM theory can be restated in this framework as the idea that in dreams the mind is not performing active inference. Delusions represent an interesting intermediate case where the DMN is stuck in a cycle of rigid active inference constrained by the goal of narrative coherence. This is why delusions are not responsive to epistemic norms: the model that constrains delusional thought is not epistemic.

## 3.   Dreaming as mindwandering

A good way to understand the role of the DMN is by considering recent work on the continuities between dreaming and so called mindwandering or daydreaming. This work takes as its target discontinuity and deficiency models of dreaming that treat dreams as the product of malfunction in cognitive systems whose role is best characterised in epistemic terms: accuracy, veracity, and consistency. A focus of these accounts is the acceptance of bizarre experiences in dreams where bizarreness refers to the juxtaposition of incongruent elements in episodes of experience (Revonsuo and Tarkko 2002, Kirberg 2022). In non-delusional waking cognition by contrast, the bizarre juxtaposition of features such as identity and appearance or spatiotemporal discontinuities are registered as requiring an explanation. So on deficiency accounts the explanation of delusion involves identifying a cognitive process whose malfunction is the result of mechanistic malfunction.

This is one way to characterise the 'unbinding' accounts of Revonsuo and Tarrko. In waking life, the stream of consciousness is organised in coherent narratives that contextualise experiences. This process of 'context-binding' is a high level metacognitive process that is intrinsically flexible allowing episodes to be combined in different though coherent patterns of association (Revonsuo and Tarkko 2002). As well as fitting experience into a coherent autobiographical history we can re-imagine life trajectories 'features of these experiences need to be de-contextualized, abstracted, and generalized to be useful in a variety of new situations that the organism might face' (Kirberg 2022: 12).

So called *feature binding* refers to the way in which perceptual elements are integrated in experience to produce a coherent image. It is a lower-level, more rigid process, which is why perceptual experience tends to remain coherent even when context binding is compromised. For example, the dreamscape continues to be composed of objects even when they appear in unusual combinations or with different features.

Unbinding theories of delusions and dreams explain bizarreness in terms of lack of context binding and (partial) feature binding. On this view, mindwandering and dreaming are on a continuum of unbinding with dreaming characterised by the complete absence of cognitive constraint and extreme bizarreness. Unbinding accounts can be assimilated to deficiency accounts since binding is treated as a cognitive process that degrades under different conditions producing epistemic deficiencies that make these states discontinuous with waking cognition (Hobson 1999).

In contrast, the dynamic simulation view treats mindwandering and dreaming as continuous aspects of the process of immersive simulation: 'Instead of asking which mechanisms bring about discontinuities in certain types of thought, we can ask what bizarreness tells us about the mechanisms that bring about continuous, non-bizarre thought' (Kirberg

2021: 23). On this view what bizarreness tells us that the same mechanisms underlie 'processes of spontaneous de-contextualization and associative re-combination of previous experiences' (Kirberg 2021: 16). And in fact when we look at mindwandering from a neutral perspective, we find more instances of bizarreness than in dreaming. In mindwandering, spatio-temporal discontinuity and vagueness are the dominant forms of bizarreness whereas in dreaming the type of bizarreness produced by perceptual and quasi perceptual unbinding of identity and appearance are more prominent. In mindwandering, we will not typically 'recognize A's sister. I am surprised by her beard. She looks much more like a man, with a beard and a big nose' (Gerrans 2012: 222) because mindwandering occurs in waking cognition, a context in which binding in the face processing system is intact. In dreams perceptual as well as contextual unbinding is common.

The continuity thesis unites work on the nature of dreaming and the role of the DMN network in different cognitive contexts with the idea that dreams are 'immersive simulations'. This fits with the often remarked feature about DMN activity: it is *self-referential*. The activity of the DMN allows the subject to represent actual or possible episodes of her life as part of a narrative, or to empathetically identify with others by imaginative projection.

It is for this reason that that DMN activity is *anticorrelated* with activity in systems that co-ordinate the processing of information that is not intrinsically subjective and or narrative. These processes are co-ordinated by the central executive network (CEN). Sometimes called System 2, Decontextualised or Executive processing, activity in these systems is probed by a variety of tasks that require the subject to detach from the perceptually-driven here and now and process information in abstract or a modal formats according to procedures that are objective or neutral (Menon 2011). Working memory or reasoning tasks are examples but the essence is processing of information in formats that do not entail the subjective perspective.

Simulation processes cannot be deficient, measured against epistemic norms, because dynamic, spontaneous, associative processing is not governed by epistemic norms. To complain that default processing is not governed by epistemic norms or represents a defective standard of reasoning is like complaining that a story is not true. Such complaints only make sense in contexts like testimony or reportage where a narrative is offered as a description of a sequence of events and as such is evaluated according to epistemic norms. Delusional subjects however are not trying to justify their delusion according to norms of empirical adequacy or rationality. They are constructing a subjectively adequate story that fits the experience.

An example of the difference between the subjectively adequate and objective representational formats is a difference between planning a journey by recalling a journey, in which case the subject recreates an episode of personal experience, and by consulting a map. If doubt arises about the accuracy of recollection (perhaps someone else recalls the journey differently) the solution is to consult a map. A map is not intrinsically linked to the subject's perspective on the world. Nor is procedural rationality. One can correct one's recollection by treating it as an empirical premise and reasoning about it. How to carve up the cognitive territory here is a work in progress, but it is important to note (i) activity in CEN and DMN is anticorrelated (ii) switching between those networks depends on activity in the Anterior Insula, the peak of the salience network (SN) (iii) a key hub of CEN activity is the dorsolateral prefrontal cortex (DLPFC) whose activity co-ordinates distributed processing that supports reflective, deliberative, abstract cognition (iv) In psychosis and in dreams, the DLPFC is hypoactive ('conspicuously deactivated' in dreams) and the DMN is strongly activated (Sridharan et al. 2008, Menon 2011, Whitfield-Gabrieli and Ford 2012). An interpretation that I will not defend further is that high levels of activity in the SN make it impossible for the subject to deactivate the DMN and activate the CEN in both delusions and dreams.

> This is consistent with the observation that dorsolateral prefrontal deactivation observed both during REM sleep and in schizophrenia seems to suppress or decrease its own functions, *including the loss or decrease of reflectiveness*, and at the same time disinhibits older subcortical structures and corresponding functions, with the exaggeration of accumbens' and amygdala nuclei's own processes: in our case, the appearance of hallucinations, delusions, bizarre thought processes, and affective disturbances.
>
> *(Gottesmann 2006: 1113)*

> Thus, there is consensus that the CEN is inactive in dreams due to the deactivation of the dorsolateral prefrontal circuitry on which it depends. 'REM [rapid eye movment] sleep may constitute a state of generalized brain activity with the specific exclusion of executive systems that normally participate in the highest order analysis and integration of neural information.'
>
> *(Braun et al. 1997: 1190)*

These facts together account for the fact that when DMN activity dominates cognition the subject is immersed in a subjective world from which she cannot easily detach.

## 4.  The AIM model and its discontents

Against this background accounts like the AIM model can be seen not as eliminative of phenomenology but as attempts to describe the fundamental mechanisms that enable the mind to fluently co-ordinate its resources for different kinds of active inference. Some of the early formulations of the AIM model have been empirically disconfirmed. The Pons, a key structure involved in sleep regulation, especially sleep paralysis, is no longer seen as essential to dreaming. The related idea that that dreaming is associated exclusively with rapid eye movement (REM) sleep is also not empirically supported (Solms 2000). However, the basic ideas of neurotransmitter theories of dreams and delusion can be restated in the active inference framework outlined above.

The AIM model is a neurotransmitter theory of dreaming and psychosis. Recall that the acronym stands for Activation, Information, Mode. It reminds us that characteristic patterns of experience depend on co-ordinated patterns of activity across the brain. The reference to Information reminds us that that activity enables the transmission and processing of information across the mind. The concept of Mode here refers to the fact that activity sustains cognition in characteristic modes. In waking life for example, we can be attentively engaged in perceptual scanning, in active intentional control of behaviour, automatically responding to environmental cues, engaged in abstract logical reasoning or personal recollection and planning or social cognition or daydreaming.

Each of these modes coordinates the information processing resources of the mind in a characteristic way. Those resources are organised in a cognitive architecture that describes the overall information processing structure of the mind. Most theories of cognition conceive of cognition for heuristic purposes as a set of *relatively discrete hierarchical interacting processes*. That conception is then modified by the evidence that signals are processed in parallel across distributed networks whose structure can be transient according to task and in which iterative and recurrent processing is influenced by higher level models. Thus, on recent views, the architecture of the mind is more like a matrix or heterarchy in which cognitive processing is performed by coalitions of neuronal assemblies constructed and maintained according to context. The concept of heterarchy expresses the idea that the integration of processing resources is horizontal, 'across' the mind, as well as vertical.

Luis Pessoa puts the idea this way, extending the concept of a neural matrix developed by Ronald Melzack to explain pain processing:

> The high degree of signal distribution and integration provides a nexus for the intermixing of information related to perception, cognition, emotion, motivation, and action. Importantly, the functional architecture consists of multiple overlapping networks that are highly dynamic and context-sensitive. Thus, how a given brain region affiliates with a specific network shifts as a function of task demands and brain state.
>
> *(Pessoa 2017: 357)*

The brain has to configure its activity to deal with information acquired in sensation. To do so, it needs some structure, transient or permanent, to produce and maintain adaptive patterns of activity across the matrix. Clearly permanent recurring problems (such as transducing photonic irradiation to produce a 3D coloured representation of the world as in visual perception) have *relatively* determinate and specialised neural substrates whose architecture is genetically canalised (the connectome as it is sometimes called). The less specific and recurrent the problem, the less rigid the architecture.

The idea of the AIM model is that basic configuration of the matrix/heterarchy for different kinds of active inference is determined by the influence of neurotransmitters. In alert waking cognition, the mind co-ordinates its resources to explore and engage with the physical and social world. This co-ordination requires the activity of the prefrontal cortex to activate and maintain activity in networks that enable attentive engagement and problem solving. It is important to note that controlled problem solving can be accomplished in different ways. When we solve problems using immersive simulation, we activate the DMN. Here a key hub of prefrontal activity is the ventromedial prefrontal cortex, which co-ordinates the assembly of episodes into coherent personally relevant narrative scenarios. In contrast when we are solving problem in more impersonal formats, the dorsolateral prefrontal cortex is active, maintaining activity across the CEN to support abstract amodal cognition.

Prefrontal networks require 'active maintenance' since the mind is (partially) decoupled from the perceptual world when they are active and activity is not driven by perceptual stimuli (O'Reilly and Munakata 2000, Pessoa 2017). These networks are large and resource-intensive and maintained by tonic serotoninergic activity. Controlled cognition comes online in waking cognition when the serotonin system maintains a steady state of tonic activation that maintains large scale distributed prefrontal-posterior networks.

Controlled cognition contrasts with forms of psychosis or dreaming, in which the cognitive components of the mind retain their integrity (depending on the degree of unbinding) but cannot be co-ordinated in the service of an epistemic cognitive or practical goal. In these cases the subject has intense perceptual and emotional experience but cannot mobilise the resources to respond adaptively because the necessary prefrontal resources are not available.

Another mode of the mind that dramatises the contrast between integration and disintegration sustained by serotoninergically-enabled prefrontal control is psychedelic experience (Letheby and Gerrans 2017, Letheby 2021). In some forms of psychedelic experience, disintegration occurs not just between but also within subsystemic components of the matrix. Thus, in psychedelic experience, objects change shape and texture and various perceptual *impossibilia* arise. It is no coincidence that psychedelic experience is the result of disruption to the serotoninergic system leading to what has been described as 'disintegration' and 'increase in entropy' across the mind. Or in the terminology of Antii Revonsuo and Krista Tarrko (2002) 'unbinding'.

The psychedelic case is another demonstration that high level cognition integration is a resource intensive process that requires the activation of the so-called CEN. A hub of this network is the dorsolateral prefrontal cortex, implicated in working memory, controlled attention and abstract forms of inference.

At the level of large scale overall cognitive organisation the CEN is one of three large networks. Another is the DMN whose properties we discussed earlier. The final large scale network is the so-called SN involved in detection, evaluation of, and response to self-relevant information. The SN co-ordinates activity in systems responsible for emotional appraisal, affective experience, and reinforcement. The highest level of the SN is the anterior insula cortex whose activity implicated in almost every form of self-referential activity. Deactivation of the AI produces loss of the sense that things matter to *me* often manifest in feelings of depersonalisation or flattened affect. Another important role of the AI seems to be in switching between activity in the DMN and CEN.

High levels of AI activation create intense forms of subjective awareness such as anxiety and distress (Craig 2009). In such cases, interestingly, subjects find it very difficult to activate the DMN to create alternative forms of immersive simulation. Someone with Social Anxiety for example cannot imaginatively inhabit a future in which their social interactions are rewarding. Instead they seem trapped in a miserable present state of foreboding that they cannot evaluate objectively (Terasawa et al. 2012, Murray et al. 2015, Gerrans and Murray 2020). Nor can they simulate an alternative with a different affective outcome (DMN). In fact when questioned, they tend to produce a rigid script attesting the inability to imaginatively inhabit alternative futures. In effect, the high levels of distress trap them in a present from which they cannot detach imaginatively or conceptually.

The network view of the mind it fits well with the idea that it functions as a heterarchical matrix whose operations are configured in a context sensitive way. Each of these networks configures the mind to deal more or less adaptively with a class of problems. Within the active inference framework, this means that each network configures the matrix to take action to verify particular types of model.

It is against this background that that the AIM model makes most sense. The table below integrates the network model above with the Cognitive Modes proposed by Hobson. Hobson was concerned to distinguish stages of the sleep cycle. He equated REM with deep dreaming characterised by bizarreness and incoherence. Non-rapid eye movement (NREM) is associated with coherent but stereotyped and repetitive scenarios such being late for an important event or searching unavailingly. When we look at activity of the DMN in waking cognition, it also exhibits different degrees of coherence. Mental time travel can be seen as a coherent form of simulation because it is a form of goal directed active inference. When not structured by a goal, the simulation process reverts to mindwandering or daydreaming.

| Global state | Wake<br>*Active inference model building* | NREM | REM |
| --- | --- | --- | --- |
| Cognition<br>Automatic processing.<br>  System1<br>Default mode<br>  processing<br>Central executive<br>  network processing | Acquisition and manipulation<br>  and evaluation of<br>  information<br>Perceptual/sensorimotor loops.<br>Affective response<br>Mental time travel. Narrative<br>  fragments. Autobiographical<br>  episodes<br>Abstract inference<br>Detection of inconsistencies,<br>Reality testing<br>Selective inhibition of<br>  lower-level processing | Iteration of<br>  information<br>Rehearsal of<br>  standard patterns<br>  of behavior and<br>  familiar scenarios | Episodic<br>  fragments |
| Phenomenology<br>Perception<br>Movement<br>Thought | External, vivid<br>Continuous, voluntary<br>(CEN)<br>Logical, coherent progressive<br>(DMN)<br>Mental time travel. Coherent<br>  associative trains of<br>  autobiographical episodes.<br>  narrative structure<br>MIndwandering. Less coherent<br>  trains of association. | Dull or absent<br>Episodic, involuntary<br>Coherent<br>  perseverative.<br>  scripts and<br>  sequences | Internal, vivid<br>Commanded<br>  but inhibited<br>Incoherent<br>  associative |
| Neurochemistry<br>5HT (serotonin),<br>  NA(Noradrenaline)<br>Cholinergic<br>DA dopamine | High<br>Low<br>Task dependent | Decreasing at end<br>  of cycle<br>Increasing at end<br>  of cycle<br>Tonic. stabilise<br>  scenarios | Low<br>High<br>Phasic |

Transitions between modes are essentially a consequence of the balance between cholinergic (acetylcholine) and aminergic (5 hydroxytryptamine/serotonin, norepinephrine and dopamine) regulation of the brain by reticular activating systems which project throughout the brain from the brainstem.

Very roughly, aminergic regulation is required for wakeful exploration of the environment and goal-directed behaviour and cognition. Amines assist the prefrontal cortical structures to communicate with posterior ones and to build and actively maintain transient distributed networks necessary for controlled processing. During active waking, characterised by slow-wave firing patterns across the brain maintained by tonic levels of 5HT in particular, the noradrenergic, serotoninergic, and cholinergic systems are firing together. During slow-wave (NREM) sleep, these three systems reduce their discharge, while during REM (rapid eye movement) sleep, the noradrenergic and 5HT systems shut off completely, as the cholinergic system resumes its firing. However, the dopamine system projecting from the nucleus accumbens remains active even during REM sleep.

Serotonin seems to enable the construction of stable patterns of activation across widely distributed neural circuits, enabling global integration of different systems for particular tasks involved in wakeful exploratory activity. The regular delivery of serotonin across the brain keeps the organism in a state of wakeful exploration, coordinating perceptual, motor, and cognitive activity to enable life-supporting activities.

Acetylcholine plays a role in maintaining patterns of activation across localised assemblies rather than the global patterns maintained by the serotonin system. It is thus an antagonist to 5HT, adaptively disrupting stable global patterns of activity and detaching local assemblies from global integration. One feature of cholinergic regulation is that when it increases in wakeful stressful episodes prefrontal activation is reduced. High levels thus produce a reversion to automatic mode. This has consequences for the understanding of many developmental disorders and stress disorders manifest in episodes of disinhibition. As with other neurotransmitters, a one-to-one correlation with a cognitive function has not been proposed. Rather, the balance with other neurotransmitters and the density and type of receptors in areas to which it projects determine how it influences cognition. However, we can note that when choline levels are high relative to amines they produce lack of prefrontally based executive supervision and reversion to automaticity.

The norepinephrine system pays a crucial role in poising the system for defensive action ('flight or fight'). Circuits it innervates control alertness, vigilance, and agonistic behavior, releasing appropriate hormones and priming visceral and somatic systems for rapid response.

Finally, the dopamine system is a crucial part of the salience system. It enables an organism to target attention and cognitive effort on relevant stimuli by accentuating activation in circuits which represent salient information. This is known as increasing the 'gain' on signals.

Of course, at any given moment, the effect of any neurotransmitter is highly context-dependent. It depends on density and type of receptors, mode of delivery, and current activation level and neurochemical state of the circuit it innervates and the representational architecture of those circuits. No monolithic interpretation of the role of a neurotransmitter is possible for this reason. This is why Hobson introduced the notion of cognitive mode. It describes the global functional integration and coordination of cognitive subsystems when the mind is in a particular neurotransmitter-mediated state. The global state of the brain (sleep, wake, explore, withdraw, automatic, controlled) is regulated by fundamental neurochemistry because that chemistry synchronises global activation patterns at different ranges and time scales.

When the balance of cholines and amines distributed across brain regions by the reticular activating systems changes in favour of cholines, prefrontal activity, and with it the capacity for metacognitive responses to experience, subsides. Simultaneously, motor expression is inhibited and early stages of perceptual and sensory processing are shut down. Alert wakefulness and REM sleep are the ends of a cycle with NREM sleep constituting an intermediate stage, neurochemically and cognitively (see table above). In NREM sleep, there is no perceptual input and metacognitive supervision is reduced. Volitional control is largely absent as a consequence of prefrontal deactivation. Consequently, standard routines or associative repertoires tend to be replayed, often accompanied by negative affect since the emotional systems remain active, but there is no top-down integration or supervision of these routines.

When serotonin is at its lowest level and the brain is cholinergically regulated, automatic processes continue without being organised externally by the environment through perceptual inputs or internally under volitional control.

'In REM sleep, the dorsolateral prefrontal cortex 'remains conspicuously deactivated' (Hobson 1999: 691) and the mind is dominated by highly salient imagery and emotional sensations. The resources to respond to inconsistencies and gaps in the narrative or to represent an overall goal for the narrative are absent due to dorsolateral deactivation, and the hyperassociation of salient imagery continues unbroken. The selective activation of dorsolateral areas for decontextualised, and ventromedial for subjective or personal, thought is a feature of waking cognition replayed in dreaming. In studies of dreaming in prefrontal lesion patients (many of whom experience intense and disturbing dreams) Mark Solms (2000) found that dreams were suppressed in ventromedial patients. In contrast, patients with dorsolateral lesions who exhibit the characteristic deficits in abstract problem solving had normal dreams.

## 5. Are delusions dreams? States of imagination? Beliefs?

Delusions are not dreams, but as in dreams, the balance of activity between DMN and CEN processing has changed. In dreams, the default system churns out highly salient simulations triggered by activity in automatic feature binding systems unmoored from the environment. The incongruities and inconsistencies of both feature and context binding are not detected or resolved. Thus, narrative incoherence as well as (a lesser degree of) feature-binding incoherence is characteristic of REM dreams. Kahn, Pace-Schott, and Hobson make a similar point:

> When the DLPFC is in poor communication with these areas as in REM sleep, the ability to perform logical inference, to recall accurately and to discern whether a premise is fact or fiction may very well be compromised
>
> *(Kahn et al. 2002: 46)*

In delusions, the simulation system is not entirely endogenously activated. Streams of subjective association are triggered by highly salient experiences that initiate activity in the simulation system. What seems to be missing in delusion is the ability to subject the resulting narrative fragment to evaluation for consistency or coherence because the CEN of delusional subjects is not playing its role.

The idea that the DMN is a simulation system accounts for the attractiveness of imaginative theories of delusion. If delusions are essentially imaginative states then their lack of epistemic constraint is straightforward to explain. To imagine being handsome, the president of Canada, intelligent, charming, and popular is not a mistake. It is only a mistake if one believes it, and only pathological if that belief introduces a significant amount of dysfunction into the subject's life. The problem for the imaginative theory of delusion is of course that subjects often incorporate the delusion, cognitively and behaviourally with a high degree of conviction. This is the attraction of doxastic theories of delusion. People act according to their (often irrational) beliefs and also rationalise, elaborate, defend, or compartmentalise them. Imaginative states do not lead to action (but see e.g Anna Ichino 2019) and can be discarded at will (at least on some folk psychological conceptions of imagination). So it is tempting to assimilate delusions to beliefs to explain their tenacity.

As well as the fact that these doxastic or imaginative accounts never line up precisely with the phenomenology a more important difficulty for any theory phrased in folk psychological terms is that folk psychology and mechanistic explanation do not dovetail. I propose the relationship between dreams and (some) delusions is ultimately best explained in terms of neurochemically-induced changes in the activity of the DMN. These changes affect the intrinsic properties of the network (the way its components interact) and its extrinsic properties (its interaction with other networks). The result is characteristic forms of immersive simulation insulated from rational evaluation.

# References

Barrett, L. F., et al. (2016). "An active inference theory of allostasis and interoception in depression." *Philosophical Transactions of the Royal Society B* **371**(1708): 20160011.

Bayne, T. (2010). "Delusions as doxastic states: Contexts, compartments, and commitments." *Philosophy, Psychiatry, & Psychology* **17**(4): 329–336.

Braun, A. R., et al. (1997). "Regional cerebral blood flow throughout the sleep-wake cycle. An H2 (15) O PET study." *Brain: A Journal of Neurology* **120**(7): 1173–1197.

Corcoran, A. W., et al. (2020). "From allostatic agents to counterfactual cognisers: Active inference, biological regulation, and the origins of cognition." *Biology & Philosophy* **35**(3): 1–45.

Craig, A. D. (2009). "How do you feel--now? The anterior insula and human awareness." *Nature Reviews Neuroscience* **10**(1): 59–70.

Currie, G. and J. Jureidini (2004). "Narrative and coherence." *Mind and Language* **19**(4): 409–427.

Domhoff, G. W. (2011). "The neural substrate for dreaming: Is it a subsystem of the default network?" *Consciousness and Cognition* **20**: 1163–1174.

Frankish, K. (2012). "Delusions, levels of belief, and non-doxastic acceptances." *Neuroethics* **5**(1): 23–27.

Gendler, T. S. (2008). "Alief in action (and reaction)." *Mind & Language* **23**(5): 552–585.

Gerrans, P. (2001). "Delusions as performance failures." *Cognitive Neuropsychiatry* **6**(3): 161–173.

Gerrans, P. (2012). "Dream experience and a revisionist account of delusions of misidentification." *Consciousness and Cognition* **21**(1): 217–227.

Gerrans, P. (2014a). *The measure of madness: Philosophy of mind, cognitive neuroscience, and delusional thought*. Cambridge, MIT Press.

Gerrans, P. (2014b). "Pathologies of hyperfamiliarity in dreams, delusions and déjà vu." *Frontiers in Psychology* **5**: 97.

Gerrans, P. and R. J. Murray (2020). "Interoceptive active inference and self-representation in social anxiety disorder (SAD): exploring the neurocognitive traits of the SAD self." *Neuroscience of Consciousness*, 2020(1).

Goldie, P. (2011). "Life, fiction, and narrative." *Narrative, emotion, and insight*, N. Carroll and J. Gibson (eds.). Pennsylvania, Pennsylvania State University Press: 8–22.

Gonçalves, L. M. and A. Tosoni (2016). "Sudden onset of Cotard's syndrome as a clinical sign of brain tumor." *Archives of Clinical Psychiatry (São Paulo)* **43**: 35–36.

Gottesmann, C. (2006). "The dreaming sleep stage: A new neurobiological model of schizophrenia?" *Neuroscience* **140**(4): 1105–1115.

Hobson, J. A. (1999). *Dreaming as delirium: How the brain goes out of its mind*, Cambridge Mass: MIT Press.

Hobson, J. A., et al. (2000). "Dreaming and the brain: Toward a cognitive neuroscience of conscious states." *Behavioral and Brain Sciences* **23**(6): 793–842.

Ichino, A. (2019). "Imagination and belief in action." *Philosophia* 47(5): 1517–1534.

Kahn, D., et al. (2002). "Emotion and cognition: Feeling and character identification in dreaming." *Consciousness and Cognition* 11(1): 34–50.

Keshavan, M. S. and M. Sudarshan (2017). "Deep dreaming, aberrant salience and psychosis: Connecting the dots by artificial neural networks." *Schizophrenia Research* 188: 178–181.

Kirberg, M. (2021). *Comparing spontaneous thoughts across the sleep-wake-cycle*. Unpublished Doctoral Thesis, Monash University.

Kirberg, M. (2022). "Neurocognitive dynamics of spontaneous offline simulations: Re-conceptualizing (dream) bizarreness." *Philosophical Psychology* 35(7): 1072–1101.

Kirchhoff, M., et al. (2018). "The Markov blankets of life: Autonomy, active inference and the free energy principle." *Journal of the Royal Society Interface* 15(138): 20170792.

Letheby, C. (2021). *Philosophy of psychedelics*, Oxford, Oxford University Press.

Letheby, C. and P. Gerrans (2017). "Self unbound: Ego dissolution in psychedelic experience." *Neuroscience of Consciousness* 2017(1): nix016.

Menary, R. (2008). "Embodied narratives." *Journal of Consciousness Studies* 15(6). 63–84.

Menon, V. (2011). "Large-scale brain networks and psychopathology: A unifying triple network model." *Trends in Cognitive Sciences* 15(10): 483–506.

Michaelian, K. (2016). *Mental time travel: Episodic memory and our knowledge of the personal past*, MIT Press.

Murray, R. J., et al. (2015). "When at rest:" Event-free" active inference may give rise to implicit self-models of coping potential." *Behavioral and Brain Sciences* 38.e114

O'Reilly, R. C. and Y. Munakata (2000). *Computational explorations in cognitive neuroscience: Understanding the mind by simulating the brain*, Cambridge, MA: MIT press.

Parr, T., et al. (2022). *Active inference: The free energy principle in mind, brain, and behavior*, Cambridge, MA: MIT Press.

Pessoa, L. (2017). "A network model of the emotional brain." *Trends in Cognitive Sciences* 21(5): 357–371.

Revonsuo, A. (2000). "The reinterpretation of dreams: An evolutionary hypothesis of the function of dreaming." *Behavioral and Brain Sciences* 23(6): 877–901.

Revonsuo, A. and K. Tarkko (2002). "Binding in dreams-the bizarreness of dream images and the unity of consciousness." *Journal of Consciousness Studies* 9(7): 3–24.

Solms, M. (2000). "Dreaming and REM sleep are controlled by different brain mechanisms." *Behavioral and Brain Sciences* 23(6): 843–850.

Sridharan, D., et al. (2008). "A critical role for the right fronto-insular cortex in switching between central-executive and default-mode networks." *Proceedings of the National Academy of Sciences* 105(34): 12569–12574.

Suddendorf, T. and M. C. Corballis (2007). "The evolution of foresight: What is mental time travel, and is it unique to humans?" *Behavioral and Brain Sciences* 30(3): 299–313.

Suddendorf, T., et al. (2009). "Mental time travel and the shaping of the human mind." *Philosophical Transactions of the Royal Society of London B: Biological Sciences* 364(1521): 1317–1324.

Terasawa, Y., et al. (2012). "Anterior insular cortex mediates bodily sensibility and social anxiety." *Social Cognitive and Affective Neuroscience* 8(3):(3), 259–266.

Whitfield-Gabrieli, S. and J. M. Ford (2012). "Default mode network activity and connectivity in psychopathology." *Annual Review of Clinical Psychology* 8: 49–76.

Windt, J. M. (2010). "The immersive spatiotemporal hallucination model of dreaming." *Phenomenology and the Cognitive Sciences* 9: 295–316.

Windt, J. M. (2015). *Dreaming: A conceptual framework for philosophy of mind and empirical research*, Cambridge, MA: MIT Press.

# 25
# DELUSION AND FOLK PSYCHOLOGY

*Dominic Murphy*

## 1.  Philosophical approaches to delusion

Philosophical discussions of delusion usually start by assuming that 'delusion' denotes a psychological kind whose basic cognitive structure can be worked out via attention to paradigm cases (see other contributions to this volume's Part 4 on *Delusion's Place in the Mind*). This project sees delusions as deficient forms of belief, with abnormal relations among components of our standard processes of belief fixation. Jennifer Radden (2011) notes the similarities between this philosophical conception of delusion and analytic epistemology. She reads the project of explaining delusion as the inversion of the familiar attempts made by modern epistemologists to define knowledge. A delusion is a false belief, just as knowledge is true belief, but, as with knowledge, philosophers do not rest there. Knowledge is true belief plus something else. So too, philosophers, cognitive scientists and psychiatrists engaged in this project are looking for that extra property of a false belief that converts it from a mere false belief into a delusion. They look for the features that, when they exist alongside a false belief, make it a delusion – not just an epistemic error but a pathology (for more on delusion and pathology see Petrolini, Chapter 1).

This conceptual program is the prelude to the development of empirical theories of delusion, which work out the physiological and information-processing basis of these states. The dominant preoccupation shaping recent philosophical discussions of delusion has been the doxastic conception of delusion, which begins from the same starting point as most clinical definitions.

The definition of delusion in the *Diagnostic and Statistical Manual of Mental Disorders* (*DSM-5*: American Psychiatric Association 2013: 87) specifies that delusions 'are fixed beliefs that are not amenable to change in the light of conflicting evidence' and goes on to list their clinical varieties. On the face of it, that is a terrible definition that includes all manner of normal beliefs, since the existence of some contrary evidence is compatible with the firm holding of a belief (for more on delusion and evidence see Flores, Chapter 12). The point, as the passage goes on to note, is that the difference between a strongly held belief and a delusion 'depends in part on the degree of conviction with which the belief is held despite clear or reasonable contradictory evidence regarding its veracity'. So, a delusion

DOI: 10.4324/9781003296386-30

is a belief held with undue conviction. This is less detailed than the previous *DSM-IV* (American Psychiatric Association 2000) characterization of delusion (2000: 821): 'A false belief based on incorrect inference about external reality that is firmly sustained despite what almost everybody else believes and despite what constitutes incontrovertible and obvious proof or evidence to the contrary'. This *DSM-IV* definition survives in the glossary of *DSM-5* (2013: 819), even though it is not entirely consistent with the revised definition in the text. You can see why philosophers would be drawn towards explicating this concept. A delusion has to be false – and we know how to write about truth. Second, delusions are in some way based on an incorrect inferences about the world. These two criteria suggest a doxastic/epistemic understanding of delusion, which is further sustained by the subsequent demand that the delusion be retained in the face of both conventional wisdom and proof of its falsehood. The problem, apparently, is that of relation to the evidence.

This doxastic conception construes delusions as a type of belief, although what this means precisely is controversial (Bortolotti 2009). Not everyone agrees: Philip Gerrans (2014), for example, sees delusions as imaginative states and is suspicious of attempts to understand delusion as a species of belief (for more on delusion and imagination see Kind, Chapter 21). Sean Gallagher (2009) draws attention to the idea of delusional realities, in which one's experiences and and orientation to the world shift in a delusional state. More broadly, exactly what it means to call a state of mind a belief is much less clear than we tend to think. Lisa Bortolotti (2009) points out that some philosophers insist on very strict criteria for beliefs as rational processes of inference attuned to evidence. This is especially acute in interpretivist philosophers of mind who take rational coherence as a condition for ascription of mental states to entities at all. If we slacken these rational standards somewhat then some states will qualify as beliefs despite being less than fully rational. Other scholars, such as Ema Sullivan-Bissett and colleagues (2017), have followed Bortolotti and persuasively argued that delusional and nondelusional beliefs differ in degree but not in kind. Nondelusional beliefs often exhibit the same epistemic shortcomings that define delusions: resistance to counterevidence, undue perseverance, and formation under the influence of bias and wishful thinking.

Another complication is that there are pathological states that are not delusions or beliefs but also exhibit some of these qualities. Robert Noggle draws attention to the implication in Obsessive Compulsive Disorder of what look like quite sophisticated contentful states of mind, such as:

> anxiety that some dreaded state of affairs might come true, along with motivation to take suitable precautions. Moreover, the compulsive motivations typically bear a clear relationship to the content of the obsession. Persons with contamination obsessions experience motivation to wash. Persons with obsessive thoughts about disasters occurring because of unlocked doors or improperly flipped switches tend to check them.
>
> *(Noggle 2016: 661)*

The natural interpretation, thinks Noggle, is that these states are 'quasi-beliefs'; belief-like states that lack some of the characteristics assigned by folk psychology to fully fledged beliefs, but nonetheless closely resemble beliefs in that they help to cause behaviour (for more on delusions in OCD see Szalai, Chapter 9). Some delusions, on the other hand, seem to be decoupled from behaviour – delusional patients don't always act as you would predict based on their avowed beliefs (for more on delusion and action see Tumulty, Chapter 18).

This brief treatment could be extended easily, but I hope the point is clear; we face a broad array of content bearing intentional states with belief-like properties. It is unclear what basis we have for judging that some of these are really beliefs, and it is also unclear how we decide which of them are delusions or otherwise pathological. In the remainder of this chapter, I will discuss one way into this problem, namely the relationship between these judgements and folk psychology as a system of psychological attribution and assessment.

## 2. Folk psychology[1]

Humans are social creatures who teach each other, cooperate, and form mutually advantageous coalitions. To do all this, we need to understand and predict the behaviour of others. In philosophy, we call this folk psychology. Like language, it is a fluent capacity that phenomenologically is a natural part of ordinary human experience. But it still needs to be explained, and, as with language, we can investigate the underlying machinery that enables it. And of course going along with co-operation is failure to co-operate. We deceive others and monitor them for signs of deceit. We are also alert to the failure of others to act as we predict not due to their malice or our errors, but because they are in some way not entirely normal or typical. Human behaviour, like biological phenomena more broadly, is prone to an unusual sort of predictive failure; sometimes we get a prediction wrong not through the misapplication of a body of knowledge, or errors in description from which a prediction is derived, but because the system being predicted is not working normally. And, of course, we are surrounded by other creatures who are also possess wills of their own; wild and domestic animals need to be understood too. For many cultures, perhaps all, so do supernatural agents.

These are truisms, but they raise a lot of issues. I have said that something about us lets us understand and predict others. What is it? And how are we able to distinguish errors in our understanding from the failure of others to conform to a correct account of normal function? I shall discuss these in turn. The first question asks about the nature of what philosophers and other theorists call *folk psychology*. It has inspired a massive literature. The second question asks about the intersection of folk psychology and philosophical psychopathology. Not as many people have tried to answer it, but there is a growing literature on the nature of human judgement about the mental states of others.

The general consensus among contemporary cognitive scientists and analytic philosophers is that normal human beings understand one another – or engage in 'mindreading' – via possession of 'commonsense' or 'folk' psychology. 'Folk psychology' is often also known as 'theory of mind.' The possession of theory of mind has become operationalized in psychology as the ability to pass the false belief test, by attributing to another person a representation of a situation that one knows is incorrect; for example, seeing that they falsely believe there are cookies in a jar that you know to be empty. The ability to pass the false belief test is taken to indicate the capacity treat people as acting on intentional states (which can misrepresent the world) rather than simply being directed at the environment. Most neurotypical children can do this by the age of four. I am going to observe a distinction in this essay between folk psychology and theory of mind, treating possession of the latter as a way to explain the former. The two are often elided, but it is useful to distinguish them, since there is a sense in which even behaviourists have a theory of mind.

We owe the contemporary debate to Wilfred Sellars (1956). Sellars imagined a distant ancestor called Jones who lives in a culture with no language for mental states. Jones proposes a theory to account for visible behaviour, positing unobservable entities just as any scientist might who wants to explain visible phenomena. Jones develops a theory for talking about inner states underlying public behaviour, and it is this theory that has come to be known by philosophers as *folk psychology*. Sellars's target was a Cartesian conception of the mental. On the Cartesian view, our knowledge of mental states comes to us via introspection and is thus, in the first place, private. Sellars's rival conception models inner processes on speech, and requires the prior possession of a language which members of the culture can use to construe thought as a form of inner speech. Sellars offers a picture of folk psychology as a culturally transmitted theory that explains the existence of our mental concepts without positing direct knowledge of inner states. For our purposes, what is important is that we can see Sellars as leaving a set of questions for later thinkers to wrangle over.

One set of questions concerns the utility and accuracy of folk psychology; if it is a hypothesis about the underlying basis of behaviour, then, like any other such hypothesis, folk psychology might not be empirically accurate. Notwithstanding its utility in predicting human behaviour, its status as a scientifically acceptable theory has been challenged on several grounds. Champions of folk psychology stress how it lets us coordinate actions over time and space, as well as predict the behaviour of others. Jerry Fodor (1987, Chapter 1), for example, argues that making inferences about people's behaviour, based on their utterances and other pieces of information, involves filling in a lot of gaps. This is achieved using information derived from our stock of knowledge about how people – including total strangers – work. The ensuing inferences look like informal, fallible scientific reasoning. Fodor also thinks that the form of folk psychology is reminiscent of a scientific theory, in that it consists of generalizations; these he takes to specify the unobservable (mental) states that cause the observable ones. Examples might include (Fodor 1987: 7): if $x$ wants $p$, and believes that not $p$ unless $q$, then $x$ will attempt to make it the case that $q$, or if $x$ is $y$'s rival, then $x$ prefers $y$'s discomfiture. Folk psychology, for philosophers like Fodor, is made up of such generalizations. They have exceptions, and so are true only ceteris paribus. But ceteris paribus laws characterize many sciences.

For Fodorians, if we treat folk psychology like a scientific theory then two further consequences follow: (a) we see that the theory is likely to be true and (b) we can learn something about the nature of the unobservables that the theory mentions. The case for (a) is that the theory is so useful that it is very likely to be true. Again the analogy is with science, in which predictive accuracy is taken to be a reason for believing in the approximate truth of a theory. The predictive accuracy of Mendelian population genetics, for example, was held to be a reason for believing in the existence of genes. Those who accept this are also likely to think that, whatever genes are made of, they are very likely to have the properties that Mendel's laws specify. Similarly, the argument for (b) is that the entities that feature in the laws of folk psychology should have the properties that the laws say they have. What this means is that mental states cause behaviour and are made true, or fulfilled, by their relation to the world. If I think there is beer in the fridge, then my belief is true just in case the fridge contains beer. If I want a beer, and intend to get one, then those states of mind are fulfilled by my having a beer.

This constitutes the realist position on folk psychology; to wit, that it is a correct theory of the mental states that cause human behaviour, not just a heuristic device. A weaker view is possible if one keeps some parts of the realist view while discarding others: Sellars, for example, seems to have been an agnostic about whether beliefs and desires really do have the properties specified by the theory, despite his contention that folk psychology was predictively accurate.

But there are many skeptics. One sceptical camp admits that folk psychology is a theory, but disputes its utility. The eliminative materialist movement has asked about the scientific credentials of the concepts of folk psychology. Paul Feyerabend (1963) raised questions about our capacity to reduce folk psychology to physiology, and argued that any successful materialist theory would undermine folk psychology, by showing that there was really nothing mental at all. Others have questioned the scientific credentials of the theory on other grounds. Paul Churchland (1981) argued that folk psychology could do nothing to explain many psychological matters, such as the nature of dreams and mental illness. He also charged folk psychology with stagnation, given that it had not changed since classical antiquity. These properties are grave defects in a scientific theory. Churchland took them to be evidence that folk psychology was overdue for replacement by a successor theory, which he assumed would come from neuroscience. Stephen Stich (1983) also argued that cognitive science would supplant folk psychology with a computational theory and employ syntactically individuated states rather than semantically characterized representations.

Our folk concepts, Stich ventured, are too vague to be scientifically useful. Stich's point here is that there are many cases in which it is unclear whether the concept of belief really applies at all. Stich's famous example is that of an elderly lady, Mrs T. Mrs T is able to state that 'McKinley was assassinated' even though she cannot, owing to memory loss due to neurodegenerative disease, say who McKinley was, whether he is alive or dead, or what assassination might be. So, does she really believe that McKinley was assassinated? The tragic yet hilarious story of Mrs. T points to vagueness in our concept of belief, but it does not support eliminativism without further assumptions from the philosophy of language, as Stich (1996, Chapter 1) was led to acknowledge. Churchland and Stich assumed that the meaning of a theoretical term is functionally defined by the theory that it features in, as the things filling the causal roles that the theory postulates. So if the laws of folk psychology are false, 'belief' is literally meaningless since the laws tell us what the nature of belief is. An alternative view is that there really are such things as beliefs, but that folk psychology is partly or largely wrong about their nature. In that case, we would be led to revise folk psychology, rather than reject it altogether. This is a hard issue to adjudicate, and turns on subtle philosophical questions in the theory of reference as well as more empirical considerations.

Other sceptics see no sense in conceding the theoretical basis of folk psychology. Matthew Ratcliffe (2007) contends not simply that folk psychology constitutes an erroneous understanding of other minds, but rather that no such understanding is, in any sense, attributable to ordinary people. Ratcliffe's view is that folk psychological descriptions are only 'commensensical' to those who have already been inculcated in intellectual disciplines where the salience of folk psychology is taken for granted, and that experimental work has assumed its existence, rather than searched for it. He argues instead that much of our understanding of others is ascertained directly through embodied interaction, and tacitly informed by an intersubjective context of shared norms and social roles. One problem with Ratcliffe's position is his assumption that folk psychology requires making explicit inferences about others; the theorists we have mentioned do not normally argue that these inferences are explicit. Explicit reasoning about others is certainly possible, but folk psychology is usually considered to be an implicit theory, rather than something we consciously entertain. Some of Ratcliffe's other arguments raise interesting questions about the phenomenology of our social cognition, but folk psychology is usually taken to be a theory of underlying psychological processes rather than conscious mental life. Like Churchland, Ratcliffe also raises issues about the scope of folk psychology, albeit with different concerns.

Another prominent disagreement occurs over whether the basis of folk psychology should be seen as possession of a theory or a capacity for simulating the minds of others. While theory-theorists understand folk psychology as the possession of a protoscientific theory of mind, simulationists argue that mind reading is a matter of cognitively modeling another person's mental states using one's own as an analogue. The theory-theory assumes that successful explanation and prediction of behaviour requires a rich body of information about human minds, encoded in a theory. Simulationist approaches, on the other hand, are information-poor. Working on the basis that other people have minds much like one's own, some philosophers argue that to predict their behaviour one should simply imagine oneself in their place (Heal 1986). On a more cognitively loaded account (Goldman 1989; Gordon 1986), the story is that one uses one's own practical decision-making systems to predict the behaviour of another, but with imaginary beliefs as input.

Last, we can ask about the scope and uses of folk psychology. Alvin Goldman (2006) distinguishes 'high-level' mind reading, which is concerned with beliefs and desires, from 'low-level' mind reading, which has to do with bodily and affective phenomena like pain, fear, and disgust. The philosophical debate outlined so far has concentrated on the ability to predict the behaviour of others in terms of their beliefs and desires and the degree to which we should see this as mastery of a theory. This issue has dominated the philosophical discussion. But our repertoire of psychological concepts is not limited to belief and desire. It is much bigger and more varied than that. Most people who read this will have been raised in cultures that explain people's behaviour not just as a product of beliefs, desires, and other propositional attitudes but also in terms of, to take some simple examples, affective states like moods and emotions, as well as relatively enduring traits of character such as piety, bravery, intelligence, or sloth. The boundaries of the mental are not easy to discern, but all of these seem to qualify. Thinkers like Tadeusz Zawidzki (2013) and Kristin Andrews (2016) argue that sophisticated propositional attitude ascription is much less pervasive than is presumed by the standard view I have outlined, and exists alongside a great variety of other folk psychological practices that draw on these other concepts. They also emphasize non-epistemic, normative goals such as the justification and regulation of other's behaviours and mental states. We can also mention in this context the attribution of mental illness (or 'folk psychiatry'), and possibly too the idea of a folk 'epistemology' that looks at the thoughts that underlie public expressions and evaluates them as sources of information (Mercier 2010; Sperber et al. 2010).

Construed broadly, then, folk psychology incorporates a great deal that has been missed by the debates we have mentioned above. In the last few years analogues of those debates have cropped up in other areas. Eliminativist arguments have been made for the common-sense understanding of several psychological phenomena, although these are less likely to dwell on the details of a commonsense theory and more likely to simply argue that science shows some of our ordinary psychology to be full of errors. Paul Griffiths (1997) suggested that the folk psychology of emotion lumped together three categories that science should keep apart, to wit: evolved, modular basic emotions (anger); nonmodular, cognitively penetrated higher emotions (envy); and socially constructed behavioural roles with affective components (hysteria). Griffiths maintained that no useful science treats all three phenomena as members of a common kind, and that 'emotion' is not a scientifically useful category.

Similarly, John Doris (2003) argues that our tendency to couch moral evaluation in terms of character traits is undermined by findings in social psychology that stress situational rather than personal causes of behaviour. Doris argues that moral psychology, especially virtue ethics, has committed what social psychologists call 'the fundamental attribution error' of explaining behaviour by inner traits rather than contextual forces. For example, we may think that somebody who accepts a bribe is especially dishonest, rather than paying attention to their social context, which makes corruption a more likely choice for anyone regardless of their character. If the virtues are enduring, causally potent traits of character then they have a place in folk psychology but virtues may not reflect any genuine, scientifically respectable category.

So, we can see that philosophical disputes about folk psychology have not just been limited to competing explanations of theory of mind – our competence at ascribing the propositional attitudes, like belief and desire does not exhaustour everyday thought about the mind. That folk thought goes far beyond the attutudes to range across other mental states, and there is a philosophical literature pertaining to these other corners of folk psychology. The question I want to pursue in the remainder of this chapter is how far we can understand the concept of delusion as an aspect of this wider folk psychology. As we have seen, belief looks like a vague concept that covers a lot of more or less rational states. Presumably, if delusion slots in as a component of folk psychology it inherits much of that vagueness. That may not help us explicate a scientifically respectable kind as the referent of 'delusion', but it might help us understand how the concept works and better grasp some of the disputes about it.

## 3.  Folk psychology and delusion

Pascal Boyer (2011) and Nick Haslam, Lauren Ban, and Leah Kaufman (2007) have suggested that the intuitive detection of mental disorder involves judging that a particular type of behaviour is so different from what one's culture expects that it is evidence that some mental systems are dysfunctional. This attribution of mental disorder depends on the principles that organize our understanding of other people's behaviour. We have noted the role that theory of mind is supposed to play in this. Boyer's suggestion fits in to the broader pattern of folk psychological explanation, though he understands theory of mind in terms of models or sets of expectations rather than a body of explicit theory. Therefore, his theory (like that of Kaufman et al.) should be acceptable to all sides in the folk psychology debates that were outlined earlier. Further articulations of this basic picture might depend on where one's commitment lie in that debate about folk psychology, however. The hypothesis we are considering is that normal adults possess intuitive expectations about the normal functioning of other people's psychology, as manifested in their observed behaviour. When these expectations are not satisfied, a dysfunction is inferred, and then understood through a folk model. This initial attribution can be overridden as more information comes in, so that initial attributions of dysfunctions may be retracted.

If Boyer's picture applies to delusion, the application is straightforward. We harbour expectations about the normal fixation of belief in others and we are alert to possible explanations if these expectations are frustrated. The evidence relevant to these expectations could take many forms. Normally, we infer beliefs based on linguistic behaviour other types of behaviour. We might also expect the world to play a role – if something catches fire in front of us and we can both see it, I will expect you to act like you believe there's a fire in the vicinity.

However, a narrow focus on truth tracking and justification of belief misses the many ways in which we acknowledge that beliefs can be caused – but not justified – by psychological processes that are epistemically much less legitimate. Beliefs are often caused by processes that do not justify them; everyday cognition is notoriously prone to wish-fulfilment, bias, and the influence of factors like class position, ideology, or loyalty to a research program. However much we deplore it, we can make sense of it according to our normal ways of understanding human nature. If you know that somebody votes a certain way you can often predict their beliefs about a range of seemingly unrelated matters (the best predictor of support for Brexit among British voters, for example, was support for the return of capital punishment). Beliefs can be related as a matter of logical consequence or as predictions from nature – if it has been raining, I can expect to believe that the streets will be wet. But beliefs can also follow one another as a matter of psychological affiliation or bias. This is one aspect of normal belief fixation that is not well captured by strongly rationalist views of belief, but it is clearly pervasive; people believe all sorts of rubbish without good reasons. People will, for example, believe propositions that they wish to be true. They may not do so where the stakes are high for them personally – your business will be better off if you make that sale, but that might not lead you to believe you have made the sale. However, you might believe that the election was stolen because you want it to be true that your candidate is the more legitimate head of state. Obviously, the fate of the nation is of more import than the health of your small business, but maybe not to you right now. So in some sense you are free to be irrational because the stakes are small for you. The claim is not that irrationality dominates human belief fixation. (I wouldn't recommend betting against that claim, but the argument being made here doesn't depend on it.) Rather, the claim is the conjunction of the familiar point that there is a good deal of non-rational belief fixation, together with the further suggestion that folk psychology, broadly construed, takes this into account. It is entirely consistent with folk psychology to make a prediction that a person is more likely to believe something if their salary depends on it. We can make sense of our readiness to accept these epistemically flawed yet fully human types of belief fixation if we admit that folk psychology expands beyond the remit of rational intentional states. If this is correct, then what should we expect if delusions are a category that folk psychology recognises?

We might not expect a category called 'delusions', though we do see commonsense uses of the term that have some overlap between with scientific uses. But we should expect to see a category of belief-like states that are marked as not predictable or explicable by folk psychology in the extended sense I have conjectured. Folk conceptions of human nature seem to recognise a variety of ways in which norms can be broken – some of these are marked as criminal or attributed to illness or incapacity. Others appear to be marked as pathological, in that we monitor and stigmatize failures to acquire and update beliefs in ways that indicate normal capacity. For Haslam, Ban, and Kaufman (2007), the attribution of deviant folk psychological states involves four main cognitive processes: first, the behaviour is unfamiliar; second, it eludes explanation; third, pathologising sees the locus of the abnormality as within the person; fourth pathologising involves not just a perception of the personas individually deviant, but as an instance of a coherent and reified type of person – an example of a category of human.

All of this could be done without an explicit concept of delusion. A simpler propensity to group deviant believers together suffices. The upshot would be a shared tendency to attribute delusions when resources for explaining deviant beliefs run out – if a belief is not explained via rational inference nor by such nonrational causes as class position or gain or wishful thinking, then we might start to think it must be the output of a pathological process rather than just a non-legitimating one.

In this context its notable that the definition of delusion in *DSM-IV*, that endures in the glossary in *DSM-5*, qualifies the epistemic understanding of delusions with the proviso that what might otherwise seem to be a delusion is in fact not a delusion if it is culturally appropriate. There is something odd about this parenthetical acknowledgement of religion, or other culturally sanctioned beliefs, as non-delusional. Why should a false, incorrectly inferred belief suddenly come to be non-delusional just because the surrounding culture goes along with it? I think we can see this as a nod to the idea that we should expect neurotypical epistemic agents to acquire beliefs that may not stand up to rational investigation but should not be regarded as outside the human norm, and hence are not proper candidates for psychiatric appraisal (for more on delusion and culture see Gold and Gold, Chapter 36).

Boyer argues that some aspects of folk psychology depend on neurocognitive systems that are, to a large degree, cross-culturally invariant and phylogenetically quite ancient. But obviously, many aspects of our understanding of others depend on local norms and ideas about how people should and do behave (Lillard 1997). This is true of both tacit folk psychology and (even more so) explicit models. Even if every culture is largely made up of people with a capacity to attribute intentional states to others and monitor the associated norms, it does not mean that the capacity or the basis for monitoring are culturally invariant, and this is a question that needs further scrutiny. Delusions may be a byproduct of standards for legitimating belief that are inescapably part of the modern world with its stress on rational norms (Murphy 2020). Such norms need monitoring and enforcing, but they may not be a pre-occupation of all cultures.

## 4.  Conclusion

The existing literature on the concept of delusion is dominated by questions about epistemology and rationality. It may be productive to reconfigure this debate by considering delusion as a concept with a home inside a broadly understood folk psychology that incorporates tendencies to judge mental states as pathological.

## Note

1  This section draws on Murphy and Donovan (2015).

## References

American Psychiatric Association (2000). *Diagnostic and Statistical Manual of Mental Disorders*, 4th edition, text revision. Washington, DC: American Psychiatric Association.
American Psychiatric Association (2013). *Diagnostic and Statistical Manual of Mental Disorders*, 5th edition. Washington, DC: American Psychiatric Association.
Andrews, K. (2016). Pluralistic folk psychology and varieties of self-knowledge: An exploration. *Philosophical Explorations*, 18(2), 282–296.
Bortolotti, L. (2009). *Delusions and Other Irrational Beliefs*. Oxford: Oxford University Press.
Boyer, P. (2011). Intuitive expectations and the detection of mental disorder: A cognitive background to Folk-psychiatries. *Philosophical Psychology*, 23, 821–844.

Churchland, P. M. (1981). Eliminative materialism and the propositional attitudes. *Journal of Philosophy*, 78, 67–90.

Doris, J. (2003). *Lack of Character*. Cambridge: Cambridge University Press.

Feyerabend, P. (1963). Mental events and the brain. *Journal of Philosophy*, 40, 295–296.

Fodor, J. (1987). *Psychosemantics*. Cambridge: MIT Press.

Gallagher, S. (2009). Delusional realities. In L. Bortolotti and M. Broome (eds.), *Psychiatry as Cognitive Neuroscience* (pp. 245–266). Oxford: Oxford University Press.

Gerrans, P. (2014). *The Measure of Madness: Philosophy of Mind, Cognitive Neuroscience, and Delusional Thought*. Cambridge, MA: MIT Press. 2014

Goldman, A. (1989). Interpretation psychologized. *Mind and Language*, 4, 161–185; reprinted in M. Davies and T. Stone (Eds.) (1995). *Folk Psychology: The Theory of Mind Debate*. Oxford: Blackwell Publishers.

Goldman, A. I. (2006). *Simulating Minds: The Philosophy, Psychology, and Neuroscience of Mindreading*. Oxford: Oxford University Press.

Gordon, R. (1986). Folk psychology as simulation. *Mind and Language*, 1, 158–171; reprinted in M. Davies and T. Stone (Eds.) (1995). *Folk Psychology: The Theory of Mind Debate*. Oxford: Blackwell Publishers.

Griffiths, P. (1997). *What Emotions Really Are*. Chicago, IL: University of Chicago Press.

Haslam, N., Ban. L., & Kaufman, L. (2007). Lay conceptions of mental disorder: The folk psychiatry model. *Australian Psychologist*, 42, 129–137.

Heal, J. (1986). Replication and functionalism. In J. Butterfield (Ed.), *Language, Mind, and Logic* (pp. 135–150). Cambridge: Cambridge University Press; reprinted in M. Davies and T. Stone (Eds.) (1995). *Folk Psychology: The Theory of Mind Debate*. Oxford: Blackwell Publishers.

Lillard, A. S. (1997). Other folks' theories of mind and behaviour. *Psychological Science*, 8(4), 268–274.

Mercier, H. (2010). The social origins of folk epistemology. *Review of Philosophy and Psychology*, 1, 499–514.

Murphy, D. (2020). Delusions across cultures. In M. Mizumoto, J. Ganeri, & C. Goddard (Eds.), *Ethno-Epistemology: New Directions for Global Epistemology* (pp. 184–200). New York: Routledge.

Murphy, D., & Donovan, C. (2015). Folk psychology. In R. L. Cautin and S. O. Lilienfeld (Eds.), *The Encyclopedia of Clinical Psychology* https://doi.org/10.1002/9781118625392.wbecp416

Noggle, R. (2016). Belief, quasi-belief, and obsessive-compulsive disorder. *Philosophical Psychology*, 29(5): 654–668.

Radden, J. (2011). *On Delusion*. London: Routledge

Ratcliffe, M. (2007). *Rethinking Commonsense Psychology: A Critique of Folk Psychology, Theory of Mind and Simulation*. New York: Palgrave Macmillan.

Sellars, W. (1956). Empiricism and the philosophy of mind. In H. Feigl & M. Scriven (Eds.), *Minnesota Studies in Philosophy of Science* (vol. 1, pp. 253–329). Minneapolis: University of Minnesota Press.

Sperber, D., Clément, F., Heintz, C., Mascaro, O., Mercier, H., Origgi, G., & Wilson, D. (2010). Epistemic vigilance. *Mind & Language*, 25, 359–393.

Stich, S. (1983). *From Folk Psychology to Cognitive Science*. Cambridge: MIT Press.

Stich, S. (1996). *Deconstructing the Mind*. Oxford: Oxford University Press.

Sullivan-Bissett, E., Bortolotti, L., Broome, M., & Mameli, M. (2017). Moral and legal implications of the continuity between delusional and non-delusional beliefs. In G. Keil (Ed.), *Vagueness in Psychiatry* (pp. 191–201). Oxford: Oxford University Press.

Zawidzki, T. (2013). *Mindshaping*. Cambridge: MIT Press.

# PART 5

# Delusion formation

# 26

# EMPIRICISM

*Federico Bongiorno and Matthew Parrott*

People develop delusions in association with a number of different conditions, including schizophrenia, dementia, multiple sclerosis, and traumatic injury to the brain (Coltheart et al. 2011). Yet none of these conditions is by itself sufficient for someone to become delusional. So why exactly do only certain people develop delusions, while others do not? Following standard diagnostic criteria, we'll assume that a significant part of what it is to be delusional is to hold a highly unusual belief, a belief that is poorly supported by any evidence, and is also retained even when its subject is vividly presented with counterevidence. On this assumption, different theories of delusion are aiming to understand what exactly leads people to hold delusional beliefs.

Since there is an enormous amount of theoretical work that addresses this topic, it has become common practice to group theories into categories based on general features they have in common. Perhaps the most influential classificatory scheme was introduced by John Campbell, who presented a distinction between what he labelled 'rationalist' and 'empiricist' approaches to explaining delusions (Campbell 2001). Campbell's scheme has been widely accepted, and a brief survey of the contemporary literature would suggest that the empiricist paradigm is now well-established as the dominant theoretical approach to explaining delusional beliefs (for further discussion, see Noordhof and Sullivan-Bissett 2021).

In the broadest sense, 'empiricism' can be understood as the view that sensory experience causally generates delusions. Yet, even though the majority of contemporary theorists would tend to identify themselves as 'empiricists', it is not clear that they share the same general theoretical commitments or methodological principles. We therefore believe that it is useful to distinguish different senses of 'empiricism'. This will be our task in the first three sections of this chapter, in which we shall lay out different ways in which someone might pursue an empiricist approach to understanding delusion formation.

Once we have the different types of empiricism in view, we shall turn to Campbell's defence of rationalism (for detailed discussion of rationalism, see Ohlhorst, Chapter 27). As we will see, Campbell's rationalism rejects the central empiricist idea that sensory experiences causally generate delusional beliefs. This may be part of the reason that few contemporary theorists identify as rationalists. Since there is experimental evidence confirming

 DOI: 10.4324/9781003296386-32

the occurrence of anomalous sensory experiences in at least certain cases of delusion (e.g., Brighetti et al. 2007; Prakash et al. 2012), rationalism may strike many as an unpromising research paradigm.

Some empiricists think that sensory experiences not only causally generate delusional beliefs but that they do so in virtue of lending some sort of (minimal) rational support to them. In this sense, they think of delusional beliefs as broadly rational responses to experience, or as based on reasons. Campbell's rationalism also rejects this idea. Yet, once we distinguish different kinds of empiricism, we will see that there are non-empiricist ways to develop the normative thesis that delusions are based on reasons, two of which we shall present in Section 4.

Contemporary discussions of delusion often tacitly assume that Campbell's disjunction of empiricism and rationalism is both exclusive and exhaustive. We think there is little to be said for this assumption. Thus, in Section 5, we briefly present two theoretical frameworks that cannot easily be categorised as either empiricist or rationalist, and one that incorporates elements of both. This does not mean that the categories of empiricism and rationalism are mistaken, or unhelpful, only that they do not exhaust the full range of possibilities for answering questions about why people develop delusions.

## 1. Normative empiricism

When Campbell introduces the idea that many theoretical approaches to understanding delusion formation are 'empiricist', he emphasises the normative or reason-giving role of sensory experience. Indeed, Campbell explicitly defines empiricism in terms of its commitment to the idea that a delusion is 'a rational response to highly unusual experiences that the subject has, perhaps as a result of organic damage' (Campbell 2001: 89; Bayne and Pacherie 2004). Thus, empiricism, for Campbell, is not simply the claim that some strange or unusual experiences figures somehow in the onset of delusional thinking, or in the establishing of a delusional belief. It is the stronger claim that certain kinds of sensory experiences, no matter how seemingly bizarre or unusual, provide warrant, or justification, or give a subject reasons for accepting a delusional belief. It is in this sense that a delusional belief is a 'rational response' to a sensory experience. On the normative conception of empiricism, delusion formation is a matter of an individual adopting a belief for broadly epistemic reasons (Bayne 2017).

This is the sort of picture of delusion formation that one finds articulated in the work of Brendan Maher. Maher insists that someone adopts a delusional belief 'because of evidence powerful enough to support it' (1974: 99), and that delusional beliefs are 'rational, given the intensity of the experiences that they are adopted to explain' (1974: 105; cf. Maher 1999). In this respect, Maher thinks delusional beliefs are formed in the same way as non-delusional beliefs. In both cases, an agent undergoes a particular sensory experience that functions as evidence for the truth of some proposition $P$, and the individual believes that $P$ on the basis of that evidence. For Maher, the only difference in cases of delusion is that the agent's sensory experiences are highly unusual and also felt to be extremely significant.

The normative empiricist approach can also be found in an extremely influential neuropsychiatric model of delusions of misidentification (Ellis and Young 1990). We can illustrate the model by considering how it explains Capgras delusion, which is the delusional belief that a familiar person or object in one's life has been replaced by an imposter

(Coltheart and Davies 2022). The central idea of this neuropsychiatric model is that face recognition is supported by two distinct neurocognitive pathways, one of which processes affect, and the other of which processes semantic information concerning identity (Ellis and Young 1990; Stone and Young 1997). According to this model, the Capgras delusion is caused by damage to the affective processing pathway, which results in a person maintaining the ability to visually recognise familiar faces, but lacking the feeling of familiarity which normally accompanies visual experiences of close friends or family members. As a result of this damage, a person will have 'an experience of seeing a face that looks just like their relative, but without experiencing the affective response that would normally be part and parcel of that experience' (Stone and Young 1997: 337).[1] This experience is then treated by the subject as a reason to adopt the delusional belief that their relative has been replaced by an imposter. As with Maher, this is a theory according to which the occurrence of an anomalous sensory experience is taken to warrant or justify the imposter belief.

Over the last 25 years or so, normative empiricism has developed along two different avenues. According to a framework that has come to be known as 'explanationism', a person forms a delusional belief in order to 'explain' her anomalous sensory experience. Explanationism is a natural extension of the idea that people frequently form novel beliefs in order to explain away or make sense of surprising evidence (Coltheart and Davies 2021). For instance, in the case of Capgras delusion, an explanationist might claim that an individual who has an anomalous experience of their mother will adopt the delusional belief that the person is an imposter because it 'provides an explanation of this unusual phenomenon' (Coltheart et al. 2011: 284). This language of 'explanation' clarifies the reason-giving relation between sensory experience and belief. It highlights how, for the explanationist, the logical structure of the relation is that of an abductive inference (rather than, for instance, some type of enumerative induction).[2]

The second direction in which normative empiricism has developed is a framework known as 'endorsement theory'. Rather than thinking that delusional beliefs are adopted in order to explain experiences, the endorsement theorist claims that they are simply the natural result of taking the content of a perceptual experience 'at face value' (Bayne and Pacherie 2004; Pacherie 2009). In contrast to the explanationist, the endorsement theorist will typically claim that the anomalous sensory experiences found in cases of delusion have the exact same contents, or perhaps very similar contents, to the contents of delusional beliefs. An endorsement account of Capgras delusion might claim, for instance, that patients have experiences with the content <that is an imposter> (Pacherie 2009: 110; cf. Bongiorno 2019) or perhaps <that looks like mum, but is not really her> (Davies et al. 2001: 50). It is natural to think of beliefs as encoding or somehow taking up the content of visual experiences. But notice that the notion of 'endorsement' is a normative concept; it is a concept that suggests that one is standing behind, or approving of the content that one believes. To 'endorse' a content is not simply to happen to believe it, but to recognise it as something that one has reason to believe. It is in this sense that the endorsement theorist is a type of normative empiricist. They think a person is *prima facie* warranted or justified in believing the contents of any vivid sensory experience, even a highly unusual one.[3]

Someone might object to the coherence of the normative empiricist approach on the grounds that delusional beliefs are manifestly irrational, and so they simply could not be warranted or justified. How, one might wonder, could a strange or anomalous experience provide any sort of reason for a delusional belief? Indeed, the sorts of experiences that one encounters in delusional subjects might seem to be too strange to justify anything at all.

Similarly, one might think that some beliefs, like the belief that one's mother is a qualitatively identical imposter, are so outlandish that no type of experience could possibly justify accepting it.[4] The worry for normative empiricism is that transitions from highly anomalous sensory experiences to delusional beliefs, even ones where we assume the two share the exact same content, could not be reason-giving (Campbell 2001).

However, a normative empiricist is not committed to the view that delusional beliefs are formed in response to *objectively* good epistemic reasons. Rather, they need only hold the weaker thesis that delusional subjects treat their experiences as reasons or justification for their beliefs, even if, from a more objective perspective, we might very well understand that this is a mistake (Pollock 1979: 109–110; compare Grice, 2001, Ch. 2).

As an analogy, suppose certain people formed beliefs in empirical generalisations in accordance with an inference rule of counter-induction. Whenever these individuals faced an enumerative series of F's that are G, rather than believing that all F's are G, or that the next F will be G, they form the belief that most F's are not-G (Van Cleve 1984). Can we really regard a subject who makes an inference to a counter-inductive conclusion as someone who is making a rational transition? Perhaps not. But even if *we* don't think counter-induction is a good rule of inference, it remains the case that a subject who treats evidence this way is treating it as a reason or as justification for believing that most F's are not-G. From a more objective point of view, we may have doubts as to whether an enumerative series could really give a reason for believing a counter-inductive conclusion, but that conclusion is nevertheless plausibly a 'rational response' from the subject's own point of view. Similarly, the normative empiricist is only committed to thinking that anomalous sensory experiences are treated by delusional subjects as reasons, or justification, or warrant for their delusional beliefs, even if, from a more objective perspective, things seem different.

## 2. Causal empiricism

The normative conception of empiricism seems natural when we think of sensory experience in normative terms, as something that grounds or justifies beliefs.[5] But the normative conception of sensory experience is not mandatory. We might think of sensory experiences not as reasons or justification, but as nothing more than causal stimuli. Indeed, Donald Davidson famously argued that sensory experiences could not be reasons for belief. He claimed that 'sensations cause some beliefs and in *this* sense are the basis or grounds of those beliefs. But a causal explanation of a belief does not show how or why the belief is justified' (1986a: 143). Davidson's conception of sensory experience recommends a *merely* causal conception of empiricism.

According to a (merely) causal empiricism, undergoing an anomalous sensory experience is causally sufficient, or causally necessary, for forming a delusional belief. This, of course, means that normative empiricism is itself a type of causal empiricism, it is just that the normative theorist insists that experiences cause beliefs in virtue of their standing in some type of reason-giving relation. But there are ways to develop causal empiricism in a non-normative direction. On these sorts of views, the relation between an anomalous sensory experience and a belief is brute causation.

For instance, causal empiricism is the theoretical paradigm accepted by theorists attracted to a so-called 'Spinozan' view of perceptual belief. The central idea of the Spinozan theory is that the contents of (some) sensory experiences are automatically believed, without critical assessment or reflective scrutiny. Thus, according to the Spinozan theory, simply apprehending the perceptual presentation of *P* generates the belief that *P*. In this sense, forming a belief is a completely automatic response to a presented content (Mandelbaum 2014).

To give a basic sense of this view, consider how it gives a clear prediction in cases of known visual illusion. Suppose that someone knows they are looking at a Ponzo illusion, an illusion in which two lines of equal length appear to be different in length. On many theories, this background knowledge would inhibit the agent's inclination to believe that the lines are different lengths, and it would normally do so by undermining the justificatory status of the visual experience. After all, the agent *knows* they are looking at an illusion. The Spinozan view recommends a different picture. It claims that when the agent is perceptually presented with an appearance of two equal lines, this immediately causes them to believe the lines are equal. The agent may be able to reflectively evaluate or reject this belief after it has been adopted, but, for the Spinozan, the experience of the lines is sufficient to cause the agent to acquire the belief.

The Spinozan conception can easily be applied to delusions (Davies and Egan 2013; Bongiorno 2022). For instance, a Spinozan theory could maintain that a person who has an anomalous experience of their mother's face would automatically believe that their mother is an imposter. For the Spinozan, simply entertaining the imposter proposition would be causally sufficient for believing it, regardless of whatever else the person might believe.[6]

The Spinozan view has some odd consequences, but it is not the only way to develop a merely causal version of empiricism. We might think, for instance, that delusional beliefs are formed on the basis of non-rational associative transitions. The basic idea would be that the psychology of a delusional subject includes stored associative structures that link together the occurrence of an anomalous experience with the content of a delusional belief. Because of these structures, the occurrence, or perhaps the repeated occurrence of, for instance, an irregular experience of their mother's face, causes the individual to think that their mother has been replaced by an imposter. In cases where the associative links are sufficiently strong, the result would be a delusional belief. This sort of account would maintain that delusional beliefs are causally generated by anomalous sensory experiences, but because associative transitions are insensitive to reasons, it would be a non-normative type of empiricism (Mandelbaum and Quilty-Dunn 2019).

As these examples illustrate, the basic paradigm of causal empiricism offers us a broader conception of the relationship between sensory experience and belief than we find in normative empiricist views. One could therefore commit to a causal empiricist framework, even if one were worried about the rationality of transitions between anomalous sensory experiences and delusional beliefs.

## 3.   Content empiricism

Both normative empiricism and (merely) causal empiricism are views primarily about the nature of the relation between sensory experience and belief. But, in the history of philosophy, empiricism is often thought of as a doctrine about meaning or reference. Hume and Locke are primarily concerned with how the content of ideas is fixed by sensory experience. Similarly, many empiricists in the early 20th century were concerned with how sensory experiences conferred meaning on some privileged class of sentences, for instance the sentences of a sense-data language (e.g., Schlick 1932; Ayer 1936). Following on from this tradition, we could interpret 'empiricism' primarily as a thesis about the meaning or content of delusional beliefs.

The primary theoretical commitment of content empiricism is the idea that delusional beliefs are meaningful, or have content, only insofar as they can be traced back to sensory experience.[7] This need not be understood in an atomic way, such that every meaningful term figuring in the content of a delusional belief must itself be grounded in some aspect of sensory experience. The content empiricist could think that something like whole propositions are the most basic unit of meaning, and therefore hold that the content of a delusional belief is meaningful if and only if the proposition that one believes is appropriately grounded in sensory experience. Content empiricism would stand in opposition to any framework according to which delusional beliefs could have meaningful contents in some way that is independent of sensory experience.

One reason to adopt the content empiricist paradigm is that it offers very clear criteria for distinguishing meaningful expressions from nonsense. This can be especially useful when we consider the verbal expression of delusional beliefs, because these have struck some theorists as nonsensical. Perhaps most prominently, Karl Jaspers is well-known for holding the view that verbal expressions of what he called 'primary delusions' are not meaningful. According to Jaspers, when we encounter a person trying to articulate a delusional experience, their experience 'remain[s] largely incomprehensible, unreal and beyond our understanding' (1913/1997: 98; Berrios 1991). Although Jaspers does concede that delusional beliefs are often meaningful to their subjects, he thinks this subjective sense of meaning undergoes what he calls a 'radical transformation', making it completely incomprehensible to others.

Many have found it difficult to accept Jaspers's conclusion in full generality. Doing so would mean that every person who tried to express a delusional belief would be speaking nonsense.[8] Content empiricism can help us to resist this conclusion. As we have seen, according to content empiricism, certain expressions may seem *prima facie* puzzling, or nonsensical, for instance utterances like 'there's been someone like my son's double' or 'I am dead', but these can nevertheless be meaningful if they are ultimately derived from sensory experience. So, in contrast to Jaspers, the content of a delusional belief can be meaningful (and thus its verbal expression can be meaningful), if it is some proposition, perhaps not the one typically associated with the utterance, that is appropriately grounded in experience.

To quickly see how this might work, consider Cotard syndrome. If we hear someone sincerely report 'I am dead', we might be inclined to think the person has lost their grip on the meaning of 'being dead'. But content empiricism lays the ground for a different response. It suggests that we might *translate* the initial expression into some other expression like 'I don't feel like I have a body' (Young and Leafhead 1996; Billon 2017). This is plausibly meaningful because its central terms all have contents determined by sensory experience, and so, if we take the translation to properly express the content of the delusional belief, then it turns out to be meaningful after all (for more on delusion and meaning see Ritunnano and Littlemore, Chapter 2).

## 4. Rationalism and reasons

There are various reasons that one might be suspicious of empiricism. One might worry about whether each and every delusion can really be traced back to some type of sensory experience. Or, one might have more general worries about the epistemology presupposed by empiricist theories. The alternative paradigm which Campbell presents he labels *rationalism*.

Campbell's rationalism departs from empiricism on two key points. First, Campbell rejects the normative claim that delusional beliefs are 'broadly rational' responses to sensory experiences. Second, Campbell rejects the causal claim that delusional beliefs are causally generated by sensory experiences. Instead, he suggests that the direction of causal explanation works in the opposite direction. Rather than thinking, as the empiricist does, that an unusual experience occurs first, which causally explains why an individual develops a delusional belief, Campbell is committed to the idea that one or more delusional beliefs occur first, and these causally explain why subjects have unusual sensory experiences.[9]

Campbell attempts to further explicate the connection between a delusional belief and sensory experience using Wittgenstein's notion of a 'framework proposition' (2001: 97). For Wittgenstein, a framework proposition is a type of proposition that is completely immune from empirical or rational scrutiny because it is 'treated' as a fundamental background assumption, one which grounds the entire practice of empirical confirmation and disconfirmation. In other words, our acceptance of framework propositions functions to establish epistemic standards, and thus underlies the reason-giving or justificatory relations which hold between the empirical beliefs we hold (for discussion of framework propositions, see Ohlhorst, Chapter 27, and Eilan 2001).

But if delusional beliefs function like framework propositions and are not caused by sensory experience, as the empiricist thinks, then where do they come from? What is it exactly that leads a person to start thinking their mother is an imposter, if not a strange experience of her face? Campbell suggests that delusional beliefs arise from what he calls an 'organic malfunction' to the brain. The thought seems to be that some kind of brain damage directly causes a person to believe, for instance, that their mother is an imposter. Then, once that belief is established as a 'framework', it has downstream causal consequences, including the attenuation of affective responses when one looks at one's mother. As Campbell says, the rationalist 'would expect there to be differences in the affective aspects of the patients perceptions of other people' (2001: 97).

Campbell presents his version of rationalism very briefly, and several philosophers have raised objections to it, which we shall not rehearse here (for discussion of these objections, see Ohlhorst, Chapter 27, and Bayne and Pacherie 2004). The one point we would like to make here is that Campbell's view is not the only theoretical alternative to empiricism. There are ways to develop alternative views which, like Campbell, reject the central doctrines of empiricism, but which do not rely so heavily on analogies with Wittgensteinian themes. In order to bring them into view, we need to keep in mind that the two theoretical commitments of Campbell's rationalism are distinct. Campbell is primarily concerned with the direction of causal explanation between anomalous sensory experiences and delusional beliefs. However, it is possible to develop a view which focuses primarily on the normative grounds of delusional beliefs, or on the reasons for which delusional beliefs are established. Indeed, one might wish to remain fairly neutral about the causal relation between experience and belief, while nevertheless holding onto the idea that delusional beliefs are 'broadly rational' responses. Campbell himself does not consider this possibility because he thinks of delusions as 'framework propositions' that lie outside the realm of normativity. But it is possible to deny the normative empiricist thesis that sensory experiences constitute reasons, or justification or warrant for delusional beliefs, while nevertheless accepting that delusions are formed for epistemic reasons.

For instance, one might adopt a view according to which the reason a person accepts a delusional belief is not because of an experience, but because of other things the person believes. That is, one might think that delusional beliefs are 'broadly rational' responses to other beliefs. This would be a sort of 'coherentist' view of rational support that Davidson thought was true of beliefs generally (Davidson 1986a). On a Davidsonian view, the reason that someone would believe, for instance, that their mother is an imposter, would need to be traced back to other things they believed, such as, for instance, the belief that one's father had colluded with the imposter to murder their mother (Brighetti et al. 2007).

One might worry that this sort of coherentist view would have the consequence that everything a delusional subject believes comes out as irrational, or as delusional, because, on this picture, there is a sense in which the entire network of a person's beliefs gives rational support to the delusional belief. But someone attracted to this sort of view can resist this worry. Given the immense complexity of the system of overlapping reason-giving relations, it seems perfectly possible that a delusional belief could be partially supported by many ordinary empirical beliefs, even if it also partially supported by some delusional or quasi-delusional ones.

A different way to avoid this concern would be to appeal to the notion of psychological fragmentation.[10] To say that a person's psychology is fragmented is just to say that it is partitioned into somewhat autonomous or independent psychological structures (Davidson 1982). Within each partition there would be a set of beliefs that stood in mutually supportive reason-giving relations, yet there would be no reason-giving relations that held across distinct partitions. Several theorists working on delusional beliefs have appealed to some conception of psychological fragmentation (e.g., Bortolotti 2009; Davies and Egan 2013). On such view, since a delusional belief would be embedded within a somewhat autonomous fragment, we would not be forced to think that everything the person thinks is irrational or delusional.

Another worry that one might have about this type of coherentist view is that it is not clear how a bizarre delusional belief could ever arise. If a person's psychological life is a rationally coherent system of beliefs prior to the onset of delusion, then what sort of thing would cause a delusional belief that fails to cohere with that body of beliefs?

This is a good question, which we unfortunately cannot pursue in this chapter. But it is worth noting that in response, Davidson himself would have sided with the causal empiricist. Davidson thought that empirical beliefs were caused by sensory experiences, even though those did not constitute evidence or reasons for them (Davidson 1986a). However, it is possible to develop a view that does not follow him on this point. To do so, one would need to conceive of the causal origins of a delusional belief as something other than sensory experience, but we have already seen one way to do this, namely Campbell's suggestion that some type of organic brain damage directly causes the formation of a delusional belief, after which it becomes embedded in a system of rationally supporting beliefs.

Someone attracted to the idea that delusional beliefs are, in some sense, responses to reasons is not forced to think that those reasons are other beliefs. Instead, one could think they are something like intuitions, or intellectual presentations. According to certain non-reductive views, intuitions are *sui generis* attitudes which present contents as true. For instance, John Bengson argues that 'in having an intuition…it is presented to one as being the case that things are a certain way' (2015: 726). That is to say that having an intuition that $P$ makes it seem to you that $P$ is true, and so therefore plausibly gives you a good reason to believe that $P$ (which may be defeated).[11] This sort of transition from intuition to belief may be how certain delusions arise. For example, one schizophrenic individual describes how it just seemed to him that the shadow of Satan was on his living room floor (Emmons et al.

1997). Similarly, John Nash, who suffered from schizophrenia, once said, 'the ideas I had about supernatural beings came to me the same way that my mathematical ideas did. So I took them seriously' (Nasar 1998: 11). We naturally think mathematical beliefs are based on intuition, and so, if we take Nash at his word, it would seem that his delusional beliefs may be as well.

## 5. Exhaustiveness and exclusivity

In philosophy, disjunctions are often presumed to be both exhaustive and exclusive. However, the disjunction of rationalist and empiricist accounts of delusional belief is neither of these. There are contemporary accounts of delusional beliefs that seem to include elements from both categories, and there are other accounts that do not fit neatly into either one. In this final section, we will briefly give examples of each in order to demonstrate that there are actually many more options for explaining delusion formation than the rationalism/empiricism disjunction might initially suggest.

Let's start with exclusivity. As we have characterised it, empiricism, in both its normative and causal forms, is committed to the direction of explanation of a delusional belief proceeding from the occurrence of an unusual experience to the formation of a delusional belief. By contrast, Campbell's rationalism is committed to the converse direction. It holds that agents first form delusional beliefs, which then cause them to develop anomalous experiences. Explanation is asymmetric and so it would be natural to think that only one of these could be correct.

Nevertheless, many computational psychiatrists are now attracted to predictive processing accounts of delusional beliefs. According to predictive processing models, delusional beliefs are formed through complex, multi-level, dynamic processes. Very briefly, the central idea of the predictive processing approach is that the brain is constantly trying to 'predict' incoming sensory stimulation by virtue of constructing probabilistic models of the immediate environment (Friston 2010; Hohwy 2013). When those models are accurate, nothing happens. Yet, when they are inaccurate, a sequence of 'error signals' is propagated through the brain so that it is able to make adjustments to its predictive model. Predictive processing theorists think that, in every domain, the brain aims to solve just one computational problem – how to best minimise error. Thus, a predictive processing explanation of delusional belief (or indeed of anything else) will consist of some kind of dynamic interaction between predictive models and the incoming sensory stimulus.[12] Although neither of these theoretical constructs are quite what rationalists or empiricists have in mind, the predictive processing approach seems to accept aspects of each of these paradigms (for more on predictive processing accounts, see Corlett, Chapter 30; Hohwy 2004).

Now for exhaustiveness. In the previous section, we looked at two different possible ways in which one could develop reasons-based theories of delusion formation, neither of which can be classified as either rationalist or empiricist. But, there are also existing theoretical accounts of delusion formation that do not fit into either of these categories. So the rationalism/empiricism disjunction does not even exhaust the range of actual theories.

For example, some researchers working on delusions have been impressed by the way beliefs function to organise social structures. These theorists claim that social processes and mechanisms are able to directly cause beliefs, including delusional ones. Thus, Vaughan Bell and colleagues write that 'social influence can form and maintain beliefs that are as epistemically irrational, affectively loaded, and strongly held as delusional beliefs' (2021: 4; Williams

2021). It isn't clear how exactly 'social influence' forms beliefs or maintains beliefs, nor is it clear exactly what a social process or mechanism is. But, on one way of understanding these claims, social factors causally influence the ways individuals process empirical evidence (Williams 2020). That seems obviously true. But it is compatible with empiricism. However, another way to understand the claim that 'social influence' forms beliefs is to hypothesise that social processes or mechanisms directly cause beliefs in ways that are insensitive to reasons or evidence. For instance, it may be that the best explanation for why someone believes that senior members of the Democratic Party are involved in sex trafficking is that everyone in their community believes it. The fact that everyone believes it is not, on this view, evidence that the belief is true or an epistemic reason in its favour. Rather, the idea is that the person forms the belief as a result of sensitivity to 'social influence'.

The social influence hypothesis might seem like a nonstarter when it comes to delusional beliefs. Even though the content of delusional beliefs often involves a person's social environment, individuals with delusions tend to be relatively isolated and detached from social groups. What group of people would be exerting influence on someone who thinks their mother is an imposter, or that they are infested with parasites? Unlike people who hold conspiratorial beliefs, or who accept bizarre ideologies, delusional individuals are not usually members of social groups of likeminded thinkers. So it is difficult to see how holding a delusional belief could possibly be the result of some kind of direct 'social influence'.

Nonetheless, the social influence hypothesis may not be a complete dead end. If, as the view suggests, there really are social processes or mechanisms that generate beliefs, then it should be possible for those to become impaired. Thus, we might hypothesise that dysfunctional or impaired social processes or mechanisms generate delusional beliefs. Although there would need to be much more discussion of how exactly a social process becomes impaired, this would be a picture according to which social factors explained the formation of delusional beliefs without lending them rational support, which would distinguish it from both rationalism and empiricism (for more on the social turn in delusions research, see Williams, Chapter 35).[13]

To briefly take just one more example, consider theorists who adopt a 'phenomenological approach' to understanding delusions. Many of those attracted to this framework insist that delusions involve fundamental disturbances to 'the most basic structure of experience', which includes such things as lived time, space, causality, felt reality status, and self-experience (Sass and Pienkos 2013: 633). Although phenomenologists do sometimes refer to 'delusional experiences', they think of these as a symptom of some crucial alteration in the framework of experience. For instance, Matthew Ratcliffe argues that certain delusions are expressions of 'existential orientations', understood here as the 'backgrounds' within which any token experience can be had. The phenomenological approach to explaining delusional beliefs therefore does not seem to be either rationalist or empiricist.

## 6.  Conclusion

Despite receiving a fair amount of attention in recent years, delusional beliefs remain poorly understood. Even in cases where there appears to be relevant experimental evidence, such as the case of Capgras delusion, there is little agreement among theorists as to the aetiology. This sort of explanatory impasse could reasonably be taken to suggest that the field is in need of a novel theoretical approach. However, there is a risk that theoretical innovation might be hindered by presupposing too rigid a picture of the logical space of theoretical options.

The primary aim of this chapter has been to highlight different ways of understanding empiricism. Since it was first articulated by Campbell, empiricism has come to dominate research programmes in cognitive neuropsychology and computational psychiatry, even in cases where researchers depart from some of its central principles. Nevertheless, it seems worthwhile to get a clear sense of different avenues along which an explanatory account of delusion could be developed. Empiricism is bound to seem like the only plausible research paradigm if we restrict our attention to monothematic delusions, like the Capgras delusion, for which there is strong experimental evidence implicating anomalous sensory experience. Yet it is not obvious that what we learn from these sorts of cases can generalise to all cases of delusion, particularly to the sorts of delusional systems found in case of schizophrenia. To fully explain these more perplexing phenomena, theorists may need to appeal to some other approach. Indeed, given the tremendous variety among cases of delusion, we think it is best to have as many options available as possible.

## Acknowledgements

Federico Bongiorno is grateful to Portuguese Funds through FCT – Fundaçao para Ciência e a Tecnologia, I.P., within the project UIDP/00310/2020, for supporting his work on this chapter. Matthew Parrott is grateful to the British Academy for generously awarding him a Mid-Career Fellowship, which supported his work on this chapter.

## Notes

1 As has been widely discussed, responses in one's autonomic nervous system do not register consciously. Yet it is plausible to think that abnormal autonomic activity could generate an unusual conscious experience, perhaps a generic sense of something being amiss with the familiar looking face. This experience would likely be odd and would prompt one to go searching for a way to explain. For further discussion, see Coltheart et al. (2010).

2 For other explanationists, the logical structure takes the form of Bayesian inference (for discussion of Bayesianism, see Davies and Egan 2013; McKay 2012; Parrott 2016, and Laukaityte and Colombo, Chapter 32).

3 An epistemological theory that would seem to support the endorsement theory would be dogmatism (Pryor 1990).

4 To take an example of this, David Lewis thought that certain beliefs, like the belief that unexamined emeralds are grue, were 'unreasonable in a strong sense' and so simply could not be justified (1986: 38–39).

5 For a detailed explication of this conception of sensory experience, see McDowell (1994).

6 A full-blown Spinozan account of delusion formation would need to explain why the delusional belief isn't immediately defeated or rejected on the basis of the available evidence. For some ideas in this direction, see Bongiorno (2022).

7 Because it is concerned with meaning or content, content empiricism is compatible with either of the previous versions of empiricism.

8 Indeed, it is not clear that Jaspers himself thinks expressions of delusional beliefs are *impossible* to understand in every single case (Eilan 2000).

9 Rather often this distinction between directions of explanation is put in terms of empiricism being a 'bottom-up' framework and rationalism being a 'top-down' framework (Bayne and Pacherie 2004; Bortolotti 2022).

10 Davidson himself appeals to fragmentation to explain self-deception (Davidson 1982, 1986b).

11 How one feels about the intuitionist view depends upon how liberal one is about what counts as 'sensory experience'. Intellectual seemings, as Bengson thinks of them, obviously do not involve sensory organs, like eyes, or ears. But in other respects, they seem very similar to paradigmatic sensory experiences. Thus, if one adopts a liberal enough conception of sensory experience, or

something like what Shoemaker (1994) calls the 'broad perceptual model', then the intuitionist view could plausibly be regarded as an empiricist view.

12 To see different ways in which a predictive processing account of delusion could be developed, see Parrott (2020).

13 To be clear, just saying that social factors cause the formation of delusional beliefs is logically compatible with the coherentist view that we considered in Section 4. For the social approach to be wholly distinct, one would need to deny that delusional beliefs were rationally supported by other beliefs. We suspect that most theorists attracted to 'social influence' views would deny this.

# References


Ayer, A. J. (1936) *Language, Truth, and Logic.* London: Dover.

Bayne, T. (2017) "Delusion and the Norms of Rationality," in T. Hung, and T. J. Lane (eds.), *Rationality: Constraints and Contexts.* Cambridge, MA: Academic Press. pp. 77–94.

Bayne, T. and Pacherie, E. (2004) "Bottom-Up or Top-Down: Campbell's Rationalist Account of Monothematic Delusions," *Philosophy, Psychiatry, and Psychology* 11 (1): 1–11.

Bell, V., Raihani, N. and Wilkinson, S. (2021) "Derationalising Delusions," *Clinical Psychological Science* 1: 24–37.

Bengson, J. (2015) "The Intellectual Given," *Mind* 124 (495): 707–760.

Berrios, G. E. (1991) "Delusions as 'Wrong Beliefs': A Conceptual History," *The British Journal of Psychiatry* 159 (S14): 6–13.

Billon, A. (2017) "Mineness First," in Adrian J. T. Alsmith and Frédérique de Vignemont (eds.), *The Subject's Matter: Self-Consciousness and the Body.* Boston, MA: MIT Press. pp. 189–216.

Bongiorno, F. (2019) "Is the Capgras Delusion and Endorsement of Experience?," *Mind and Language* 35 (3): 293–312.

Bongiorno, F. (2022) "Spinozan Doxasticism about Delusions," *Pacific Philosophical Quarterly* 103 (4): 720–752.

Bortolotti, L. (2009) *Delusions and Other Irrational Beliefs.* Oxford: Oxford University Press.

Bortolotti, L. (2022) "Delusions," In E. N. Zalta (ed.), *The Stanford Encyclopedia of Philosophy.* https://plato.stanford.edu/entries/delusion/

Brighetti, G., Bonifacci, P., Borlimi, R., and Ottaviani, C. (2007) "'Far From the Heart, Far from the Eye': Evidence from the Capgras Delusion," *Cognitive Neuropsychiatry* 1 (3): 189–197.

Campbell, J. (2001) "Rationality, Meaning, the Analysis of Delusion," *Philosophy, Psychiatry and Psychology* 8 (2–3): 89–100.

Coltheart, M., and Davies, M. (2021) "How Unexpected Observations Lead to New Beliefs: A Peircean Pathway," *Consciousness and Cognition* 87: 103037.

Coltheart, M., and Davies, M. (2022) "What Is Capgras Delusion?," *Cognitive Neuropsychiatry* 27: 69–82.

Coltheart, M., Menzies, P., and Sutton, J. (2010) "Abductive Inference and Delusional Belief," *Cognitive Neuropsychiatry* 15: 261–287.

Coltheart, M., Langdon, R., and McKay, R. (2011) "Delusional Belief," *Annual Review of Psychology* 62: 271–298.

Davidson, D. (1982) "Paradoxes of Irrationality," in D. Davidson (ed.), *Problems of Rationality.* Oxford: Oxford University Press. pp. 169–188.

Davidson, D. (1986a) "A Coherence Theory of Truth and Knowledge," in D. Davidson (ed.), *Subjective, Intersubjective, Objective.* Oxford: Oxford University Press. pp. 137–158.

Davidson, D. (1986b) "Deception and Division," in D. Davidson (ed.), *Problems of Rationality.* Oxford: Oxford University Press. pp. 199–212.

Davies, M., Coltheart, M.. Langdon, R. and Breen, N. (2001) "Monothematic Delusions: Towards a Two-Factor Account," *Philosophy, Psychiatry and Psychology* 8: 133–58.

Davies, M. and Egan, A. (2013) "Delusion: Cognitive Approaches – Bayesian Inference and Compartmentalisation," in K. W. M. Fulford, M. Davies, and R. G. T. Gipps, G. Graham, J. Z. Sadler, G. Stanghellini, and T. Thornton (eds.), *The Oxford Handbook of Philosophy and Psychiatry.* Oxford: Oxford University Press. pp. 689–727.

Eilan, N. (2000) "On Understanding Schizophrenia," in D. Zahavi (ed.), *Exploring the Self: Philosophical and Psychopathological Perspectives on Self-Experience.* Amsterdam: John Benjamins Publishing. pp. 97–113.

Eilan, N. (2001) "Meaning, Truth, and the Self: Commentary on Campbell and Parnas and Sass," *Philosophy, Psychiatry, and Psychology* 8 (2): 121–132.

Ellis, H., and Young, A. (1990) "Accounting for Delusional Misidentifications," *The British Journal of Psychiatry* 157 (2): 239–248.

Emmons, S., Geiser, C., Kaplan, K., and Harrow, M. (1997) *Living with Schizophrenia*. London: Taylor and Francis.

Friston, K. (2010) "The Free-Energy Principle: A Unified Brain Theory?," *Nature Reviews Neuroscience* 11 (2): 127–138.

Grice, P. (2001) *Aspects of Reason*. Oxford: Clarendon Press.

Hohwy, J. (2004) "Top-Down or Bottom-Up in Delusion Formation," *Philosophy, Psychiatry, Psychology* 11 (1): 65–70.

Hohwy, J. (2013) *The Predictive Mind*. Oxford: Oxford University Press.

Jaspers, K. (1913/1997) *General Psychopathology*. Baltimore, MD: Johns Hopkins University Press.

Lewis, D. (1986) *On the Plurality of Worlds*. London: Wiley-Blackwell.

Maher, B. (1974) "Delusional Thinking and Perceptual Disorder," *Journal of Individual Psychology* 30 (1): 98–113.

Maher, B. (1999) "Anomalous Experience in Everyday Life: Its Significance for Psychopathology," *The Monist* 82 (4): 547–570.

Mandelbaum, E. (2014) "Thinking Is Believing," *Inquiry* 57 (1): 55–96.

Mandelbaum, E. and Quilty-Dunn, J. (2019) "Non-Inferential Transitions: Imagery and Association," in T. Chan and A Nes (eds.), *Inference and Consciousness*. London: Routledge.

McDowell, J. (1994) *Mind and World*. Cambridge: Harvard University Press.

McKay, R. (2012) "Delusional Inference," *Mind & Language* 27(3): 330–355.

Nasar, S. (1998) *A Beautiful Mind*. New York: Simon and Schuster.

Noordhof, P. and Sullivan-Bissett, E. (2021) "The Clinical Significance of Anomalous Experience in the Explanation of Monothematic Delusions," *Synthese* 199 (3–4): 10277–10309.

Pacherie, E. (2009) "Perception, Emotions and Delusions: Revisiting the Capgras delusion," in T. Bayne and J. Fernandez (eds.), *Delusions and Self-Deception*. Hove: Psychology Press. pp. 107–126.

Parrott, M. (2016) "Bayesian Models, Delusional Beliefs, and Epistemic Possibilities," *The British Journal for the Philosophy of Science* 67 (1): 271–296.

Parrott, M. (2020). "Delusional Predictions and Explanations," *British Journal for the Philosophy of Science* 72 (1): 325–353.

Pollock, J. (1979) "A Plethora of Epistemological Theories," in G. Pappas (ed.), *Justification and Knowledge*. Dordrecht: Springer. pp. 98–113.

Prakash, J., Shashikumar, R., Bhat, P. S., Srivastava, K., Nath, S., and Rajendran, A. (2012) "Delusional Parasitosis: Worms of the Mind," *Indian Journal of Psychiatry* 21 (1): 72–74.

Pryor, J. (1990) "The Skeptic and the Dogmatist," *Nous* 34 (4): 517–549.

Sass, L. A., and Pienkos, E. (2013) "Varieties of Self-experience: A Comparative Phenomenology of Melancholia, Mania, and Schizophrenia, Part 1," *Journal of Consciousness Studies* 20 (7–8): 103–130.

Schlick, M. (1932) "Positivism and Realism," in A. J. Ayer (ed.), *Logical Postivism*. New York: The Free Press. pp. 82–107.

Shoemaker, S. (1994) "Self-Knowledge and 'Inner Sense': Lecture 1: The Object Perception Model," *Philosophy and Phenomenological Research* 54 (2): 249–269.

Stone, T., and Young, A. W. (1997) "Delusions and Brain Injury: The Philosophy and Psychology of Belief," *Mind and Language* 12 (3–4): 327–364.

Van Cleve, J. (1984) "Reliability, Justification, and the Problem of Induction," *Midwest Studies in Philosophy* 9 (1): 555–567.

Williams, D. (2020) "Socially Adaptive Belief," *Mind and Language* 36 (3): 333–354.

Williams, D. (2021) "Signalling, Commitment, and Strategic Absurdities" *Mind and Language* 37 (5): 1011–1029.

Young, A. W., and Leafhead, K. M. (1996) "Betwixt Life and Death: Case Studies of the Cotard Delusion," in P. Halligan and J. Marshall (eds.), *Method in Madness: Case Studies in Cognitive Neuropsychiatry*. London: Routledge. pp. 147–171.

# 27
# RATIONALISM

*Jakob Ohlhorst*

## 1.  Introduction

Rationalism about delusions is the theory that the root of delusions lies in a *cognitive* disturbance. The idea is quite simple: delusions are disturbed thoughts and consequently the subject's *thinking* must be the source of the disturbance. Rationalism contrasts with empiricism about delusions (see Bongiorno and Parrott, Chapter 26) which posits that delusions are the products of a disturbed *experience*. In a way, rationalism and empiricism about delusions are the extension of traditional rationalism and empiricism – the extension from theories about the sources of our knowledge into theories about the sources of our delusions.

Rationalism was originally proposed by John Campbell in his 'Rationality, Meaning, and the Analysis of Delusion' (2001). The distinction between rationalist and empiricist accounts of delusions has proven highly influential in the debate. Following Campbell's terminology, on the empiricist account, delusions are also described as 'bottom-up' where the experience's content is the cause of the delusion. On rationalist accounts, delusions are 'top-down' and the delusional cognitive content informs the content of the subject's disturbing experience (Campbell 2001: 95–96; Hohwy 2004).

In this chapter, I will first give an account of Campbell's argument for rationalism about delusions as well as his theory of delusion. Second, I will present the most prominent challenges to rationalism about delusions and respond on behalf of the rationalist. Third, I will present developments of the rationalist account and how they may address these challenges. Rationalism is a niche position in the epistemology of delusions, but due to its alignment with Wittgensteinian hinge epistemology, it has profited from the latter's growing popularity in recent years.

## 2.  Campbell's argument

Campbell (2001: 89) presents delusions in light of the problem of radical interpretation (Quine 1960; Davidson 1968). Namely, if we want to meaningfully ascribe any mental state – beliefs, hopes, emotions – to some agent, then we are forced to assume that they

DOI: 10.4324/9781003296386-33

are rational. We cannot meaningfully describe a person as believing something if we do not think that they are subject to rationality, i.e. that they are not constrained by coherence and some kind of reasons.[1]

Delusions *are ascribed as beliefs*, but at the same time, they are also described as un-understandable, beyond rationality, and constituting a *breakdown* of rationality. This gives us two options: either we treat a person who exhibits delusions as absolutely arational and lacking what we would be willing to describe a mental life with beliefs, hopes, and desires or we grant that the person has meaningful beliefs, hopes and desires, i.e. a mental life. We grant that they exhibit some kind of rationality, and we take delusions to be meaningful doxastic states.

Like many others, Campbell (2001: 89) opts for the latter option – subjects with a delusion have a describable mental life. But this then raises the question: How can a person exhibiting such strange beliefs and being insensitive to all sorts of reasons possess any rationality? The subject is often not understandable by the ordinary routes that we use to understand each other, they cannot give convincing reasons for their delusions, and they fail to appreciate the force of reasons we would give against their delusions – hence the appearance of a- or irrationality (for more on delusion and rationality see Bradley and Gibson, Chapter 14).

Campbell suggests that there are two ways the subject can acquire these apparently arational and un-understandable beliefs: They come 'bottom-up' and are the product of strange, un-understandable, and disturbing experiences on whose basis the delusional beliefs are formed because the delusional content appears to be the best explanation available for the subject (Stone and Young 1997). Campbell (2001: 89) calls this approach *empiricism*. He criticises the view by noting that strange experiences are not sufficient[2] to rationally explain why the subject would for instance hold such strange delusions like *I am dead* with Cotard's syndrome. After all, rationally speaking, I can never have evidence for my own death because, once I am dead, I am unable to have beliefs and possess evidence. The most reasonable response to an unsettling and strange experience would arguably be to recognise that it is pathological.

As an alternative solution, he proposes, that delusions are produced 'top-down' by our belief system. That is, what is at the heart of a delusion is the formation of strange beliefs which are the delusions, and these subsequently influence and shape the subject's experience. Campbell (2001: 89) calls this view *rationalism* about delusions.

Some authors are convinced by Campbell's argument against empiricism but less by his positive rationalist proposal. Consequently they opt for a third option, injecting empiricism with a rationalist second factor (Hohwy 2004: 66). Such two-factor theories argue that strange and unsettling experiences are interpreted by some defective top-down cognitive mechanism to form a delusion. I will examine one such two-factor theory that shares a considerable overlap with Campbell's rationalism further below. But most two-factor theories do not involve a rationalist element – instead their top-down mechanism is a bias or a cognitive error, i.e. a kind of irrationality (for more on two-factor theories, see Davies and Coltheart, Chapter 29).

How can we then make sense of delusions rationalistically, i.e. as a top-down phenomenon? Coming back to the problem of radical interpretation, if someone uses language in an apparently irrational and un-understandable way, while we nevertheless assume that this person is rational and has a mental life that can in principle be interpreted, then the only reasonable inference is that this person uses language differently from us. That is, the subject is not arational and insensitive to reasons, but rather they mean something altogether different than what we understand from their utterances. For instance, the delusion 'I am dead' in the case of Cotard syndrome is compatible with the person still holding beliefs or breathing because the words 'I', 'am', and 'dead' work differently in this case. It is worth noting that Campbell only focuses on monothematic delusions, namely the Cotard and Capgras syndromes. Monothematic delusions are limited to the content of a single delusion while polythematic delusions connect several different delusions.

But how would a subject with a delusion come to such a profound transformation in their language? Campbell (2001: 96) proposes that Ludwig Wittgenstein's *On Certainty* (1969) can shed light on this shift. Namely, Campbell suggests that delusions are the product of a shift in our 'framework', or *hinge*, propositions.

Hinge propositions have their name from the metaphor that 'If I want the door [of our epistemic life] to turn, the hinges must stay put' (Wittgenstein 1969: §343) just as a framework must be fixed for a canvas to be stretched on it. That is, hinge propositions enable our rational epistemic life, our having beliefs, our investigating, and our giving reasons, like a hinge enables a door to turn. They are the presuppositions that we need to share in order to understand each other, or as Annalisa Coliva (2015) puts it: they are constitutive of our rationality. Our hinges are the unmovable commitments that give meaning and doxastic force to our ordinary beliefs and the language that we use to describe them – they are the framework on which our belief system hangs. A further important notion is the idea of an *animal hinge* as proposed by Danièle Moyal-Sharrock (2004): animal hinges are the standing certainties which enable us to live our lives normally. For instance, the hinge proposition 'I have a body' is presupposed in almost everything that I do; I do not try to walk through walls, I simply pick up objects without even considering whether this is possible, etc. This shows how deep our hinges run and that they are mostly implicit. Note that the hinge rationalist is in no way wedded to the entirety of Wittgenstein's philosophy.

What happens if our hinges nevertheless shift or diverge? If epistemic communities have divergent hinges, then they *deeply disagree* (Fogelin 1985; Ranalli 2020) and cannot rationally come to an accord. The divergent hinges mean that the disagreeing parties mean different things by what they are talking about because they understand the underlying concepts differently. Take for example a physicalist atheist having the hinge that there is no god but only physics and a dualist theist with the contradictory hinge arguing about whether something was a miracle. They mean something altogether different by 'miracle': the former takes miracles to be definitionally impossible while the latter takes them to be normal occurrences. They talk past each other about miracles.

If a single individual has a divergent hinge, and the hinge is sufficiently incompatible with the individual's community, then this looks a lot like a delusion as Campbell (2001: 96) suggests.[3] For the subject with Cotard, it is not an open question whether they are dead. Instead it is the hinge on which their other beliefs turn – just as it is a hinge for you that you are alive. This would colour the subject's experience of everything – given that you are dead, everything is meaningless. The shift in hinges also translates into a shift of the subject's language: 'My life is over' means something else if you have the hinge, i.e. presuppose, that *I am dead*, than if you presuppose that you are alive. Your hinges determine how you use certain terms and what inferential roles you assign them – for instance 'I am dead' does not entail 'I stopped breathing and moving' anymore. Thus, the subject's expression of the delusion appear un-understandable and bizarre. Campbell (2001: 98) compares this to a paradigm shift (Kuhn 1996) across which communication is not possible because the theoretical frameworks are incommensurable. Campbell consequently suggests that delusions may be divergent hinges that are produced top-down by an organic malfunction which have the far-reaching reverberations that manifest as delusional symptoms because they are hinges.

The key point regarding this rationalist account of delusions is that it gives us an avenue to at least attempt to understand the subject's belief system even though they have a delusion. If we find which hinges have shifted, we may at least try to model what the subject is believing and trying to say. Thus, the benefit of the rationalist perspective is two-fold: First, it allows us to still ascribe a meaningful mental life to the subject with a delusion even though it may at first appear inscrutable to us. Second, it gives us a wedge to at least attempt to grasp what the subject with a delusion is trying to express. This is possible without having to take recourse to even more inscrutable strange experiences, as the empiricist must, especially because it is often hard to see how a strange experience would rationally support the specific content of a delusion over non-delusional alternatives like 'I am hallucinating' or 'I am mentally ill'.

## 3.  Criticisms of rationalism

The most prominent and stringent critics of Campbell's rationalism are Tim Bayne and Elisabeth Pacherie (2004). First, they defend empiricism against Campbell's criticisms (Bayne and Pacherie 2004: 2–7). I will bracket this defence of empiricism here. Second, they directly criticise the tenability of Campbell's theory.

Bayne and Pacherie (2004: 7) make an interesting and important observation about Campbell's account: There are two logically separate aspects that we can examine each on their own merit. First, there is the idea that delusions are produced aetiologically top-down through a defectively formed belief that produces the further symptoms of delusion. Second, there is the epistemological idea that delusions are Wittgensteinian hinges which epistemically explain the delusion. Bayne and Pacherie criticise both these aspects one after the other. I agree that the two aspects should be distinguished; I suggest calling the former part of Campbell's account his *aetiological top-down account*, while I would call the latter his *rationalist hinge account*. The account of delusion defended in Campbell (2001) is then the conjunction of the aetiological top-down account and the rationalist hinge account.

### 3.1  *Against the top-down model*

What are the objections against an aetiological top-down model of delusion? First, Bayne and Pacherie (2004: 8) raise the worry that top-down delusion appears even less rational than an empiricist account. Namely, the empiricist bottom-up account gives the subject at least their experience to point to as a reason for their delusion. But if the delusion is simply the product of a top-down cognitive defect, this is completely arational and would not make the subject more understandable. Campbell can grant the point that the acquisition of the delusion is completely un-understandable, because what he is aiming at is not the understandability of the acquisition of the delusion, but rather the interpretability of the solidified delusional belief system. To ascribe a person with a delusion a mental life, we do not need to understand how she acquired the delusion, but we need to understand the delusional state. Also we ourselves sometimes discover that we just acquired a belief for no apparent reason – what is key for understandability is whether we maintain it also against defeaters.

The second kind of worry about the top-down account is about its aetiological nature (Bayne and Pacherie 2004: 8): If delusional beliefs are the direct product of brain damage, then why aren't there as many topics of delusions as there are topics of beliefs? And inversely, how could a supposed cognitive defect cause defects to non-cognitive autonomic systems as they occur in Capgras syndrome for instance? These aetiological worries are, I think, the weak point of the cognitive top-down account (see also Hohwy 2004). An initial response is to note that there are more kinds of delusions with more diverse topics; especially delusional disorder (WHO 2018: 6A24) can involve delusions about almost any topic. The second, albeit weaker, response is to note that, differently from Cotard and Capgras, the hypothesised aetiologies for other kinds of delusions are much less clear.

Indeed, I think that limiting ourselves to Cotard and Capgras is not helpful when theorising about delusions as an epistemological phenomenon. Plausibly, there is no unified aetiology for our delusions: some may be top-down, others bottom-up, most will be mixed – depending on what caused the delusion (Hohwy 2004: 67–68). It would be surprising if drugs, schizophrenia, depression, neural damage, etc. created delusions all through the exactly same mechanism – be it top-down or bottom-up. Gerrans (2013: 87) indeed complains that the rationalist hinge part of Campbell's theory does not give us any neurocognitive explanation because it does not pinpoint any causal processes that lead to the formation of the delusion. Demanding such explanations, however, means misunderstanding the theoretical goals of rationalist or empiricist epistemologists – in this case, the goal is to integrate delusions with our epistemology and to explain how it relates to knowledge, doubt, certainty, and so on.

## 3.2  *Against the rationalist account*

I want to argue that delusions are all unified by their epistemology – namely, all delusions are rationalist hinges. Consequently, I will defend the rationalist hinge part of Campbell's theory more stridently in what remains of this chapter. A broad complaint that Bayne and Pacherie (2004: 8) have about the rationalist thesis is that the Wittgensteinian hinge framework is not very well-developed – and indeed in 2001, hinge epistemology was in its infancy. Since then, a lot has happened, and hinge epistemology has come to be a field in its own right. Prominent contributions have been (Moyal-Sharrock 2004; Coliva 2015; Pritchard 2016). These developments also allow us to better respond to the worries that Bayne and Pacherie raise about rationalism about hinges.

Bayne and Pacherie (2004: 8) agree that delusions have one key feature of hinge beliefs: They are extraordinarily resistant against counterevidence, and subjects reject ordinary hinge beliefs rather than their delusion. For instance, someone with Cotard Syndrome and the hinge *I am dead* might reject the ordinary fundamental conviction that 'dead people do not breathe', given that they take themselves to be dead but breathing. This is exactly how hinges are supposed to work. It is not even considered that the hinge certainty might be mistaken – instead the other beliefs are adapted to the hinge.

However, Bayne and Pacherie (2004: 8) suggest that it is nevertheless implausible that delusions are hinges because subjects with delusions frequently recognise the bizarreness of their delusion's content. Namely, if you ask them what they would think of someone else telling them a story analogous to their delusions with different protagonists, they would frequently consider it to be bizarre and absurd, and they may admit that their delusion is hard to believe. Consequently, their delusion cannot be a hinge because, if it were, that would arguably normalise the delusion's content for the subject.

The rationalist can respond that we need to pay careful attention to *what* the delusional hinge is. Note that delusions are often very subject-specific: they are *about* the subject – the subject is the delusion's protagonist. Consequently also the corresponding hinge is *about* the subject – the delusional content limitedly only applies to the subject. That is, a subject with persecutory delusion does not have the hinge that *people, including or like me, are being persecuted*, but specifically that *I am persecuted*. Similarly, Cotard syndrome is not based on the hinge that *some dead people still move, speak, and breathe*. Instead, it has the hinge that *I am dead*, notwithstanding the fact that I still move, speak, and breathe. It is more epistemically conservative to take one's individual (hinge) case to be an exception – and to maintain that other dead people stay dead without breathing – conserving one's old hinges as much as possible. Consequently, the meaning of 'dead' would only undergo a subject-centric change.

This point relates to Bayne and Pacherie's (2004: 9) second worry: they point out that delusions are fairly encapsulated. Monothematic delusions especially often have rather limited consequences for the subject's epistemic and practical life. The delusion may manifest mostly in linguistic behaviour and not engender many revisions in the subject's belief system. Thornton (2008: 162) makes this point especially vivid, and a telling illustration of this is the phenomenon of double bookkeeping (Fuchs 2020: 76) where the subject maintains a normal epistemic and practical life but also has a delusional world-view in parallel which is kept insulated and separated from the former (for more on delusion and double bookkeeping see Porcher, Chapter 13). If our delusions were hinges, then we would expect them to have far-reaching implications because they are our presuppositions about everything else.

I hinted already above that these delusional hinges are highly specific in their content: They are specifically only about the individual who has a delusion, and they ascribe the individual a particular status, e.g. being dead. This specificity in content arguably blocks the spread of far-reaching epistemic and practical consequences. Consider for example the epistemic, semantic, and practical consequences of the delusion *I am chosen by god* – it is a hinge about me specifically and it does not imply that other people might also be chosen. My being chosen might even speak against other people's being so. Such encapsulated delusions are what Danièle Moyal-Sharrock (2004: 102) calls *personal hinges* which are mostly about the holder of the hinge – Wittgenstein's (1969, §486) example of a personal hinge is 'my name is L.W.' Note also that as Bayne and Pacherie (2004: 6) themselves admit that even such specific delusions can have (horrific) practical consequences.[4]

The third worry that Bayne and Pacherie (2004: 9) raise is the semantic role of hinges. They criticise Campbell's suggestion that our delusions *qua* hinges have semantic consequences. If the subject with a delusion has aberrant hinges, e.g., *my spouse was replaced by an impostor*, then the constituents of the hinge, what 'impostor' and 'replaced' mean, shifts in meaning because the hinge – given its fundamentality – starts working like a definition for its constituent parts. We cannot understand anymore what the subject means when talking about impostors, because the meaning of 'impostor' has now changed to include that their spouse is an impostor as well as the delusion's other far-reaching implications. Replace 'impostor' with any delusional content you like. Intuitively, however, the content of the delusion seems quite transparent: 'What does the Capgras subject believe if not that his wife has been replaced by an impostor?' (Bayne and Pacherie 2004: 9) The threat is then that a rationalist hinge account exaggerates the semantic effects of a delusion.

I agree with Bayne and Pacherie that delusions arguably do not have the far-reaching semantic consequences that Campbell appears to suggest. The subject with a delusion does not speak a profoundly different incommensurable language. Meanwhile, I do not think that such stark semantic consequences need to follow from rationalism about delusions. As argued above, the limited content of our delusions arguably also has limited semantic consequences. That is, a subject with a delusion does use some terms differently than the majority does, but this difference in use mostly manifests in differences of entailments which are limited to the consequences of the highly specific content of the delusion. What may occur in such a case is not a total linguistic incommensurability, but rather local incommensurability (Carey 2009: 367).

### 3.3 *Wittgensteinian criticisms*

A second, less prominent critique of Campbell's hinge rationalism is made by Thornton (2008). His argumentative target is, very limitedly, that a rationalist hinge account of delusions cannot provide us *any* epistemic access to understand a person with a delusion thereby undermining the Davidsonian motivation for the rationalist hinge view. He motivates this with more broadly Wittgensteinian considerations about linguistic intelligibility, notably from the *Philosophical Investigations* (Wittgenstein 1958).

Thornton's (2008: 166) first point is that it is impossible to consider and understand false propositions as hinges because we do have our own set of hinges – note that delusional hinges need not necessarily be false. They would just be 'nonsensical sense', empty contradictions to our most fundamental certainties. I think this idea underestimates our capacities for modelling. For instance, our hinge framework is arguably Euclidian, and *space does not bend* is a hinge, nevertheless we are capable of doing non-Euclidian geometry. Bracketing our own hinges or limiting their reach just requires some imagination – we do it in mathematics and philosophy (Coliva and Doulas 2022), why should we not be able to do it in psychiatry?

Thornton's (2008: 170) second argument is analogously that we are incapable of conceiving of delusions as abnormal framework propositions because this would be incommensurable with our linguistic practice. He considers two options: First, that delusions generate a totally alien and globally incommensurable hinge framework. He rejects this by appealing to Davidson and McDowell without elaboration; I think we can reject the global incommensurability because some limited communication with subjects who have a delusion is arguably still possible on topics unrelated to the delusion. They do not become completely isolated but still communicate about everyday issues – total breakdown of communication is not part of the symptoms of delusion.

Second, he considers the option – that I appealed to above – that delusional hinges are very local and narrow. Thornton (2008: 177) argues that hinges work just like grammatical rules (cf. Coliva 2015). His key idea appears to be that grammatical rules essentially need to be socially shared in order to function as grammatical rules – if they are not, then the grammar breaks down and there are no rules left at all. Consequently, hinges also need to be shared in order to function as hinges, otherwise they are not hinges. Given that delusions are, definitionally, not shared, they cannot be hinges that could be understood.

To this, the rationalist can respond that Thornton confuses philosophy of language with epistemology. Social epistemic practice, i.e. the sharing and transmission of knowledge, obviously is very central to epistemology, but it is not the case that epistemic activity completely breaks down if sharing breaks down. Language's constitutive function is the sharing of information; meanwhile there is a legitimate individual epistemology – internalism is not dead yet. In that sense, Thornton's analogy between grammatical rules of language and epistemological hinge rules falls short. While the linguistic function of grammatical rules is completely undermined by not being shared, the function of epistemic hinge rules is only damaged and reduced if they are not shared, because their social epistemic function is undermined. Nevertheless, delusions that form hinges which are not shared are simply dysfunctional but not completely undermined.

To illustrate this point: if you are very, very smart (I am not), then you could play chess against yourself just in your head – and thereby follow the rules of chess. You would be playing chess, even though Wittgenstein and Thornton would complain that it is meaningless to talk about such an internal game of chess because a rule can only be followed publicly – but *talking about it* is not the same as *playing the game.*

Still, the worry remains that hinges that are not locally shared would completely undermine the understandability, i.e. social epistemological aspects, of the delusional hinge belief system. The ordinary shareability of beliefs is undermined; a subject's testimony fails given the discrepancies in the speaker's and hearer's respective frameworks. I reiterate my point above: our imagination is not that limited – just as we can model alternative hinge frameworks in philosophy or geometry, we can do so in psychiatry in order to salvage some meaning from the subject's testimony (see also Henriksen 2013).

As third and final objection, Thornton (2008: 172–173) argues against Eilan's (2000) rationalist hinge account, which I will present below, that we cannot be considered to believe our hinges.[5] Many authors agree with Thornton that hinges cannot be believed because they are not reasons-sensitive or knowledge-apt (Coliva 2015: 44; Pritchard 2016: 92). Note, however, that delusions should not be considered to be beliefs in this sense either – they are also not reasons-sensitive or knowledge-apt. The question whether we believe hinges and delusions is vexed (see Nordhoof, Chs. 19 and 20), but it appears likely that if you fall on one side of the question for hinges, then you will fall on the same side for delusions and vice versa. Consequently, if hinges cannot be believed, this gives us reason to also be non-doxasticists about delusions rather than giving us any reason to reject rationalism.

## 3.4  Summary

In sum, we can split Campbell's (2001) view into two parts: the aetiological top-down account about what produces or causes delusions, and the rationalist account about the epistemic role that delusions play in a subject's belief system. While some cases of delusion may be produced top-down, the bottom-up role of experience cannot be denied.[6] Consequently, the top-down account of delusions does not apply generally. However, I have suggested that the rationalist hinge account of delusions applies to all cases of delusions, and on this view delusions are unified by being pathological hinge certainties. As we will see below, this rationalist hinge account has been quite attractive to theorists in the last two decades.

This hinge rationalism about delusions has two principal theoretical consequences: First, we can make predictions about how delusions, *qua* hinges, relate to other beliefs. Namely our ordinary beliefs should be interpreted in the light of the delusion, ordinary beliefs should be rejected or relativised if they contradict a delusion, and the delusion is simply presupposed and taken for granted, not requiring any argument. Second, if delusions are hinges, then beliefs that may appear to be delusions but which do not play the functional role of hinges do not count as full-blown delusions. Instead they would simply be irrational, and maybe pathological, beliefs. We will now examine how Campbell's original proposal has been developed by other authors.

## 4.  Developments of rationalism

### 4.1  *Wittgenstein meets Jaspers*

The first development of rationalism about delusions appeared roughly at the same time as Campbell's (2001). Namely, Naomi Eilan (2000) examines the epistemic status of schizophrenic delusions and the problem of radical interpretation that this raises. Her starting point is a puzzle that Karl Jaspers' account of delusions generates because Jaspers emphasises the un-understandability or utter bizarreness of schizophrenic delusions while at the same time wanting to ascribe a mental life to subjects with a delusion.[7] Eilan (2000: 106–107) considers the empiricist route but argues that not all schizophrenic delusions could be boiled down to strange and unsettling experiences. Eilan therefore looks to Campbell's work, going with rationalism.

She points out that someone with divergent hinges would appear to be mad, because they have such an alien take on the world (Eilan 2000: 103). However they would not become completely un-understandable. Namely, Eilan emphasises that while delusions as hinges explain *prima facie* why they are un-understandable, the hinge account also allows us to 'fall in, to an extent, with a deluded subject's reasoning' (Eilan 2000: 109) by imagining a delusion's content to be a hinge certainty.

Further, Eilan (2000: 112) suggests that what makes a particular strange belief into a delusional hinge is an emotional loading of the proposition with significance. For instance, in the case of morbid jealousy (Kingham and Gordon 2004), the belief that *my partner cheats on me* gets loaded by the emotion of jealousy which transforms the testable and refutable belief into an incontrovertible hinge certainty which colours all my further beliefs and experiences. Consequently, Eilan does not endorse the top-down account of delusion because she also looks to emotion as a causal factor, nevertheless she is a rationalist because she takes delusions to be hinges.

### 4.2  *Stark and pedestrian delusions*

Another prominent early development of Campbell's rationalism was Klee's (2004) suggestion that delusions split into *pedestrian* and *stark* delusions. Pedestrian delusions are cases that are tractable and fit within our shared epistemic framework, e.g. litigious delusions that *the state has been treating me unjustly*. Klee (2004: 29) explains them as instances of a Davidsonian fragmented belief set where the different fragments do not interact epistemically. Meanwhile, stark delusions are the extreme cases that are un-understandable, e.g. claims that *external forces insert thoughts into my mind* or that *I am dead*. These, Klee suggests, are instances of the subject having acquired a different set of hinges from us – thereby making subjects with stark delusions un-understandable.

Hohwy (2004: 66–67) argues that the line between stark and pedestrian delusions is much harder to draw than Klee suggests. Notably, the distinction seems to cut across particular types of delusions. For instance, some paranoid delusions are very pedestrian – *the*

*NSA is wiretapping my phone calls* – while others are completely out of this world and unexpected – *the Spanish Inquisition is monitoring my every thought*. I agree with Hohwy. Additionally, I think that even clearly pedestrian delusions can be explained by delusional hinges with a very narrow content. Consequently, a pure hinge rationalism is more economical than Klee's mixed view. In this vein, Bardina (2018) develops an account of the broad range of possible kinds of delusions of varying starkness by relying on Moyal-Sharrock's (2004) typology of different kinds of hinges – personal hinges, animal hinges, etc.

### 4.3   Delusion as a loss of hinges

A prominent alternative account of the role of hinges for delusions is by Gipps and Rhodes (2008, 2011). Instead of describing delusions as hinge certainties like Campbell, they emphasise the subject's loss of the ordinary hinges that we all share. Thus, a delusion is a lack of shared hinges, which permits the subject to have such strange beliefs as 'I am setting the sun'. An interesting recent elaboration on this idea is by Jeppsson (2021) who reports that she experienced her own delusional episodes as the loss of the bedrock of her hinge beliefs. She also points out that endorsing scepticism involves a suspension of our fundamental hinge certainties – e.g. 'there is an external world' or 'there are other minds' – and suffering from a delusion feels, according to her, a lot like being in the throes of scepticism.

Bortolotti (2011: 83) objects to Rhodes and Gipps's proposal on the grounds that it does not explain the fixedness of our delusions. If we lacked fundamental hinge certainties nailing our beliefs down, should our delusions not become florid and constantly change? Delusion do not usually behave like this, consequently this is an insufficient explanation.

An indirect response to this objection can be found in Fuchs's (2020). He rejects the rationalist label because he misinterprets Campbell's account as involving irrational thinking errors and because he rejects the top-down model (Fuchs 2020: 71). However, he endorses the rationalist hinge framework, integrating it into an enactivist two-factor account. Fuchs suggests that schizophrenic delusions develop in two stages: first, as proposed by Gipps and Rhodes (2008) and Jeppsson (2021), our hinge certainties become inoperative, and our perception stops being structured by our animal hinges (Fuchs 2020: 67). However, this is not yet the full-blown delusion, but a mere precursor. Second, the subject attempts to reorder their unhinged epistemic life by settling for new hinge certainties – the full blown delusional hinge which integrates the subject's unsettled experience again (Fuchs 2020: 68).

Fuchs has an additional reason why he rejects the 'rationalist' label for his hinge account. Namely, he argues similarly to Coliva (2015), that abandoning our ordinary hinges, which are constitutive of rationality, means abandoning rationality entirely. Note that Bortolotti (2005) argues *contra* Campbell's motivation for rationalism and empiricism that we can ascribe subjects beliefs even though the subject is patently irrational. Coliva's view of rationality is relying on a very narrow and fundamental range of hinges which guarantee classical logic and a minimal common-sense world view. I believe that many delusions remain at least partially within the bounds of this minimal framework because subjects with a delusion do not start rejecting logical or mathematical reasoning per se.

### 4.4   Delusion as certainty

Finally, in Ohlhorst (2021), I develop an epistemological rationalist account of delusions. Notably, the paper gives a positive epistemological argument that delusions really are (hinge) certainties. It shows that dysfunctional hinge certainties are the best available epistemic candidate for delusions by examining and rejecting the proposed alternative accounts of the epistemology of delusions. A key idea is that delusions are taken to be dysfunctional hinges – that is delusions pervert the function of hinge certainties just as autoimmune diseases pervert the function of our immune system. As a weaker option, it also suggests that delusions are just certainties that the subject cannot doubt, and not hinge certainties. Meanwhile, the account remains silent on the aetiological roots of delusions and does not defend a top-down account; instead defending a rationalist hinge theory of delusions.

## 5.  Conclusion

Campbell's rationalism has proven to be very influential. Principally, it has served as a foil for its opponents – especially discussion on the top-down/bottom-up distinction has proven very fruitful. Meanwhile, also the rationalist hinge aspect of Campbell's account has played an influential role. The basic Wittgensteinian idea that delusions are defective hinges has seen many interesting developments which leaves hinge rationalism about delusions as a distinct epistemological position in the philosophical debate about delusions.

## Notes

1 Bortolotti (2005) attacks this Davidsonian view of mental life, arguing that delusions are beliefs, even though the subject is patently irrational.
2 Empiricists would reject that they are committed to the claim that strange experiences are sufficient for a delusion. I explain below, how two-factor theorists modified their account in response to Campbell's challenge, but even empiricist one-factor theorists would not necessarily accept it (Sullivan-Bissett 2022).
3 Bortolotti and Broome (2008: 835) suggest that the fact that a person with a delusion proffers different and incompatible reasons than the common-sense majority speaks against their delusion being a hinge. This presupposes a view of hinges as essentially socially anchored and shared institution to enable reason-giving. This would just be a confirmation of the rationalist thesis that the un-understandable delusion has replaced the ordinary common-sense hinge – doxastically, it functions like a hinge for the individual. I treat this concern which has also been raised by Thornton further below.
4 In Ohlhorst (2021), I argue for a weaker thesis that delusions are just psychologically indubitable certainties rather than hinge certainties. They consequently have weaker implications.
5 Similarly, Henriksen (2013: 112) suggests that we only assume hinges – but assumptions are easily defeated by counter-evidence, so hinges cannot be assumptions.
6 I personally do not think that a pure empiricist account can get off the ground because we arguably also want to distinguish delusions from ordinary mistaken beliefs based on hallucinations. Consequently, some top-down mechanism must play a role.
7 I am simplifying Jasper's account here, he distinguishes different possible kinds of understanding.

## References

Bardina, S. (2018) "Abnormal Certainty: Examining the Epistemological Status of Delusional Beliefs," *International Journal of Philosophical Studies*, 26(4), pp. 546–560. doi: 10.1080/09672559. 2018.1497072.
Bayne, T. and Pacherie, E. (2004) "Bottom-Up or Top-Down: Campbell's Rationalist Account of Monothematic Delusions," *Philosophy, Psychiatry, & Psychology*, 11(1), pp. 1–11.
Bortolotti, L. (2005) "Delusions and the Background of Rationality," *Mind and Language*, 20(2), pp. 189–208. doi: 10.1111/j.0268-1064.2005.00282.x.

Bortolotti, L. (2011) "Continuing Commentary: Shaking the Bedrock," *Philosophy, Psychiatry, & Psychology*, 18(1), pp. 77–87.

Bortolotti, L. and Broome, M. R. (2008) "Delusional Beliefs and Reason Giving," *Philosophical Psychology*, 21(6), pp. 821–841. doi: 10.1080/09515080802516212.

Campbell, J. (2001) "Rationality, Meaning, and the Analysis of Delusion," *Philosophy, Psychiatry, & Psychology*, 8(2), pp. 89–100.

Carey, S. (2009) *The Origin of Concepts*, Oxford: Oxford University Press.

Coliva, A. (2015) *Extended Rationality*, Basingstoke: Palgrave Macmillan.

Coliva, A. and Doulas, L. (2022) "What Philosophical Disagreement and Philosophical Skepticism Hinge on," *Synthese*, 200(3), p. 251. doi: 10.1007/s11229-022-03735-6.

Davidson, D. (1968) "On Saying That," *Synthese*, 19(1/2), pp. 130–146.

Eilan, N. (2000) "On Understanding Schizophrenia," in Zahavi, D. (ed.), *Exploring the Self. Philosophical and Psychopathological Perspectives on Self-Experience*, Amsterdam: John Benjamins Publishing Company, pp. 97–113. doi: 10.1075/aicr.23.09eil.

Fogelin, R. (1985) "The Logic of Deep Disagreements," *Informal Logic*, 7(1), pp. 1–8.

Fuchs, T. (2020) "Delusion, Reality and Intersubjectivity: A Phenomenological and Enactive Analysis," *Phenomenology and Mind*, 18(1), pp. 120–143. doi: 10.17454/pam-1810.

Gerrans, P. (2013) "Delusional Attitudes and Default Thinking," *Mind & Language*, 28(1), pp. 83–102. doi: 10.1111/mila.12010.

Gipps, R. G. T. and Rhodes, J. (2008) "The Background Theory of Delusion and Existential Phenomenology," *Philosophy, Psychiatry, & Psychology*, 15(4), pp. 321–326.

Gipps, R. G. T. and Rhodes, J. (2011) "Delusions and the Non-epistemic Foundations of Belief," *Philosophy, Psychiatry, & Psychology*, 18(1), pp. 89–97.

Henriksen, M. G. (2013) "On incomprehensibility in Schizophrenia," *Phenomenology and the Cognitive Sciences*, 12(1), pp. 105–129. doi: 10.1007/s11097-010-9194-7.

Hohwy, J. (2004) "Top-Down and Bottom-Up in Delusion Formation," *Philosophy, Psychiatry, & Psychology; Psychology*, 11(1), pp. 65–70. doi: 10.1353/ppp.2004.0043.

Jeppsson, S. (2021) "Psychosis and Intelligibility," *Philosophy, Psychiatry and Psychology*, 28(3), pp. 233–249. doi: 10.1353/ppp.2021.0036.

Kingham, M. and Gordon, H. (2004) "Aspects of Morbid Jealousy," *Advances in Psychiatric Treatment*, 10(3), pp. 207–215.

Klee, R. (2004) "Why Some Delusions Are Necessarily Inexplicable Beliefs," *Philosophy, Psychiatry, & Psychology*, 11(1), pp. 25–34.

Kuhn, T. (1996) *The Structure of Scientific Revolutions*, Chicago, IL: The University of Chicago Press.

Moyal-Sharrock, D. (2004) *Understanding Wittgenstein's On Certainty*, Basingstoke: Palgrave Macmillan.

Ohlhorst, J. (2021) "The Certainties of Delusion," in Moretti, L. and Pedersen, N. J. L. L. (eds.), *Non-Evidentialist Epistemology*, Leiden: BRILL, pp. 211–229. doi: 10.1163/9789004465534_012.

Pritchard, D. (2016) *Epistemic Angst*, Princeton, NJ: Princeton University Press.

Quine, W. V. O. (1960) *Word and Object*, Cambridge: MIT Press.

Ranalli, C. (2020) "Deep Disagreement and Hinge Epistemology," *Synthese*, 197(11), pp. 4975–5007. doi: 10.1007/s11229-018-01956-2.

Stone, T. and Young, A. W. (1997) "Delusions and Brain Injury: The Philosophy and Psychology of Belief," *Mind and Language*, 12(3–4), pp. 327–364. doi: 10.1111/j.1468-0017.1997.tb00077.x.

Sullivan-Bissett, E. (2022) "Against a Second Factor," *Asian Journal of Philosophy*, 1(1), pp. 1–10. doi: 10.1007/s44204-022-00036-0.

Thornton, T. (2008) "Why the Idea of Framework Propositions Cannot Contribute to an Understanding of Delusions," *Phenomenology and the Cognitive Sciences*, 7(2), pp. 159–175. doi: 10.1007/s11097-007-9079-6.

WHO (ed.) (2018) *ICD-11 for Mortality and Morbidity Statistics (ICD-11 MMS)*. Available at: https://icd.who.int/browse11/l-m/en.

Wittgenstein, L. (1958) *Philosophical Investigations*, Oxford: Blackwell.

Wittgenstein, L. (1969) *Über Gewissheit – On Certainty*, Oxford: Blackwell.

# 28

# THE ONE-FACTOR THEORY

*Ema Sullivan-Bissett*

This chapter will consider the one-factor approach to delusion formation. I begin by examining what is meant by *factor*, since this is obviously crucial to a proper discussion of the approach's merits, particularly as part of a wider debate with a rival theory which argues for two factors. I then consider delusional beliefs as *explanations* of anomalous experiences (a claim shared by one- and two-factor theorists), before identifying the point of disagreement: the one-factor theory's claim that such explanations are *normal* ones. The idea of delusional beliefs as normal explanations naturally gives rise to concerns regarding hypothesis selection, that is, selection of the delusional hypothesis might indicate the need for a second factor. I discuss this in the service of properly understanding the commitments and resources of the one-factor theory. Finally, I turn to the most common objection to the view: the objection from dissociation. I offer two responses before concluding that the one-factor approach should be the default approach to understanding the genesis and maintenance of monothematic delusions.

## 1.  Preliminaries

One-factor theories of delusion formation are a branch of a wider view, *empiricism*, according to which anomalous experiences are part of the causal story for the formation of a delusion (see Bongiorno and Parrott, Chapter 26). One-factor versions of empiricism have it that the anomalous experience is the only factor to which we need to appeal to explain why someone forms or maintains a delusional belief. Two-factor theories also fall under the empiricist umbrella, accepting the story so far, but adding a second factor to explain delusion in the form of a reasoning bias, deficit, or performance error (see Davies and Coltheart, Chapter 29). This chapter will focus on the one-factor approach, with particular emphasis on how its resources have been underestimated by its opponents. I will focus on *monothematic* delusions (hereafter simply 'delusions'), because the recent debate between one- and two-factor theorists has taken place in this context (two-factor theorists also restrict their remits in this way, see e.g. Davies et al. 2001: 137, Coltheart et al. 2011: 282; Coltheart 2013: 103, Coltheart and Davies 2021: 225–226).[1] I will also take for granted doxasticism about delusion, that is, I take it that delusions are *beliefs*. Here again, I am following the

DOI: 10.4324/9781003296386-34

convention set by the debate within empiricism (for defences of doxasticism see Bayne and Pacherie 2005, Bortolotti 2009, and Noordhof, Chapter 19).

## 2.    Factors and abnormality

It is, of course, crucial to be precise regarding what is meant by *factor* in a piece discussing factors in delusion. In turn, it will be equally crucial to be precise about what is meant by *abnormality*.

One- and two-factor accounts take themselves to be identifying features of the context that are explanatorily relevant to *delusional* belief formation and maintenance in particular. The task isn't to identify all the background features and cognitive contributions of everyday belief formation, *and then* add in whatever other versions of those things are also required to explain belief which is properly characterised as *delusional*. Rather, one- and two-factor theorists alike begin with a shared background of ordinary belief formation, and then take their task to be one of identifying what *else* we need to explain the genesis and maintenance of belief of a particular kind. All sides can agree that in the ordinary case of garden variety beliefs about cats on mats and grass being green, we are zero-factor theorists. When we turn to delusion, those extra ingredients required in our explanation are the *factors*, and the disagreement lies in how many of those we need.

Factors then are not merely causal contributions. The task is not to create an inventory of everything to which we need to appeal in order to explain delusional belief. Even in everyday cases, if that were the task, the inventory would be substantial. We would need to appeal to the subject having oxygen in her environment, having suitably developed cognitive capacities to form beliefs, being in such-a-such a place $p$ at such-and-such a time $t$ to receive evidence $e$, and so on. Background conditions are not factors. Nor, importantly, are various quirks of cognition that might go into an explanation of why folk have particular beliefs. My Uncle Mark's belief that *the earth is flat* can be in part explained by appeal to the epistemic bubbles and chambers in which he is immersed (Nguyen 2020), as well as the exercise of, say, intentionality bias (Brotherton 2015: 188–189) or need for uniqueness (Imhoff and Lamberty 2017). My Auntie Eileen's belief that *the positions of celestial bodies influence the trajectory of human relationships* can be in part explained by her preference for non-naturalistic explanations of various phenomena, and her engagement with numerous astrological media. My Grandmother's belief that *poltergeists inhabit her home* can be in part explained by high intuitive and low analytical thinking (Lindeman and Aarnio 2006). These idiosyncrasies are also not factors. They are simply part of the wide catalogue of quirks and tendencies in human psychology. If our task were a causal inventory, they would make an appearance. But that is not our task.

How then should a factor be understood if mere causal contribution is not what we mean? In addition to causally contributing to the formation or maintenance of a delusional belief, the term *factor* picks out a contribution which is *abnormal*. Two-factor theorists have often recognised this. Tony Stone and Andrew Young talk of delusional reasoning being 'abnormal' and 'differences between people with and without delusions' (Stone and Young 1997: 342). Martin Davies and colleagues characterise the second factor as 'a departure from what is normally the case' (Davies et al. 2005: 228). Ryan McKay and colleagues characterise the deficit two-factor approach as one which 'conceptualises delusions as involving dysfunction or disruption in ordinary cognitive processes' (McKay et al. 2010: 316–317). Finally, in discussing how to defend the one-factor approach,

Philip Gerrans suggests showing the second factor to in fact be describing 'a rationalization process which is within the normal range' (Gerrans 2002: 48). This wouldn't be a defence of the one-factor approach if the second factor were not proposed to constitute an abnormality.[2]

Of course, understanding *factor* as picking out a causal contribution to delusion which is *abnormal* raises a new question: how should we understand *normality*? There are broadly two ways: functionally or statistically. Take *functional normality* to be picking out the property of being within the range of reasoning styles between which evolutionary selection has not distinguished, and *functional abnormality* the opposite. Take *statistical normality* to be picking out the property of occurring in non-delusional populations, and *statistical abnormality* the opposite. Often these notions of normality will not characterise different sets of belief, that is, where we find functional normality we also find statistical normality, and vice versa. But they are separable, and it's important to be clear on which is in play when we're seeking to adjudicate between one- and two-factor theories. For example, suppose that a particular style of reasoning $R$ were functionally normal, but occurred in all and only people with delusions. Were we working with a statistical notion of abnormality, $R$ would be a factor. Were we working with a functional notion of abnormality, it would not. In what follows, I will understand two-factor theorists as seeking to identify a functional abnormality against a statistical assumption (i.e., functional abnormalities purported to be involved in delusion are also taken to be statistical abnormalities).[3]

Now that we know how to understand what is meant by *factor*, we can be more precise in stating the commitments of the one- and two-factor approaches. One-factor theories have it that to explain the formation or maintenance of a delusion, along with a range of background conditions, we can[4] appeal to an abnormal anomalous experience. Two-factor theories add the requirement of an abnormality in belief formation or evaluation in light of such an experience.

## 3.  Delusions as explanations of experience

As already noted, subjects with delusions often undergo some profoundly anomalous experiences, and it is the recognition that these experiences are explanatorily relevant to the project of understanding the formation and maintenance of these beliefs that is the backbone of the empiricist approach. Let us see some examples to get a sense of what subjects may be labouring under.

A subject with perceptual delusional bicephaly (the belief that *one has a second head*) may hallucinate a second head on her shoulder (Ames 1984). Not all anomalous experiences are hallucinatory in this way, that is, they do not all present objects and properties in the world that are not really there. In Capgras delusion (the belief that *someone familiar*, often a loved one, *has been replaced by an imposter*), the experience has been understood as the *absence* of something expected. In particular, the subject has reduced affective response to familiar faces traceable to ventromedial prefrontal cortex damage (Tranel, Damasio, and Damasio 1995. In the case of Cotard delusion (the belief that *one is dead* or *has ceased existing*), similar damage has been found and it has been suggested that these subjects have no emotional feelings regarding their environment (Young et al. 1992: 800).

Coltheart and colleagues identify the key point of the one-factor theory to be the claim that 'delusional beliefs are normal attempts to explain abnormal perceptual or affective phenomena' (Coltheart et al. 2011: 284). They trace this idea back to William James, their evidence for doing so is given in the following quotation:

The delusions of the insane are apt to affect certain typical forms, very difficult to explain. But in many cases they are certainly theories which the patients invent to account for their bodily sensations.

*(James 1890: chapter XIX, 114, fn. 122)*

Coltheart and colleagues take Brendan Maher to be the inheritor of the view, capturing it as the claim that '[a] delusion is a hypothesis designed to explain unusual perceptual phenomena' (Maher 1974: 103). However, these quotations from James and Maher in fact only get us to the idea that delusional beliefs are explanations of anomalous experience. This is consistent with the two-factor theory. Two-factor theorists can accept the insight from James and Maher that delusions arise from attempts to explain abnormal data, but they build on that insight by insisting that we need another factor to explain why the explanation is taken up in belief, or why the belief is maintained.

What distinguishes the one-factor theory is the claim that the ways in which these explanations of experience are formed and maintained is *normal*. That is, whatever cognitive influences are involved in the formation or maintenance of a delusion, they are within the normal range for human psychology. All sides can accept the idea of delusional hypotheses as explanations of experience, the point of divergence is on whether we need to appeal to any abnormality to explain the adoption and maintenance of those hypotheses (or even their generation, see discussion in next section). The two-factor account says that we do. The one-factor account says that we do not. Let us turn to Maher's view to further elucidate this key idea.

## 4. Delusions as *normal* explanations for experience

Maher defended the idea that delusions are adopted as explanations for experience and are 'developed in much the same way that normal beliefs are' (Maher 1988: 22). As Coltheart notes, although Maher's view was primarily concerned with explaining the adoption of delusions of reference (and usually in the context of schizophrenia), his approach can nevertheless be explored in the context of monothematic delusions (Coltheart 2011: 284).

Maher draws an analogy with science, suggesting that delusional hypotheses are best thought of as like scientific theories – both 'serve the purpose of providing order and meaning for empirical data obtained by observation' (Maher 1988: 20). The individual with a delusion is presented with a puzzle in their anomalous experience, which they come up with a theory to explain. Delusional hypotheses can become tenacious, and seemingly insensitive to counterevidence (for more on delusion and evidence see Flores, Chapter 12).[5] Maher claims that this is analogous to scientific theory change:

As in science, a coherent theory is only overthrown by a better theory and the chances that this can be done successfully by a clinician are reduced when the patient has found a generally satisfactory theory of his own.

*(Maher 1974: 107)*

Of course, better theories are sometimes resisted because they conflict with a scientist's commitment to her own theory.

Let us see whether Maher's account can answer the two questions which structure the opposing account. The two-factor theory seeks to answer two questions regarding the genesis and maintenance of delusional belief:

> The first question is, what brought the delusional idea to mind in the first place? The second question is, why is this idea accepted as true and adopted as a belief when the belief is typically bizarre and when so much evidence against its truth is available to the patient?
>
> *(Coltheart et al. 2011: 271)*

One- and two-factor theorists alike have a fairly straightforward answer to the first question – they can appeal to the anomalous experience that the delusion is taken to explain. We have seen above what this looks like for Maher – the delusional hypothesis is prompted by the anomalous experience, and, via abductive inference, is taken to explain that experience. The second question is taken by two-factor theorists to be unanswerable without appeal to a second factor (Davies 2009: 72). Can we explain why a bizarre belief is adopted in the face of evidence against it which is available to the subject? This is where a bit of pressure is often thought to apply to the one-factor theory: why does the subject opt for such a poor explanation of the data generated by the anomalous experience? How can the one-factor theory explain why the explanation opted for is so flawed?

Some theorists have gone further, suggesting that it is not that delusional explanations are merely *poor*, they are 'unintelligible' (Nie 2023, cf. Sullivan-Bissett and Noordhof 2024: 3–5), or 'nonstarters', and 'the explanations of the delusional patients are nothing like explanations as we understand them' (Fine et al. 2005b: 160). Matthew Parrott, in the context of assessing predictive processing accounts of delusion (see Corlett, Chapter 30), argues that the implausibility of delusional explanations is so extreme that we should posit impaired or disrupted mechanisms of hypothesis generation (Parrott 2021: 342). This kind of concern can of course be levelled against the one-factor approach which understands delusions as normal explanations of experience.

However, if, as Parrott puts it, 'simply *considering* an implausible delusional hypothesis as a candidate explanation manifests a clear departure from ordinary cognition' (Parrott 2021: 342, my emphasis), we might well be in the realms of a more general objection to the empiricist research programme, rather than something which could help us adjudicate between the one- and two-factor versions thereof. After all, some versions of the two-factor theory relate the second factor to belief *evaluation* rather than formation, and so if there is a problem concerning hypothesis generation, it is one which is equally pressing for two-factor theorists. Parrott speculates that some proposed second factors (cognitive biases) might influence hypothesis generation in such a way that a two-factor account could explain why nonstarter hypotheses are even entertained by subjects. But he notes that without a more developed model of hypothesis generation, we're not yet in a position to determine the prospects for such an approach (Parrott 2021: 344, fn. 24).

Let us move from the non starter problem to the less extreme nearby problem: delusional explanations are *really poor* explanations. This has been taken to be a problem for the one-factor approach in particular. Indeed, Davies and colleagues have it that the idea that delusions arise from the subject's 'normal construction and adoption of an explanation' for an anomalous experience is problematic because 'delusional patients construct explanations that are not plausible and adopt them even when better explanations are available' (Davies et al. 2001: 147). More recently, Coltheart and Davies have argued that given that delusions are 'often bizarre or outlandish', the subject's conflicting knowledge or other beliefs ought to function as disconfirmatory evidence leading to the rejection of the delusional hypothesis (Coltheart and Davies 2021: 222).

I make two points in reply. First, constructing implausible explanations instead of better explanations is hardly unique to delusions. Beliefs in conspiracy theories and the paranormal will often share these features, and yet it is rare to find the suggestion that we have clinically abnormal belief formation or evaluation in these cases. Everyday irrationalities are seen as perfectly well-suited to carry the explanatory burden (Noordhof and Sullivan-Bissett 2021: 10302–10303, 2023: 92–94). This needn't be to deny that there are important differences between delusional beliefs and beliefs of these other kinds (as Chenwie Nie interprets Noordhof and Sullivan-Bissett (2021) [2023: 16, see Sullivan-Bissett and Noordhof 2024: 7 in reply]), but the latter do demonstrate that the charge of poor hypothesis selection is very far from a charge uniquely applicable to delusional explanations. Far more needs to be said before that feature of delusion gives us grounds for a second factor. Furthermore, in these other cases of poor hypothesis selection, it can be more difficult to make excuses on behalf of the subject's seemingly poor judgement. Although (some) conspiracy beliefs or paranormal beliefs may enjoy limited social support, they are not responses to highly anomalous and repeated experiences which are often the basis of delusions.[6] As I have noted elsewhere in a discussion of paranormal beliefs:

> When psychologists studying subjects with delusions become convinced that there needs to be a second factor involving clinical irrationality, they don't keep in firm view just how bizarre the beliefs of subjects in the normal range are, which are formed on the basis of less profound anomalous experiences with socially supported paranormal interpretation. If clinical irrationality is not required here, then it is not required for delusional beliefs.
>
> *(Noordhof and Sullivan-Bissett 2023: 96)*

Second, we can also question the implicit assumption that alternative explanations are *available* in the relevant respect. Let us distinguish three kinds of unavailability of alternatives: *strict* (where the alternative is inaccessible to the subject, perhaps because it is based on information opaque to introspection or otherwise irretrievable); *motivational* (where the alternative is inhibited or inaccessible due to motivational factors); and *explanatory* (where the alternative strikes the subject as implausible enough to not be regarded as a genuine contender) (for more on these notions of unavailability see Sullivan-Bissett 2018: 925–926). Speculatively, strict unavailability of alternatives might be bound up with anomalous experience, although this would need to be reconciled with case reports of people with delusions recognising the bizarre nature of their belief (see e.g. Alexander et al. 1979: 335).[7]

With respect to motivational unavailability, it is commonplace to recognise that beliefs can be formed with some assistance from motivational influences, and indeed, that alternative beliefs can be kept at bay by influences of this kind.[8] Delusions too. Most obviously perhaps in the case of motivational delusions, where the content believed is also the content desired (for example, erotomania or Reverse Othello delusion). But even in delusions which have unwelcome contents, significant relief from the distress caused by anomalous experience may be had for a subject upon forming the delusional belief and *figuring things out*. In addition, the alternative hypothesis that one's experience arises from a problem with oneself is hardly motivationally neutral – in the case of Capgras, accepting that one's imposter experience is neurobiological is 'not a particularly uplifting prospect' (Bortolotti 2023: 59, see also 107). Furthermore, as Maher puts it, 'the social costs and consequences of major decisions made under the influence of the delusion may create a situation in which it is very difficult for the patient to re-examine the belief and publicly reject it' (Maher 2006: 182). (See also Lisa Bortolotti's discussion of delusional persistence and identity, 2023: 83.)

*Explanatory unavailability* may also have something to offer. Maher takes the psychological and epistemic weight of anomalous experience very seriously, describing delusions as developed 'via evidence powerful enough to support [them]' and anomalous experiences as ones which cannot be 'reasoned away' (Maher 1974: 99). Maher's point here is not the obvious one that argument cannot make experience cease, but rather that the experience has epistemic import not easily undercut by claims about its veridicality. Such epistemic import may go some way towards explaining why delusional hypotheses are preferred to non-delusional ones: the experiences may strike one as better explained by the former. As Maher puts it, 'asking patients to prefer a naturalistic theory to their own' would be 'tantamount to asking them to trust the evidence of other people's senses in preference to their own', which, although 'not impossible', is also 'not readily done by most people' (Maher 1988: 25).

In addition, alternative explanations might simply strike the subject as less good than the delusional explanation, insofar as they are being offered by those in poorer epistemic positions:

> Surely, we know our mother or spouse better than anybody else and can tell the subtle differences between the original and the imposter while the people around us are more likely to be fooled by substitution.
>
> *(Bortolotti 2023: 42, see also Reimer 2009: 679–680)*

In discussing the nature of delusional explanations, we have seen the range of resources available to the one-factor theorist. I have been brief but the take-home point is that we can approach poor hypothesis selection in much the same way as we do elsewhere. That is not to deny that it is perfectly interesting to investigate the range of cognitive influences which might contribute to the selection of the less good explanation, indeed, huge swathes of research in psychology and cognitive science seek to do this for other kinds of belief (religious, conspiratorial, paranormal). But since these influences are decidedly not *factors*, that project ought to be kept separate from the one engaged in by one- and two-factor theorists. At this point, we have been given no reason to suppose that the explanatory toolbox usually employed in explanations of other strange beliefs would be inadequate when turning to delusion.[9]

I turn now to discuss an extremely common objection to the one-factor approach, which will reveal the range of explanatory resources available to it.

## 5.   The objection from dissociation

The objection from dissociation has been repeatedly levelled against Maher's one-factor approach. A very clear statement of it is found in Davies and colleagues (2001). In reflecting on experiences that could lead to eight types of delusion, they say:

> On Maher's view, simply suffering from any one of these experiences would be sufficient to produce a delusion, because a delusion is the normal response to such unusual experiences. It follows that anyone who has suffered neuropsychological damage that reduces the affective response to faces should exhibit the Capgras delusion; anyone with a right hemisphere lesion that paralyzes the left limbs and leaves the subject with a sense that the limbs are alien should deny ownership of the limbs; anyone with a loss of the ability to interact fluently with mirrors should exhibit mirrored-self misidentification, and so on. However, these predictions from Maher's theory are clearly falsified by examples from the neuropsychological literature.
>
> *(2001: 144)*

Davies and colleagues proceed to survey several cases of dissociation. This objection has been raised again and again. Indeed, to my knowledge, all two-factor theorists argue that if a one-factor theory were true, then every subject who had the relevant anomalous experience would have the delusional belief. But, since this is not the case, there must be a second factor (see e.g. Chapman and Chapman 1988: 174, Garety 1991: 15, Garety et al. 1991: 194–195, Davies and Coltheart 2000: 11–12, Young and De Pauw 2002: 56, Davies et al. 2005: 224–225, Fine et al. 2005a: 145, Coltheart et al. 2011: 284–285, Coltheart 2015: 23, Miyazono 2018: 39, Coltheart and Davies 2021: 213ff, Nie 2023: 9–10).

There are broadly two ways to respond to the objection. The first is to deny that there are any such cases, and the second is to accept that there are, but show that this is consistent with the one-factor approach. I consider these in turn.

### 5.1   *Denying dissociation*

There are two ways of denying dissociation. The first is to contest the validity of the supposed empirical observation (Davies and colleagues themselves note this with respect to some of their cases [2001: 145]). Consider the case of Capgras delusion, its associated anomalous experience, and purported cases of dissociation. Coltheart has argued that the absence of autonomic response taken to be indicative of anomalous experiences in Capgras subjects is also present in subjects with ventromedial lesions, but the latter subjects do not have the Capgras delusion (Tranel et al. 1995, Coltheart 2007: 1048–1049). However, Sam Wilkinson points out that the lesions are in different areas. Whilst Capgras subjects tend to have right lateral temporal lesions and dorsolateral prefrontal damage, those subjects taken to constitute examples of dissociation have ventromedial prefrontal damage (Wilkinson 2015: 18, see also Corlett 2019 for discussion of the Tranel and colleagues study and its implications for two-factor theories).

The second way to deny dissociation is to distinguish between experiences leading to delusions and those, apparently identical, experiences, which do not. In considering the potential problem of dissociation, Maher suggests that, compared to experience in the healthy population, 'the kinds of anomalous experience that deluded patients have appeared to be much more intense and prolonged' (Maher 1999: 566), and are 'repeated or continue over an extended period' (Maher 2006: 182). If that were right, then anomalous experience (at the requisite intensity and length) would be sufficient for delusion – apparent cases of the same experience would in fact be cases of experience of a more modest nature. To support this idea, Maher draws on Torsten Ingemann Nielsen's (1963) study in which subjects displayed signs of delusion-like thinking having undergone artificially induced anomalous experiences in a laboratory setting (for discussion see Maher 2006: 182, Noordhof and Sullivan-Bissett 2021: 10281–10282). The lesson drawn is that if delusion-like explanations can be prompted by even brief and unrepeated anomalous experiences, then when such experiences are 'more intense and prolonged', they are sufficient for delusion formation. Dissociation is not explained by appeal to a second factor, but rather debunked by appeal to differences in experience.[10]

Davies and colleagues reply to both the claims of duration and intensity. On *duration*, they note that in general, delusions do not arise only after a prolonged period of the subject labouring under an anomalous experience. On *intensity* they say that it is unclear how it is that we could quantify the intensity of an experience (2001: 146). However, they draw on experimental data from Connie Cahill and colleagues (1996) showing that normal subjects and subjects with schizophrenia responded differently to an anomalous experience of hearing their own voice pitch-distorted. Normal subjects were able to identify the voice as their own, despite the distortion, whilst those subjects with schizophrenia often identified the voice as coming from another agent. The frequency of attributing a voice to another agent was correlated both with severity of delusion and the degree of pitch distortion (Cahill et al. 1996: 207). Cahill and colleagues take their findings to suggest that

> the 'hallucination-like' reports elicited by our paradigm resulted from an interaction between an unusual perceptual experience (distorted auditory feedback) and an abnormal mechanism for belief formation present in deluded patients.
>
> *(Cahill et al. 1996: 201)*

I make two points here. First, the study participants had schizophrenia. Davies and colleagues open their paper by contrasting monothematic delusions with 'the polythematic and elaborated delusions or delusional systems that are characteristic of some schizophrenia patients' (Davies et al. 2001: 135). Their two-factor theory is tagged explicitly to monothematic delusions arising from brain injury in particular (although they note an ambition for it to extend to monothematic delusions in psychiatric patients [Davies et al. 2001: 137]). Given this, we must be wary of appealing to experimental data on subjects with delusions in the context of schizophrenia to inform our account of monothematic delusion.[11]

Second, the experimental data are consistent with Maher's claim that cases of dissociation are cases of different experience with respect to duration and/or intensity. Even granting that Cahill and colleagues achieved sameness of experience with respect to intensity across their participants, dissociation of anomalous experience in the laboratory need not suggest the possibility of dissociation of *delusional* experience outside of it. It is consistent with the claim that a particular kind of experience (meeting the relevant thresholds of length and intensity) is sufficient for delusion formation, that we find dissociation in interpretation of experiences which do not have these features to the relevant threshold. The participants underwent 13 trials (each with difference pitch distortion) which were presented in a random order. The experience then, understood as *hearing voice x at pitch y* was not repeated

(Cahill et al. 1996: 206). Were the experiences as *intense* as those associated with delusions? It is hard to deny that the intensity of an experience could be affected by the broader context (taking place in a laboratory, knowing the genesis even if not the source), and the possibility of cognitive penetration resulting from this background knowledge could well make one's experience less intense than the experiences associated with delusion. Cahill and colleagues may have demonstrated a difference in response to experience without a difference in intensity, but there are reasons to doubt that such experience is a good model for the anomalous experience to which deluded subjects are responding outside of the laboratory. (For further critique of the relevance of Cahill and colleagues' study for understanding the nature of anomalous experience, see Reimer 2009: 679.)

## 5.2 Embrace dissociation

The second response to the objection from dissociation is to show that the observation of dissociation is consistent with the one-factor approach. That is, let us proceed without questioning any further the claim that there are cases of *same experience*, but only some of those experiences lead to delusion. Let us instead turn to the *sufficiency claim*, that is, the claim that anomalous experience is *sufficient* for delusion formation. The force of the objection from dissociation comes from taking Maher to endorse the sufficiency claim, without which, dissociation would be unproblematic. I suggest that (1) it is *probably* a mistake to understand Maher as a proponent of the sufficiency claim, but in any case (2) it is *definitely* a mistake to understand the one-factor approach as requiring it.

Davies and colleagues characterise Maher's view as one which holds that 'delusions are false beliefs that arise as normal responses to experiences' (Davies et al. 2001: 133), and in outlining Maher's account, they quote the four hypotheses constituting his model:

- Delusional beliefs, like normal beliefs, arise from an attempt to explain experience.
- The processes by which deluded persons reason from experience to belief are not significantly different from the processes by which non-deluded persons do.
- Defective reasoning about actual personal normal experience is not the primary contributor to the formation of delusional beliefs.
- The origins of anomalous experience may lie in a broad band of neuropsychological anomalies.

(Maher 1999: 550–551, cited in Davies et al. 2001: 138)

Nothing in the characterisation of Maher's position here suggests an endorsement of the sufficiency claim. Maher is rather interested in *normality*. In earlier work he had it that the cognitive activity of people with delusions is 'essentially indistinguishable' from that employed by non-delusional people, and talks of delusions being developed 'through the operation of *normal cognitive processes*' (Maher 1974: 103, my emphasis). Later he argued that 'the cognitive processes by which delusions are formed are in no important respect different from those by which normal beliefs are formed' (Maher 1992: 262). And in the above outline of his view, the first two points concern normal processes of belief formation directed at strange experience. Not only does nothing in these claims suggest that anomalous experience is sufficient for delusion formation, they suggest quite the opposite! Normal cognitive processes, in addition to anomalous experiences, are also clearly implicated in a delusion's genesis. *Normal* cognition will tolerate a range of responses to particular experiences. It could thus even be a prediction of the one-factor approach, and indeed utterly unremarkable, that some people will have a given anomalous experience but not go on to develop a delusion.

Davies and colleagues move from something's being *normal*, to something's being *sufficient*. This move is evident when they say 'on Maher's view, simply suffering from any one of these experiences would be sufficient to produce a delusion, *because* a delusion is the normal response to such unusual experiences' (Davies et al. 2001: 145, my emphasis). But the key point for Maher was that whatever cognitive quirks or intellectual styles we find to be involved in the move from experience to belief formation and maintenance, they do not constitute clinical abnormalities.

All of that said, though, there are two places that Maher hints at the sufficiency claim, which is why I say that he was only *probably* not committed to it. The first is when he cites Graham Reed:

> Given the necessary information, the observer can empathise with the subject; If he himself were to have such an unusual experience he would express beliefs about it which would be just as unusual as those of the subject.
>
> *(Reed 1974: 154, cited in Maher 1999: 551)*

The second hint at the sufficiency claim comes later in the same paper where Maher turns to pre-empt the objection from dissociation (Maher 1999: 566). He responds by denying dissociation, and appealing to duration and intensity as the relevant experiential difference makers (as discussed in the previous sub-section).

So did Maher endorse the sufficiency claim? If he did, it was certainly not central to his approach. When we look at the various outlines of his model, the sufficiency claim or anything equivalent is missing (see for example the commitments of the model given in Maher 1992: 262–264, 1999: 550–551, 2006: 181–182). Where there is some evidence that he endorsed sufficiency (in quoting Reed and responding to the problem of dissociation, Maher 1999), he concludes that same paper in a way unfriendly to the sufficiency claim:

> It is entirely possible that delusions, like normal beliefs, arise from heterogenous sources. [...] the study of delusions [...] highlights the cognitive processes that typically emerge in the attempt to find meaning in the presence of uncertainty.
>
> *(Maher 1999: 567)*

It is hard to reconcile the idea that delusions arise from heterogenous sources and a range of cognitive processes with the idea that anomalous experiences are *sufficient* for delusion formation. Maher's quoted conclusion here does not suggest that it is his view that an experiential anomaly would – whatever else might be going on with the subject cognitively – produce or sustain a delusion. There is, then, limited evidence that Maher endorsed the sufficiency claim. And yet, such a perceived endorsement has been the main grounds on which his view has been rejected.

However, even if Maher were a one-factor theorist of the sufficiency kind, this is not the only way of being a one-factor theorist, and the overall prospects of the approach have been vastly underestimated when this is not recognised. The key point of the one-factor approach is that there is one clinical abnormality involved in the genesis and maintenance of a delusional belief. As Gerrans put it, for the one-factor theorist, delusions are 'rationalizations of anomalous experiences via reasoning strategies that are not, in themselves abnormal' (Gerrans 2002: 47). As I note elsewhere, 'nothing in the statement of this approach suggests that anybody who has the definitive anomalous experience must have the delusional belief as well' (Noordhof and Sullivan-Bissett 2021: 10297). The two-factor theorist is mistaken in expecting the one-factor theorist to identify an anomaly which would, whatever the psychology, give rise to delusion. As Maher puts it:

> Normal beliefs appear to be acquired in many different ways. [...] We do not seek to find a single cause of normal beliefs. Nor should we assume that manifestly similar clinical phenomena necessarily arise from a pathway that began with a single specific pathology.
>
> *(Maher 1992: 267)*

The empirical observation of different beliefs arising from the same experience is simply not relevant in assessing the merits of the one-factor view, since the key point is not that delusional beliefs have a single cause, but rather that, of the range of causes of delusional beliefs, only one of them has the feature of being abnormal.

Now, it might be accepted that, strictly speaking, dissociation is not inconsistent with the one-factor theory – the observation that some non-delusional people have the experience implicated in delusion is, technically, no mark against the account. However, it might nevertheless be thought that cases of dissociation lend support to two-factor theories, who take such cases as their starting point for identifying a second factor. A natural question to ask in the face of dissociation cases is *what explains the difference* between those who have the experience and become delusional, and those who have the experience and do not? Two-factor theorists have a ready-made answer in their pockets: what explains the difference is the second factor, present in the person who becomes delusional, and absent in the person who does not. Does the one-factor account have anything to offer here?

The one-factor theorist can help herself to the many resources of cognitive science, social psychology, epistemology, philosophy of mind, and so on in explaining cases of dissociation. Everyday irrationalities, or idiosyncrasies, can bear the weight of the explanatory burden. This kind of project, though, need not be taken to be within the remit of a one-factor theorist's task. Her task is to identify the number of factors needed to explain delusional belief, *not* to explain the various other causal contributions in this context.

## 6.   Concluding remarks

In this chapter, I have overviewed Maher's one-factor approach. I explicated its virtues and explanatory resources by considering hypothesis selection, and a key objection from dissociation. We have seen that the one-factor account is not put under pressure by the idea that delusions are poor explanations, or the (apparent) observation of cases of dissociation.

The two-factor theory has been advertised as able to fill the explanatory gaps charged to be left by the one-factor theory. This is based on an underestimation of the resources available to the one-factor theory. I haven't spoken to the positive case for the two-factor theory (although I have done some of this work elsewhere, see Noordhof and Sullivan-Bissett 2021). I have not, then, shown that there is no case to be made for a two-factor theory, only that it ought not be motivated by the misperceived inadequacies of a one-factor approach. For my money, the one-factor approach should be the default hypothesis.

I finish with a couple of methodological remarks. I have argued elsewhere that the research trajectory of researchers seeking a second factor is different from that of researchers investigating alien abduction beliefs (Sullivan-Bissett 2020), paranormal beliefs (Noordhof and Sullivan-Bissett 2023), and conspiracy beliefs (Ichino and Sullivan-Bissett *manuscript*). Now that we can see the shape of the one-factor theory, it is my view that these methodological differences in our approaches to understanding delusions as compared to other bizarre, evidence-resistant beliefs, is not justified.

Finally, a temptation is to identify some cases where it does look proper to appeal to two factors. Particular cases may well involve abnormalities of the kind two-factor theorists appeal to. But that does not justify generalising from particular cases to the nature of delusions simpliciter. And the claim of the two-factor theorist is strong, as Coltheart and Davies have recently put it: 'a delusion will *only* result when a second factor is also present' (2021: 215, my emphasis), and in several places Coltheart, Davies, and their collaborators have suggested that their approach is intended to apply to *all* monothematic delusions (see e.g. Coltheart et al. 2011: 285). But it is a mistake to generalise from particular cases to a claim about the nature of monothematic delusion simpliciter. If we're in the market for a theory of monothematic delusions as a kind, the one-factor account strikes me as a good place to start.

## Acknowledgements

I acknowledge the support of the Arts and Humanities Research Council (*Deluded by Experience*, grant no. AH/T013486/10). I am grateful to Carolina Flores, Eleanor Palafox-Harris, and Sam Wilkinson for comments on an earlier draft of this chapter. Thanks go also to Paul Noordhof with whom I have previously developed many of the ideas presented here.

## Notes

1 Paul Francheschi (2008) has argued for a one-factor approach to polythematic delusions, understanding them as rising from *apophenia*, helped along by common errors of reasoning.
2 Sometimes this characterisation of a factor is not kept firmly in view. For example, Max Coltheart and Davies have recently defended a two-factor theory of the Koro delusion (the belief that *one's penis is shrinking into one's abdomen in a way that might be fatal*) (2024). The 'factors' they appeal to are, by their own lights, perfectly ordinary experiences, together with culturally normal background beliefs, limited formal education, and/or sociocultural factors. However, the explanatory power of factor-talk is lost when we divorce it from picking out abnormalities, since the explanatory role of e.g. limited formal education in an explanation of a belief is not a role relevant to an explanation of *delusional* belief in particular. Theories identifying the various normal range contributions to delusions are of course interesting and important, but talk of factors in this context obscures the special explanatory role played by particular kinds of contribution (those which are abnormal).
3 Although factors are often associated with neuropsychological damage, two-factor theorists have been clear that they need not be (see e.g. Coltheart et al. 2011: 291). Functional abnormalities need not always be realised by neuropsychological damage, but where functional abnormality remains hard to make out, theorists could fall back on statistical abnormality to capture the relevant anomalies. Since this is a taxonomical difficulty for all involved, I put this complication aside.
4 I say *can* because I do not want to rule out delusions arising as explanations of experiences which need not be abnormal (erotomania might be such a case, see also discussion in Bell et al. 2008). Understanding the one-factor approach as an *at most* claim may well be idiosyncratic, but the key point is that we certainly do not need a second factor. This flexibility may allow us to tell a story about alien

abduction beliefs which could be properly characterised as delusions, even though the experience which prompts them may be shared among healthy subjects and so is not a statistical abnormality (Sullivan-Bissett 2020). We might also characterise the Koro belief as a delusion, even though the experiences which might prompt the hypothesis are everyday (illness, urination, ejaculation) and so do not constitute a functional abnormality (see Coltheart and Davies 2024 for discussion).

5 For reasons of space, I do not consider the relationship between delusion and evidence, and how that bears on the plausibility of the one-factor account. I have done so elsewhere (see Noordhof and Sullivan-Bissett 2021, 2023. For arguments that delusions are evidence-responsive see Flores (2021).

6 Garry Young has argued that, at least in the case of Capgras delusion, in light of the anomalous experience, 'the subject feels justified in broadening the scope of what he feels is epistemically possible, as he looks to explain what is happening' (Young 2023: 161).

7 In their discussion of Parrott's objection that predictive processing theories cannot explain non starter hypothesis generation, Federico Bongiorno and Philip Corlett draw on Jakob Hohwy who has it that 'those more probable alternatives are not selected because they are unable to explain away aberrant prediction errors at the right spatiotemporal fineness of grain' (2013: 161, cited in Bongiorno and Corlett *forthcoming*).

8 One way of motivational influences having this effect is through evidence avoidance, something taken to be key to the development and maintenance of self-deceptive beliefs, and even more everyday cognitive failings like the application of confirmation bias (Flores 2021: 6309).

9 So often the one-factor theory earns itself a bad reputation because it is mistaken to be overly generous. Indeed, some folk have even understood Maher to claim that forming a delusional belief on the basis of an anomalous experience is *rational response* to that experience (Davies and Coltheart 2000: 8, Bentall et al. 2001: 1149, Bortolotti 2009: 57). It has long been recognised that this is not the claim of the one-factor approach (Gerrans 2002: 48).

10 Marga Reimer takes forward this idea suggesting that, in the case of Capgras at least, the neurological damage 'causes both an affective deficit in face processing and some other experiential abnormality', and suggests that the resulting experience could be sufficient to generate Capgras (Reimer 2009: 678). The second experiential abnormality would explain the special intensity or vividness of the anomalous experience. B. S. Lana Frankle has recently made a similar argument. She notes that two subjects (one delusional, one not) can have perfect overlap in the information they share, by which she means that someone with delusional experience could, in theory, articulate that experience in a way that it is fully captured and understood by a non-delusional subject. However, to explain dissociation she speculates that we can posit a 'fundamental qualia about certain altered perceptual experiences that is beyond the realm of explicit knowledge' (Frankle 2021: 7). And so, even though experiences that prompt delusions may resemble experiences which do not prompt delusions, the addition of a particular kind of qualia in the case of the former can explain why delusions are prompted. This hypothesis is destined to remain in the realms of speculation; Frankle gives no theoretical or empirical justification for it, and although it is friendly to the one-factor account, no one not already committed to such an approach would have any new grounds to accept it.

11 Although Davies and colleagues note that the relationships between monothematicity and circumscription on the one hand, and polythematicity and elaboration on the other are not exceptionless (Davies et al. 2001: 135), their focus is nevertheless on monothematic delusions, and not delusions as they occur in the broader context of schizophrenia.

# References

Alexander, M. P., Stuss, D. T., and Benson, D. F. 1979: 'Capgras Syndrome: A Reduplicative Phenomenon'. *Neurology*. Vol. 29, pp. 334–339.

Ames, David 1984: 'Self-Shooting of a Phantom Head'. *The British Journal of Psychiatry*. Vol. 145, no. 2, pp. 193–194.

Bayne, Tim and Pacherie, Elisabeth 2005: 'In Defence of the Doxastic Conception of Delusion'. *Mind and Language*. Vol. 20, no. 2, pp. 163–188.

Bayne, Tim and Pacherie, Elisabeth 2004: 'Bottom-Up or Top-Down: Campbell's Rationalist Account of Monothematic Delusions'. *Philosophy, Psychiatry, and Psychology*. Vol. 11, no. 1, pp. 1–11.

Bell, Vaughan, Halligan, Peter W., and Hadyn, Ellis. 2008: 'Are Anomalous Perceptual Experiences Necessary for Delusions?' *The Journal of Nervous and Mental Disease*. Vol. 196, no. 1, pp. 3–8.

Bentall, Richard P., Corcoran, Rhiannon, Howard, Robert, Blackwood, Nigel, and Kinderman, Peter 2001: 'Persecutory Delusions: A Review and Theoretical Integration'. *Clinical Psychology Review*. Vol. 21, no. 8, pp. 1143–1192.

Bongiorno, Federico and Corlett, Philip *forthcoming*: 'Delusions and the Predictive Mind'. *Australasian Journal of Philosophy*. doi: 10.1080/00048402.2023.2293825

Bortolotti, Lisa 2009: *Delusions and Other Irrational Beliefs*. Oxford: Oxford University Press.

Bortolotti, Lisa 2023: *Why Delusions Matter*. London: Bloomsbury.

Brotherton, Rob 2015: *Suspicious Minds. Why We Believe Conspiracy Theories*. London: Bloomsbury Sigma.

Cahill, Connie, Silbersweig, David, and Frith, Chris 1996: 'Psychotic Experiences Induced in Deluded Patients Using Distorted Auditory Feedback'. *Cognitive Neuropsychiatry*. Vol. 1, no. 3, pp. 201–211.

Chapman, Loren J. and Chapman, Jean P. 1988: 'The Genesis of Delusions'. In Oltmanns, T. F. and Maher, B. A. (eds.) *Delusional Beliefs*. Wiley, pp. 167–183.

Coltheart, Max 2007: 'Cognitive Neuropsychology and Delusional Belief'. *The Quarterly Journal of Experimental Psychology*. Vol. 60, no. 8, pp. 1041–1062.

Coltheart, Max 2013: 'On the Distinction between Monothematic and Polythematic Delusions'. *Mind & Language*. Vol. 28, no. 1, pp. 103–112.

Coltheart, Max 2015: 'From the Internal Lexicon to Delusional Belief'. *AVANT*. Vol. 3, pp. 19–29.

Coltheart, Max and Davies, Martin 2021: 'Failure of Hypothesis Evaluation as a Factor in Delusional Belief'. *Cognitive Neuropsychiatry*. Vol. 26, no. 4, pp. 213–260.

Coltheart, Max and Davies, Martin 2024: 'Koro: A Socially-transmitted Delusional Belief'. *Cognitive Neuropsychiatry*. Vol. 29, no. 1, pp. 10–28.

Coltheart, Max, Langdon, Robyn, and McKay, Ryan 2011: 'Delusional Belief'. *Annual Review of Psychology*. Vol. 62, no. 1, pp. 271–298.

Corlett, Philip 2019: 'Factor One, Familiarity and Frontal Cortex, a Challenge to the Two-Factor Theory of Delusions'. *Cognitive Neuropsychiatry*. Vol. 24, no. 3, pp. 165–177.

Davies, Martin 2009: 'Delusion and Motivationally Biased Belief. Self-Deception in the Two-Factor Framework'. In Bayne, Tim and Fernández, Jordi (eds.) *Delusion and Self-Deception*. New York: Psychology Press, pp. 71–86.

Davies, Martin and Coltheart, Max 2000: 'Introduction: Pathologies of Belief'. *Mind and Language*. Vol 15, no. 1, pp. 1–46.

Davies, Martin, Coltheart, Max, Langdon, Robyn, and Breen, Nora 2001: 'Monothematic Delusions: Towards a Two-Factor Account'. *Philosophy, Psychiatry, & Psychology*. Vol. 8, no. (2–3), pp. 133–158.

Davies, Martin, Davies, Aimola Anna, and Coltheart, Max 2005: 'Anosognosia and the Two-Factor Theory of Delusions'. *Mind and Language*. Vol. 20, no. 2, pp. 209–236.

Fine, Cordelia, Craigie, Jillian and Gold, Ian 2005a: 'Damned If You Do; Damned If You Don't: The Impasses in Cognitive Accounts of the Capgras Delusion'. *Philosophy, Psychiatry, and Psychology*. Vol. 12, no. 2, pp. 143–151.

Fine, Cordelia, Craigie, Jillian and Gold, Ian 2005b: 'The Explanation Approach to Delusion'. *Philosophy, Psychiatry, and Psychology*. Vol. 12, no. 2, pp. 159–163.

Flores, Carolina 2021: 'Delusional Evidence-Responsiveness'. *Synthese*. Vol. 199, pp. 6299–6330.

Francheschi, Paul 2008: 'A Logical Defence of Maher's Model of Polythematic Delusions'. *Philosophiques*. Vol. 25, no. 2, pp. 451–475. English translation used here, available: https://core.ac.uk/download/pdf/14897.pdf

Frankle, B. S. Lana 2021: 'In Defense of the One-Factor Doxastic Account: A Phenomenal Account of Delusions'. *Consciousness and Cognition*. Vol. 94, p. 10381.

Garety, Philippa 1991: 'Reasoning and Delusions'. *British Journal of Psychiatry*. Vol. 159, no. 14, pp. 14–19.

Garety, Philippa A., Hemsley, David R., and Wessely, Simon. 1991: 'Reasoning in Deluded Schizophrenic and Paranoid Patients Biases in Performance on a Probabilistic Inference Task'. *The Journal of Nervous and Mental Disease*. Vol. 179, pp. 194–201.

Gerrans, Philip 2002: 'A One-Stage Explanation of the Cotard Delusion'. *Philosophy, Psychiatry, and Psychology*. Vol. 9, no. 1, pp. 47–53.

Hohwy, Jakob 2013: *The Predictive Mind*. Croydon: Oxford University Press.

Ichino, Anna and Sullivan-Bissett, Ema *manuscript*: 'Conspiracy Beliefs and Monothematic Delusions: A Case for De-Patholigizing'.

Imhoff, Roland and Lamberty, Pia Karoline 2017: 'Too Special to Be Duped: Need for Uniqueness Motivates Conspiracy Beliefs'. *European Journal of Social Psychology*. Vol. 47, no. 6, pp. 724–734.

James, William 1890: *The Principles of Psychology*. Volume Two. New York: Henry Holt and Company.

Lindeman, Marjaana and Aarnio, Kia 2006: 'Paranormal Beliefs: Their Dimensionality and Correlates'. *European Journal of Personality*. Vol. 20, pp. 585–602.

Maher, Brendan 1974: 'Delusional Thinking and Perceptual Disorder'. *Journal of Individual Psychology*. Vol. 30, no. 1, pp. 98–113.

Maher, Brendan 1988: 'Anomalous Experience and Delusional Thinking: The Logic of Explanations'. In Oltmanns, Thomas and Maher, Brendan (eds.) *Delusional Beliefs*. New York: John Wiley and Sons, pages 15–33.

Maher, Brendan 1992: 'Delusions: Contemporary Etiological Hypotheses'. *Psychiatric Annals*. Vol. 22, no. 5, pp. 260–268.

Maher, Brendan 1999: 'Anomalous Experience in Everyday Life: Its Significance for Psychopathology'. *The Monist*. Vol. 82, no. 4, pp. 547–570.

Maher, Brendan 2006: 'The Relationship between Delusions and Hallucinations'. *Current Psychiatric Reports*. Vol. 8, pp. 179–183.

McKay, Ryan, Langdon, Robyn, and Coltheart, Max 2010: '"Sleights of Mind": Delusions, Defences and Self-deception'. *Cognitive Neuropsychiatry*. Vol. 10, no. 4, pp. 305–326.

Miyazono, Kengo 2018: *Delusions and Belief*. Oxon: Routledge.

Nguyen, C. Thi 2020: 'Echo Chambers and Epistemic Bubbles'. *Episteme*. Vol. 17, no. 2, pp. 141–161.

Nie, Chenwei 2023: 'Revising Maher's One-Factor Theory of Delusion'. *Neuroethics*. Vol. 16, article no. 15, pp. 1–16.

Nielsen, Torsten Ingemann 1963: 'Volition: A New Experimental Approach'. *Scandanavian Journal of Psychology*. Vol. 4, pp. 225–230.

Noordhof, Paul and Sullivan-Bissett, Ema 2021: 'The Clinical Significance of Anomalous Experience in the Explanation of Delusion Formation'. *Synthese*. Vol. 199, pp. 10277–10309.

Noordhof, Paul and Sullivan-Bissett, Ema 2023: 'The Everyday Irrationality of Monothematic Delusion'. In Henne, Paul and Murray, Sam (eds.) *Advances in Experimental Philosophy of Action*. London: Routledge, pp. 87–111.

Parrott, Matthew 2021: 'Delusional Predictions and Explanations'. *The British Journal for the Philosophy of Science*. Vol. 72, no. 1, pp. 325–353.

Reed, Graham 1974: *The Psychology of Anomalous Experience: A Cognitive Approach*. Boston, MA: Houghton Mifflin.

Reimer, Marga 2009: 'Is the Imposter Hypothesis Really So Preposterous? Understanding the Capgras Experience'. *Philosophical Psychology*. Vol. 22, no. 6, pp. 669–686.

Stone and Young 1997: 'Delusions and Brain Injury: The Philosophy and Psychology of Belief'. *Mind and Language*. Vol. 12, no. 3–4, pp. 327–364.

Sullivan-Bissett, Ema 2018: 'Monothematic Delusion: A Case of Innocence from Experience'. *Philosophical Psychology*. Vol. 31, no. 6, pp. 920–947.

Sullivan-Bissett, Ema 2020: 'Unimpaired Abduction to Alien Abduction: Lessons on Delusion Formation'. *Philosophical Psychology*. Vol. 33, no. 5, pp. 679–704.

Sullivan-Bissett, Ema and Noordhof, Paul 2024: 'Revisiting Maher's One-Factor Theory of Delusion, Again'. *Neuroethics*. Vol. 17, no. 17, pp. 1–8.

Tranel, Daniel, Damasio, Hanna and Damasio, Antonio R. 1995: 'Double Dissociation between Overt and Covert Face Recognition', *Journal of Cognitive Neuroscience*. Vol. 7, no. 4, pp. 425–432.

Wilkinson, Sam 2015: 'Delusions, Dreams and the Nature of Identification'. *Philosophical Psychology*. Vol. 28, no. 2, pp. 203–226.

Young, Andrew W. and De Pauw, Karel W. 2002: 'One Stage Is Not Enough'. *Philosophy, Psychiatry, and Psychology*. Vol. 9, no. 1, pp. 55–59. Young, Andrew W., Robertson, Ian H., Hellawell, Deborah J., de Pauw, Karel W., and Pentland, Brian 1992: 'Cotard Delusion after Brain Injury'. *Psychological Medicine*. Vol. 22, 799–804.

Young, Garry 2023: 'The Capgras Delusion: An Interactionist Approach Revisited'. In Sullivan-Bissett, Ema (ed.) *Belief, Imagination, and Delusion*. Oxford: Oxford University Press, pp. 151–182.

29

# THE TWO-FACTOR THEORY

*Martin Davies and Max Coltheart*

## 1. Introduction

The starting point for the two-factor theory of delusion is that an explanation of any case of monothematic delusional belief requires answers to two questions. The first question is:

What initially prompted the delusional idea or hypothesis?

William James proposed that delusional ideas arise as putatively explanatory hypotheses prompted by bodily sensations: 'The delusions of the insane are apt to affect certain typical forms, often very hard to explain. But in many cases they are certainly theories which the patients invent to account for their abnormal bodily sensations' (1890, Volume 2: 114). Brendan Maher made a similar proposal: 'Strange events, felt to be significant, demand explanation. [A] delusion is a hypothesis designed to explain unusual perceptual phenomena' (1974: 103).

We think that James and Maher were broadly correct about our first question: delusional ideas arise as possible explanations of unpredicted phenomena. The trigger for the generation of a delusional idea or hypothesis is a prediction error (failed prediction) and the two-factor theory has been a prediction-error theory since its inception (Langdon & Coltheart 2000; also see Coltheart 2005a: 73, 2005b: 155; for more on prediction error accounts, see Corlett, Chapter 30). It is clear, however, that an answer to the first question—an account of what prompted a delusional idea or hypothesis—would not yet provide an explanation of a case of delusion. The reason is that a delusional idea or hypothesis is not yet a delusion. It is not a belief—let alone a 'fixed belief [that is] not amenable to change in light of conflicting evidence' (*DSM-5*, 2013: 87). Thus, an explanation of a case of delusion also requires an answer to a second question:

Why was the delusional idea or hypothesis adopted and maintained as a belief rather than being rejected—as it should have been—on the basis of available evidence and background knowledge that counted against it?

DOI: 10.4324/9781003296386-35

430

An answer to the first question indicates a first factor in the explanation of a case of delusion—a factor that prompts hypothesis generation—whereas an answer to the second question indicates a second factor—resulting in a failure of hypothesis evaluation.

Plausible answers to our first question have been identified for cases of several monothematic delusions, including mirrored-self misidentification, Capgras delusion, Cotard delusion, Fregoli delusion, somatoparaphrenia, and the delusion of alien control (see Table 29.1).[1] In these cases, the first factors have been neuropsychological in nature and (as Table 29.1 illustrates) first factors vary from delusion to delusion and may also vary between cases of the same delusion (e.g., mirrored-self misidentification). As a result of the first-factor neuropsychological impairment, the person observes or encounters an unpredicted phenomenon—a surprising fact or event—and this, in turn, prompts the delusional idea or hypothesis (see Table 29.1, columns 1–3).

*Table 29.1* Six types of delusional condition

| Delusional condition | Unpredicted phenomenon | Delusional hypothesis | Non-delusional cases in which the unexpected phenomenon is present |
|---|---|---|---|
| Mirrored-self misidentification (e.g., Breen et al. 2000: case FE) | Failure to recognise the face one sees when looking into a mirror as one's own face. | The person I see when I look in the mirror is a stranger, not me. | Many people with prosopagnosia are not delusional. |
| Mirrored-self misidentification (e.g., Breen et al. 2000: case TH) | Mirror agnosia present, so mirrors treated as windows. The seen person appears to be in the space behind the glass. | The person I see when I look in the mirror is a stranger, not me. | Binkofski and colleagues (1999): mirror agnosia without delusion. |
| Capgras delusion (e.g., Edelstyn and Oyebode 1999) | Failure of autonomic response to familiar faces (e.g., face of spouse). | This person I am looking at is a stranger, not my spouse. | Following neurosurgery to treat intractable epilepsy, a patient reported that there was something different about her mother—'it didn't feel like her'; but the patient had no delusion (Turner and Coltheart 2010). |
| Cotard delusion (e.g., Young et al. 1992) | Depersonalisation (e.g., de-emotivity, derealisation, de-somatisation). | I am dead. | Many people with depersonalisation symptoms do not have Cotard delusion.[a] |
| Fregoli delusion (e.g., Langdon, Connaughton, and Coltheart 2014) | Presence of autonomic response even to unfamiliar faces.[b] | People with whom I am familiar are present in my environment, disguised. | Vuilleumier and colleagues (2003): strong autonomic responses to unfamiliar faces (we presume) but no delusion. |

*(Continued)*

*Table 29.1* (Continued)

| Delusional condition | Unpredicted phenomenon | Delusional hypothesis | Non-delusional cases in which the unexpected phenomenon is present |
|---|---|---|---|
| Somatoparaphrenia (e.g., Vallar and Ronchi 2009) | Paralysis and loss of kinaesthetic and proprioceptive feedback from the arm. | This limb (the paralysed limb) is not mine, it is someone else's. | Many people with a paralysed limb and without kinaesthetic and proprioceptive feedback are not delusional. |
| Passivity delusion ('alien control') (e.g., Stirling, Hellewell, and Quraishi 1998) | Failure of cancellation of feedback from motor response by efference copy. | Other people can cause my limbs to move without my volition. | In 'haptic deafferentation', the patient gets no sensory feedback from actions performed (Fourneret et al. 2002). But no delusion present. |

For each type of delusional condition, the table shows the specific unpredicted phenomenon associated with the delusion, the delusional hypothesis which would explain this phenomenon, and cases where the specific unexpected phenomenon associated with the delusion is present in people who are nevertheless not delusional.

[a] A diagnosis of depersonalisation disorder requires that reality testing is intact. Patients describe their experiences in 'as if' terms.

[b] Here, we adopt a suggestion by Ramachandran and Blakeslee (1998: 171). But we also note that Langdon and colleagues (2014) argue, against this suggestion, that 'the Fregoli delusional content is generated when hyperexcitation from the cognitive system to the PINs [person identity nodes] causes a known person to be identified as present, even when no matching face is also present' (2014: 628).

Here are two examples. First, as a result of significantly impaired face processing (Breen et al. 2001), patient FE encountered the unpredicted phenomenon of seeing in the mirror a face that he did not recognise as his own face, and this prompted the idea that the person that he saw in the mirror was not himself. Second, as a result of disconnection of the face processing system from the autonomic nervous system, a person with Capgras delusion encounters an unpredicted phenomenon—the absence of the predicted autonomic response to a familiar face (e.g., the spouse's face). The person (consciously) observes only that there is something odd about the viewed individual but, by unconscious processes that draw on the information that the faces of strangers do not evoke autonomic responses, the unpredicted phenomenon prompts the idea that the individual is a stranger.

Delusional ideas or hypotheses should be rejected on the basis of available evidence and background knowledge that counts against them but, in every case of delusion, a delusional hypothesis is adopted and maintained as a belief. This failure to reject the hypothesis is not explained by the first factor (indicated by the answer to the first question) but by a second factor (indicated by an answer to the second question). Earlier expositions of the two-factor theory have typically argued the need for a second factor by presenting cases in which the first factor is present but the corresponding delusion is absent. This is not a matter of presenting, for each delusion, a single case of dissociation: first factor without delusion. Rather, there are large numbers of people who have the first factor impairment, and observe or encounter the unpredicted phenomenon that prompts the delusional idea, but who do not have the delusion. This shows that the first factor (and the resulting unpredicted phenomenon) does not, by itself, explain the delusion; there must be at least one explanatory factor in addition to the first factor. (For arguments against the need for a second factor, see Noordhof and Sullivan-Bissett, 2021; Sullivan-Bissett, 2022; and Sullivan-Bissett, Chapter 28. Note that arguments for or against a second factor in delusions may depend on how the notion of a 'factor' is understood.)

The question might be raised, however, why this shows that there must be, not just some additional factor or other but, specifically, a second factor that results in a failure of hypothesis evaluation. In earlier expositions of the argument for a second factor, there has been an implicit assumption that the delusional idea comes to the minds of all people who have the first factor impairment and observe or encounter the resulting unpredicted phenomenon. Given this assumption, all people with the first factor but not the corresponding delusion have entertained the delusional hypothesis and have rejected it as false—or, at least, have declined the opportunity to adopt and maintain it as a belief. These non-delusional people demonstrate that having the first factor and generating the delusional hypothesis does not inevitably lead to the delusion. By comparison with the non-delusional people, the people who adopt and maintain the delusional hypothesis as a belief show a failure of hypothesis evaluation. (We shall return to this point in Section 4, below.)

There is some reason to propose that, in the cases under discussion (in which the first factor is neuropsychological in nature), the second factor—resulting in failure of hypothesis evaluation—is also neuropsychological, with a neural basis in damage to, or hypoactivation of, right dorsolateral prefrontal cortex (rDLPFC). Max Coltheart (2007, 2010) reviewed evidence supporting this proposal and Coltheart and colleagues (2018) found that repetitive transcranial magnetic stimulation (rTMS) to rDLPFC (but not rTMS to left DLPFC) resulted in healthy subjects being less likely to reject the false hypotheses embodied in hypnotic suggestions.

In the early development of the two-factor theory of delusion, the methodology of the (then) emerging discipline of cognitive neuropsychiatry (David 1993; Halligan & David 2001) was adopted. That is, the methods of cognitive neuropsychology were applied to psychiatric disorders—specifically, to delusions (for discussion, see Young 2000). Questions about the scope of the theory were explicitly addressed (e.g., Coltheart 2005a). One option would have been to limit the scope of the theory to neuropsychological cases of delusion and to leave it to some other theory to explain other cases. The option that was actually adopted was

> to explore the idea that, in any delusion, there is a factor that explains where the idea came from in the first place and a second factor that explains why the idea becomes an enduring belief rather than being rejected; but these factors are not always neuropsychological deficits.
>
> *(2005a: 75)*

## 2.   The two-factor theory and the Peircean pathway model

According to the two-factor theory of delusion, the first factor results in the person observing or encountering an unpredicted phenomenon—a surprising fact or event—and this prompts the delusional hypothesis. In early expositions of the theory, rather little was said about the process of hypothesis generation that brings the delusional hypothesis to mind.

The second factor results in a failure of hypothesis evaluation but, again, rather little was said about the processes that are involved in hypothesis evaluation and how they might fail. It has proved illuminating to consider the two-factor theory against the background of an eight-step model of the normal pathway from surprising facts to new beliefs, based on the work of the American pragmatist philosopher Charles Sanders Peirce (1839–1914)—the Peircean pathway model (see Figure 29.1).[2] As John Marshall and Peter Halligan (1996) remarked:

> One would … hope that theories of normal belief-formation will eventually cast light on both the content of delusions and on the processes by which the beliefs came to be held.
>
> *(1996: 8)*

Peirce used the term 'abduction' for the process by which explanatory hypotheses are generated from surprising observations:

> Long before I first classed abduction as an inference it was recognized by logicians that the operation of adopting an explanatory hypothesis,—which is just what abduction is,—was subject to certain conditions. Namely, the hypothesis cannot be admitted, even as a hypothesis, unless it be supposed that it would account for the facts or some of them. The form of inference therefore is this:
> The surprising fact, $C$, is observed;
> But if $A$ were true, $C$ would be a matter of course.
> Hence, there is reason to suspect that $A$ is true.
>
> *(Peirce 1903/1998: 231)*

This three-line inference, set out in Peirce's 1903/1998 *Harvard Lectures on Pragmatism*, is commonly considered to be his canonical rendering of the logical form of abductive inference.

We can see how Peirce's work on abduction—and, particularly, his abductive inference— might shed light on the processes implicated in the formation of delusional beliefs if, for example (see Table 29.1, case FE), we take Peirce's surprising fact $C$ to be:

> I do not recognise the face that I see when looking into the mirror as my own face.

and his hypothesis $A$ to be:

> The person I see when I look in the mirror is a stranger, not me.

The three-line abductive inference would then be:

> The surprising fact $C$, 'I do not recognise the face that I see when looking into the mirror as my own face', is observed;
> But if $A$, 'The person I see when I look in the mirror is a stranger, not me', were true, $C$ would be a matter of course.
> Hence, there is reason to suspect that 'The person I see when I look in the mirror is a stranger, not me' is true.

Step 1 along the Peircean pathway is observation of a surprising fact and Step 2 is generation of a hypothesis that putatively meets the critical criterion that if the hypothesis were true, the surprising fact would follow as a matter of course. If hypothesis generation is understood as an empirical—not necessarily ideal—process, then it would be as well to confirm (i) that the generated hypothesis actually met the critical criterion. In some of his work (e.g., 1901/1998: 106–110), Peirce proposed additional desiderata: the hypothesis should be (ii) testable and (iii) reasonably economical. Here, the notion of economy encompassed both efficient deployment of limited resources—time, energy and money—and explanatory virtues such as breadth, depth, simplicity and naturalness—the features of a hypothesis that contribute to its 'loveliness' in the terminology of Peter Lipton (2004).[3] Thus, Step 3 along the Peircean pathway is a threefold assessment of the generated hypothesis. If the hypothesis does not satisfy the critical criterion and the additional desiderata then the system must return to Step 2 and generate a new hypothesis that might satisfy the three requirements. If, on the other hand, the hypothesis generated at Step 2 does satisfy the critical criterion and the additional desiderata at Step 3 then it is passed on to Step 4—the step of abductive inference.

How are we to understand the conclusion of the abductive inference: 'There is reason to suspect that *A* is true'? It is important that the conclusion is not that hypothesis *A* provides the best explanation of surprising fact *C*—Peirce's abduction is *not* inference to the best explanation. Nor is the conclusion that hypothesis *A* is true, nor even that *A* is probably true. Peirce, himself, said: 'Abduction is the process of forming an explanatory hypothesis. ... Abduction merely suggests that something *may be*. ... It merely offers suggestions' (1903/1998: 216–217). We interpret the conclusion of the abductive inference along the lines that hypothesis *A* is a candidate or 'suspect' for being the true explanation of the surprising fact *C*.

The abductive inference at Step 4 has three premises, taking account of Peirce's additional desiderata:

The surprising fact, *C*, is observed;
But if the hypothesis *A* were true, *C* would be a matter of course.
The hypothesis *A* is testable and reasonably economical.

The conclusion is:

The hypothesis *A* can be considered a pursuit-worthy candidate for being the true explanation of the surprising fact *C*.

Following the step of abductive inference, the hypothesis—or candidate-for-belief—must be tested. Step 5 along the Peircean pathway is deductive inference of predictions from the candidate-for-belief and Step 6 is the testing of these predictions. Peirce usually focused on experimental testing of predictions but predictions can also be tested by observations or by drawing on available background knowledge. Step 7 is then assessment of the candidate-for-belief in the light of the results of the Step 6 testing. If the predictions are falsified then the candidate-for-belief is rejected and the system must return to Step 2 and generate a new hypothesis. If the predictions are supported then the candidate-for-belief may be adopted as a belief at Step 8. (Peirce referred to this process of testing and confirmation as 'induction', so that the pathway comprised abduction, deduction and induction.)

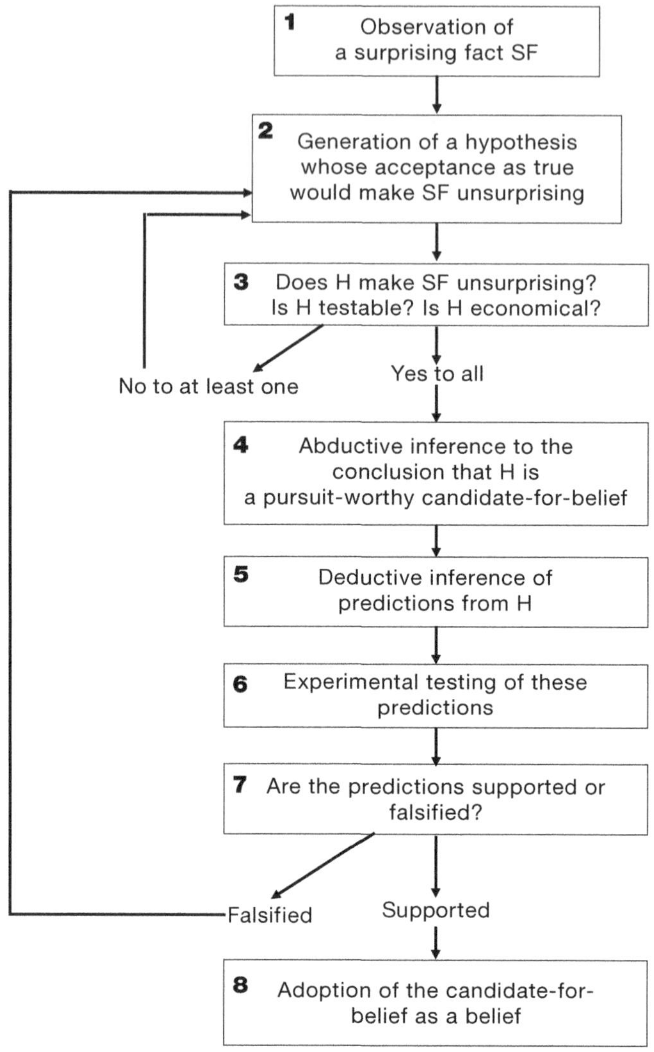



*Figure 29.1* Peircean pathway model of the adoption of a new belief in response to the observation of a surprising fact (Davies and Coltheart 2020; Coltheart and Davies 2021a, 2021b, 2022). Reprinted from Coltheart & Davies (2022: 76), by permission of the publisher.[4]

When we consider a case of delusion, the first factor results in observation of a surprising fact at Step 1 of the Peircean pathway and this triggers a process of hypothesis generation at Step 2. Pre-testing assessment of the generated delusional hypothesis at Step 3 is then followed, at Step 4, by adoption of the hypothesis, *not* as the *true* explanation of the surprising fact or as a *belief*, but as a *possible* explanation of the surprising fact and as a *candidate-for-belief*. The person commits no error in considering the delusional hypothesis as a candidate-for-belief, but the candidate should be rejected and an alternative hypothesis should be generated. The person's adoption and maintenance of the delusional hypothesis as a belief demonstrates a failure of hypothesis evaluation at one or more of Steps 5–7—resulting from the second factor.

In the following four sections, we shall consider in more detail the processes of hypothesis generation (Step 2) and of hypothesis evaluation (Steps 5–7).

### 3.   Individual differences in hypothesis generation

Concerning Step 2, Peirce said:

> The inquiry begins with pondering these [surprising] phenomena in all their aspects, in the search of some point of view whence the wonder shall be resolved. At length a conjecture arises that furnishes a possible Explanation.
>
> *(1908/1998: 441)*

Peirce also referred to 'the whole series of mental performances between the notice of the wonderful phenomenon [C] and the acceptance of the hypothesis [A]' (1908/1998: 441). He wrote about psychological—particularly, associative—processes and he conducted psychological experiments. But he did not provide a fully satisfactory account of the psychological processes by which a hypothesis is generated.

Drawing on hints from Peirce and work by Steven Pinker (2005) and Matthew Rellihan (2009), Max Coltheart and Martin Davies (2021a) proposed that hypothesis generation is an associative heuristic procedure that takes advantage of two features of spreading-activation networks: direct access to content-addressable memory (rather than potentially exhaustive serial search) and pattern completion. There is, however, a residual concern arising from the fact that, for a given surprising fact, there will be many hypotheses with the property that, if the hypothesis were true, the surprising fact would follow as a matter of course. In fact, as Peirce remarked, 'the possible explanations of our facts may be strictly innumerable' (1901/1998: 107). Having Step 2 pass innumerably many hypotheses to Step 3 for assessment cannot be an aspect of a realistic account of human cognitive processes. In response to this concern, we can note that, on any associative account, the time taken to generate a hypothesis will vary as a function of the strength of its association with the observed surprising fact. So hypothesis generation will be asynchronous and, for any given surprising fact, one hypothesis will be generated first—at which point the operation of Step 2 could be paused. In fact, Coltheart and Davies (2021a) proposed that, from Step 2 onwards along the Peircean pathway, 'only one hypothesis is being entertained at any one time' (p. 7).

Research using the Alternative Uses paradigm (Guilford 1971; Guilford et al. 1978) casts further light on the nature of associative evocation of hypotheses. In this paradigm, participants are asked to generate as many alternative uses for a familiar object as they can; for example, 'What can you do with a brick?'. Ken Gilhooly and colleagues (Gilhooly et al. 2007) reported: 'First responses tend to be based on contextualized personal experience stored as episodic or more generalized autobiographical memories' (p. 623) and they provided an example: 'I remember my father used a brick to stop a car rolling away' (p. 615). Some later responses were based on 'retrieval of one or more properties of the target object and a search of semantic memory for uses or functions which have as a requirement the retrieved property or properties' (p. 618). An example of an alternative use for a pencil was: 'A pencil is sharp so can be used to poke holes in paper' (p. 615).

Associative evocation of explanatory hypotheses draws on autobiographical memory and semantic memory (available knowledge of facts) no less than does performance of the Alternative Uses task. Furthermore, it is beyond dispute that there are individual differences in autobiographical memory (not everyone remembers their father using a brick to stop a car rolling away) and in semantic memory (different people know different facts). It follows that hypothesis generation at Step 2 of the Peircean pathway is a locus of individual differences. For example, a patient with Cotard delusion gave an account—after her recovery—of how, when she was in the acute phase of catatonia (of which immobility is a frequent symptom), the idea that she was dead came to mind: 'she thought that she was dead because of the feeling that time was passing extremely slow, and because she could not talk or move despite her will' (Ramírez-Bermúdez et al. 2021: 67). A doctor specialising in the diagnosis, treatment, and neurological nature of catatonia—with quite different background knowledge from the patient—might one day experience the same unpredicted phenomena as the patient but not generate the Cotard delusional hypothesis, 'I am dead'. The doctor's feeling that time was passing slowly and his inability to talk or move might, instead, evoke the hypothesis, 'I am suffering from catatonia'.

## 4.  Individual differences and the argument for a second factor

If a large number of individuals observe or encounter the same surprising fact or event at Step 1 then we should predict that there will be some variation in the explanatory hypotheses that are generated at Step 2. This certainly calls into question the implicit assumption (mentioned toward the end of Section 1, above) that the same delusional idea comes to the minds of all people who have the same first factor and observe or encounter the resulting unpredicted phenomenon.

It might seem that if the implicit assumption is called into question then the argument for a second factor (specifically, a second factor that results in a failure of hypothesis evaluation) is also called into question—but that would not be correct. The argument for a second factor depends on there being people of two kinds. There are people with the first factor who, having generated the delusional hypothesis, evaluate it and reject it and are not delusional; and there are other people with the first factor who, having generated the same delusional hypothesis, adopt and maintain it as a delusional belief. The implicit assumption had the consequence that *all* people with the first factor who are not delusional are of the first kind: they generated the delusional hypothesis and then evaluated and rejected it. Without the assumption, we must allow that there might be people with the first factor who are not delusional simply because they did not generate the delusional hypothesis. Nevertheless, provided there were still people of the first kind, the argument would proceed in just the same way.

People of the first kind demonstrate that having the first factor and generating the delusional hypothesis does not inevitably lead to the delusion. So, concerning any person of the second kind, we can ask (our second question) why the delusional hypothesis was not rejected. What explains this person's failure of hypothesis evaluation? The second factor is whatever is indicated by the answer to that question. In order to resist the argument for a second factor, a critic of the two-factor theory must argue that there are no people of the first kind; the only way to avoid delusion is not to generate a delusional hypothesis in the first place. Thus, the critic must claim that the possibility that a person with the first factor might generate the delusional hypothesis and then evaluate and reject it can be excluded. The onus would be on the critic to justify that claim.

Might the needed justification be provided by a Spinozan account of belief formation? As James summarised this account, 'all propositions are believed through the very fact of being conceived' (1890, Volume 2: 290) and, as Daniel Gilbert (1991) explained, 'Spinoza argued that to comprehend a proposition, a person had implicitly to accept that proposition' (p. 108). (For an extended defence of the Spinozan account, see Mandelbaum, 2014.) On such an account it would, indeed, be impossible for a person to evaluate a generated hypothesis before believing it. Consequently, there would be no people of the first kind—no people who, having generated a delusional hypothesis, evaluated and rejected it rather than believing it.

Adoption of a Spinozan account would not, however, allow a critic to resist the argument for a second factor. A Spinozan account excludes evaluation of a hypothesis before it is initially adopted as a belief—evaluation that would lead either to acceptance or else to rejection of the hypothesis. But evaluation is re-located to a point after initial acceptance of a hypothesis as a belief. This post-acceptance evaluation leads either to certification or else to unacceptance of the belief (see Gilbert 1991: 109, Figure 1; also see Mandelbaum 2014: 62, Figure 2). If a Spinozan account is assumed, then the second factor in the two-factor theory does not, strictly speaking, result in a failure of hypothesis evaluation but rather in a failure of belief evaluation. In this new setting, the argument for a second factor depends, once again, on there being people of two kinds. There are people with the first factor who, having generated the delusional hypothesis and initially accepted it as a belief, evaluate it and unaccept it and are not delusional; and there are other people with the first factor who, having generated the same delusional hypothesis and initially accepted it as a belief, certify and maintain the delusional belief.

People of the first kind demonstrate that having the first factor, generating the delusional hypothesis and initially accepting it as a belief does not inevitably lead to the delusion. By comparison with these non-delusional people, any person of the second kind—who certifies and maintains the delusional belief—shows a failure of belief evaluation, and we can ask what explains that failure. Again, the second factor is whatever is indicated by the answer to that question. To resist the argument for a second factor given a Spinozan account, the critic must claim that the possibility that a person with the first factor might generate the delusional hypothesis, initially accept it as a belief, and then evaluate and unaccept the delusional belief can be excluded. Once again, the onus would be on the critic to justify that claim.

The Peircean pathway model (see Figure 29.1) assumes that a generated hypothesis is adopted at Step 4 as a research question to be investigated and that the hypothesis is adopted as a belief at Step 8 only if 'prediction after prediction ... is verified by experiment' (1901/1998: 97). Peirce did allow, however, that sometimes—perhaps if the hypothesis was considered to be especially pursuit-worthy at Step 4—a subject might not just express the hypothesis 'in the interrogative mood', but might have an 'uncontrollable inclination to believe' it (1908/1998: 441). We interpret this to mean that a subject might proceed directly from Step 4 to Step 8, altogether omitting Steps 5–7. A belief that is adopted as the result of uncontrollable inclination still stands in need of evaluation and, as the Peircean pathway model is configured, this post-adoption evaluation would require a return from Step 8 to Step 5. If a Spinozan account of belief were adopted then the model could be reconfigured to have the generated hypothesis initially accepted as a belief at Step 4 (or, even earlier, at Step 3), with post-acceptance testing at Steps 5–7. The belief would be unaccepted if was refuted, or certified at Step 8 if it was supported.

## 5.  Failure of hypothesis evaluation and the BADE paradigm

Concerning the steps to be taken after Step 4, the step of abductive inference when the generated hypothesis is adopted as a candidate-for-belief, Peirce said:

> That which is to be done with the hypothesis is to trace out its consequences by deduction, to compare them with results of experiment …, and to discard the hypothesis, and try another, as soon as the first has been refuted.
>
> *(Peirce 1901/1998: 107)*

The Peircean pathway model's identification of three steps between adoption of the generated hypothesis as a candidate-for-belief (Step 4) and adoption of the hypothesis as a belief (Step 8) provides a structure in which to investigate the cognitive nature of the failure of hypothesis evaluation that results from the second factor. There could be a failure at Step 5 to derive predictions from the delusional hypothesis; or a failure at Step 6 to test derived predictions by experiment or observation or by drawing on available background knowledge; or a failure at Step 7 to recognise that the results of testing have falsified the predictions, to reject the refuted hypothesis and to generate an alternative. Whereas the first factor—and the resulting unpredicted phenomenon and the associatively evoked delusional hypothesis—inevitably varies from delusion to delusion, the second factor always results in a failure of hypothesis evaluation. In principle, however, the two-factor theory allows that the precise nature of this failure of hypothesis evaluation—and its location at Step 5, 6, or 7—might vary from case to case.

Coltheart and Davies (2021b) examined several published cases of delusion to find out whether Steps 5 and 6 were executed properly. In some cases, predictions were clearly derived (Step 5) and tested (Step 6). For example, patient YY (Brighetti et al. 2007) had Capgras delusion and believed, 'This person is not my father, but a stranger'. From the Capgras delusional hypothesis, patient YY derived predictions, such as 'This person will not be able to answer questions about my childhood', and tested these predictions (e.g., by asking the person questions). Given the results of this testing (e.g., patient YY's father answered the questions correctly), patient YY should have recognised that the predictions were falsified, rejected the refuted hypothesis and generated an alternative; but that is not what happened. There was a failure of hypothesis evaluation at Step 7. In other cases, people derived from their delusional hypothesis predictions that were falsified by background knowledge that was already available—even without experiment or observation. But, again, there was a failure of hypothesis evaluation at Step 7. They did not reject the refuted hypothesis.

There may be other cases of delusion in which one or other (or both) of Steps 5 and 6 are not properly executed but it seems that, in at least some cases, there is a failure of hypothesis evaluation at Step 7. One possibility to consider is that this failure is not specific to the delusional hypothesis but results from a more general failure to reject—or, at least, to reduce credence in—hypotheses in the face of counter-evidence. There is a substantial body of research using the BADE paradigm to investigate a bias against disconfirmatory evidence in individuals with schizophrenia (e.g., Sanford et al. 2014).

In the BADE paradigm, subjects rate the plausibility of four possible interpretations of a scenario that is presented in three consecutively-presented statements (see Table 29.2). After the first statement is presented (and then after each successive statement), the subject

*Table 29.2* Two examples from the BADE paradigm

| | *Scenario* | |
|---|---|---|
| | STATEMENT 1 | STATEMENT 1 |
| | *Amy doesn't like high waves* | *Jenny can't fall asleep* |
| | STATEMENT 2 | STATEMENT 2 |
| | *Amy has already been under water for a few minutes* | *Jenny can't wait until it is finally morning* |
| | STATEMENT 3 | STATEMENT 3 |
| | *It is Amy's job to be at the beach*[a] | *Jenny wonders how many presents she will find under the tree*[b] |
| | *Interpretation* | |
| 1 | Amy is learning wind-surfing | Jenny is nervous about her exam the next day |
| 2 | Amy witnessed the tsunami catastrophe in Thailand | Jenny is worried about her ill mother |
| 3 | Amy is afraid that fish might bite her on the nose | Jenny loves her bed |
| 4 | Amy is a lifeguard | Jenny is excited about Christmas morning |

[a] See Veckenstedt and colleagues (2011: 178).
[b] See Sanford and colleagues (2014: 2730).

rates each interpretation on a scale from 0 (implausible) to 10 (very plausible). Two 'lure' interpretations seem plausible after the first statement but are disconfirmed by later statements. An absurd interpretation seems implausible after the first statement and remains implausible. A true interpretation does not seem to be the most plausible after the first statement but is confirmed by the third statement. A bias against disconfirmatory evidence is demonstrated by the subject's failure to reduce the ratings of the initially plausible 'lure' interpretations as they are shown to be implausible. (A bias against confirmatory evidence would be demonstrated by failure to increase the rating of the true interpretation.)

In their study of 214 subjects, of whom 164 had a diagnosis of schizophrenia (or schizo-affective disorder), Nicole Sanford and colleagues (2014) found that 'evidence integration' scores (a composite score for bias against disconfirmatory evidence and bias against confirmatory evidence) were significantly higher in highly delusional individuals with schizophrenia than in low-delusional individuals with schizophrenia, people with obsessive-compulsive disorder, and healthy control subjects. In a meta-analysis of eight studies using the BADE task, Benjamin McLean, Julie Mattiske, and Ryan Balzan (2017) found a stronger bias against disconfirmatory evidence in schizophrenia patients with delusions than in schizophrenia patients without delusions and healthy control subjects. These findings are consistent with the proposal that a general cognitive bias against disconfirmatory evidence 'may underlie maintenance of delusions in the face of counter-evidence' (Sanford et al. 2014: 2729), but we know of no research using the BADE paradigm to investigate people with delusions but without a psychiatric diagnosis.

## 6. Bias against disconfirmatory evidence in patients with anosognosia

There is some evidence of a bias against disconfirmatory evidence in patients with anosognosia for their left-side motor impairments following right-hemisphere stroke. Anosognosia is a delusion but the delusional hypothesis ('I can move my left arm and leg') is not newly generated, and so the early steps of the Peircean pathway model are not relevant. The answer to our first question, 'What initially prompted the delusional idea or hypothesis?', is that it has been true throughout the patient's life—until the brain injury that resulted in the patient's motor impairments. First factor neuropsychological impairments in anosognosia do not result in observation of a surprising fact or event. Instead, they prevent the patient from observing the surprising fact of their motoric failure when they try to move their arm or leg and, in some cases, they result in an illusion of motoric success—illusory limb movements (Davies et al. 2005, 2024). There is still a mass of available evidence against the delusional hypothesis: patients cannot stand up from their chair or walk upstairs unaided and cannot perform bimanual tasks such as tying a knot or picking up a tray of glasses. The answer to our second question, 'Why was the delusional idea or hypothesis maintained as a belief rather than being rejected—as it should have been—on the basis of available evidence against it?', is the same as before: a second factor results in a failure of hypothesis evaluation at one or more of Steps 5–7.

Is there a failure, specifically, at Step 7 in patients with anosognosia? Roland Vocat and colleagues (2013) used a riddle task in a study of right hemisphere stroke patients—with or without anosognosia—and healthy control subjects. Subjects were given five successively more informative clues and, after each clue, they were asked to guess the target word (see Table 29.3). The first clue was sufficiently uninformative to create doubt in healthy subjects, while the final clue was intended to leave no doubt about the correct answer. The measure of bias against disconfirmatory evidence was the number of times (across ten riddles) the subject proposed the same incorrect guess following two consecutive clues in the same riddle.

Patients with anosognosia were no less likely than the other two groups to respond with the correct target word after the final clue, but were more than twice as likely as the other two groups to repeat the same incorrect guess.

> This suggests that anosognosics had no general problem in reasoning but required a repeated signal of errors, or a larger incongruence between a new clue and the previous guess, in order to prompt a re-appraisal of their preceding responses and to trigger a new solution.
>
> *(Vocat et al. 2013: 1778)*

In other words, the patients with anosognosia showed a bias against disconfirmatory evidence.

The proposal that, in at least some cases of delusion, the failure of hypothesis evaluation resulting from the second factor may take the form of a bias against disconfirmatory evidence is broadly consistent with the earlier proposal (at the end of Section 1) that the second factor has its neural basis in damage to, or hypoactivation of, rDLPFC). In fact, Vocat and colleagues (2013) suggested (citing Coltheart 2010) that the anosognosia patients' failure to update current beliefs despite the presence of incongruent information 'might reflect damage to prefrontal cortical areas' (p. 1778)—and, of course, these patients had only right hemisphere damage. Also, in a study of patients with focal lesions who performed the Wisconsin Card Sorting Task, Jan Gläscher, Ralph Adolphs, and Daniel Tranel (2019) found that lower rates of hypothesis updating in response to disconfirmatory evidence were associated with lesions 'located primarily in the right PFC [prefrontal cortex] reaching from

*Table 29.3* Two examples from the riddle task

| Clue | Target word | |
|---|---|---|
| | *Carrot* | *Heart* |
| 1 | I am a food | My weight is approximately 300 g |
| 2 | I am very cultivated | I produce a regular sound |
| 3 | I am a vegetable | Sport makes me feel excited |
| 4 | I am usually orange | I am usually on the left rather than on the right side |
| 5 | The rabbits adore me | Lovers often draw me |

dorsolateral PFC to the frontal pole and mostly focused in the underlying white matter' (p. 5). Finally, in an fMRI study of schizophrenia patients—with or without delusions— and healthy control subjects, Katie Lavigne, Mahesh Menon, and Todd Woodward (2020) found that reduced activity in a cognitive evaluation network including rDLPFC, during integration of disconfirmatory evidence in a novel task, was associated with poorer performance on the BADE task (outside the scanner) and with delusions in individuals with schizophrenia.

## 7.   Delusion without neuropsychological impairment

The two-factor theory of delusion has mainly been applied to cases of delusion in which the first factor is neuropsychological in nature; and we have seen that there is some support for the proposal that, in such cases, the second factor (that results in failure of hypothesis evaluation) is also neuropsychological. It is, nevertheless, not part of the two-factor theory that one or both of the two factors must be a neuropsychological impairment. The theory allows that observing or encountering an unpredicted phenomenon that does not result from a neuropsychological impairment might prompt a delusional hypothesis, and also that the second factor might not be neuropsychological—for example, it might be motivational. To put this point another way: answers to the two questions which are at the heart of the two-factor theory of delusion (What initially prompted the delusional idea? Why was the delusional idea adopted and maintained as a belief rather than being rejected, as it should have been?) do not inevitably require an appeal to neuropsychology.

There are three examples where the two-factor theory has been applied to the explanation of delusion without appeal to neuropsychology: folie à deux delusion, a particular form of somatic delusion, and alien abduction delusion. We discuss each in turn.

### 7.1   *Folie à deux*

In folie à deux, a delusional belief of one individual (the 'primary') is subsequently adopted by another (the 'secondary') via social contact between the two (for a review, see Arnone et al. 2006). Sometimes there is more than one secondary and, typically, the primary and secondary or secondaries are members of the same family. Robyn Langdon (2013) and Olav Nielssen and colleagues (Nielssen, Langdon, and Large 2013) have offered an account of folie à deux—specifically, of the secondary's delusion—in terms of the two-factor theory.

What initially prompted the secondary's delusional idea? It did not arise in the secondary's mind endogenously, as a hypothesis generated to explain an unpredicted phenomenon.

Rather, it arose exogenously, as an idea communicated to the secondary by the primary. Thus, folie à deux is an example of socially-transmitted delusion. (Koro is another example—see Coltheart and Davies 2024, Li 2010.)

Why did the secondary adopt and maintain this idea as a belief, rather than rejecting it? Langdon (2013) distinguished two kinds of answer to this question. The second factor might be endogenous and relatively permanent—perhaps 'a neuropathological vulnerability' (p. 76)—or exogenously imposed and temporary—contingent on the relationship between the secondary and the primary.

Nielssen and colleagues (2013) retrospectively analysed five cases of folie à deux and concluded that all six secondaries were delusional and had a significant impairment of hypothesis evaluation (see 2013: 397, Table 2). In three secondaries, this impairment was judged to be explained by neuropathy associated with schizophrenia or schizoaffective disorder. In the other three secondaries, it was at least partly explained in terms of the relationship with a dominant primary (sister, wife, or brother), whose beliefs were accepted uncritically. For two of these three secondaries, subsequent separation from the primary resulted in remission of the delusion. For one of these two secondaries, there was 'no obvious neuropathological basis' (p. 404) for the impairment of hypothesis evaluation—a particularly clear case of a non-neuropsychological second factor.

## 7.2   *A non-neuropsychological somatic delusion*

A person described by Coltheart and Langdon (2019) believed that his gums were rotting, even though he had visited oral pathologists on numerous occasions and all had informed him that his gums were normal. What initially prompted his delusional idea?

Coltheart and Langdon (2019) reported that he had not been accepted into University—though other members of his ambitious family had succeeded—and that this had triggered depression and despondency. Perhaps the first possible explanation of his not going to university that came to his mind was that he had been rejected because he lacked certain abilities. If that triggered depression and despondency, he might have set himself to generate an *alternative* explanation. His having an unpleasant physical condition that he did not want other people to see would explain why he was not going to university, but why was it the rotting gums explanation, specifically, that came to mind? Coltheart and Langdon could only speculate, but the person told them that his gum disease started in his late teens after he had cut his gum while eating. Recollection of such events might have prompted the rotting gums idea.

There was no evidence of any neuropsychological abnormality in this young man. So, why did he adopt and maintain the rotting gums delusional idea as a belief rather than rejecting it? Coltheart and Langdon (2019) suggested a motivational explanation: 'his adoption of the belief about his gums allowed him to interpret his not going to University as something that did not imply a personal rejection' (p. 84). So here the failure of hypothesis evaluation occurred because it was motivated by a personal benefit.

We have argued that the failure of hypothesis evaluation resulting from the second factor may take the form of a bias against disconfirmatory evidence (Coltheart and Davies 2021b; also see Sections 5 and 6). Individuals who are strongly motivated to adopt and maintain a particular hypothesis as a belief may establish an exceptionally high threshold for accepting that disconfirmatory evidence falsifies the hypothesis—or even for accepting that the evidence warrants reducing their credence in the hypothesis.

### 7.3  *Alien abduction delusion*

This is the belief that one has been abducted by extraterrestrial beings and subsequently returned to Earth. What might bring such an idea to mind? A plausible proposal (Holden and French 2002) is that the idea comes to mind as a result of an experience of sleep paralysis—inability to perform voluntary movements of the trunk and limbs at sleep onset or on waking. Sleep paralysis may be accompanied by hallucinations of three main kinds: (i) a sensed presence and visual, auditory and tactile sensations as if there were an intruder in the room; (ii) breathing difficulties, feelings of pressure on the chest and of suffocation; and (iii) feelings of floating, flying or falling, and out-of-body experiences.

Many people sometimes have these experiences as they wake. For example, Brian Sharpless and Jacques Barber (2011) found that 7.6 per cent of the general population, 28.3 per cent of students and 31.9 per cent of psychiatric patients experienced at least one episode of sleep paralysis. But most of these people do not believe that they have been abducted by aliens. Why is it that in a subset of people who have these experiences, the idea 'I am being abducted by aliens' comes to mind and is adopted as a belief?

Richard McNally and Susan Clancy (2005) reported that 'abductees' entertained 'a wide range of "New Age" beliefs' (120) and McNally (2012) provided some detail: 'belief in foretelling the future/tarot cards (70% [*versus* 8% in the control group]), astrology (60% [*vs* 25%]), ghosts (70% [*vs* 42%]), bioenergetic healing therapies (70% [*vs* 17%]), and alternative/herbal remedies (80% [*vs* 58%])' (p. 7). Christopher French and colleagues (2008) reported that people who claimed to have had extraterrestrial contact scored significantly higher than control subjects on two scales measuring beliefs about, and experiences of, paranormal phenomena.

The presence of these unorthodox beliefs may help explain, not only why the alien abduction idea came to mind, but also why it was adopted and maintained as a belief. Acceptance of unorthodox beliefs may indicate 'a susceptibility to uncritically accept beliefs' (Nielssen et al. 2013: 399). The literature on alien abduction delusion provides some evidence of reduced cognitive ability to carry out hypothesis evaluation (McNally et al. 2004; French et al. 2008; Cheyne & Pennycook 2013) and also of strong motivation to maintain the alien abduction belief (Clancy 2005; McNally 2012). There is, however, no suggestion of neuropsychological impairment. (For a one-factor account of alien abduction delusion, see Sullivan-Bissett 2020. We note again that arguments for or against a second factor may depend on how the notion of a 'factor' is understood.)

## 8.  Conclusion

In the two-factor theory of delusion, the first factor explains why a delusional idea or hypothesis came to mind in the first place and the second factor explains why the hypothesis was adopted and maintained as a belief rather than being rejected—as it should have been—on the basis of available evidence and background knowledge that counted against it.

It has proved illuminating to consider the two-factor theory against the background of an eight-step model of the normal pathway from surprising facts to new beliefs—the Peircean pathway model. This has allowed a more substantive account of the associative processes by which a delusional hypothesis is generated. One consequence of the account is that hypothesis generation is a locus of individual differences. The model also provides a structure in which to investigate the cognitive nature of the failure of hypothesis evaluation. One proposal is that this is a bias against disconfirmatory evidence.

The two-factor theory has been applied to cases of monothematic delusion in which the first factor has been a neuropsychological impairment. There is some reason to propose that, in these cases, the second factor is also neuropsychological, with a neural basis in damage to, or hypoactivation of, rDLPFC. It is not, however, part of the two-factor theory that the two factors must be neuropsychological. The delusional hypothesis might be socially transmitted, for example, and the failure of hypothesis evaluation might result from a motivated bias against disconfirmatory evidence. In recent work, the two-factor theory has been applied to provide explanations of folie à deux, a somatic delusion, and alien abduction delusion—without appeal to neuropsychology.

## Notes

1 For reviews, see Coltheart (2007, 2010), Coltheart, Langdon, and McKay (2011), Coltheart, Menzies, and Sutton (2010), Davies et al. (2001), Langdon and Coltheart (2000).
2 For discussion of the Peircean pathway model, see Coltheart and Davies (2021a, 2021b, 2022), Davies and Coltheart (2020).
3 In Lipton's (2004) terminology, the *loveliest* hypothesis or candidate explanation is the one that would 'provide the most understanding', whereas the *likeliest* is the one that is 'best supported by the evidence' (p. 57).
4 Figure 29.1 appeared in 'What is Capgras delusion?' by Max Coltheart and Martin Davies, published in *Cognitive Neuropsychiatry*, Volume 27, Issue 1 (2022: 69–82). It is reprinted here by permission of the publisher Taylor & Francis Ltd, http://www.tandfonline.com.

## References

American Psychiatric Association (2013). *Diagnostic and Statistical Manual of Mental Disorders: DSM-5*. Washington, DC: American Psychiatric Association.

Arnone, D., Patel, A., & Tan, G. M-Y. (2006). The nosological significance of Folie à Deux: A review of the literature. *Annals of General Psychiatry*, 5:11, 1–8.

Binkofski, F., Buccino, G., Dohle, C., Seitz, R. J., & Freund H.-J. (1999). Mirror agnosia and mirror ataxia constitute different parietal lobe disorders. *Annals of Neurology*, 46, 51–61.

Breen, N., Caine, D., & Coltheart, M. (2001). Mirrored-self misidentification: Two cases of focal onset dementia. *Neurocase*, 7, 239–254.

Breen, N., Caine, D., Coltheart, M., Roberts, C., & Hendy, J. (2000). Towards an understanding of delusions of misidentification: Four case studies. *Mind & Language*, 15, 74–110.

Brighetti, G., Bonifacci, P., Borlimi, R., & Ottaviani, C. (2007). "Far from the heart far from the eye": Evidence from the Capgras delusion. *Cognitive Neuropsychiatry*, 12, 189–197.

Cheyne, J. A., & Pennycook, G. (2013). Sleep paralysis postepisode distress: Modeling potential effects of episode characteristics, general psychological distress, beliefs, and cognitive style. *Clinical Psychological Science*, 1, 135–148.

Clancy, S. A. (2005). *Abducted: How People Come to Believe They Were Kidnapped by Aliens*. Cambridge, MA: Harvard University Press.

Coltheart M. (2005a). Delusional belief. *Australian Journal of Psychology*, 57, 72–76.

Coltheart, M. (2005b). Conscious experience and delusional belief. *Philosophy, Psychiatry, & Psychology*, 12, 153–157.

Coltheart, M. (2007). The 33rd Bartlett Lecture: Cognitive neuropsychiatry and delusional belief. *Quarterly Journal of Experimental Psychology*, 60, 1041–1062.

Coltheart, M. (2010). The neuropsychology of delusions. *Annals of the New York Academy of Sciences*, 1191, 16–26.

Coltheart, M., Cox, R., Sowman, P., Morgan, H., Barnier, A., Langdon, R., Connaughton, E., Teichmann, L., Williams, N., & Polito, V. (2018). Belief, delusion, hypnosis, and the right dorsolateral prefrontal cortex: A transcranial magnetic stimulation study. *Cortex*, 101, 234–248.

Coltheart, M., & Davies, M. (2021a). How unexpected observations lead to new beliefs: A Peircean pathway. *Consciousness and Cognition, 87*:103037, 1–13.

Coltheart, M., & Davies, M. (2021b). Failure of hypothesis evaluation as a factor in delusional belief. *Cognitive Neuropsychiatry, 26*, 213–230.

Coltheart, M., & Davies, M. (2022). What is Capgras delusion? *Cognitive Neuropsychiatry, 27*, 69–82.

Coltheart, M., & Davies, M. (2024). Koro: A socially-transmitted delusional belief. *Cognitive Neuropsychiatry, 29*, 10–28.

Coltheart, M., & Langdon, R. (2019). Somatic delusions as motivated beliefs? *Australian & New Zealand Journal of Psychiatry, 53*, 83–84.

Coltheart, M., Langdon, R., & McKay, R. (2011). Delusional belief. *Annual Review of Psychology, 62*, 271–298.

Coltheart, M., Menzies, P., & Sutton, J. (2010). Abductive inference and delusional belief. *Cognitive Neuropsychiatry, 15*, 261–287.

David, A. S. (1993). Cognitive neuropsychiatry? *Psychological Medicine, 23*, 1–5.

Davies, M., Aimola Davies, A. M., & Coltheart, M. (2005). Anosognosia and the two-factor theory of delusions, *Mind & Language, 20*, 209–236.

Davies, M., & Coltheart, M. (2020). A Peircean pathway from surprising facts to new beliefs. *Transactions of the Charles S. Peirce Society, 56*, 400–426.

Davies, M., Coltheart, M., Langdon, R., & Breen, N. (2001). Monothematic delusions: Towards a two-factor account. *Philosophy, Psychiatry & Psychology, 8*, 133–158.

Davies, M., McGill, C. L., & Aimola Davies, A. M. (2024). Anosognosia for motor impairments as a delusion: Anomalies of experience and belief evaluation. In A. L. Mishara, M. Moskalewicz, M. A. Schwartz and A. Kranjec (Eds.), *Phenomenological Neuropsychiatry: How Patient Experience Bridges the Clinic with Clinical Neuroscience* (pp. 175–197). New York: Springer.

Edelstyn, N. M. J., & Oyebode, F. (1999). A review of the phenomenology and cognitive neuropsychological origins of the Capgras syndrome. *International Journal of Geriatric Psychiatry, 14*, 48–59.

Fourneret, P., Paillard, J., Lamarre, Y., Cole, J., & Jeannerod, M. (2002). Lack of conscious recognition of one's own actions in a haptically deafferented patient. *NeuroReport, 13*, 541–547.

French, C. C., Santomauro, J., Hamilton, V., Fox, R., & Thalbourne, M. A. (2008). Psychological aspects of the alien contact experience. *Cortex, 44*, 1387–1395.

Gilbert, D. T. (1991). How mental systems believe. *American Psychologist, 46*, 107–119.

Gilhooly, K. J., Fioratu, E., Anthony, S. H., & Wynn, V. (2007). Divergent thinking: Strategies and executive involvement in generating novel uses for familiar objects. *British Journal of Psychology, 98*, 611–625.

Gläscher, J., Adolphs, R., & Tranel, D. (2019). Model-based lesion mapping of cognitive control using the Wisconsin Card Sorting Test. *Nature Communications, 10*:20, 1–12.

Guilford, J. P. (1971). *The Nature of Human Intelligence*. New York: McGraw-Hill.

Guilford, J. P., Christensen, P. R., Merrifield, P. R., & Wilson, R. C. (1978). *Alternate Uses: Manual of Instructions and Interpretations*. Orange, CA: Sheridan Psychological Services.

Halligan, P. W., & David, A. S. (2001). Cognitive neuropsychiatry: Towards a scientific psychopathology. *Nature Reviews Neuroscience, 2*, 209–215.

Holden, K. J., & French, C. C. (2002). Alien abduction experiences: Some clues from neuropsychology and neuropsychiatry. *Cognitive Neuropsychiatry, 7*, 163–178.

James, W. (1890). *The Principles of Psychology* (in two volumes). New York: Henry Holt and Company.

Langdon, R. (2013). Folie à deux and its lessons for two-factor theorists. *Mind & Language, 28*, 72–82.

Langdon, R., & Coltheart, M. (2000). The cognitive neuropsychology of delusions. *Mind & Language, 15*, 183–216.

Langdon, R., Connaughton, E., & Coltheart, M. (2014). The Fregoli delusion: A disorder of person identification and tracking. *Topics in Cognitive Science, 6*, 615–631.

Lavigne, K. M., Menon, M., & Woodward, T. S. (2020). Functional brain networks underlying evidence integration and delusions in schizophrenia. *Schizophrenia Bulletin, 46*, 175–183.

Li, J. (2010). Koro endemic among school children in Guangdong, China. *World Cultural Psychiatry Research Review, 5*, 102–105.

Lipton, P. (2004). *Inference to the Best Explanation* (Second Edition). London: Routledge.

Maher, B. A. (1974). Delusional thinking and perceptual disorder. *Journal of Individual Psychology, 30*, 98–113.

Mandelbaum, E. (2014). Thinking is believing. *Inquiry, 57*, 55–96.

Marshall, J. C., & Halligan, P. W. (1996). Towards a cognitive neuropsychiatry. In P. W. Halligan and J. C. Marshall (Eds.), *Method in Madness: Case Studies in Cognitive Neuropsychiatry* (pp. 3–12). Hove: Psychology Press.

McLean, B. F., Mattiske, J. K., & Balzan, R. P. (2017). Association of the jumping to conclusions and evidence integration biases with delusions in psychosis: A detailed meta-analysis. *Schizophrenia Bulletin, 43*, 344–354.

McNally, R. J. (2012). Explaining 'memories' of space alien abduction and past lives: An experimental psychopathology approach. *Journal of Experimental Psychopathology, 3*, 2–16.

McNally, R. J., & Clancy, S. A. (2005). Sleep paralysis, sexual abuse, and space alien abduction. *Transcultural Psychiatry, 42*, 113–122.

McNally, R. J., Lasko, N. B., Clancy, S. A., Macklin, M. L., Pitman, R. K., & Orr, S. P. (2004). Psychophysiological responding during script-driven imagery in people reporting abduction by space aliens. *Psychological Science, 15*, 493–497.

Nielssen, O., Langdon, R., & Large, M. (2013). Folie à deux homicide and the two-factor model of delusions. *Cognitive Neuropsychiatry, 18*, 390–408.

Noordhof, P., & Sullivan-Bissett, E. (2021). The clinical significance of anomalous experience in the explanation of monothematic delusions. *Synthese, 199*, 10277–10309.

Peirce, C. S. (1901/1998). On the logic of drawing history from ancient documents, especially from testimonies. In Peirce Edition Project (Eds.), *The Essential Peirce, Volume 2 (1893–1913)* (pp. 75–114). Bloomington: Indiana University Press.

Peirce, C. S. (1903/1998). *Harvard Lectures on Pragmatism (1903), Lecture 7: Pragmatism as the logic of abduction.* In Peirce Edition Project (Eds.), *The Essential Peirce, Volume 2 (1893–1913)* (pp. 226–241). Bloomington: Indiana University Press.

Peirce, C. S. (1908/1998). A neglected argument for the reality of God. In Peirce Edition Project (Eds.), *The Essential Peirce, Volume 2 (1893–1913)* (pp. 434–450). Bloomington: Indiana University Press.

Pinker, S. (2005). So how *does* the mind work? *Mind & Language, 20*, 1–24.

Ramachandran, V. S., & Blakeslee, S. (1998). *Phantoms in the Brain: Probing the Mysteries of the Human Mind.* New York: William Morrow.

Ramírez-Bermúdez, J., Bustamante-Gomez, P., Espinola-Nadurille, M., Kerik, N. E., Dias Meneses, I. E., Restrepo-Martínez, M., & Mendez, M. F. (2021). Cotard syndrome in anti-NMDAR encephalitis: Two patients and insights from molecular imaging. *Neurocase, 27*, 64–71.

Rellihan, M. J. (2009). Fodor's riddle of abduction. *Philosophical Studies: An International Journal for Philosophy in the Analytic Tradition, 144*, 313–338.

Sanford, N., Veckenstedt, R., Moritz, S., Balzan, R. P., & Woodward, T. S. (2014). Impaired integration of disambiguating evidence in delusional schizophrenia patients. *Psychological Medicine, 44*, 2729–2738.

Sharpless, B. A., & Barber, J. P. (2011). Lifetime prevalence rates of sleep paralysis: A systematic review. *Sleep Medicine Reviews, 15*, 311–315.

Stirling, J. D., Hellewell, J. S. E., & Quraishi, N. (1998). Self-monitoring dysfunction and the schizophrenic symptoms of alien control. *Psychological Medicine, 28*, 675–683.

Sullivan-Bissett, E. (2020). Unimpaired abduction to alien abduction: Lessons on delusion formation. *Philosophical Psychology, 33*, 679–704.

Sullivan-Bissett, E. (2022). Against a second factor. *Asian Journal of Philosophy, 1*:33, 1–10.

Turner, M., & Coltheart, M. (2010). Confabulation and delusion: A common monitoring framework. *Cognitive Neuropsychiatry, 15*, 346–376.

Vallar, G., & Ronchi, R. (2009). Somatoparaphrenia: A body delusion. A review of the neuropsychological literature. *Experimental Brain Research, 192*, 533–551.

Veckenstedt, R., Randjbar, S., Vitzthum, F., Hottenrott, B., Woodward, T. S., & Moritz, S. (2011). Incorrigibility, jumping to conclusions, and decision threshold in schizophrenia. *Cognitive Neuropsychiatry, 16*, 174–192.

Vocat, R., Saj, A., & Vuilleumier, P. (2013). The riddle of anosognosia: Does unawareness of hemiplegia involve a failure to update beliefs? *Cortex, 49*, 1771–1781.

Vuilleumier, P., Mohr, C., Valenza, N., Wetzel, C., & Landis, T. (2003). Hyperfamiliarity for unknown faces after left lateral temporo-occipital venous infarction: A double dissociation with prosopagnosia. *Brain, 126*, 889–907.

Young, A. W. (2000). Wondrous strange: The neuropsychology of abnormal beliefs. *Mind & Language, 15*, 47–73.

Young, A. W., Robertson, I. H., Hellawell, D. J., de Pauw, K. W., & Pentland, G. (1992). Cotard delusion after brain injury. *Psychological Medicine, 22*, 799–804.

# 30

# THE PREDICTION ERROR THEORY

*Philip Corlett*

Delusions – the fixed false beliefs that characterize psychotic illnesses like schizophrenia (but also bipolar disorder, depression, neurological and autoimmune illnesses) represent profound departures from consensual reality. They have yet to yield entirely to empirical investigation, and, whilst they appear to be readily treated with antipsychotic drugs that block dopamine $D_2$ receptors, many patients (up to 50 per cent) do not experience symptom resolution. Furthermore, we lack a coherent account that connects the phenomenology of delusions (what it is like to experience them) with the mental and neural processes that underwrite them, and the social factors that form and foment them. That is the promise of computational psychiatry (Corlett and Fletcher 2014). It has begun to deliver, but there is substantial distance yet to cover.

This chapter will address the development of the prediction error model of delusions through a series of phases. It will conclude with current challenges and future directions for this work. Central to this chapter is an appreciation of cross-species and cross-disciplinary translation: from the bench (preclinical work in rodents and primates) to the bedside (in patients and along the continuum from health to illness) and back again, via advances in engineering and computer science and their application to neuroscience.

## 1. Roots in cognitive neuropsychiatry

The prediction error account of delusions is deeply indebted to, and grounded within, cognitive neuropsychology and the neuroscience of perception and belief. Termed *cognitive neuropsychiatry*, this fundamental framework strives to explain hallucinations and delusions as mutations of, or deviations from, normal cognitive and perceptual processes (Halligan and David 2001).

The logic is as follows: if a person hears voices in their head, we should be able to investigate that phenomenon by leveraging what is known of hearing, speech processing, and the location of percepts in space, for example. The inner speech account of voices – that they represent mischaracterization of one's own inner speech (our internal monologue) as external speech, and the two-factor theory of delusions (which lays blame for delusions in faulty perception and aberrant belief evaluation, see Davies and Coltheart Chapter 29) – are key

DOI: 10.4324/9781003296386-36

cognitive neuropsychiatric models (see Corlett 2019 and Corlett et al. 2019 and below for critiques of these models).

These models were largely cast at the level of human cognitive science. One advance, facilitated by computational psychiatry, has been the fractionation of these higher-level, perhaps human-specific, processes (belief, speech-perception) into component mechanisms more amenable to modeling in non-human animals – like expectation, learning, and inference. The benefits are at least two-fold; first, the molecular and circuit mechanisms of these building blocks are more amenable to investigation, and thus, there are more potential discoveries to be translated into the clinic. Second, these more basic processes can be readily studied in patients, even those who suffer cognitive deficits and motivational problems that might confound investigations of psychotic symptoms using more complex procedures.

## 2.    The aberrant salience hypothesis

Perhaps the most influential prototypical computational psychiatry explanations of psychosis is Shitij Kapur's perspicuous aberrant incentive salience hypothesis, which leverages work in the preclinical behavioural neuroscience of addiction suggesting that dopamine in the nucleus accumbens is responsible for attributing incentive salience to drug-related cues. Cues with incentive salience grab attention and drive goal directed action. In psychosis, then, delusions involve the attribution of inappropriate salience to stimuli, thoughts, and percepts that are coincident with elevated accumbal dopamine (Kapur 2003) (for more on delusion and salience see McKenna Chapter 31). This model was extremely generative of new work, but its predictions have been disconfirmed; the locus of dopamine dysfunction in the striatum is the associative striatum rather than the accumbens (Kegeles et al. 2010), and behavioural tasks of incentive salience attribution do not correlate with delusion severity.

## 3.    Getting precise about salience

The British statistician George Box famously quipped that 'all models are wrong, but some are useful'. The aberrant salience model inspired attempts to link phenomenology to biology in psychosis by replacing incentive salience with other bridging processes. Dopamine in the meoscortical and mesostriatal pathways may instead signal a prediction error – a mismatch between expectation and experience, that garners attention and new learning.

In perhaps the paradigmatic example of computational neuroscience, Wolfram Schultz has demonstrated in a series of studies that the prediction error signals that drive conditioning are generated in midbrain dopamine neurons (Waelti et al. 2001). The signals are communicated to the striatum and prefrontal cortex via glutamate co-release (Lavin et al. 2005), where they have a role in ascribing salience to coincident stimuli, thoughts and percepts (Kapur 2003) and determining agency for important events (Redgrave and Gurney 2006). It is argued that the dopamine signals in the ventral tegmental area (VTA) do respond to expectancy violations; however, their role in the behaviour is one of agency attribution – did I cause that surprising event to happen with my actions and is it something I want to happen again? This is achieved by discerning whether the VTA prediction error was coincident with forward-models of action, reverberating representations of intended actions in the striatum (Redgrave and Gurney 2006). When predictions and prediction errors are disrupted, agency for actions can be misattributed externally, leading to delusions of alien control or passivity (feeling that one's actions are under the control of an external agent) (Redgrave and Gurney 2006). Since speech is a motor act, it, too, may be generated and attributed via prediction error mechanisms, and through similar mechanisms, inner speech may be externalized (Feinberg 1978). Despite lacking speech per se, experimental animals can provide model systems for studying these signals. Forward models for motor control and eye-movements have been mapped in exquisite detail in the cerebellum, mediodorsal thalamus, and frontal eye-fields in primates (Crapse and Sommer 2008). The findings from this model system have enriched our understanding of psychotic symptoms in human participants (Ford et al. 2007). However, the path from these signals to psychological constructs like salience is less clear.

## 4.　From salience to psychosis?

Instead of incentive salience, perhaps the blame for psychosis lies in attentional salience or associability (the readiness with which cues enter associative relationships); in this way, aberrant associations can be formed and can influence perception, cognition, and comportment, without appeal to the accumbens or incentives per se. The aberrant incentive salience model paved the way for the aberrant prediction error account (though see pathbreaking work from Jeffery Gray and David Hemsley (Gray et al. 1995) that pre-dated Kapur).

In this phase of development, the prediction error account, like other cognitive neuropsychiatric accounts, was formal (in that it appealed to a model description, sometimes an equation) but more metaphorical: things that looked like prediction error signals in the brain were inappropriately engaged in people with delusions and correlated with the severity of delusions (Corlett et al. 2007b). Delusions might form under the influence of aberrant prediction error signals, registered independent from cue or context, which drive attention and learning toward irrelevant stimuli and garner belief formation to explain the inappropriate salience of those features (Corlett et al. 2010). This idea puts formal meat on the bones of Brendan Maher's influential one-factor (perceptual) account of delusions (Maher 1974) (for more on the one-factor theory see Sullivan-Bissett Chapter 28).

Functional neuroimaging data support the single factor prediction error account. In people with delusional beliefs, brain markers of prediction errors are inappropriately registered to events that ought not be surprising, and the magnitude of these aberrant signals correlates with delusion severity across participants (Corlett et al. 2007b). Similar relationships have been observed in many task contexts as well as in model psychoses wherein people are administered a drug that transiently and reversibly engenders a psychotic state. In these settings, again aberrant prediction errors have been observed, and again the magnitude of these aberrant signals correlates with the severity of delusion-like beliefs that participants experience (Corlett et al. 2006, 2007a).

One key phenomenon that emphasizes the role of prediction error in learning is the Kamin blocking effect (Kamin 1969). When a novel cue (e.g., a tone) is paired with a stimulus (e.g., a light) that already predicts an outcome (electric shock) – the pre-trained cue – the light – 'blocks' new learning about the novel cue – the tone. This is clearly a problem for contiguity-based theories of association since the tone occurs alongside the outcome, and yet learning is attenuated because there is no prediction error during the blocking trials (when light and tone occur together). This is not the case in people prone to delusional beliefs, who evince brain prediction error signals during the blocking trials and learn about the blocked cue (Corlett and Fletcher 2012). Likewise, in rodents, optogenetic (Steinberg et al. 2013) and chemogenetic (Yau and McNally 2015) techniques can be employed to induce prediction error signals at the time of blocking trials in the midbrain and dorsomedial prefrontal cortex, respectively, engendering learning about the blocked cue. Such learning also occurs with behavioural pharmacological model psychoses in rats (O'Tuathaigh et al. 2003).

## 5. Model fitting

The next phase of development of the prediction error model involved fitting computational models to participants behavioural data, inverting those models, and estimating key parameters and quantities; asking which values would these metrics need to have to explain behaviour and how might they differ between groups of participants? Estimating temporal difference prediction errors (mismatches in the temporally precise prediction of reward) in individuals with psychosis suggested again that those signals occurred to events that ought not garner prediction errors (Murray et al. 2008). However, those signals did not correlate with symptom severity (Murray et al. 2008, Romaniuk et al. 2010), though simpler, trial-based, prediction errors did. Again, this suggested alternative experiments and models: temporal difference signals are not the only kind of prediction error, and prediction errors are not solely the purview of reward learning. Rather, they may represent a basic mode of brain function, driving learning and belief updating in the cognitive, perceptual, and social domains (Corlett et al. 2022).

These broader accounts began again as metaphors, although they were often accompanied by simulations – formalized thought experiments sweeping across model parameter values seeking to capture features of delusions or hallucinations that were not baked into the equations, as a means of garnering empirical support for the account, in the absence of data acquired from behaving organisms (Adams et al. 2013). A key advantage of these methods is that they demand extremely precise definitions of concepts that can have varied semantic meaning (like salience or precision). When we adopt a Bayesian approach – which incorporates notions of prior beliefs, prediction errors and their precision-weighted trade off – to symptom theories, it is possible to conceive of a set of prior beliefs that would yield specific behaviours and symptoms. It is critically important that we gather data and test whether those priors obtain.

## 6. Hierarchy

One key innovation here – beyond temporal difference reinforcement learning accounts – is the appeal to hierarchy. Sensory systems appear to be arranged hierarchically, with fast feedforward signals and slower, modulatory feedback signals. Motor and cognitive systems may also share these anatomical motifs. In a landmark paper in 2005, Karl Friston argued that this arrangement is consistent with casting perception (and later action and cognition) as Bayesian inference across the hierarchical levels of the brain (Friston 2005b). Higher layers in the hierarchy send predictions to the layer below regarding expected inputs. Those predictions are compared with actual inputs. Any mismatch – the prediction error – may be communicated upwards, updating future predictions. This communication depends on the precision of the prediction error, relative to the predictions. If prediction errors are precise (i.e. their inverse variance is low), they will drive belief updating. However, if the top-down prior is more precise, prediction error will be discounted and ignored as noise or coincidence. This dialogue, between beliefs and evidence, via prediction errors, is the heart of the prediction error model of delusions. If prediction errors are too precise, delusions form. They are maintained by a compensatory increase of prior precision which blocks future updating (Corlett and Fletcher 2021).

Attempts have been made to cast this account in two-factor terms (Miyazono and McKay 2019). The suggestion is that prediction error is factor one and its precision is factor two, and one needs both to get fixed delusions. This relies on an inappropriate assumption of the independence of prediction error from precision-weighting. Put simply, if prediction errors are aberrant, they will have errant precision. The two are not dissociable features. The hybrid account is a one-factor, prediction error account, and not a two-factor account.

## 7.  Testing the models

The next phase of prediction error theory involved empirical tests. It focused on the continuum of delusion-like belief and showed that healthy people who harbor unusual beliefs with conviction are more susceptible to the influence of suggested expectations on their current perceptual inferences (Schmack et al. 2013). The effect may however be different in patients with schizophrenia, especially those who are medicated (Valton et al. 2019). Medicated patients seemed less likely to learn statistical regularities in moving dot stimuli and therefore hallucinated those stimuli less frequently in the task.

## 8.  Volatility

The altered sensitivity to volatility (the rate of change of the state of the task or the world) during learning in patients with psychosis has also been explored using a probabilistic reversal learning task. Given a choice between three options for points reward (or loss) people with schizophrenia tend to switch choices even after a win. This suboptimal behaviour is particularly prevalent in people who are paranoid. Using the same hierarchical modeling approach, people who are paranoid seemed to expect more volatility but learned poorly from the volatility that they experience. The same patterns of behaviour and model parameters were observed in rats treated with chronic methamphetamine (a pharmacological inducer of paranoia in humans) (Reed et al. 2020). With the same paradigm, the impact of the evolving COVID-19 pandemic and attendant uncertainty and volatility on behaviour and beliefs could be tracked. When paranoia increased, erratic choices and beliefs about volatility increased. However, these effects were modulated by local policies to which people were subjected; when people were re-entering the world, mask mandates caused an increase in paranoia, erratic task behaviour, and volatility beliefs. This was driven by an interaction with local culture and perceived rule following – paranoia flourished when there was a rule, in places where people usually follow rules, but where people were typically not following the rule (Suthaharan et al. 2021). More broadly, these results underline the potential for computational approaches to inform not just the biological and psychological aspects of psychosis but also the social and cultural processes that contribute.

## 9.  Why are psychotic symptoms social?

At issue here is the extent to which evolved social specific processing contributes to psychosis. There was no differential impact of framing the belief updating socially, rather than as a non-social card-game. However, it may be that the social task was not social enough. Follow up work examined the impact of group-identity on social suggestion in high and low paranoia participants. We find that group-membership (whether playing with a colleague or a competitor) changes prior beliefs about the reliability of advice, but no effect of paranoia on that process. Instead, paranoid people take advice from in- and out-group members, driven by a sense that their own judgments are unreliable. In a more clearly social task, the roots of paranoia are distinctly non-social (Rossi-Goldthorpe et al. 2021) – since the same effects were observed in a relatively non-social species (rats) during a non-social task under the influence of amphetamine. That is not to say that humans do not have exquisite social cognition, but rather that paranoia may not be the purview of such bespoke coalitional mechanisms. Instead, paranoia seems to reflect the aberration of low-level learning mechanisms, which, when perturbed leads individuals to blame other agents for internally-generated perceptions.

## 10   Delusion contents

Beyond their social phenomenology – that they are concerned with other people/agents and one's relationships to them – delusions have somewhat characteristic and circumscribed contents. The two-factor theory deals with these by appealing to specific neurocognitive deficits that confer the content (and reflect the malfunction of evolved domain-specific modules, like familiarity processing in the case of Capgras delusion). This specificity has already been challenged for Capgras delusion (the control cases [with lesions to orbito-frontal cortex, as well as dorsolateral prefrontal damage] show aberrant responses to a host of salient stimuli, not just familiar conspecifics (Corlett 2019)). Recently, two-factor theorists have updated their account of Cotard delusion (Davies and Coltheart 2022). Previously, they suggested that for Cotard, factor one (present in non-delusional control patients) was a complete loss of affective responses, as in affective agnosia. Cotard patients would have this same deficit (manifested for example as a lack of GSR responses to any salient stimuli – rather like that actually observed in the Capgras controls (Corlett 2019)). However, this lack of responsivity in Cotard patients has not been empirically confirmed. Instead, two-factor theorists have updated their view on factor one for Cotard (Davies and Coltheart 2022). They now implicate depersonalization as the first factor (Davies and Coltheart 2022). Depersonalization includes the sense that the self no longer exists, or only does so in a disembodied sense. People can report such experiences in the absence of believing that they have died or completely disintegrated (the Cotard delusion). Two-factor theorists maintain that a further deficit is necessary – one of belief evaluation (factor two) in order for delusions to arise. However, depersonalization cannot confer the specific content of Cotard delusions if it is also reported in other monothematic delusion cases. Like Capgras for example. The delusions can occur at the same time in the same people, they can also wax and wane sequentially. Depersonalization and derealization (as well as doubling of self, not just other) seem to co-occur with Capgras (Wright et al. 1993, Young et al. 1994). These observations are problematic for the latest two-factor explanation. Whilst the two-factor theory seems to have a clear explanation of unique delusion contents, better than that proffered by prediction error accounts, the advantage is not at all clear, and does not seem to stand up to empirical scrutiny.

How then does prediction error theory explain delusion contents?

We dealt with paranoia above. Paranoia arises under domain general volatility beliefs, which, given that other humans are often causes, and their intentions are hard to infer, such volatility is often ascribed to them. It is also reassuring to have an enemy on which to blame experiences of uncertainty and contingency (Sullivan et al. 2010). This is, ironically, quite similar to the two-factor explanation of paranoia (although I reject the need for a second factor and suggest that the difference between non-delusional and delusional cases is the extent of the aberrant uncertainty, caused by inappropriate prediction error signals) (Langdon et al. 2008).

An early attempt at a prediction error based account of paranoia, misidentification, passivity, parasitosis, and somatoparaphrenia has been made (Corlett et al. 2010). While it is possible to imagine a possible prediction error deficit that would give rise to each of these delusions, the empirical data are still lacking, and, insisting on a content providing prediction error dysfunction seems rather similar to the content-providing first factor in two-factor theory. Perhaps that is satisfactory – we would instead argue that the prediction error deficit had not yet ascended the hierarchy enough in the non-delusional control cases (Corlett 2019). That the difference between them and the people with delusions is one of degree of deficit, rather than kind (Corlett 2019). We have argued recently that the data on which two-factor theory is predicated license this sort of single association (rather than a double dissociation, in which belief and perception are independently impaired in separate cases, which would warrant independent factors (Corlett 2019)).

## 11.    Why that odd belief? Individual differences in delusion susceptibility

While some psychotic patients get paranoid, others experience passivity, others still have multiple bizarre delusions. We posit a single factor, prediction error dysfunction for delusion formation and maintenance (Corlett et al. 2007a, 2009, Fletcher and Frith 2009). We have applied this single factor account to explain the range of phenomenological effects of pharmacologically distinct psychotomimetic drugs from dopamine agonist amphetamines, to NMDA antagonists, cannabinoids and serotonergic hallucinogens (Corlett et al. 2009). We believe the same explanation may be possible for the individual differences in susceptibility to different delusional themes observed in patients with schizophrenia.

Different delusional themes are characteristic following the administration of different psychotomimetic drugs; paranoia is more intense following cannabis administration (D'Souza et al. 2009) whereas ketamine engenders delusions of reference (Krystal et al. 1994, Oye et al. 1992, Pomarol-Clotet et al. 2006), although the two themes are by no means mutually exclusive (Startup and Startup 2005). Are there any empirical data to support of our contention that delusions with different themes are mediated by distinct (but overlapping) neural circuits?

Patients suffering from dementia with Lewy bodies experience delusions (Nagahama et al. 2007, 2009) like Capgras (Hirono and Cummings 1999) (for more on delusions in the disorders of old age see Hughes, Chapter 11). Nagahama and colleagues used factor analysis to classify psychotic symptoms in dementia with Lewy bodies. They found that hallucinations, misidentification experiences and delusions were independent symptom domains (Nagahama et al. 2007). More recently they replicated this factor structure in an independent group of patients and assessed the neural correlates of those factors by regressing factor scores onto resting state neuroimaging data across subjects (Nagahama et al. 2009).

Patients suffering from misidentification had hypo-perfusion in left hippocampus, insula, inferior frontal gyrus, and nucleus accumbens compared to patients without those symptoms. Individuals who had visual hallucinations of person or a feeling of presence had hypo-perfusion in bilateral parietal and left ventral occipital gyrus. Patients with persecutory delusions showed significant hyperactivity in right cingulate sulcus, bilateral middle frontal gyri, right inferior frontal gyrus, left medial superior frontal gyrus, and left middle frontopolar gyrus. These distinct circuits tend to support our predicted delusion circuits; that is, paranoia involves a frontal hyperactivity; delusions that potentially involve hyper salience of own body representations (e.g. hallucinations of people and feeling of presence) involve a parietal dysfunction and reduplications of person and place involve a predictive memory impairment; impaired familiarity processing and fronto-hippocampal as well as fronto-striatal dysfunction.

Lewy bodies appear to accumulate in the space between bands of cortex; occupied by afferent or efferent connections with different cortical sites or with subcortical regions, that is, they have a laminar distribution (Armstrong et al. 2001). Depending on which layer, they preferentially influence the feedforward (prediction error specifying) connections originating in laminae I-III and terminating in granular lamina IV of the adjacent lobe (Armstrong et al. 2001). Alternatively, Lewy bodies may accumulate in the feedback fibers (responsible for specifying prior expectations and attentional modulation) which originate in laminae V and VI (and to some extent III) and terminate in lamina I (De Lacoste and White 1993). Why the feedforward and feedback pathways of one particular circuit would be more sensitive to Lewy body inclusions than another circuit (conferring a particular delusion content) has yet to be determined, however, the disconnection that they engender within particular circuits is consistent with the putative disconnections invoked to explain the symptoms of schizophrenia (Friston 2005a, Friston and Frith 1995).

Patients with delusions secondary to neurological damage often have lesions in right frontal cortex but, according to two-factor theories, the theme of the belief is conferred by damage to a second structure; for example the fusiform face area in Capgras delusion. There is some evidence for this sort of distinction, although it does not rise to the level of a double dissociation of factors one and two. Darby and colleagues applied an ingenious lesion-network mapping approach (Darby et al. 2017). First, they catalogued the locations of lesions which gave rise to *de novo* delusions in Capgras patients, and a group of patients with other delusions (as a comparator group). Then they created seeds from those lesion-locations and, in a large resting-state functional neuroimaging dataset gathered in healthy participants, they explored the connectivity of these lesion locations. This yielded maps of the circuits involved in Capgras and other delusions. All delusions seemed to involve damage to regions that were connected to right frontal cortex. However, Capgras was associated with damage to regions that connected to the retrosplenial cortex, which delusions with other contents did not. Ironically, this pattern of results was embraced by both two-factor theorists and prediction error theorists as consistent with their accounts (Corlett 2019, McKay 2019).

There are two important issues to consider here. First, functional connectivity analyses tell us nothing about the directions of information processing between the regions whose activity is correlated (Corlett 2019). If the dorsolateral prefrontal cortex (DLPFC) is coupled to retrosplenial cortex and driving its aberrant engagement in Capgras patients, that would be a problem for the two-factor theory, since, under the two-factor theory, belief processing cannot influence perception (Corlett 2019). The direction of influence between regions can only be discerned using effective connectivity analyses which have not been applied to these data so far (Corlett 2019).

Second, our map of prediction error processing in the human brain is now much more complete since the publication of this lesion-network analysis. We conducted a meta-analysis of all prediction error studies using human fMRI and were able to examine the circuits engaged by prediction errors (regardless of content) – a domain general circuit – as well as putative domain specific circuits (in visual processing (in visual cortices) and perhaps social processing in dorsomedial prefrontal cortex) (Corlett et al. 2022). However, the specific circuits were hardly encapsulated, as might be necessary for a two-factor account to work (Corlett et al. 2022). This observation was also made at the single neuron level in humans – there are dorsomedial prefrontal cortex neurons whose prediction error responses are induced by both social and non-social surprises (Jamali et al. 2021). Again, some effective connectivity analyses will clarify the direction of interaction between general and specific circuits. However, one can imagine at least two distinct possibilities that would give content specific delusions under a prediction error account:

1  Aberrant prediction errors arise in the domain general circuitry. When they are temporally coincident with activity in domain-specific regions, that specific domain is invoked to explain away the prediction error, and the delusion forms.
2  Aberrant prediction errors arise in the domain specific circuitry and augur belief updating in the more general circuitry – by contributing to a global sense of uncertainty and unpredictability – a delusional mood – which is resolved by explaining away the initial content specific prediction error.

These possibilities can only be resolved with data gathered from patients experiencing delusions of different contents.

The data we have so far confirm aberrant prediction errors in the domain-general circuit. Others have hypothesized that passivity delusions might arise due to misalignment of domain general prediction errors from the ventral tegmental area and pedunculopontine tegmentum (which signal that a surprising event has occurred) with motor plan representations in the striatum – leading to the conclusion that an action took place without an intention (Redgrave and Gurney 2006).

Clearly this is an issue that will only fully yield to explanation with more data. However, the key point is that delusions with specific contents can arise under prediction error theory.

A key interim analysis would be to examine the overlap between the prediction error meta-analysis and the lesion-network maps of delusions. On visual inspection, the anterior insula seems key, both to domain general prediction error, and delusions. The retrosplenial cortex does not seem to be key feature of the domain-specific perceptual circuit (and again, even there, there are general signals too). However, this may be because the majority of fMRI studies of visual prediction errors are dealing with the presence or absence of some visual stimulus, and not the prediction error over affective responses to familiar faces.

The empirical data addressing prediction error and delusions continues to build. Armed with such data, it will be possible to clarify whether encapsulated modularity and one-way information flow (from perception to belief) are present, and, if they are not, a two-factor theory cannot pertain.

## 12.   From symptoms back to syndromes

Another key challenge for prediction error theory and cognitive neuropsychiatry more broadly is to move beyond the individual symptom approach and tackle syndromic presentation. Patients with schizophrenia often have hallucinations as well as delusions. However, the computational psychiatry of delusions could be seen as at odds with that of hallucinations. Aberrant prediction errors arise in the absence of constraining beliefs. Hallucinations seem to entail stronger beliefs. One possibility is that paranoia and hallucinations both represent aberrantly strong beliefs about different environmental features (prior perceptual beliefs relate to hallucinations, prior beliefs about volatility relate to paranoia). Extending this idea further, it may be that some delusions (passivity, infestation) are more hallucination-like than others and that there is likewise more or less reliance on prior beliefs that tracks these differences in phenomenology. Computational psychiatry and phenomenology are natural allies. Changes in world-making are readily explicable in terms of the generative models at the center of computational approaches to psychosis. I suspect that these fields will further align going forwards.

Ongoing work is attempting to use measures of prior belief and volatility to predict whom from the clinical high-risk state will convert to psychotic illness, with promising initial results (Gold et al. 2020). Furthermore, it may be possible to match individuals to treatments based on the computational metrics derived from their behaviour. Since cognitive behavioural therapy – particularly aimed at worry – seems effective against paranoia (Freeman et al. 2015), it may be that those with higher volatility beliefs might benefit most. Preliminary work in patients with schizophrenia suggests that the relationship between volatility beliefs and paranoia may be mediated by worry (Sheffield et al. 2022). Using these metrics to track therapeutic trajectories will be a key focus in the future. Grounding our understanding in the basic neuroscience of belief updating may inspire novel treatments – perhaps combining new opportunities for learning with pharmacological interventions that enhance the retention and consolidation of that learning (Gottlieb et al. 2011). More broadly, falsification of our hypotheses – about behavioural and computational correlates of psychosis – with empirical evidence will guide the development of the theory and practice, lest we stick rigidly to our beliefs about delusions.

# References


Adams, R. A., Stephan, K. E., Brown, H. R., Frith, C. D. & Friston, K. J. 2013. The computational anatomy of psychosis. *Front Psychiatry*, 4, 47.

Armstrong, R. A., Cairns, N. J. & Lantos, P. L. 2001. What does the study of the spatial patterns of pathological lesions tell us about the pathogenesis of neurodegenerative disorders? *Neuropathology*, 21, 1–12.

Corlett, P. R. 2019b. Factor one, familiarity and frontal cortex: a challenge to the two-factor theory of delusions. *Cogn Neuropsychiatry*, 24(3), 165–177.

Corlett, P. R. & Fletcher, P. 2021. Modelling delusions as temporally-evolving beliefs. *Cogn Neuropsychiatry*, 26, 231–241.

Corlett, P. R. & Fletcher, P. C. 2012. The neurobiology of schizotypy: fronto-striatal prediction error signal correlates with delusion-like beliefs in healthy people. *Neuropsychologia*, 50, 3612–3620.

Corlett, P. R. & Fletcher, P. C. 2014. Computational psychiatry: a Rosetta Stone linking the brain to mental illness. *Lancet Psychiatry*, 1(5), 399–402.

Corlett, P. R., Frith, C. D. & Fletcher, P. C. 2009. From drugs to deprivation: a Bayesian framework for understanding models of psychosis. *Psychopharmacology (Berl)*, 206(4), 515–530.

Corlett, P. R., Honey, G. D., Aitken, M. R., Dickinson, A., Shanks, D. R., Absalom, A. R., Lee, M., Pomarol-Clotet, E., Murray, G. K., Mckenna, P. J., Robbins, T. W., Bullmore, E. T. & Fletcher, P. C. 2006. Frontal responses during learning predict vulnerability to the psychotogenic effects of ketamine: linking cognition, brain activity, and psychosis. *Arch Gen Psychiatry*, 63, 611–621.

Corlett, P. R., Honey, G. D. & Fletcher, P. C. 2007a. From prediction error to psychosis: ketamine as a pharmacological model of delusions. *J Psychopharmacol*, 21, 238–252.

Corlett, P. R., Horga, G., Fletcher, P. C., Alderson-Day, B., Schmack, K. & Powers, A. R., 3rd. 2019. Hallucinations and strong priors. *Trends Cogn Sci*, 23, 114–127.

Corlett, P. R., Krystal, J. K., Taylor, J. R. & Fletcher, P. C. 2009. Why do delusions persist? *Front Human Neurosci* (in press), 3, 12.

Corlett, P. R., Mollick, J. A. & Kober, H. 2022. Meta-analysis of human prediction error for incentives, perception, cognition, and action. *Neuropsychopharmacology*, 47(7), 1339–1349.

Corlett, P. R., Murray, G. K., Honey, G. D., Aitken, M. R., Shanks, D. R., Robbins, T. W., Bullmore, E. T., Dickinson, A. & Fletcher, P. C. 2007b. Disrupted prediction-error signal in psychosis: evidence for an associative account of delusions. *Brain*, 130, 2387–2400.

Corlett, P. R., Taylor, J. R., Wang, X. J., Fletcher, P. C. & Krystal, J. H. 2010. Toward a neurobiology of delusions. *Prog Neurobiol*, 92, 345–369.

Crapse, T. B. & Sommer, M. A. 2008. Corollary discharge circuits in the primate brain. *Curr Opin Neurobiol*, 18, 552–557.

D'Souza, D. C., Sewell, R. A. & Ranganathan, M. 2009. Cannabis and psychosis/schizophrenia: human studies. *Eur Arch Psychiatry Clin Neurosci*, 259, 413–431.

Darby, R. R., Laganiere, S., Pascual-Leone, A., Prasad, S. & Fox, M. D. 2017. Finding the imposter: brain connectivity of lesions causing delusional misidentifications. *Brain*, 140, 497–507.

Davies, M. & Coltheart, M. 2022. Cotard delusion, emotional experience and depersonalisation. *Cogn Neuropsychiatry*, 27, 430–446.

De Lacoste, M. C. & White, C. L., 3RD 1993. The role of cortical connectivity in Alzheimer's disease pathogenesis: a review and model system. *Neurobiol Aging*, 14, 1–16.

Feinberg, I. 1978. Efference copy and corollary discharge: implications for thinking and its disorders. *Schizophr Bull*, 4, 636–640.

Fletcher, P. C. & Frith, C. D. 2009. Perceiving is believing: a Bayesian approach to explaining the positive symptoms of schizophrenia. *Nat Rev Neurosci*, 10, 48–58.

Ford, J. M., Roach, B. J., Faustman, W. O. & Mathalon, D. H. 2007. Synch before you speak: auditory hallucinations in schizophrenia. *Am J Psychiatry*, 164, 458–466.

Freeman, D., Dunn, G., Startup, H., Pugh, K., Cordwell, J., Mander, H., Cernis, E., Wingham, G., Shirvell, K. & Kingdon, D. 2015. Effects of cognitive behaviour therapy for worry on persecutory delusions in patients with psychosis (WIT): a parallel, single-blind, randomised controlled trial with a mediation analysis. *Lancet Psychiatry*, 2, 305–313.

Friston, K. 2005a. Disconnection and cognitive dysmetria in schizophrenia. *Am J Psychiatry*, 162, 429–432.

Friston, K. 2005b. A theory of cortical responses. *Philos Trans R Soc Lond B Biol Sci*, 360, 815–836.

Friston, K. J. & Frith, C. D. 1995. Schizophrenia: a disconnection syndrome? *Clin Neurosci*, 3, 89–97.

Gold, J. M., Corlett, P. R., Strauss, G. P., Schiffman, J., Ellman, L. M., Walker, E. F., Powers, A. R., Woods, S. W., Waltz, J. A., Silverstein, S. M. & Mittal, V. A. 2020. Enhancing psychosis risk prediction through computational cognitive neuroscience. *Schizophr Bull*, 46(6), 1346–1352.

Gottlieb, J. D., Cather, C., Shanahan, M., Creedon, T., Macklin, E. A. & Goff, D. C. 2011. D-cycloserine facilitation of cognitive behavioral therapy for delusions in schizophrenia. *Schizophr Res*, 131, 69–74.

Gray, J. A., Feldon, J., Rawlins, J. N. P. & Hemsley, D. R. 1995. The neuropsychology of schizophrenia. *Behav Brain Sci*, 14, 1–20.

Halligan, P. W. & David, A. S. 2001. Cognitive neuropsychiatry: towards a scientific psychopathology. *Nat Rev Neurosci*, 2, 209–215.

Hirono, N. & Cummings, J. L. 1999. Neuropsychiatric aspects of dementia with Lewy bodies. *Curr Psychiatry Rep*, 1, 85–92.

Jamali, M., Grannan, B. L., Fedorenko, E., Saxe, R., Baez-Mendoza, R. & Williams, Z. M. 2021. Single-neuronal predictions of others' beliefs in humans. *Nature*, 591, 610–614.

Kamin, L. 1969. Predictability, surprise, attention, and conditioning. In: Campbell, B. A., Church, R. M. (eds.) *Punishment and Aversive Behavior*. New York: Appleton-Century-Crofts.

Kapur, S. 2003. Psychosis as a state of aberrant salience: a framework linking biology, phenomenology, and pharmacology in schizophrenia. *Am J Psychiatry*, 160, 13–23.

Kegeles, L. S., Abi-Dargham, A., Frankle, W. G., Gil, R., Cooper, T. B., Slifstein, M., Hwang, D. R., Huang, Y., Haber, S. N. & Laruelle, M. 2010. Increased synaptic dopamine function in associative regions of the striatum in schizophrenia. *Arch Gen Psychiatry*, 67, 231–239.

Krystal, J. H., Karper, L. P., Seibyl, J. P., Freeman, G. K., Delaney, R., Bremner, J. D., Heninger, G. R., Bowers, M. B., Jr. & Charney, D. S. 1994. Subanesthetic effects of the noncompetitive NMDA antagonist, ketamine, in humans. Psychotomimetic, perceptual, cognitive, and neuroendocrine responses. *Arch Gen Psychiatry*, 51, 199–214.

Langdon, R., Mckay, R. & Coltheart, M. 2008. The cognitive neuropsychological understanding of persecutory delusions. In: Freeman, D., Garety, P. & Bentall, R. (eds.) *Persecutory Delusions: Assessment, Theory and Treatment*. Oxford: Oxford University Press.

Lavin, A., Nogueira, L., Lapish, C. C., Wightman, R. M., Phillips, P. E. & Seamans, J. K. 2005. Mesocortical dopamine neurons operate in distinct temporal domains using multimodal signaling. *J Neurosci*, 25, 5013–5023.

Maher, B. A. 1974. Delusional thinking and perceptual disorder. *J Individ Psychol*, 30, 98–113.

Mckay, R. 2019. Measles, magic and misidentifications: a defence of the two-factor theory of delusions. *Cogn Neuropsychiatry*, 24, 183–190.

Miyazono, K. & Mckay, R. 2019. Explaining delusional beliefs: a hybrid model. *Cogn Neuropsychiatry*, 24, 335–346.

Murray, G. K., Corlett, P. R., Clark, L., Pessiglione, M., Blackwell, A. D., Honey, G., Jones, P. B., Bullmore, E. T., Robbins, T. W. & Fletcher, P. C. 2008. Substantia nigra/ventral tegmental reward prediction error disruption in psychosis. *Mol Psychiatry*, 13(239), 267–276.

Nagahama, Y., Okina, T., Suzuki, N. & Matsuda, M. 2009. Neural correlates of psychotic symptoms in dementia with Lewy bodies. *Brain*, 133(2), 557–67.

Nagahama, Y., Okina, T., Suzuki, N., Matsuda, M., Fukao, K. & Murai, T. 2007. Classification of psychotic symptoms in dementia with Lewy bodies. *Am J Geriatr Psychiatry*, 15, 961–967.

O'Tuathaigh, C. M., Salum, C., Young, A. M., Pickering, A. D., Joseph, M. H. & Moran, P. M. 2003. The effect of amphetamine on Kamin blocking and overshadowing. *Behav Pharmacol*, 14, 315–322.

Oye, I., Paulsen, O. & Maurset, A. 1992. Effects of ketamine on sensory perception: evidence for a role of N-methyl-D-aspartate receptors. *J Pharmacol Exp Ther*, 260, 1209–1213.

Pomarol-Clotet, E., Honey, G. D., Murray, G. K., Corlett, P. R., Absalom, A. R., Lee, M., Mckenna, P. J., Bullmore, E. T. & Fletcher, P. C. 2006. Psychological effects of ketamine in healthy volunteers. Phenomenological study. *Br J Psychiatry*, 189, 173–179.

Redgrave, P. & Gurney, K. 2006. The short-latency dopamine signal: a role in discovering novel actions? *Nat Rev Neurosci*, 7, 967–975.

Reed, E. J., Uddenberg, S., Suthaharan, P., Mathys, C. D., Taylor, J. R., Groman, S. M. & Corlett, P. R. 2020. Paranoia as a deficit in non-social belief updating. *Elife*, 26(9), e56345.

Romaniuk, L., Honey, G. D., King, J. R., Whalley, H. C., Mcintosh, A. M., Levita, L., Hughes, M., Johnstone, E. C., Day, M., Lawrie, S. M. & Hall, J. 2010. Midbrain activation during Pavlovian conditioning and delusional symptoms in schizophrenia. *Arch Gen Psychiatry*, 67, 1246–1254.

Rossi-Goldthorpe, R. A., Leong, Y. C., Leptourgos, P. & Corlett, P. R. 2021. Paranoia, self-deception and overconfidence. *PLoS Comput Biol*, 17, e1009453.

Schmack, K., Gomez-Carrillo de Castro, A., Rothkirch, M., Sekutowicz, M., Rossler, H., Haynes, J. D., Heinz, A., Petrovic, P. & Sterzer, P. 2013. Delusions and the role of beliefs in perceptual inference. *J Neurosci*, 33, 13701–13712.

Sheffield, J., Suthaharan, P. & Leptourgos, P. 2022. Belief Updating and Paranoia in Individuals with Schizophrenia. *Biol Psychiatry Cogn Neurosci Neuroimaging*, 7(11), 1149–1157. https://psyarxiv.com/3gyde/.

Startup, M. & Startup, S. 2005. On two kinds of delusion of reference. *Psychiatry Res*, 137, 87–92.

Steinberg, E. E., Keiflin, R., Boivin, J. R., Witten, I. B., Deisseroth, K. & Janak, P. H. 2013. A causal link between prediction errors, dopamine neurons and learning. *Nat Neurosci*, 16, 966–973.

Sullivan, D., Landau, M. J. & Rothschild, Z. K. 2010. An existential function of enemyship: evidence that people attribute influence to personal and political enemies to compensate for threats to control. *J Pers Soc Psychol*, 98, 434–449.

Suthaharan, P., Reed, E., Leptourgos, P., Kenney, J., Uddenberg, S., Mathys, C., Litman, L., Robinson, J., Moss, A., Taylor, J., Groman, S. & Corlett, P. 2021. Paranoia and belief updating during the COVID-19 crisis. *Nat Hum Behav*, 5(9), 1190–1202.

Valton, V., Karvelis, P., Richards, K. L., Seitz, A. R., Lawrie, S. M. & Series, P. 2019. Acquisition of visual priors and induced hallucinations in chronic schizophrenia. *Brain*, 142, 2523–2537.

Waelti, P., Dickinson, A. & Schultz, W. 2001. Dopamine responses comply with basic assumptions of formal learning theory. *Nature*, 412, 43–48.

Wright, S., Young, A. W. & Hellawell, D. J. 1993. Sequential Cotard and Capgras delusions. *Br J Clin Psychol*, 32, 345–349.

Yau, J. O. & Mcnally, G. P. 2015. Pharmacogenetic excitation of dorsomedial prefrontal cortex restores fear prediction error. *J Neurosci*, 35, 74–83.

Young, A. W., Leafhead, K. M. & Szulecka, T. K. 1994. The Capgras and Cotard delusions. *Psychopathology*, 27, 226–231.

# 31

# DELUSION AND SALIENCE

*Peter McKenna*

> I would overhear a conversation where I could barely make out the words, and yet it seemed to me that the speakers were of course talking about me. I once came out of my apartment building and a police officer was parked in his car just beyond the stairs. I started to approach him because, surely, he was there for something having to do with me. Fortunately, I thought twice about confronting him and I walked away. In talking to others who have had delusions of reference, I am always flabbergasted that we have shared the perplexing experience of having the television or radio talk directly to us. From the time my acute psychotic episode began to the time when the delusions of reference dissipated were about 2 months. In this time, I experienced: my own television in my single room occupancy making fun of me; the personalities on the television in the hospital carrying on a conversation with me through subtle aspects of body language; the radio on the rides from my board and care to my outpatient program broadcasting messages that were clearly derived from reading the contents of my mind; and, the television in my room at my board and care constantly addressing me and clearly knowing things about me that implied mind reading.
>
> *(Arner 2022)*

The above quote, taken from a first person account by a patient in a state of acute psychosis, illustrates a phenomenon that is particularly relevant to the subject of this chapter, *delusions of reference and misinterpretation*. The central feature of this class of delusion is that all manner of neutral events in the environment become imbued with personal significance for the patient. A closely related type of delusion is *delusional mood*: this typically occurs at the beginning of a psychotic illness and is characterized by a free-floating feeling that something strange or suspicious is going on and that events are charged with an as yet amorphous sense of new meaning. Many other forms of delusions are also seen, typically in schizophrenia, but also in other disorders such as delusional disorder and psychotic forms of major affective disorder. These include the well-known *persecutory or paranoid delusions*, where the sufferer comes to believe that they are the subject of plots and conspiracies against them involving particular individuals or organizations such as the Mafia, the Freemasons, or the Catholic Church, among many others. In *grandiose delusions*, individuals



DOI: 10.4324/9781003296386-37

feel they have unusual talents or abilities, or that they have special powers, or that they are important people such as royalty or saints. A good example here is the Nobel prize-winning mathematician John Nash (subject of the film *A Beautiful Mind*), who at the beginning of his schizophrenic illness wrote to a colleague declining an offer of a Chair on the grounds that he was about to made emperor of Antarctica (Nasar 1998). Also common in schizophrenia and other psychotic illnesses are *hypochondriacal delusions*, ideas about illness and bodily change. Here patients say things like their bones are softening, or that they have a wine glass in their stomach, or that rays are turning their liver to gold. Frequently bizarre, as in these examples, delusions may sometimes defy common sense even at its most elementary; patients with such *fantastic delusions* believe that they have visited other planets, are immortal, have multiple sets of parents, or remember being present at the birth of King Charles (despite not having been born at the time).

Unlike referential delusions and delusional mood, these latter delusions do not on the face of it involve the attribution of significance to neutral events. One of the classical writers on delusions, Schneider (1949/1974), referred to them (or more accurately some of them) as delusional intuitions:

> Like delusional perceptions [a term that in Schneider's hands broadly corresponded to referential delusions], delusional intuitions are also often special, momentous or supernatural in nature, as if they come from 'another dimension'. We may speak here again of 'special significance', but we must make it clear that the word 'significance' is now being used a very different sense from that given to it in our discussion of delusional perception. We must be careful not to lapse into mere equivocation. In delusional intuition 'special significance' means only that the intuition is of special importance to the person in question, i.e., it carries special weight.
>
> *(Schneider 1949/1974: 37–38 [in 1974 translation])*

More recently, these non-significance-bearing delusions have been collectively termed *propositional delusions* (McKenna 2017) or *thematic delusions* (Rosen et al. 2022) (henceforward the former term will be used). As it turns out, accounting for this type of delusion is a topic of some importance for the aberrant salience theory.

## 1.  Theories of delusions

Proposals as to why individuals with schizophrenia and other psychotic disorders come to hold erroneous beliefs with conviction and imperviousness to counter-argument – or even entertain them in the first place – have been proposed intermittently since the middle of the last century. Mostly, they have not fared very well. One early approach was Brendan Maher's (Maher 1974; Maher & Ross 1984) proposal of 'the deluded patient as naïve scientist'. This maintained that delusions were the result of essentially normal reasoning processes being applied to abnormal input in the shape of perceptual experiences such as hallucinations or strange physical sensations. The result, according to the theory, would be an explanation that was also abnormal, i.e., a delusion. Maher's theory faced an immediate stumbling block in that it failed to address the issue of why all individuals with abnormal sensory experiences do not develop delusions – patients with tinnitus and the phantom limb syndrome, for example, remain entirely rational about their symptoms. This problem may not be as damaging as it at first seems (for example see Noordhof & Sullivan-Bissett, 2021, and Sullivan-Bissett, Chapter 28); however, another difficulty is that the theory does not explain how patients can develop delusions in the absence of hallucinations or other abnormal perceptual experiences. This undoubtedly occurs in schizophrenia (not all patients have hallucinations), and patients with delusional disorder by definition have delusions as their only symptom. Maher recognized this problem and dealt with it by proposing that in such cases, there was something he called a 'central neuropathology', which caused abnormal significance to be attributed to normal experiences, and this experience then interacted with the same intact hypothesis testing machinery to generate delusions.

Maher's theory was never subjected to any kind of experimental test, and remains in some ways a historical curiosity. Nevertheless, as will be seen, its influence continues to be felt.

Two more theories of delusions are Philippa Garety and coworkers' (e.g. Garety & Freeman, 1999, 2013) proposal that probabilistic reasoning bias underlies at least some classes of delusions (see Davies & Coltheart, Chapter 29), and Chris Frith's (1992) suggestion that persecutory and referential delusions might be due to theory of mind impairment. The former theory proposes that, when making judgements under conditions of uncertainty, patients with delusions require less evidence than usual to arrive at a decision; in other words they 'jump to conclusions'. The latter argues that deluded patients have an inability to make inferences about others's mental states. Unlike patients with autism, whose lifelong inability to infer mental states means that they do not try to make such inferences, the difficulty in patients with delusions is acquired – they had normal theory of mind abilities before they became ill and continue to make inferences about others's mental states but now make many errors. In the words of Frith:

> They will 'see' intentions to communicate when none are there (delusions of reference). They may start to believe that people are deliberately behaving in such a way as to disguise their intentions. They will deduce that there is a general conspiracy against them and that people's intentions towards them are evil (paranoid delusions).
>
> *(Frith 1992: 105)*

Unlike Maher's proposal, both these latter theories of delusions have been tested, in fact quite extensively. It has been very well demonstrated that patients with schizophrenia show a tendency to jump to conclusions (for reviews see Garety & Freeman 2013 and Bora, Yucel, & Pantelis 2009). However, attempts to show that jumping to conclusions is related to delusions – i.e., that it is present in patients in delusions but not in those without delusions, or that it correlates with the severity of delusional symptoms – have been less successful. The present author (McKenna 2017) reviewed the literature and found that out of 13 studies that examined the relationship between jumping to conclusions and delusions, only two found evidence of an association, and in both cases, this was only seen in one of two experimental conditions employed. On the other hand, a meta-analysis of a slightly larger database of studies (Dudley et al. 2016) (a meta-analysis mathematically combines the results of studies and can yield positive effects when individual studies fail to do so) had more encouraging findings with respect to the association with delusions, although the effect was still modest. The pattern of findings the theory of mind is similar – clear evidence of impairment in schizophrenia (e.g., see meta-analysis by Bora, Yucel, & Pantelis 2009), but no strong evidence for an association with delusions (for a review see McKenna 2017).

In recent years, a new theory of delusions has appeared on the scene and has generated considerable excitement. This is the idea that delusions might reflect an abnormality in the brain mechanisms of learning, specifically involving the way in which reward is processed. An abnormality here, it is argued, interferes with the process whereby stimuli in the environment that are repeatedly associated with reward acquire 'salience', i.e., motivational value and the ability to reinforce learning in their own right. It is a theory that neatly accounts for the phenomenon of neutral events seeming significant to the patient that is at the heart of the class of referential delusions. Its application to propositional delusions is more challenging, but progress has been made here too. Most importantly, it is a theory that can be and has been tested, principally by means of the high-tech methodology of functional brain imaging.

## 2.   Origins of the aberrant salience theory

The aberrant salience theory has its roots in two lines of evidence dating from the latter half of the 20th century. One was the dopamine hypothesis of schizophrenia – the proposal that there is a functional excess of this brain transmitter in the disorder. This was originally based on two complementary findings, that all antipsychotic drugs exert their therapeutic effects by blocking postsynaptic dopamine D2 receptors (Creese, Burt, & Snyder 1976; Peroutka & Synder 1980; Seeman 1987), and that amphetamine and other stimulant drugs (which act to increase dopamine among other pharmacological actions) can cause a psychotic state essentially indistinguishable from schizophrenia.

The other line of evidence concerned the involvement of dopamine in reward signalling in the brain. Research here began with James Olds and Peter Milner's (1954) demonstration that electrical stimulation of certain brain regions could act to reinforce learning in rats. This was followed by a series of experiments which established first that catecholamine neurotransmitters (which comprise dopamine and noradrenalin) were crucially involved in the effect (Wise 1978), and then that dopamine rather than noradrenalin was the important transmitter (Mason 1984).

Research in this latter area took a leap forward in 1997 when Wolfram Schultz and co-workers (Schultz, Dayan, & Montague 1997) recorded neuronal activity from dopamine cell bodies in the midbrain of awake monkeys while they learned a task. They were able to show that 75–80 per cent of such neurons switched from their usual pattern of tonic activity to phasic bursts when the animal received a reward, for example, touching a morsel of food or receiving a drop of fruit juice. Importantly, when a stimulus such as a light or a tone that reliably preceded reward was introduced into the experimental environment, the phasic activity to the reward itself progressively decreased and was replaced by phasic activity in response to the stimulus. Ultimately, increased activity to the reward no longer occurred, although it could be re-instated if the reward was delivered unassociated with the stimulus.

The significance of this finding was that brain dopamine signalling appeared to be following the rules of a mathematical theory of reward learning elaborated several decades earlier, the so-called Rescorla and Wagner model (see Glimcher 2011). According to this model, the strength of the association between a natural reward and a stimulus associated with it is not simply a function of how many times the two have been paired, but instead takes into account the degree to which the natural reward is greater or less than expected on any given trial, the so-called reward prediction error. Thus, when an animal first encounters, say, a large unexpected amount of food in a particular environment, this generates a large positive reward prediction error signal which then causes learning to start to take place, as part of which environmental stimuli associated with the reward begin to acquire salience. Ultimately, there comes a point where there will be no difference between the reward that is predicted to occur and the reward that is actually received, and so no further learning (and salience attribution) takes place. If for some reason, the reward then stops being provided, a negative reward prediction error begins to be generated, and everything that was previously learnt starts to be unlearnt.

The first author to combine the concept of a functional dopamine excess in schizophrenia and this neurotransmitter's role in reward signalling to delusions was Richard Beninger (1983). He speculated that overstimulated dopamine function might have the consequence that patients with the disorder would lose their ability to ignore irrelevant stimuli in the environment, and that paranoia or delusions of grandeur could represent cognitive elaborations of the apparent meaningfulness that such stimuli had erroneously acquired. A few years later, the present author proposed something similar, arguing that the role of dopamine in reward meant that a functional dopamine excess might result in significance being wrongly acquired by stimuli that did not in fact signal anything, and that such a state would likely have the features of delusional mood (McKenna 1987). A decade or so later, Andreas Heinz (2002) refined the same idea, now placing it in the context of Schultz and colleagues' (1997) findings in monkeys:

> [A] chaotic or stress-induced overactivation of phasic dopamine release may focus attention on stimuli that carry no relevant information and bear no specific significance for other persons. Such an over-attribution of meaning to otherwise irrelevant cues may play an important role in the pathogenesis of delusional mood in the early course of schizophrenia.
>
> *(Heinz 2002: 13)*

The stage was set for a fully-fledged salience theory of delusions, one that addressed not only referential but also what this chapter terms propositional delusions.

## 3.  Kapur's aberrant salience theory

The Canadian psychiatrist and researcher, Shitij Kapur (2003), argued that the occurrence of pathologically increased dopamine transmission in schizophrenia would lead to a release of dopamine outside the proper context, and this, by inappropriately signalling reward prediction error, would cause neutral stimuli to inappropriately acquire significance for behaviour, or in his words, aberrant salience. The result of saliences being created where they ought not to be would then be the subjective experience of events that were in reality of little or no significance to the individual acquiring exaggerated importance. Kapur drew attention here to descriptions that schizophrenic patients gave of the earliest stages of their illness, like 'I developed a greater awareness of….My senses were sharpened. I became fascinated by the little insignificant things around me' (Bowers & Freedman 1966), and 'My senses seemed alive….Things seemed clearcut, I noticed things I had never noticed before' (Bowers 1968). Often, patients interpreted these experiences as reflecting something in the world around them changing, leaving them puzzled and looking for an explanation: 'I felt that there was some overwhelming significance in this' (McDonald 1960) and 'I felt like I was putting a piece of the puzzle together' (Bowers 1968). Kapur was describing in all but name the symptom of delusional mood.

Kapur regarded delusions of reference and misinterpretation as an attempt to explain the persistent experience of aberrant salience. It drove the patient to search for further confirmatory evidence, 'in the glances of strangers, in the headlines of newspapers, and in the lapel pins of newscasters' (Kapur 2003: 16). He did not rule out the possibility that other factors might also contribute to the process whereby a fully formed referential framework developed out of the initially amorphous experience of aberrant salience. These could include a jumping to conclusions cognitive style and poorly developed theory of mind skills, and perhaps personality factors as well.

Delusions – by which Kapur meant propositional delusions in the sense the term is used in this chapter – were also proposed to be the result of the individual's effort to make sense of the experience of aberrant salience as it was repeated over days, months, or years:

> Delusions in this framework are a 'top-down' cognitive explanation that the individual imposes on these experiences of aberrant salience in an effort to make sense of them. Since delusions are constructed by the individual, they are imbued with the psychodynamic themes relevant to the individual and are embedded in the cultural context of the individual. This explains how the same neurochemical dysregulation leads to variable phenomenological expression: a patient in Africa struggling to make sense of aberrant saliences is much more likely to accord them to the evil ministrations of a shaman, while the one living in Toronto is more likely to see them as the machinations of the Royal Canadian Mounted Police.
>
> *(Kapur 2003: 15)*

## 4. Strengths and weaknesses of the aberrant salience theory

The strength of the salience theory is obvious: it forges a direct, intuitive, and plausible link between a putative disturbance of brain function in schizophrenia, namely functional dopamine excess, and a symptom of the disorder, delusional mood. It is only a short step to extend the proposal to other classes of delusion whose central phenomenological feature is an abnormal feeling of significance, i.e., delusions of reference and misinterpretation. This could be via the individual's effort to make sense of the persistent experience of aberrant salience, as Kapur proposed. Alternatively, it is possible to imagine a simpler process involving little or no cognitive mediation.

But at the same time is clear that the theory has a weakness. This is that it provides no obvious mechanism whereby propositional delusions might arise. Kapur's proposal that these are the result of the individual's struggle to make sense of all that he or she is experiencing is vague to the point of hand-waving. This part of the theory is also similar to Maher's (Maher 1974; Maher & Ross 1984) proposal from over 50 years ago, and suffers from some of the same explanatory shortcomings.

The application of Kapur's theory also faces a further difficulty in that it predicts that the development of propositional delusions should always be preceded by delusional mood and/or delusions of reference and misinterpretation. The classical writers on schizophrenia Emil Kraepelin (1913) and Eugen Bleuler (1911) certainly accepted that referential delusions could be the starting point for the development of persecutory delusions, which finally – sometimes only after years – crystallized as an explanation of all that had been happening to the patient. However, they were clear this was not necessarily the case. Bleuler (1911, 1924), in particular, observed that the sudden experience of sharply formulated abnormal ideas by patients could be the first symptom of schizophrenia; in other patients, delusions appeared in consciousness all at once as finished products. At the clinical level, it seems, there is a partial dissociation between referential and propositional delusions.

## 5.  The Fletcher/Frith/Corlett modification of the aberrant salience theory

The weakness of salience theory in accounting for propositional delusions has been addressed by a group of researchers that includes Frith, Paul Fletcher and Philip Corlett, and others such as Karl Friston and Rick Adams (Corlett, Frith, & Fletcher 2009; Fletcher & Frith, 2009; Corlett et al. 2010; Adams et al. 2013). Their approach hinges on the fact that reward prediction error does not exist in a vacuum, but instead is inextricably bound up with a second process that takes place in learning – the making of predictions. Thus, during learning, predictive models are formed about those aspects of the environment which are associated with reward; these models generate prediction errors when they are violated; and these prediction errors in turn modify the predictive model.

How might this additional component of reward-based learning apply to delusions? With respect to the initial formation of delusions, Corlett and colleagues agreed with Kapur that

> during the earliest phases of delusion formation aberrant novelty, salience or prediction error signals drive attention toward redundant or irrelevant environmental cues, the world seems to have changed, it feels strange and sinister...
>
> *(Corlett et al. 2010: 347)*

But now, the occurrence of erroneous prediction errors also leads to a modification of the relevant predictive model about the world:

> Such signals and experiences provide an impetus for new learning which updates the world model inappropriately, manifest as a delusion.
>
> *(Corlett et al. 2010: 347)*

Fletcher and Frith (2009) made the additional point that the new model of the world can never be successful because it can never eliminate the prediction error. The rogue signal persists however many attempts are made to accommodate it, and so the predictive model deviates more and more from reality. Working within a hierarchical model of central nervous system organization proposed by Friston and co-workers (Friston 2005; Friston, Kilner, & Harrison 2006) where prediction errors from lower levels form the input to higher levels of analysis, they argued:

> These [false prediction] errors require higher levels of the hierarchy to adjust their models of the world. However, as the errors are false, these adjustments can never fully resolve the problem. As a result, prediction errors will be propagated even further up the system to ever-higher levels of abstraction
>
> *(Fletcher and Frith 2009: 55).*

With this modification, the aberrant salience theory becomes a complete account of delusions, one that can in principle explain both referential and propositional delusions. It should be noted that the problem of the theory predicting that the development of propositional delusions will always be preceded by delusional mood (or referential delusions if the above broadening of Kapur's original argument is accepted) remains. However, the fact that there are now two processes at work – erroneous attribution of reward prediction error and progressive subversion of predictive models – might give the theory some room for manoeuvre here. Some speculations on this issue are offered in the concluding remarks (see also Corlett, Chapter 30).

## 6.   Testing the aberrant salience theory

Salience theory rests ultimately on something that is an article of faith among many biological schizophrenia researchers, that there is a functional excess of dopamine in the disorder. As described above, this view is supported by highly suggestive circumstantial evidence. The road to proof of the dopamine hypothesis, however, has proved to be arduous. The first candidate abnormality was pathologically increased numbers of postsynaptic dopamine receptors (strictly speaking one class of these, D2 receptors), something that would act to multiply the effects of a normal level of the transmitter at synapses. This possibility was ruled out in the 1990s, when all but one of a series of brain imaging studies using radioactively labelled compounds that bind to dopamine D2 receptors (i.e. antipsychotics) failed to find increases in dopamine D2 receptor numbers in never-treated ('drug naïve') patients with schizophrenia (for a review see Weinberger and Laruelle 2001). (Drug naivety is important because antipsychotic drug treatment itself is known to induce increases in post-synaptic D2 receptor numbers.) Findings concerning two further dopaminergic abnormalities in schizophrenia, increased synthesis and increased synaptic release of dopamine, have subsequently been explored, with promising but not fully consistent results (for a review see Jauhar, Johnstone, & McKenna 2022). It is not too much to say that, after more than 50 years of investigation, the dopamine hypothesis of schizophrenia remains in limbo, neither definitively proved or disproved.

Even if the dopamine hypothesis is eventually confirmed, this does not automatically mean that the salience theory of delusions is correct. For this, it would have to be shown firstly that patients with schizophrenia show alterations in reward processing, secondly, that this is present in patients with delusions, but not (or less so) in patients without delusions, and finally, that the abnormality affects reward prediction error rather than other aspects of reward processing. It seems like a tall order, but in fact developments in brain imaging have made testing of all these proposals feasible.

By the end of the 1990s, functional imaging studies had demonstrated that the experience of reward, ranging from receiving a small amount of fruit juice or seeing attractive faces at one end of the spectrum, to viewing erotic videos or being administered cocaine at the other, was accompanied by a pattern of activation in the brain (McClure, York, and Montague 2004). The regions activated were broadly similar to those established as involved in reward by single cell recording studies in animals, and included importantly the ventral striatum (a heavily dopamine innervated part of the basal ganglia) and an area encompassing the orbitofrontal and ventromedial prefrontal cortex (which also receives dopamine innervation, along with the rest of the cerebral cortex).

Then, slightly over 20 years ago, a functional magnetic imaging (fMRI) task, the monetary incentive delay task (Knutson et al. 2000), was developed which enabled different aspects of the brain response to rewarding stimuli (in this case money) to be examined in more detail. A representation of the paradigm is shown in Figure 31.1. While in an fMRI scanner, subjects perform a task (pressing a button as quickly as possible when they see e.g., a white square before it disappears), whose difficulty is individually adjusted during a previous training phase outside the scanner so that they are successful approximately two-thirds of the time. On some trials, the task is preceded by a cue, e.g., a circle, which signals that the participants will win a certain amount of money if they perform the task within the allotted time. Other trials are preceded by a different cue, e.g., a triangle, which signals that successful performance will not be followed by reward. Often, the value of the potential reward varies from trial to trial, which is indicated, as shown in Figure 31.1, by the number of bars superimposed on the cue. Feedback about whether money has been won is presented immediately after the response has been made.

Comparison of brain activations to the reward signalling cue compared to the non-reward-signalling cue during the period immediately after presentation but before feedback is given provides a measure of reward anticipation, something that equates to the extent to which the stimulus has acquired salience. Activations at the time information about whether money has been won on a particular trial is given provide a measure of the brain's response to receipt of the reward (generally referred to as reward feedback or delivery). There are many variations of the monetary incentive delay task: in some, rather than being pretrained, the subjects have to learn the predictive values of the cues by trial and error while being scanned; in others there is no interpolated reaction time task; and in still others the stimuli reverse or are regularly replaced with new ones during the scanning session. Some of these modifications make it possible to measure reward prediction error.

Joaquim Radua and colleagues (2015) meta-analysed studies of the monetary incentive delay task in schizophrenia. These studies were carried out on patients with established forms of the disorder, who would typically be on antipsychotic treatment, as well as samples of first-episode patients some or all of whom would be drug free or drug naïve, and also in subjects at high risk of developing schizophrenia (e.g., by virtue of having a family history of the disorder), who would typically never have received treatment. Radua and colleagues (2015) focused on studies using the so-called region of interest (ROI) approach, i.e., that reported the average activation in a prespecified area, in this case the dopamine-rich, heavily reward implicated ventral striatum. In 23 studies examining activations during reward anticipation, activation was found to be significantly reduced in patients compared to healthy controls. Significantly reduced activation was also found in the reward feedback/ delivery phase in nine studies. Radua and colleagues were able to find eight studies that measured reward prediction error and here the finding was once again of significant reduction in activation, although the size of the effect was smaller. There was no evidence of an association between ventral striatal activation and positive schizophrenic symptoms, the group of symptoms encompassing delusions, hallucinations, and formal thought disorder (the incoherence of speech seen in a proportion of patients with the disorder) – although as the authors noted, the number of relevant studies was small and there was considerably heterogeneity among them.

Clearly, these findings are not what one would hope to see from the point of view of finding support for salience theory, indicating as they do that ventral striatal activation in patients during the phase of reward anticipation (i.e., when salience is being experienced) is reduced rather than showing an increase as the theory predicts. Nevertheless, ROI studies, as meta-analyzed by Radua and colleagues (2015), are not the whole story; it is also possible, and in many ways methodologically preferable, to map task-related activations across the entire brain, an approach that generates clusters of activation which exceed

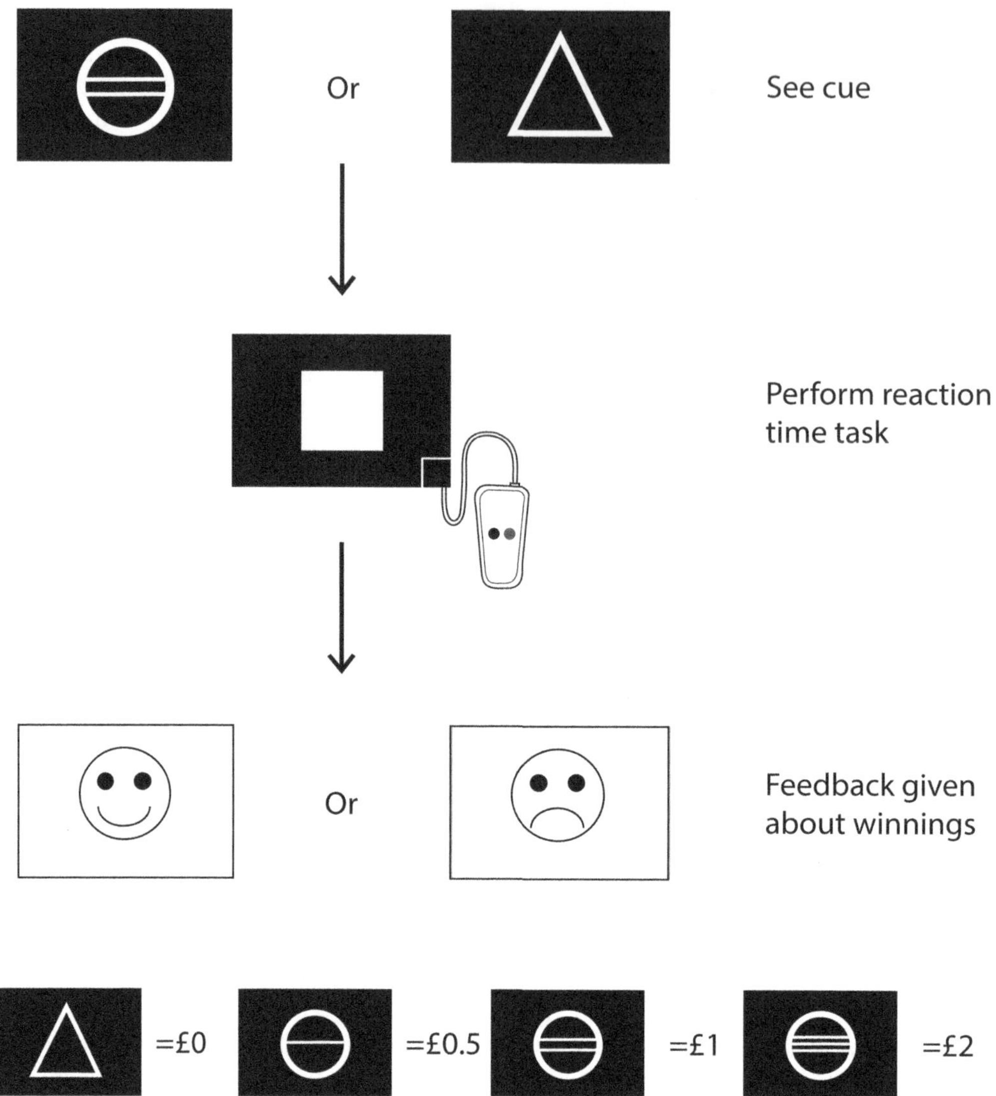



*Figure 31.1*   The monetary incentive delay task.

*Source*: Reprinted from (McKenna 2017: 130), by permission of the publisher.

a predefined (usually conservative) statistical threshold. Jianguang Zeng and colleagues (2022) meta-analysed 17 studies of this latter type using the monetary incentive delay task in patients with schizophrenia. Like Radua and colleagues (2015), they found reduced activation during reward anticipation, this time in a cluster involving a large portion of the basal ganglia, not just its ventral striatal sector, with reduced activation also being seen in the amygdala and a range of cortical regions. During reward feedback/delivery, in contrast, there was a pattern of increased activation in the patients, affecting the striatum, the amygdala, and the hippocampus, plus various cortical regions. This finding is of some interest because the reward prediction error signal is generated at the moment feedback about reward is received. However, areas of reduced activation were also seen in the ventromedial frontal cortex and the dorsolateral frontal cortex.

What about reward prediction error itself? Here the results have been less than encouraging. In a meta-analysis of 10 studies of schizophrenia patients and 15 studies of healthy controls (the greater number of studies in controls reflected that fact that the authors also investigated studies of depression and employed the healthy control groups from these in the comparison with schizophrenia), Zachary Yaple and colleagues (2021) failed to find any clear evidence of differences between the two groups.

## 7.   Concluding remarks

There can be no doubt that aberrant salience is an attractive and even powerful theory of delusions. It can account for the phenomenon of referential delusions, where significance is attached to neutral events, for which it provides a highly intuitive account. As modified by Fletcher, Frith, Corlett, and their co-workers, the theory is also able to handle delusions where there is no discernible component of abnormal significance. Fletcher and Frith's (2009) point that predictive models generated by aberrant reward prediction error will be inherently unstable because the rogue signal can never be eliminated adds further value here, as it provides a mechanism whereby abnormal beliefs can depart further and further from reality, forming a not-implausible basis for the bizarre or even fantastic qualities that delusions can sometimes have, something no other theory can account for.

Despite this, the aberrant salience theory cannot as yet be considered completely successful at the conceptual level. This is because, even as modified by Fletcher, Frith and Corlett, it makes the clear prediction that propositional delusions will always be preceded by delusional mood and/or delusions of reference and misinterpretation. This goes against the clinical reality that, although propositional delusions (especially when they are persecutory) may grow out of the experience of referentiality, sometimes they seem to develop in the absence of such antecedents, arising as it were out of the blue. Conceivably, the Fletcher/ Friston/Corlett modification could act to dilute this problem – for example, it is possible to envisage a circumstance where abnormal reward prediction error occurs so subtly and unobtrusively that it is not enough to provoke the clinical experience of referentiality but is still sufficient to progessively subvert predictive modelling; or conversely a situation where reward prediction error signalling becomes so rapidly and severely uncontrolled that its effect on predictive modelling swamps its more subtle salience-inducing manifestations which effectively have no time to develop. Neither of these possibilities, it has to be said, is wholly convincing.

Whatever its theoretical strengths, the harsh fact is that salience theory is not currently supported by experimental evidence. Functional imaging using the monetary incentive delay task has found decreased instead of increased activation in schizophrenia during reward anticipation, the period when aberrant salience attribution would be expected to be most on display. According to current meta-analytic evidence, activations to reward delivery are increased in schizophrenia – intriguingly, since this is the time when the reward prediction error signal is generated – but there is currently no convincing evidence for abnormal signalling of reward prediction error itself in the disorder. With only ten or so studies to date, it is entirely possible that the position with respect to reward prediction error will change as more studies are carried out. It can also be pointed out that mixed, contradictory and overall unclear findings are almost the rule in biological schizophrenia research: several findings that are now widely accepted had to be established painstakingly over the course of many years marked by both positive and negative findings, and in some cases only emerged with the assistance of meta-analysis.

If the salience theory of delusions does ultimately turn out to be correct, it will represent an important advance: arguably the first time that a schizophrenic symptom has been linked to an underlying brain dysfunction. It will also provide something of a vindication for the views on delusions of the 20th century psychiatrist and philosopher, Karl Jaspers (1959). Based on a careful consideration of patients' descriptions of their abnormal beliefs, a method he called 'phenomenology' (not to be confused with the sense of the term in existential philosophy), he concluded that delusions showed the characteristics of being immediate and unmediated, and were in some sense experiential (though not in the sense of perception, which remained normal); they represented something that 'comes before thought, although it becomes clear to itself only in thought' (for a succinct review of Jaspers's views on delusions see Walker 1991). Jaspers (1959) identified this process as involving a change the way that meaning was perceived, which was radically transformed so that it became immediate and intrusive. After making the obvious application of this analysis to delusional mood and delusions of reference and misinterpretation, however, Jaspers went further, arguing that all delusions – in other words propositional delusions as well – were characterized by the same changed awareness of meaning. His reasoning here may not have been entirely clear or convincing – Walker (1991), for example, was skeptical about it – but the parallels with salience theory are striking, to the point that Jaspers could almost be considered to have explicitly foreshadowed it.

# References


Adams, R. A., Stephan, K. E., Brown, H. R., Frith, C. D., & Friston, K. J. (2013). "The computational anatomy of psychosis," *Frontiers in Psychiatry, 4,* 47.

Arner, M. (2022). "The Quest for Reality," *Schizophrenia Bulletin,* sbac115, https://doi.org/10.1093/schbul/sbac115.

Beninger, R. J. (1983). "The role of dopamine in locomotor activity and learning," *Brain Research, 287,* 173–196.

Bleuler, E. (1911). *Dementia Praecox or the Group of Schizophrenias* (translated by J. Zinkin, 1950). New York: International Universities Press.

Bleuler, E. (1924). *Textbook of Psychiatry* (translated by A.A. Brill, 1951). London: George Allen and Unwin.

Bora, E., Yucel, M., & Pantelis, C. (2009). "Theory of mind impairment in schizophrenia: meta-analysis," *Schizophrenia Research, 109,* 1–9.

Bowers, M. B., Jr. (1968). "Pathogenesis of acute schizophrenic psychosis. An experimental approach," *Archives of General Psychiatry, 19,* 348–355.

Bowers, M. B., Jr., & Freedman, D. X. (1966). "'Psychedelic' experiences in acute psychoses," *Archives of General Psychiatry, 15,* 240–248.

Corlett, P. R., Frith, C. D., & Fletcher, P. C. (2009). "From drugs to deprivation: a Bayesian framework for understanding models of psychosis," *Psychopharmacology, 206,* 515–530.

Corlett, P. R., Taylor, J. R., Wang, X. J., Fletcher, P. C., & Krystal, J. H. (2010). "Toward a neurobiology of delusions," *Progress in Neurobiology, 92,* 345–369.

Creese, I., Burt, D. R., & Snyder, S. H. (1976). "Dopamine receptor binding predicts clinical and pharmacological potencies of antischizophrenic drugs," *Science, 192,* 481–483.

Dudley, R., Taylor, P., Wickham, S., & Hutton P. (2016). "Psychosis, delusions and the 'jumping to conclusions' reasoning bias: a systematic review and meta-analysis," *Schizophrenia Bulletin, 42,* 652–665.

Fletcher, P. C., & Frith, C. D. (2009). "Perceiving is believing: a Bayesian approach to explaining the positive symptoms of schizophrenia," *Nature Reviews Neuroscience, 10,* 48–58.

Friston, K. (2005). "A theory of cortical responses," *Philosophical Transactions of the Royal Society of London. Series B, Biological Sciences, 360,* 815–836.

Friston, K., Kilner, J., & Harrison, L. (2006). "A free energy principle for the brain," *Journal of Physiology, Paris, 100,* 70–87.

Frith, C. D. (1992). *The Cognitive Neuropsychology of Schizophrenia.* Hove: Erlbaum (UK) Taylor & Francis.

Garety, P. A., & Freeman, D. (1999). "Cognitive approaches to delusions: a critical review of theories and evidence," *British Journal of Clinical Psychology, 38 (Pt 2),* 113–154.

Garety, P. A., & Freeman, D. (2013). "The past and future of delusions research: from the inexplicable to the treatable," *British Journal of Psychiatry, 203,* 327–333.

Glimcher, P. W. (2011). "Understanding dopamine and reinforcement learning: the dopamine reward prediction error hypothesis," *Proceedings of the National Academy of Sciences U S A, 108*(Suppl 3), 15647–15654.

Heinz, A. (2002). "Dopaminergic dysfunction in alcoholism and schizophrenia--psychopathological and behavioral correlates," *European Psychiatry, 17,* 9–16.

Jaspers, K. (1959). *General Psychopathology* (transated by J. Hoenig and M.W. Hamilton, 1963). Manchester: Manchester University Press.

Jauhar, S., Johnstone, M., & McKenna, P. J. (2022). "Schizophrenia," *Lancet, 399,* 473–486.

Kapur, S. (2003). "Psychosis as a state of aberrant salience: a framework linking biology, phenomenology, and pharmacology in schizophrenia," *American Journal of Psychiatry, 160,* 13–23.

Knutson, B., Westdorp, A., Kaiser, E., & Hommer, D. (2000). "fMRI visualization of brain activity during a monetary incentive delay task," *NeuroImage, 12,* 20–27.

Kraepelin, E. (1913). *Dementia praecox and Paraphrenia* (translated by R.M. Barclay, 1919). Edinburgh: Livingstone.

Maher, B., & Ross, J. S. (1984). "Delusions". In H. E. Adams & P. B. Sutker (Eds.), *Comprehensive Handbook of Psychopathology* (pp. 383–410). New York: Plenum.

Maher, B. A. (1974). "Delusional thinking and perceptual disorder," *Journal of Individual Psychology, 30,* 98–113.

Mason, S. T. (1984). *Catecholamines and Behaviour.* Cambridge: Cambridge University Press.

McClure, S. M., York, M. K., & Montague, P. R. (2004). "The neural substrates of reward processing in humans: the modern role of fMRI," *Neuroscientist, 10,* 260–268.

McDonald, N. (1960). "Living with schizophrenia," *Canadian Medical Association Journal, 82,* 218–221.

McKenna, P. (2017). *Delusions: Understanding the Un-understandable.* Cambridge: Cambridge University Press.

McKenna, P. J. (1987). "Pathology, phenomenology and the dopamine hypothesis of schizophrenia," *The British Journal of Psychiatry, 151,* 288–301.

Nasar, S. (1998). *A Beautiful Mind: a Biography of John Forbes Nash, Jr., Winner of the Nobel Prize in Economics, 1994.* New York: Simon & Schuster.

Noordhof, P., & Sullivan-Bissett, E. (2021). "The clinical significance of anomalous experience in the explanation of monothematic delusions," *Synthese, 199,* 10277–10309.

Olds, J., & Milner, P. (1954). "Positive reinforcement produced by electrical stimulation of septal area and other regions of rat brain," *Journal of Comparative and Physiological Psychology, 47,* 419–427.

Peroutka, S. J., & Synder, S. H. (1980). "Relationship of neuroleptic drug effects at brain dopamine, serotonin, alpha-adrenergic, and histamine receptors to clinical potency," *American Journal of Psychiatry, 137,* 1518–1522.

Radua, J., Schmidt, A., Borgwardt, S., Heinz, A., Schlagenhauf, F., McGuire, P., & Fusar-Poli, P. (2015). "Ventral striatal activation during reward processing in psychosis: a neurofunctional meta-analysis," *JAMA Psychiatry, 72,* 1243–1251.

Rosen, C., Harrow, M., Humpston, C., Tong, L., Jobe, T. H., & Harrow, H. (2022). "'An experience of meaning': A 20-year prospective analysis of delusional realities in schizophrenia and affective psychoses," *Frontiers in Psychiatry, 13,* 940124.

Schneider, K. (1949/1974). "The concept of delusion". In S. R. Hirsch & M. Shepherd (Eds.), *Themes and Variations in European Psychiatry* (pp. 33–39). Bristol: Wright.

Schultz, W., Dayan, P., & Montague, P. R. (1997). "A neural substrate of prediction and reward," *Science, 275,* 1593–1599.

Seeman, P. (1987). "Dopamine receptors and the dopamine hypothesis of schizophrenia," *Synapse, 1,* 133–152.

Walker, C. (1991). "Delusion: what did Jaspers really say?," *British Journal of Psychiatry, 159, Supplement 14,* 94–103.

Weinberger, D. R., & Laruelle, M. (2001). "Neurochemical and neuropharmachological imaging in schizophrenia," In K. l. Davis, D. Charney, J. T. Coyle, & C. Nemeroff (Eds.), *Neuropsychopharmacology - The Fifth Generation of Progress,* pp. 833–855. Baltimore, MD: Lippincott Williams Wilkins.

Wise, R. A. (1978). "Catecholamine theories of reward: a critical review," *Brain Research, 152,* 215–247.

Yaple, Z. A., Tolomeo, S., & Yu, R. (2021). "Abnormal prediction error processing in schizophrenia and depression," *Human Brain Mapping, 42,* 3547–3560.

Zeng, J., Yan, J., Cao, H., Su, Y., Song, Y., Luo, Y., & Yang, X. (2022). "Neural substrates of reward anticipation and outcome in schizophrenia: a meta-analysis of fMRI findings in the monetary incentive delay task," *Translational Psychiatry, 12,* 448.

32

# DELUSION AND INFERENCE

*Urte Laukaityte and Matteo Colombo*

## 1.  Introduction

Delusions are commonly defined as beliefs 'based on incorrect inference about external reality' (APA 1994: 765; APA 2013: 819; Berrios 1991). Delusions can be based on *incorrect* inferences in virtue of a *jumping to conclusion* bias, where a conclusion is drawn hastily from insufficient evidence (Huq, Garety, & Hemsley 1988; Dudley et al. 2016; Tripoli et al. 2021), a bias *against disconfirming evidence*, where information inconsistent with one's beliefs is neglected, under-weighed or misinterpreted (Woodward et al. 2006), or *over-weighing of new sensory evidence*, which can lead one to over-interpret and give too much significance to meaningless events and coincidences, resulting in outlandish explanations (Maher 1974; Corlett, Frith, & Fletcher 2009; Jardri & Denève 2014).

If delusions are based on incorrect inferences, then they can redound badly on a subject's *rational* standing. In fact, both psychiatrists and philosophers often qualify delusions as odd, irrational beliefs that are incomprehensible to other members of one's community (Jaspers 1913/1963: 95–96; Foucault 1965: Ch. 4; Bermúdez 2001). Assuming that delusions are based on incorrect inferences about external reality also suggests that cognitive-behavioural therapies and reasoning training could prevent, or at least reduce delusions (Garety et al. 2011; 2015).

Although widespread, however, the assumption that delusions are nothing but beliefs is contentious (Gallagher 2009; Feyaerts et al. 2021). And similarly contentious is the assumption that delusions are 'incorrect', 'false', or 'irrational' inferences about external reality (Sanati & Kyratsous 2015; Bortolotti 2020; Garson 2022).

Drawing on phenomenological analyses and patients' reports about their overall sense of unreality, some psychiatrists and philosophers emphasise the experiential, perceptual, and affective dimensions of delusions rather than their cognitive aspects (Ratcliffe 2013; Sass et al. 2017). Some delusions seemingly arise spontaneously from anomalous experiences, involving pervasive shifts in mood, attention, and perception (Feyaerts et al. 2021). But if delusions cannot be understood as just odd beliefs, then it is not obvious they are based on inference either, since paradigms of inference ordinarily involve thoughts and beliefs rather than affectively valenced perceptual experiences. And if delusions were not based on

477      DOI: 10.4324/9781003296386-38

inference, then it would be unclear that they can redound badly on one's rational standing and that therapies aimed at weakening one's reasoning and learning biases would be effective treatment aids (Hayes & Hofmann 2017; Sass 2019).

In evaluating and trying to resolve this disagreement about the nature of delusion and its relationship with inference, one problem is that the term 'inference' is used in different fields with a lot of variation. Here, to address this problem, we put forward a minimalist definition of *inference*, which can productively be used to scout intriguing theoretical and empirical implications of thinking of delusion as inferentially based. Specifically, we begin by showing that our minimalist working definition of inference fits diverse examples of delusion without the additional requirements that such inference must involve propositional content, conscious deliberation or epistemic standards of appraisal (Section 2). Next, following our definition, we explore the possibility that not just humans, but many kinds of systems, from basal organisms to collective agents, can perform incorrect inferences issuing in delusions (Sections 3 and 4). There is a short conclusion (Section 5).

## 2.  Inferences: the (non)propositional, the (un)conscious, and the (non)epistemic

Inference is a rationally evaluable psychological transition between informational states, where some informational states functioning as premises in the inference provide reasons for drawing another informational state constituting the conclusion of the transition. This working definition, though minimalistic, can productively advance a cross-disciplinary understanding of delusion. It can help us distinguish delusions from other mental states, taxonomise different kinds of delusions based on the sorts of informational states, transitions, and standards of rational evaluation that they involve, and – as we'll see in the next sections – to explore the possibility that delusions can affect not only humans, but also more basic, non-human cognitive systems, as well as human group agents.

Let's start by considering these two examples of delusion:

A patient walking up the staircase to his psychiatrist's office, noticed through a window, a canvas with intense blue color, among some furniture stabled in the yard. Seeing the painting with its blue color, the patient became aware of being insane.
*(Blankenburg 1965: 289; also cited in Feyaerts et al. 2021: 239, Panel 2:*
*'Clinical illustrations of primary delusions')*

Ramona, the representative of Mars, was angry with me since I had conquered the devil. The devil was an energy supplier to Mars. So now I thought Ramona wanted to kill me. I thought she entered my body, and she was very strong.

*(Meijer 2017: 1147)*

The term 'delusion' can refer to a belief-like mental state that purports to present things as they are or could be. In the first example, the belief-like mental state 'I am now aware of being insane' would be an example of delusion in this sense; likewise, the belief-like mental state 'Ramona wanted to kill me' is another example. But 'delusion' can also be used more broadly to refer to a temporally extended mental process ushering in belief-like mental states, anomalous experiences, and attitudes, which constitute a 'delusional atmosphere' colouring one's engagement with the environment. In the first example, the process going from the patient's noticing the canvas through the window to the patient's becoming aware of being insane would be an example of a delusional process in this second sense. Likewise, the process described in the second example going from thoughts about Ramona's being angry to the thoughts about Ramona's entering the patient's body, along with their accompanying experiences and attitudes, would be another example of delusion in this broader sense.

If the delusions described in these two examples are based on inferences, then the first consists in a transition from an affectively valenced perceptual experience to a true belief; this transition does not comply with the schema of a formal rule such as a rule in deductive logic; and the standards for its appraisal refer not only to truth and error avoidance, but also to affectively-laden, practical needs that contribute to the thriving and functioning of the patient in his social environment. The second example consists in a transition from seemingly false beliefs to another seemingly false belief; this transition is logically structured and can fit the schema of a formal rule in deductive logic; and the standards for its appraisal are more naturally understood in purely epistemic terms, where the conclusion inherits the epistemic ill-foundedness of the premises in the inference.

Now suppose we strengthen our definition in three ways, by saying that, firstly, all informational states in inference must be propositions; secondly, every inference must involve conscious deliberation; and thirdly, the relevant standards for evaluating inferences can only be epistemic. One consequence is that the first example will not count as a delusion anymore, since the experiences ushering in the belief-like state that the patient is insane do not obviously have propositional contents, the informational transition involved is unconscious, and should be appraised with respect to not exclusively epistemic standards. While the second example might more clearly fit those three additional requirements, it would still remain opaque why it should count as an example of *incorrect* inference. A moment ago, we said that the epistemic standards for its appraisal refer to the ill-foundedness of the informational states that enter the inference. In a way, though, those informational states do support the conclusion that 'Ramona wanted to kill me', since the transition to this conclusion can be reconstructed as a monotonic deductively valid argument. To clarify what exactly might be 'incorrect' with this transition, it is plausible to refer to non-epistemic standards concerning the statistical *normality* and social *acceptability* of the patient's beliefs in her community.

These preliminary observations indicate that strengthening our minimalistic definition of inference will probably *not* help us make better sense of diverse examples of delusion. But one immediate worry is that our definition is too weak, as it might not allow us to distinguish delusions from other kinds of mental states or from non-mental processes. Let's then revisit the two examples with this worry in mind.

According to the first requirement, inference must be a transition between *propositional thoughts* (Currie 1987; Wright 2004). May-May Meijer's (2017) conclusion that Ramona wanted to kill her involves a thought with propositional content, and the premises supporting that conclusion also involve thoughts with propositional content. But the first example, where the patient concludes that he is ill from his perceptual experiences of a blue painting, is not well described as movement between thoughts with propositional content, since the inference here goes from perceptual experiences without propositional content to a thought. So, the requirement that inferences can only occur between propositional thoughts would rule out any case – like the one in our first example – where a delusion is inferred from perceptual experiences with non-propositional content.

Fortunately, there are good reasons to believe that inferences are transitions that can involve affectively laden perceptual experiences, and not only thoughts and beliefs with propositional content (Hatfield 2002; Siegel 2016). If perceptual experiences do not always have propositional content, then the inferential structure of at least some delusions should not be explicated in terms of semantic or logical relationships between propositions. And if we drop the requirement that inferences must always involve propositions, then human infants, organisms much simpler than humans, as well as certain artificial systems, might be capable of drawing inferences; and some of their inferences might produce delusions. In general, there is no compelling reason to assume that the informational states in an inference should always be isomorphic with words or propositions expressed in some natural language.

According to the second requirement, inferences must be *conscious*. Paul Boghossian (2014), for instance, suggests that inferring a conclusion from an informational state requires that the inferrer *takes* the informational state to support the conclusion. This requirement displays inference as a form of 'personal-level, conscious and voluntary' kind of reasoning (Boghossian 2014: 3). If the inferrer did *not* take the informational states functioning as premises in an inference to support the inferred conclusion, we could not explain in virtue of what rational considerations the inferrer draws that conclusion, and we would thereby lose the grounds for rationally appraising their inference as correct or incorrect.

This requirement plausibly fits the second example, where Meijer (2017) seems to consciously take the premises that Ramona is angry with her to support the conclusion that Ramona wants to kill her. Less clear is that the first case involves any conscious deliberation at all. Conscious deliberation, then, might not be an adequate requirement for describing all examples of delusion. Some inferences involve conscious deliberation. But most inferences are performed without taking, consciously, certain premises to support a conclusion; and if we drop this requirement, then non-human animals, artificial agents, and sub-personal systems might perform inferences (Buckner 2019; Colombo & Fabry 2021).

According to the third requirement, the standards of rationality for the appraisal of inferences should only be epistemic, where 'inferences are local and it is short-term transitions that determine epistemic status of the output – not the status of the cognitive engines overall' (Siegel 2018). That is, in inferring a conclusion, the sole basis for the rational appraisal of the inference would consist of the evidential support of the conclusion and the reliability or ill-foundedness of the processes and states from which the conclusion is inferred. So, if the informational states on which a subject relies to draw a conclusion are ill-founded, provide weak or irrelevant evidence for the conclusion, or, though relevant, are inaccessible from memory and thus bypassed, the subject should not believe the conclusion.

The inference in our first example of delusion might be aptly characterised as epistemically flawed, because it produces a belief unsupported by the subject's perceptual evidence. In the second example, the conclusion the subject draws might inherit the ill-foundedness of the premises, or bypass pertinent background information, which the subject possesses about the existence of demons and the inhabitants of Mars. This background information would remain insulated from the other bodies of information, which the subject uses in her inference; and so, she fails to respond to it.

However, for an adequate appraisal of the inferences in both examples, and in delusion more generally, we should also consider the role of inferences in supporting long-term, affectively-laden, and action-involving processes that manifest the extent to which the subject is sensitive to new information that could further, or rather thwart, their thriving and social functioning. We should also rely, that is, on *norms of agency*. After all, the examples of delusions above involve inferences leading the subject to lose touch with reality. This in turn involves a breakdown of the subject's action-involving, affectively laden grasp of the physical and social world they inhabit. What also matters for the appraisal of inferences issuing in delusion is 'their role in guiding temporally extended cycles of perception and action' that allow a subject to flexibly infer correct solutions to practical problems contributing to their thriving, which might require negotiation and interaction with other agents and the material environment (Clark 2018: 747).

Our definition is minimalistic, but it can nevertheless distinguish inferences from brute causal transitions and from other non-inferential mental processes. For example, suppose somebody taps the tendon in my knee with a hammer, which causes my leg to rise. This is a non-rational, inflexible, reflexive causal transition, which goes from a non-informational state to a bodily movement. Or, you tell me 'It ain't hard to see, my seeds need God-degree' and I reply 'I got mouths to feed, unnecessary beef is more cows to breed'. Here, I move from one informational state to another because the words used to express the former rhyme with the latter. It is not an inferential transition. Again, suppose that I observe that the faces of my audience are increasingly bored and I make the free association that I will go to a concert tonight. The association between my observation and my belief involves informational states, but their relationship is not inferential: it is associative.

Most interestingly, our working definition of inference allows us to explore questions about inference and delusion in very different kinds of systems from just individual humans. Both phenomena have traditionally been considered to characterise exclusively human mental processes; but if inferences can be performed without requiring conscious, propositional reasoning, then the bounds of delusion can be more malleable as well. We can ask empirically tractable questions about the nature, mechanisms, and impact of delusional processes in systems at multiple scales of complexity. Exploring these questions is independently warranted in light of research in *basal cognition*, which has stimulated gradualist (re)-conceptualisations when it comes to a whole range of phenomena that have previously been thought to uniquely define the domain of human psychology. It is basal cognition, and its potential bearing on delusion, to which we turn next.

## 3.   Deluded inferences in basal, artificial, and other non-human systems

The basal cognition framework has prompted a rethink of a whole range of assumptions that have underlied our conceptions of cognitive phenomena as well as the sorts of material systems that can manifest goal-directedness and intelligence, and that could hence also show systematic breakdowns of interest to psychiatry. We primarily focus on delusion here, but the implications are much broader and more wide-ranging than any single symptom or condition.[1]

Part of the impetus for expanding the use of psychiatric terms like delusion comes from taking the implications of evolutionary gradualism seriously, whereby 'large-scale changes that involve the origin of complex new traits occur gradually, in a broad sense of that term; they do not jump into existence as wholes' (Godfrey-Smith 2020: 201). Importantly, we maintain it is possible to acknowledge the relative novelty that emerges as a result of major transitions in evolution without losing sight of the extent to which such novel features or capacities are nonetheless expanding and building on what was already there.

As basal cognition research is increasingly demonstrating, it is not only more empirically fruitful but also more accurate to stress comparability across the multiple scales of biological organisation when it comes to instantiating such cognitive abilities as perception, learning, memory, communication, decision making, and so on (Levin 2019; 2021a; 2021b; Lyon et al. 2021; Shapiro 2021). In light of this, the basal cognition framework is often also referred to as 'cognition all the way down' or 'mind everywhere'. Crucially, this should not be read as an a priori pronouncement as to where cognition is found – rather, the relevant hypotheses are meant to be empirically testable, tested and retested.

The upshot of the research paradigm can be understood as the claim that all intelligences are collective intelligences. Namely, there is an important sense in which evolution, on its way to multicellularity, did not have unicellular organisms lose their agency and cognitive capacities – instead, they got scaled up to accommodate and pursue larger multicellular organism-level goals. Each cognitive system – as a collective intelligence – will ordinarily have multiple nested selves on different scales, defined by a computational boundary across which information can flow between (sub)units integrated by close (bioelectric) communication. In brief, 'each cell is integrated, via physiological signaling, into a coherent swarm intelligence with system-level (anatomical) goals' (Levin 2019: 6).

A helpful case to illustrate this point is the phenomenon of cancer, which is what happens when, due to a breakdown in integrative intercellular communication, a still independently capable cell scales back its goals from those of the larger system and starts reproducing independently, moving to areas with better nutrition resources and otherwise exploiting its environment. If the 'cognition all the way down' approach is on the right track, it would comprise a strong basis for widening the scope of the kinds of organisms or agentic systems in which the relevant capacities may also break down in systematic ways. Furthermore, at least prima facie, it seems plausible that certain types of disruption in function of this kind might be broadly in line with (human) organism-level breakdown, and hence relevant for psychiatric theorising and research.

To motivate this argumentative move further, we will briefly describe the potential relevance of single cell research for manic depression, since some of the underlying physiology is better understood in this instance as compared to delusion. In particular, disruptions in ion channel permeability (primarily calcium signalling) seem to be causally implicated in bipolar disorder. The result has been found ex vivo in a whole range of cell lines cultured from people with manic depression – some neuronal but also platelets, leukocytes, lymphoblasts, and so on (Warsh, Andreopoulos, & Li 2004). Moreover, cell culture hyperexcitability does not depend on the affective state of the source patient, but is strongly affected by whether they are taking lithium and their degree of responsiveness to it. Crucially, the claim is not that a bipolar person's blood cell should be thought of as manic depressive on the same level of complexity as that which emerges on the scale of the human organism. But if we accept the picture of 'cognition all the way down', then we may also have to seriously consider the possibility of 'bipolar all the way down', which could yield new pathways to generate hypotheses as well as develop and test various treatments.

In light of this suggestive example, we will put forward some preliminary avenues to at least start thinking about potential delusional phenomena in various basal systems, non-human organisms, and other entities.[2] In order to do so, it is first of all important to establish whether such systems may be able to infer. There is much work within, for instance, the active inference framework to suggest that even the simplest organisms need to rely on inference to resist thermodynamic dissolution and remain viable (Parr, Pezzulo, & Friston 2022). Levin (2019) thinks of cognitive selves as goal-directed computational agents with their particular spatiotemporal 'area of concern'. A unicellular organism can 'infer, store, and operate with respect to a small subset of the patterns existing in its environment'

(Levin 2019: 11) – a capacity that is extended in more complex metazoan creatures. Indeed, prediction error minimisation implemented by inferential processes has been put forward as the explanation for the emergence and function of somatic multicellularity in the first place (Fields & Levin 2019). The sort of inference this would involve is non-epistemic, operates on informational states with non-propositional content, and in most cases bypasses conscious deliberation.

A helpful example in this context is morphogenesis, which can be understood as an instance of collective basal intelligence, since the process reliably and flexibly yields complex target anatomical structures despite interference (Levin 2019). The features of tadpoles with scrambled 'Picasso' faces will end up moving to the right locations in completely novel paths, salamander tails attached to their flank will become limbs, and so on – in each case stopping as soon as target morphology is achieved (Levin 2021b). Léo Pio-Lopez and colleagues (2022) point out a way to analyse not only various psychiatric conditions, but also disorders of morphogenesis as 'disorders of inference' by employing the same set of active inference tools used in psychopathology research. The authors provide three simulations of aberrant morphogenesis, one of which corresponds to the so-called positive symptoms of schizophrenia, including delusions. In particular, Pio-Lopez and colleagues (2022: 3) note that in this condition, 'the cells have a strong (rigid) belief that they have to be this [intestinal] type of cell and therefore won't take into account contrary sensory evidence', leading to dysfunctional development in that the cells fail to effectively migrate to the target location and do not fully differentiate. Crucially, they also conducted a real-life proof of principle study, in which *Xenopus laevis* tadpoles showed developmental defects as a result of disrupted dopamine signalling, which is thought to be involved in belief formation and strength.

In light of evolutionary gradualism, the mechanisms of cellular communication in neural and non-neural structures do not seem to be merely functionally similar but are shared in a meaningful sense (Fields et al. 2020). Specifically, evolutionary homologues of ion channels, electrical synapses, and neurotransmitters predate neurons, are found in non-neural cells and unicellular organisms (Martinac, Saimi, & Kung 2008), and could thus show comparable breakdowns as well as potential treatment responsiveness we may want to investigate further.

The same principles that ground goal-directedness and cognitive capacities in the simplest living organisms allow for a range of other systems to be viewed as inherently cognitive too, including artificial systems. Indeed, there has been a recent explosion in work on soft robotics and bio-inspired artificial intelligence (AI) that is very much in line with the basal cognition research paradigm (Kaspar et al. 2021) and is calling into question a number of long-cherished distinctions such as those between the living and the non-living, the cognitive and the non-cognitive, and others.

Even in the context of deep reinforcement learning, some AI systems that attempt to acquire complex human-like capacities, such as playing intricate games, classifying pictures, and driving cars, have been described as delusional. For example, AlphaGo was the first AI system to defeat a professional human player at the game of Go (Silver et al. 2016). In learning how to play, AlphaGo performs inferences about the state in the game and the next moves to make. Some of its inferences could lead to it losing touch with its environment and goals. One of its creators called this loss of touch a *delusion*—that is, 'games in which AlphaGo would systematically misunderstand the board in a manner that could persist for many moves' despite the available evidence.[3] Its delusional cycles of perception and action sealed it off from reality-testing engagements, which could support successful interaction with the environment. AlphaGo's delusional atmosphere led it to persistent long-term *mis*valuations of board positions, thwarting its performance. Getting out of this required *not* more hard-wired knowledge of the game of Go, but a capacity for learning to learn, which could help AlphaGo bootstrap itself out of the delusional atmosphere hampering its play.

However, there have been proposals that, despite widespread excitement as well as alarm, such methods are unlikely to lead to artificial general intelligence (AGI) and the field should seriously consider a pivot to the more embodied bio-inspired AI systems developed within soft robotics and similar approaches (Harrison, Rorot, & Laukaityte 2022). It could hence be helpful to think through the relationship between such constructed agentic systems and delusional inference. The capacities of Xenobots might provide a useful example to consider here. Xenobots are formed by *Xenopus laevis* frog developing skin and muscle cells which end up comprising novel non-neural systems capable of rudimentary communication, coherent movement, action, and even self-replication (Kriegman et al. 2021). Such simple forms already rely on some of the same mechanisms (such as calcium signalling) seen in biotic organisms and advances in synthetic bioengineering are bound to result in the creation of biobots of increasing complexity, likely involving neural tissue as well (Levin 2021a). Again, we suggest there may plausibly be circumstances in which such biobots could be induced to manifest delusions in the minimalist sense we have outlined (e.g. by manipulating the chemical properties of the Petri dish substrate) for some of the same reasons that apply in the case of basal (micro)organisms. More generally, soft robots might yield 'intelligent matter' (Kaspar et al. 2021) with cognitive properties that could be liable to break down in systematic and informative ways.

Instances of psychopathology have been observed in a range of non-human animals (Braitman 2013) and, though still contested, the idea is increasingly making headway. An intriguing subset of animal cognition research in this context concerns collective agents such as eusocial insect colonies, which show enhanced cognitive capacities beyond those of the individuals that form the group. As a result of being so highly integrated and functioning as a single unit in many ways, they are often referred to as cohesive superorganisms (Sasaki & Pratt 2018). To the extent that their decision-making, learning, and other cognitive abilities rely on inference involving group-level informational states, insect colonies would be vulnerable to collective delusional inference as well.

There is already a research programme studying irrational decision-making in such superorganisms (ibid.); and, although not couched in terms of psychopathology, it could be built upon to study persistent colony-level inferential beliefs resistant to contrary evidence – delusions. Of special relevance here could be their reliance on positive feedback, which helps the colony communicate efficiently and strengthen weak signals, but can also end up amplifying noise, leading to error. Hypothetically, provided a colony persistently failed to update its inferences, despite evidence to the contrary, it could yield an interesting case of collective delusion detrimental to the survival of the colony.

A further reason to consider psychiatric categories to be potentially applicable to collective agents of this kind is the fact that their functioning has increasingly been argued to be parallel with that of individual (human) brains, calling for the use of psychological science tools to analyse insect colony cognition (ibid.), and the insect colony findings, in turn, to be applied to brains (Navas-Zuloaga, Pavlic, & Smith 2022). Human brains are prime suspects in cases of psychopathology; and so, if the parallel holds, such collective agents may well exhibit comparable breakdowns in cognitive functioning. Furthermore, parallels have also been drawn between invertebrate collective intelligence and human collective intelligence (Krause, Ruxton, & Krause 2010), which we hence turn to addressing in the next section.

## 4.  Deluded inferences in collective human agents

Social processes are relevant to inference and delusion in at least three ways. First, social processes can partly determine when a mental state based on inference counts as 'irrational' or when an inference counts as 'incorrect'. Second, social processes such as aberrant testimonies can partly explain the formation of some delusions. Third, social processes can ground the possibility of delusional collective agents in institutions, other types of groups, or even societies (for more on delusion and the social turn in research on it, see Williams, Chapter 35).

First, social evidence from testimony often helps us learn the social norms governing interactions in a community. Social norms are bound up with rich interpretative practices for predicting others' behaviour, making sense of it, and holding them rationally accountable. Social norms are patterns of mutual (descriptive and normative) expectations about certain behaviours or mental states (in)appropriate in a given context (Colombo 2014), and so they might contribute to determining which candidate states of a subject should count as delusions (Wilkinson 2020).

Delusions are sometimes characterised as *bizarre* mental states incomprehensible to other community members (Jaspers 1913/1963), which suggests that delusions are *abnormal* partly because, regardless of their content, they are at variance from those of the rest of the community. Thus, an individual who holds that the devil entered her body might be considered delusional unless she is a member of a community who view this belief as acceptable and sufficiently widespread – say, as part of a religious or cultural system – independently of how bizarre it may appear to outsiders (for more on delusion and culture see Gold and Gold, Chapter 36, and for delusion and religion see Bentall, Chapter 38).

Second, at least some delusions are best explained in terms of inferences recruiting *social evidence*. Kengo Miyazono and Alessandro Salice (2021), for example, emphasise the distinctive roles that testimony can play in the formation of some delusions. Testimonial evidence produced by peers, experts, or individuals with higher status is routinely used by humans, as well as other animals and systems to form or change their mental states. According to Miyazono and Salice (2021), delusions should partially be explained by *testimonial abnormalities* consisting of a lack of communication with others – and so, a disregard or insensitivity to testimonial evidence, which is often due to social isolation – or an inappropriate weighing of, and response to, one's testimonial evidence, where somebody's word is given too much or too little weight.

Aberrant testimonies have also been found to amplify the *jumping to* conclusion *bias*. When a subject is in a social environment where others collect scant evidence before making judgements, the subject will also tend to collect insufficient evidence, and thus jump to conclusions (Sulik, Efferson, & McKay 2021). Aberrant testimonial processes underlying this sort of contagion might explain 'shared psychotic disorders' like *folie à deux*, where a delusion – that, say, one is about to be harmed by a persecutor – gets transmitted and increasingly amplified between two individuals (Lasègue & Falret 1877; Shimizu et al. 2007).

The amplification and transmission of delusions, and of ill-founded mental states more generally, can be boosted by inferences occurring in communication networks in a community, from which relevant bodies of information are filtered out or certain sources systematically discredited. Such situations may produce *epistemic bubbles*, where one misses out on contrary views, wrongly estimates certain views to enjoy a high degree of agreement, and runs into excessive self-confidence. Or they may produce *echo chambers*, where one is systematically misled about whom to trust, suffers from emotional isolation, and tends to be devoted to select gurus (see Hendricks & Hansen 2016; Nguyen 2020). Delusions spreading via echo chambers and epistemic bubbles differ from religious creeds and popular folk beliefs partly because they are not sanctioned by social norms in the wider population.

In *Extraordinary popular delusions and the madness of crowds*, Charles Mackay (1852/1932) vividly describes several examples of how these kinds of social processes, jointly with exaggerated feelings of danger towards (often) imaginary threats, can produce sinister outcomes, such as economic crises, witch hunts, totalitarian, oppressive political regimes, and mass suicides. Mackay's examples of 'popular delusions' include economic bubbles like the South Sea Bubble of the early 18th century, beliefs in witchcraft in 16th- and 17th-century Western Europe, and histories of alchemy, mesmerism, and fortune-telling. But *folie à deux* and the sorts of delusions described by Mackay (1852/1932) concern individual humans' delusions, albeit spreading in collectives of people; they are not held by a group agent.

Some social processes can also play a third role in delusion – they can ground the possibility of collective agency, and particularly of deluded inferences in group agents. A group agent is an organised collectivity that is unified over time (despite possible changes in its members) and possesses informational states, which it can deploy to intervene suitably in the environment. Typical examples of such potential agents could include governments, juries, corporations, scientific communities, orchestras, football teams, as well as possibly cultures and nation states. Genuine collective agents have abilities and mental states irreducible to those of their members – even though the former still depend on the latter (List & Pettit 2011).

Human group agents have been argued to perform distributed computation (Chater 2022) and, in cases of aberrant inference, could thus potentially form 'collective delusions'. The notion of 'the collective brain' is increasingly employed in group contexts (Muthukrishna & Henrich 2016). When ascribing collective delusions to a group usefully and robustly enables us to predict, explain, and rationally appraise the behaviour of the group as a whole, we have good reason for deeming that group as a genuine subject of cognitive processes (Huebner 2014), not unlike the sorts of systems covered in the previous section. After all, basal cognition points to multicellular organisms themselves being collective intelligences. Several features in particular make it the case that cell cognition can be scaled up to self-organise into a more complex metazoan organism: there is (a) a high level of integration by means of tight (bioelectric) communication, which enables the system to track and process (b) non-local more spatiotemporally distant flows of information, leading to the pursuit of (c) larger organism-level goals beyond those of any individual (often specialised) member. There has been research to suggest that analogous conditions could be met by human collective agents, who may hence, we propose, be usefully studied within the context of psychopathology as well.

Philip Pettit's (2014) account of group agents requires that such agents have sufficiently reliable information states, reflecting the relevant features of the distal environment (see (b) in the previous paragraph), which they use to pursue a set of coherent system-level goals (i.e. (c) above). Moreover, in his view, group agents proper are conversable, i.e., they have spokespersons who reflect a robust pattern of goals and information states back to the collectivity, which is organised in such a way that it is bound ordinarily to keep faith with it, despite shifting membership. This seems to be one way to ensure close communication-based integration in collective human agents (analogous with (a) above). Pettit (2014) offers commercial companies, political parties, religious organisations, protest movements, and nation states as examples of true group agents, whereas, say, the bond market or generation X would not be. Although the stringent criterion of explicit conversability may not be the only way to establish a high degree of integration in a human group agent, there would need to be some unifying mechanism. There might also be various ways for such collective agents to manifest persistent delusional inferences, impervious to contrary evidence, as well as for them to be treated.

## 5.  Conclusion

In sum, to the extent that an agentic entity exhibits goal-directedness and cognition, it can also possibly exhibit systematic disruptions of those same capacities in ways that may be of relevance to psychiatry. In other words, provided one finds the empirical picture emerging from the 'cognition all the way down' approach credible, we submit that one might be compelled to extend one's concepts of psychopathology as well – both all the way down to the simplest organisms and artificial systems, as well as potentially up to human group agents. As research within basal cognition increasingly demonstrates, moving away from exclusively neuro- and homo-centric conceptions of mental function as well as illness can yield fruitful empirical methods and theoretical insights across the board. Adopting a more minimalist reading of inference and delusion not only is more in line with evolutionary gradualism but can also open up newly productive pathways, generate testable theoretical hypotheses across multiple scales as well as novel ways to develop and test treatment options. After all, the current conception of delusion as circumscribed to contexts like schizophrenia or manic depression already misses a range of intriguing cases outside of those limited settings, such as lone delusional beliefs in otherwise fully functional people with no accompanying psychopathology, calling for at least some sort of extension either way. It is still too early to tell in which directions the field might develop exactly, following such a broadening of psychiatric notions driven by the exciting work undertaken within the life and mind sciences. As a result, with this chapter, we aim to start the conversation and encourage further basal cognition-informed investigation, especially in relation to psychopathology.

## Acknowledgements

We thank Ema Sullivan-Bissett, Matthew Sims, Wiktor Rorot, and Eamon Duede for their generous feedback on a previous version of this manuscript. We are also grateful to audiences at the University of Cincinnati, the University of Michigan, and members of the Levin Lab, Tufts University for their constructive criticisms and suggestions. Urte Laukaityte is thankful to David Harrison and Taylor Beck for helpful discussions.

## Notes

1 This is not to imply that all (currently individuated) psychiatric phenomena are liable to work in the same way – some may well emerge at higher levels of organisation. More generally, the classification in use will likely eventually require restructuring with some conditions merging, splitting, or even being removed altogether. However, we submit these are all empirical questions, which should be investigated without premature restrictions on their scope.
2 A potential objection may be that delusions are intentional states and thus could not be found in very simple or basal cognitive systems. We suggest there is a useful broader biogenic reading of intentionality, too (see Sims 2021 for an argument in support of a continuum of intentionality).
3 This example should not give readers the impression that the architecture and kinds of algorithms of systems like AlphaGo are generally sufficient to give rise to delusions. Whether ascriptions of delusion in such examples should be taken literally is obviously contentious. But, here, our purpose in highlighting this and other suggestive cases is to demonstrate that psychiatric predicates – and psychological predicates more generally – are actually used in an expansive way by ordinary people and scientists alike to motivate moving away from an unquestioningly anthropocentric view of delusion.

## References

American Psychiatric Association (1994). *Diagnostic and statistical manual of mental disorders* (4th Edition). Washington: American Psychiatric Association.

American Psychiatric Association (2013). *Diagnostic and statistical manual of mental disorders* (5th Edition). Washington: American Psychiatric Association.

Bermúdez, J. L. (2001). Normativity and rationality in delusional psychiatric disorders. *Mind & Language*, 16(5), 493–457.

Berrios, G. E. (1991). Delusions as "wrong beliefs": A conceptual history. *The British Journal of Psychiatry*, 159(S14), 6–13.

Blankenburg, W. (1965). Zur Differentialphänomenologie der Wahrnehmung. Eine Studie über abnormes Bedeutungserleben. *Nervenarzt*, 36, 285–298.

Boghossian, P. (2014). What is inference? *Philosophical Studies*, 169(1), 1–18.

Bortolotti, L. (2020). *The epistemic innocence of irrational beliefs*. Oxford: Oxford University Press.

Braitman, L. (2013). *Animal madness: A natural history of disorder*. PhD Thesis, Massachusetts Institute of Technology.

Buckner, C. (2019). Rational inference: The lowest bounds. *Philosophy and Phenomenological Research*, 98, 1–28.

Chater, N. (2022). The computational society. *Trends in Cognitive Sciences*, 26(12), 1015–1017.

Clark, A. (2018). Priors and prejudices: Comments on Susanna Siegel's *The Rationality of Perception*. *Res Philosophica*, 95(4), 741–750.

Colombo, M. (2014). Two neurocomputational building blocks of social norm compliance. *Biology & Philosophy*, 29, 71–88.

Colombo, M., Fabry, R. E. (2021). Underlying delusion: Predictive processing, looping effects, and the personal/sub-personal distinction. *Philosophical Psychology*, 34(6), 829–855.

Corlett, P. R., Frith, C. D., Fletcher, P. C. (2009). From drugs to deprivation: A Bayesian framework for understanding models of psychosis. *Psychopharmacology*, 206(4), 515–530.

Currie, G. (1987). Remarks on Frege's conception of inference. *Notre Dame Journal of Formal Logic*, 28(1), 55–68.

Dudley, R., Taylor, P., Wickham, S., Hutton, P. (2016). Psychosis, delusions and the "jumping to conclusions" reasoning bias: A systematic review and meta-analysis. *Schizophrenia bulletin*, 42(3), 652–665.

Feyaerts, J., Henriksen, M. G., Vanheule, S., Myin-Germeys, I., Sass, L. A. (2021). Delusions beyond beliefs: A critical overview of diagnostic, aetiological, and therapeutic schizophrenia research from a clinical-phenomenological perspective. *The Lancet Psychiatry*, 8(3), 237–249.

Fields, C., Bischof, J., Levin, M. (2020). Morphological coordination: A common ancestral function unifying neural and non-neural signaling. *Physiology*, 35, 16–30.

Fields, C., Levin, M. (2019). Somatic multicellularity as a satisficing solution to the prediction-error minimization problem. *Communicative & Integrative Biology*, 12(1), 119–132.

Foucault, M. (1965). *Madness and civilization. A history of insanity in the age of reason*. New York: Random House.

Gallagher, S. (2009). Delusional realities. In Bortolotti, L., Broome, M. (eds.). *Psychiatry as cognitive neuroscience: Philosophical perspectives*, 245–268. Oxford: Oxford University Press.

Garety, P., Freeman, D., Jolley, S., Ross, K., Waller, H., Dunn, G. (2011). Jumping to conclusions: The psychology of delusional reasoning. *Advances in Psychiatric Treatment*, 17(5), 332–339.

Garety, P., Waller, H., Emsley, R., Jolley, S., Kuipers, E., Bebbington, P., … Freeman, D. (2015). Cognitive mechanisms of change in delusions: An experimental investigation targeting reasoning to effect change in paranoia. *Schizophrenia Bulletin*, 41(2), 400–410.

Garson, J. (2022). *Madness: A philosophical exploration*. Oxford: Oxford University Press.

Godfrey-Smith, P. (2020). Gradualism and the evolution of experience. *Philosophical Topics* 48(1), 201–220.

Harrison, D., Rorot, W., Laukaityte, U. (2022). Mind the matter: Active matter, soft robotics, and the making of bio-inspired artificial intelligence. *Frontiers in Neurorobotics*, 16:880724, 1–19.

Hatfield, G. (2002). Perception as unconscious inference. In Heyer, D., Mausfeld, R. (eds.). *Perception and the physical world: Psychological and philosophical issues in perception*, 113–143. New York: Wiley.

Hayes, S. C., Hofmann, S. G. (2017). The third wave of cognitive behavioral therapy and the rise of process-based care. *World Psychiatry*, 16(3), 245–246.

Hendricks, V. F., Hansen, P. G. (2016). *Infostorms: Why do we 'like'? Explaining individual behavior on the social network*. Göttingen: Copernicus.

Huebner, B. (2014). *Macrocognition: A theory of distributed minds and collective intentionality*. Oxford: Oxford University Press.

Huq, S. F., Garety, P. A., Hemsley, D. R. (1988). Probabilistic judgements in deluded and non-deluded subjects. *The Quarterly Journal of Experimental Psychology Section A*, 40(4), 801–812.

Jardri, R., Denève, S. (2014). Circular inferences in Schizophrenia. *Brain*, 136(11), 3227–3241.

Jaspers, K. (1913/1963). *General psychopathology*. Manchester: Manchester University Press.

Kaspar, C., Ravoo, B. J., van der Wiel, W. G., Wegner, S. V., Pernice, W. H. P. (2021). The rise of intelligent matter. *Nature*, 594, 345–355.

Krause, J., Ruxton, G. D., Krause, S. (2010). Swarm intelligence in animals and humans. *Trends in Ecology & Evolution*, 25(1), 28–34.

Kriegman, S., Blackiston, D., Levin, L., Bongard, J. (2021). Kinematic self-replication in reconfigurable organisms. *PNAS USA*, 118, e2112672118.

Lasègue C., Falret, J. (1877). La folie à deux. *Annales Médico-psychologiques*, 18, 321–355.

Levin, M. (2019). The computational boundary of a "self": Developmental bioelectricity drives multicellularity and scale-free cognition. *Frontiers in Psychology*, 10, 2688.

Levin, M. (2021a). Life, death, and self: Fundamental questions of primitive cognition viewed through the lens of body plasticity and synthetic organisms. *Biochemical and Biophysical Research Communications*, 564, 114–133.

Levin, M. (2021b). Bioelectric signaling: Reprogrammable circuits underlying embryogenesis, regeneration, and cancer. *Cell*, 184(8), 1971–1989.

List, C., Pettit, P. (2011). *Group agency*. Oxford: Oxford University Press.

Lyon, P., Keijzer, F., Arendt, D., Levin, M. (2021). Reframing cognition: Getting down to biological basics. *Philosophical Transactions of the Royal Society B*, 376, 20190750.

Mackay, C. (1852/1932). *Extraordinary popular delusions and the madness of crowds*. Boston: Page.

Maher, B. A. (1974). Delusional thinking and perceptual disorder. *Journal of individual psychology*, 30(1), 98–113.

Martinac, B., Saimi, Y., Kung, Ch. (2008). Ion channels in microbes. *Physiological Reviews*, 88(4), 1449–1490.

Meijer, M.-M. (2017). #PeaceAndLove: The second phase of my psychoses. *Schizophrenia Bulletin*, 43(6), 1145–1147.

Miyazono, K., Salice, A. (2021). Social epistemological conception of delusion. *Synthese*, 199(1), 1831–1851.

Muthukrishna, M., Henrich, J. (2016). Innovation in the collective brain. *Philosophical Transactions of the Royal Society B*, 317, 20150192.

Navas-Zuloaga, M. G., Pavlic, T. P., Smith, B. H. (2022). Alternative model systems for cognitive variation: Eusocial-insect colonies. *Trends in Cognitive Sciences*, 26(10), 836–848.

Nguyen, C. T. (2020). Echo chambers and epistemic bubbles. *Episteme*, 17(2), 141–161.

Parr, T., Pezzulo, G., Friston, K. J. (2022). *Active inference: The free energy principle in mind, brain, and behavior*. Cambridge, MA: MIT Press.

Pettit, P. (2014). How to tell if a group is an agent. In Lackey, J. (ed.). *Essays in collective epistemology*, 97–121. Oxford: Oxford University Press.

Pio-Lopez, L., Kuchling, F., Tung, A., Pezzulo, G., Levin, M. (2022). Active inference, morphogenesis, and computational psychiatry. *Frontiers in Computational Neuroscience*, 16, 988977.

Ratcliffe, M. (2013). Delusional atmosphere and the sense of unreality. In Stanghellini, G., Fuchs, T. (eds.) *One century of Karl Jaspers' general psychopathology*, 229–244. Oxford: Oxford University Press.

Sanati, A., Kyratsous, M. (2015). Epistemic injustice in assessment of delusions. *Journal of Evaluation in Clinical Practice*, 21(3), 479–485.

Sasaki, T., Pratt, S. C. (2018) The psychology of superorganisms: Collective decision making by insect societies. *Annual Review of Entomology*, 63, 259–275.

Sass, L. (2019). Three dangers: Phenomenological reflections on the psychotherapy of psychosis. *Psychopathology*, 52(2), 126–134.

Sass, L., Pienkos, E., Skodlar, B., Stanghellini, G., Fuchs, T., Parnas, J., Jones, N. (2017). EAWE: Examination of anomalous world experience. *Psychopathology*, 50(1), 10–54.

Shapiro, J. A. (2021). All living cells are cognitive. *Biochemical and Biophysical Research Communications*, 564, 134–149.

Shimizu, M., Kubota, Y., Toichi, M., Baba, H. (2007). Folie à deux and shared psychotic disorder. *Current Psychiatry Reports*, 9(3), 200–205.

Siegel, S. (2016). *The rationality of perception*. Oxford: Oxford University Press.

Siegel, S. (2018). Perception as guessing vs. perception as knowing: Replies to Clark and Peacocke. *Res Philosophica*, 95, 761–784.

Silver, D., Huang, A., Maddison, C. J., Guez, A., Sifre, L., Van Den Driessche, G., ... & Hassabis, D. (2016). Mastering the game of Go with deep neural networks and tree search. *Nature*, 529(7587), 484–489.

Sims, M. (2021). A continuum of intentionality: Linking the biogenic and anthropogenic approaches to cognition. *Biology & Philosophy*, 36, 51.

Sulik, J., Efferson, C., McKay, R. (2021). Collectively jumping to conclusions: Social information amplifies the tendency to gather insufficient data. *Journal of Experimental Psychology: General*, 150(11), 2309–2320.

Tripoli, G., Quattrone, D., Ferraro, L., Gayer-Anderson, C., Rodriguez, V., La Cascia, C., ..., Di Forti, M. (2021). Jumping to conclusions, general intelligence, and psychosis liability: Findings from the multi-centre EU-GEI case-control study. *Psychological Medicine*, 51(4), 623–633.

Warsh, J. J., Andreopoulos, S., Li, P. P. (2004). Role of intracellular calcium signaling in the pathophysiology and pharmacotherapy of bipolar disorder: Current status. *Clinical Neuroscience Research*, 4(3–4), 201–213.

Wilkinson, S. (2020). Expressivism about delusion attribution. *European Journal of Analytic Philosophy*, 16(2), 59–77.

Woodward, T. S., Moritz, S., Cuttler, C., Whitman, J. C. (2006). The contribution of a cognitive bias against disconfirmatory evidence (BADE) to delusions in schizophrenia. *Journal of Clinical and Experimental Neuropsychology*, 28(4), 605–617.

Wright, C. (2004). Intuition, entitlement, and the epistemology of logical laws. *Dialectica*, 58(1), 155–175.

# 33

# DELUSION AND HYPNOSIS

*Michael H. Connors*

## 1.  Introduction

Hypnosis can produce compelling alterations in subjective experience (Kihlstrom 1985; 2008). Specific suggestions can cause participants to perceive sensations in the absence of any sensory input; recall memories that are not based on actual events; and act in ways that seem compulsive and involuntary (Kihlstrom 1985; 2008). Importantly, suggestions can also cause participants to believe temporarily in the external and physical reality of these experiences (Bryant & Mallard 2003; Woody & Szechtman 2011). This subjective conviction in the reality of what is suggested distinguishes hypnosis from mere compliance and role-playing (Orne 1959; Hilgard 1965; Kihlstrom 2007). As this subjective conviction conflicts with external reality, hypnotised participants have been described as temporarily deluded (Sutcliffe 1961; Kihlstrom & Hoyt 1988). This feature has been used by researchers to model clinical delusions (Connors 2015) and create 'virtual patients' (Oakley & Halligan 2009: 266), temporary analogues that can be studied for insights into the disorders themselves. This chapter examines the relevance of hypnosis to delusions and is organised in five sections. First, the chapter provides a brief overview of hypnosis for readers unfamiliar with the topic. Second, the chapter describes the range and features of hypnotic delusions. Third, the chapter reviews attempts to use hypnosis to model and study clinical delusions' underlying processes. Fourth, the chapter compares hypnotic and clinical delusions and discusses differences between them. Finally, the chapter evaluates the implications of this research for understanding delusions more broadly.

## 2.  Hypnosis

Hypnosis occurs in the context of a social interaction between a hypnotist and a participant or group of participants (Kihlstrom 1985; 2008). As such, hypnosis involves two aspects: 'hypnosis-as-procedure' – what the hypnotist does – and 'hypnosis-as-product' – what participants experience (Nash 2005). Hypnosis-as-procedure usually involves a standardised sequence of steps. First, the hypnotist establishes rapport with participants and briefly explains what the session will involve. Next, the hypnotist administers a hypnotic induction to participants. This induction usually guides participants to close their eyes, relax, and

    DOI: 10.4324/9781003296386-39

focus their attention. After the induction is completed, the hypnotist may offer specific suggestions for different imaginative experiences. These include suggestions for simple physical movements (ideomotor suggestions) or for more complex cognitive experiences such as hallucinations and delusions (cognitive-delusory suggestions). After this, the hypnotist cancels the suggestion, which signals to the participants that the particular hypnotic effect should cease. Sometimes, the hypnotist may give participants a posthypnotic suggestion, which is a suggestion to experience a hypnotic effect after the hypnosis session is terminated, when a particular cue is presented. Regardless of whether a posthypnotic suggestion is given or not, the hypnotist proceeds to administer a deinduction, which signals the end of the hypnosis session. If a posthypnotic suggestion was given, the hypnotist triggers the relevant cue, observes the participants' response, and cancels the posthypnotic suggestion.

These various steps can be performed by an individual on themselves (so-called 'self-hypnosis'). The steps can also be performed without a formal hypnotic induction. Some researchers refer to this latter scenario as 'direct verbal suggestion' and reserve the term 'hypnosis' more narrowly to the use of a formal hypnotic induction (Oakley & Halligan 2009; Oakley et al. 2021). Others, however, conceptualise hypnosis more broadly as suggestions within a social relationship that is understood by participants as being 'hypnotic' (Kihlstrom 1985; 2008). In any case, research has found that the presence of a hypnotic induction results in a relatively small increase in responsiveness to suggestion, though this appears to vary somewhat with the type of suggestion. For ideomotor suggestions, only small increases in responsiveness are apparent (Hull 1933; Hilgard 1965). For suggestions involving delusions, a hypnotic induction has been associated with a much larger increase in responsiveness (Connors et al. 2012a; Connors et al. 2013), faster onset (McConkey et al. 2001), and more vivid experience (Cox & Barnier 2009a) than the same suggestions given without a hypnotic induction.

Regardless of procedure, however, hypnosis-as-product depends mainly on individual participants (Hilgard 1965). The extent to which participants experience what is suggested to them reflects their hypnotisability, a stable trait of susceptibility to hypnotic suggestion. Hypnotisability is measured using standardised scales that assess the number of different hypnotic suggestions participants respond to (Hilgard 1965; Woody & Barnier 2008). Norms indicate that approximately 10–15 per cent of participants are 'high hypnotisable' (passing most or all items on standardised scales), approximately 70–80 per cent are 'medium hypnotisable' (passing some items but not others), and approximately 10–15 per cent are 'low hypnotisable' (passing only a few items or none at all; Hilgard 1965). Hypnotic suggestions also vary in their difficulty: Cognitive-delusory suggestions are typically more difficult than ideomotor ones. Only high hypnotisable participants experience the most difficult suggestions, which include the majority of delusion items.

Research has found that hypnotisability is remarkably stable over time (Piccione et al. 1989) and is distributed fairly similarly across different cultures, locations, and languages (Laurence et al. 2008). Research has also found that hypnotisability is unrelated to broad individual differences in intelligence or personality (Laurence et al. 2008). In fact, the most reliable correlate of hypnotisability is absorption, a tendency to allow one's attention to be fully engaged in experience, and even this correlation is only moderate (Roche & McConkey 1990). For the purposes of experimental research, therefore, it is necessary to screen participants' hypnotisability using standardised measures beforehand. This screening usually involves two separate measures of hypnotisability (Kihlstrom 2008; Woody & Barnier 2008). As a result, hypnosis research can be both resource and time intensive.

## 3.  Hypnotic delusions

The capacity for hypnosis to produce alterations in belief is evident in many suggestions that do not explicitly involve belief. This can be illustrated with examples involving perception, memory, and action respectively. For perception, suggestions for hallucinations can result in compelling experiences that participants attribute to external reality. In one experiment, high hypnotisable participants given suggestions for visual hallucinations rated their experiences as being as real and vivid as real stimuli (Bryant & Mallard 2003). For memory, suggestions for age regression – to return to a younger age and vividly recall memories from that period – can similarly produce highly convincing experiences. Many participants accept the reality of these memories despite clear evidence of their falsity (Nash 1987). For action, suggestions for involuntary movements can likewise lead participants to misattribute their experiences to an external source. In one experiment, participants were attached to a pulley system and given a suggestion that the pulley would move their arms, although, in reality, the pulley was not used (Blakemore et al. 2003). Participants moved their arm themselves but misattributed the action to the experimenter. Across these different suggestions, the alterations in belief evident reflect the vividness and subjective reality of the hypnotic experiences for responsive participants.

Hypnotic suggestion can also be explicitly used to produce delusional beliefs (Connors 2015). Hypnotic suggestions have been used, for example, to create the belief that one has changed sex. Across several seminal studies, high hypnotisable participants given such suggestions endorsed the suggested sex; offered a different first name to fit their suggested sex; and maintained their conviction in their sex change despite being challenged by the experimenter (e.g. being shown a video of themselves; Sutcliffe 1961; Noble & McConkey 1995; Burn et al. 2001; McConkey et al. 2001). Afterwards, participants described vivid experiences; in one experiment, participants commented, 'it was so real it was disgusting' and 'I could actually feel myself changing' (Noble & McConkey 1995: 72). Importantly, very high hypnotisable participants showed different responses to simulators, low hypnotisable participants instructed to fake hypnosis, with the hypnotist being blinded to participants' hypnotisability and condition. This indicates that these hypnotic delusions cannot be accounted for solely in terms of compliance or demand characteristics (aspects of the experimental procedure that invite certain responses from participants; Orne 1979; Kihlstrom 2002).

Given this ability to alter belief, researchers have used hypnotic suggestion to model many different clinical delusions (Connors 2015). Using this approach, researchers have recreated features of mirrored-self misidentification (the belief that one's reflection in the mirror is not oneself; Barnier et al. 2008; Barnier et al. 2011; Connors et al. 2015); reverse intermetamorphosis (the belief that one has changed identity; Cox & Barnier 2009a); Fregoli delusion (the belief that strangers are known people in disguise; Elliott et al. 2016); somatoparaphrenia (the belief that one's limb is not one's own; Rahmanovic et al. 2012); alien control delusion (the belief that one's limb is being controlled by an external agent; Cox et al. 2014); erotomania (the belief that one is loved from afar by another person; Attewell et al. 2012); and folie à deux (delusions that are shared between two or more people; Freeman et al. 2013). In each of these cases, researchers gave participants an explicit suggestion for the respective delusional belief. Across suggestions, a large proportion of high hypnotisable participants adopted the hypnotic delusions, maintained the delusions despite challenges, and showed striking similarities to the clinical condition in terms of both subjective reports and outward behaviour (for a more detailed review, see Connors 2015).

## 4.  Modelling underlying processes

A key advantage of using hypnosis to model delusions in this way is the ability to isolate and manipulate hypothesised contributory factors within the hypnotic model (Kihlstrom 1979; Woody & Szechtman 2011). This permits researchers to study psychological dysfunction with a degree of experimental control that is not possible with actual clinical patients (Oakley & Halligan 2009). Such an approach has been used to examine cognitive and neural underpinnings of delusion. With respect to cognition, current theories suggest that delusional ideas can arise from attempts to explain anomalous sensory data. According to some theories, a second factor – a deficit in belief evaluation – is necessary to explain why certain patients come to accept the delusional idea and maintain it as belief while others who encounter the same anomalous sensory data do not (Coltheart et al. 2011; see also Connors & Halligan 2020; Connors et al. 2024; Davies & Coltheart, Chapter 29; cf. Sullivan-Bissett, Chapter 28). Hypnosis and suggestion have been used to produce anomalous experiences and manipulate belief evaluation to recreate delusions from their hypothesised component factors.

In an early experiment, researchers used hypnotic suggestion to produce paranoia (Zimbardo et al. 1981). According to one theory of paranoia, deafness without insight can lead people to think that those around them are whispering to conceal information and conspire against them. To test this, the researchers gave high hypnotisable participants a posthypnotic suggestion for partial deafness with amnesia for the cause of their deafness. They gave other participants either the same suggestion without amnesia or an unrelated suggestion to scratch their ear. All participants completed a task while two confederates talked between themselves and the cue for the posthypnotic suggestion was triggered. As expected, participants given the suggestion for deafness with amnesia reported more hostility, agitation, and paranoia than participants in the control groups. Although not strictly examining delusional belief, the experiment demonstrated how hypnotic suggestion could be used to generate anomalous experiences that, in turn, lead to delusional ideation.

Other research has focused on mirrored-self misidentification delusion. According to an influential theory, either impaired face processing (and hence a difficulty recognising oneself in the mirror) or mirror agnosia (an inability to use mirror knowledge when interacting with mirrors) can lead to the idea that there is a stranger in the mirror (Factor 1; Connors & Coltheart 2011). A second factor – a deficit in belief evaluation – explains why some patients with Factor 1 accept this delusional hypothesis and others do not (Factor 2; Coltheart et al. 2011). Adopting this perspective, a series of experiments used hypnotic suggestion to recreate the delusion from these component factors. Specific suggestions were used to recreate either impaired face processing or mirror agnosia (Factor 1). A hypnotic induction – which itself has been shown to alter reality testing – and/or an additional suggestion were used to disrupt belief evaluation (Factor 2).

Using this approach, researchers were able to recreate many features of the mirrored-self misidentification delusion (Connors et al. 2015). High hypnotisable participants reported seeing a stranger in the mirror and maintained this belief when challenged. Participants, for example, were asked to compare the appearance of the person they saw in the mirror to themselves; touch their nose while looking in the mirror; and, when the hypnotist shifted position to stand next to them, explain how they could see the hypnotist in the mirror but not themselves. In interviews afterwards with independent experimenters, participants confirmed the vividness of their experience (e.g., reporting that they thought it was 'obvious' that their reflection was someone else and not understanding why the hypnotist was asking questions about this; Connors et al. 2012b).

A series of experiments found that a hypnotic induction was necessary for the analogue; the hypnotic induction itself could act as Factor 2 without the need for a further suggestion; and that suggestions for Factor 1 (impaired face processing or mirror agnosia) were similarly effective at producing the delusion as suggestions that directly specified seeing a stranger (Connors et al. 2012a; 2012b; 2013; 2014a; 2014b). Another experiment found differences between the responses of high hypnotisable participants and low hypnotisable simulators, which suggested that the responses of hypnotised participants could not be explained in terms of compliance or demand characteristics alone (Connors et al. 2013). Altogether, the findings indicate that it is possible to use hypnotic suggestion to model a clinical delusion from its putative underlying cognitive factors.

Other research attempted to recreate somatoparaphrenia (the belief that one's limb is owned by someone else) and alien control delusion (the belief that one's limb is being controlled by someone else) from their hypothesised components in a similar way. Researchers used a suggestion for limb paralysis and amnesia to model Factor 1 in somatoparaphrenia (Rahmanovic et al. 2012) and a suggestion for loss of control over one's limb to model Factor 1 in alien control delusion (Cox et al. 2014). In both cases, however, researchers were unsuccessful and unable to recreate the delusional belief. This could be because the suggestions offered did not sufficiently approximate Factor 1 of the clinical condition. Somatoparaphrenia, for example, is often accompanied by anosognosia (denial of impairment) and it is possible that this may play an important role in generating delusional content (Rahmanovic et al. 2012). It is also possible, though, that aspects of the experimental procedure influenced the results. The paralysis or loss of control after these suggestions, for example, was relatively brief, limited to the hypnotic context, and much less emotional significant than what clinical patients encounter. Such differences could have affected how participants interpreted their experience and encouraged alternative non-delusional explanations (Connors 2015). Further work is needed to clarify this.

With respect to neural underpinnings, an independent program of research used hypnotic suggestion to model delusions involving altered self-agency whilst participants underwent neuroimaging. In one experiment, researchers used hypnotic suggestions to independently induce a loss of control over movements (reflecting alien control delusion) and a loss of awareness over movements (reflecting beliefs about being 'possessed'; Deeley et al. 2013). The researchers found these disruptions were associated with distinct neural areas, indicating the separability of seemingly related phenomena of altered self-agency. A subsequent experiment used hypnotic suggestions to examine different attributions for altered agency (Deeley et al. 2014). The researchers compared suggestions for external personal control (alien control delusion), external impersonal control (control by a machine), and internal personal control (possession). They found that suggestions for both external and internal personal alien control were associated with similar brain activity, indicating that similar neural systems could underpin these two delusions.

Further experiments on neural underpinnings used suggestions to model automatic writing. The researchers used separate suggestions to produce the motor experiences – related to alien control – and cognitive experiences – related to thought insertion – of the phenomena (Walsh et al. 2014; 2015). The researchers found that these two types of suggestion lead to distinct subjective experiences and brain activation despite similar changes in handwriting. This likewise implies the separability of these two phenomena that otherwise might appear outwardly very similar. Altogether, this set of studies highlight the versatility of hypnotic suggestion and its capacity to help identify experiential processes and cognitive and neural mechanisms that might underlie clinical delusions.

## 5. Evaluating hypnotic models

Hypnotic delusions show many similarities to clinical delusions. As already noted, hypnotised participants report strong subjective conviction in the reality of their beliefs despite counter-evidence and explicit challenging (Connors 2015). Hypnotised participants, like clinical patients, also tend to rationalise and confabulate to support their delusional belief. Participants with hypnotic mirrored-self misidentification, for example, identified facial features of their reflection that they claimed differed from their own and sometimes provided specific details about who the other person was. In their responses, hypnotised participants exhibited much of the heterogeneity evident in clinical patients. Participants with hypnotic mirrored-self misidentification, like clinical patients, varied in their emotional reaction to the stranger; who they identified the stranger to be; how closely they thought the stranger resembled themselves; whether they showed signs of covert self-recognition (e.g., reaching for a mark placed on their face without their knowledge when the mark became visible in the mirror); whether they recognised other people in the mirror; and whether they recognised themselves in other visual media, such as photographs (Connors et al. 2015).

In a similar way, hypnotised participants show alterations in their memory recall consistent with the suggested delusion. Participants with hypnotic sex change (Burn et al. 2001) and identity delusions (Cox & Barnier 2009b) selectively recalled information from pre-recorded stories that was relevant to their suggested belief, rather than their actual identity. Such changes are consistent with theories of memory and identity (Conway 2005), including the expected impact of delusion on recall (Connors & Halligan 2015). In addition, hypnotised participants often act on their delusions, albeit in benign ways within the confines of the experimental setting. Participants given suggestions for sex change and identity delusions, for example, offered names other than their own when asked and responded to questioning from the perspective of their suggested identity (Sutcliffe 1961; Noble & McConkey 1995; Cox & Barnier 2009a).

A further similarity between hypnotic and clinical delusions is the general proclivity of some participants and patients to hold unusual beliefs beyond that of their core delusion. One experiment measured participants' delusion proneness – the tendency to endorse sub-clinical delusional ideation within the ordinary population (Peters et al. 2004) – on a separate occasion prior to hypnosis (Connors et al. 2014c). The researchers found that higher levels of delusion proneness predicted which high hypnotisable participants experienced a hypnotic Fregoli delusion. This supports the notion that delusion proneness might reflect participants' general ability and willingness to entertain other unusual beliefs, which is also elevated in delusional patients (Peters et al. 2004). The findings likewise highlights possible commonality between hypnotic and clinical delusions in terms of underlying traits and vulnerabilities (Connors et al. 2014c).

Other aspects of clinical delusions not already discussed can be readily modelled with hypnosis. Some clinical patients, for example, show evidence of double-booking – simultaneously entertaining both delusional and non-delusional accounts of reality despite the apparent contradiction (Parnas et al. 2021; see Porcher, Chapter 13). Hypnosis has an analogous phenomena known as 'trance logic', whereby some hypnotised participants engage in both their suggested experiences and objective reality without attempting to resolve the incongruity (Orne 1959; Kihlstrom 2007). Some clinical patients also fluctuate in their delusional beliefs and level of insight (Connors & Coltheart 2011). This variation could be readily produced in hypnosis using specific suggestions, such as for a 'hidden observer', a suggestion for a part of the individual to be aware of physical reality while they are experiencing a hypnotic effect (Hilgard 1977; Kihlstrom 2007).

Despite such similarities, clinical and hypnotic delusions differ in several important ways (Oakley & Halligan 2009; Cox & Barnier 2010; Bortolotti et al. 2012; Connors 2015). First, clinical and hypnotic delusions have different aetiologies. Whereas some clinical delusions develop with neurological damage and specific neuropsychological deficits, hypnotic delusions originate from suggestion and require participants' active cooperation. Second, clinical and hypnotic delusions differ in their duration and environment. Whereas clinical delusions can endure across time and across different environmental contexts, hypnotic delusions are relatively short-lived and confined to the hypnosis laboratory. Third, clinical and hypnotic delusions differ in some aspects of their experience. In particular, clinical delusions may involve significant distress, preoccupation, functional impairment, and behavioural consequences that are not present in the hypnotic model. It might be possible to recreate some of these features to some degree: Other hypnosis experiments have been able to produce posthypnotic effects lasting several months (Barnier & McConkey 1998), induce distressing intrusive memories (Hill et al. 2010), and encourage antisocial and self-injurious behaviours (Orne & Evans 1965). Ethical concerns, however, limit further study of these features and attempts to produce a closer approximation of the clinical condition.

Furthermore, it remains to be seen whether hypnotic analogues can recreate the neural mechanisms involved in clinical delusion (Connors 2015). Research on the neural correlates of hypnotic agency delusions notwithstanding, there is currently insufficient data from both hypnotised participants and clinical patients to be able to reach a verdict. Such convergence, however, is not necessary for hypnotic models to be worthwhile. Hypnotic models are intended to capture only certain features of clinical disorders that are relevant for study. As such, the criterion for successful models are their ability to generate and test hypotheses, rather than produce exact replicas of clinical conditions (Woody & Szechtman 2011). In any case, delusions, like most psychiatric disorders, are defined by the subjective reports and outward behaviour of patients, rather than by neurobiological mechanisms or biomarkers. The ability of hypnotic suggestion to recreate the subjective experience and outward features means that it is able to generate an analogue with sufficient similarity to the clinical condition for it to be useful for a variety of research purposes (Oakley & Halligan 2009; 2013).

## 6.  Implications

As illustrated by these comparisons, hypnotic models raise more fundamental questions about the nature of delusions and belief (Bortolotti et al. 2012). With hypnotised participants reporting similar conviction and content as some clinical patients with delusions, albeit only temporarily, the level of this equivalence remains uncertain and open to debate. Hypnotic models also highlight the extent to which social influence and cognitive processes can distort experience and belief. The dramatic alterations evident occur after relatively simple verbal suggestions in susceptible, though otherwise ordinary, individuals. Such effects raise questions about whether similar processes could occur in other contexts. Shared delusions, for example, usually occur within close relationships and could potentially involve aspects of suggestion in addition to other social dynamics. The cognitive strategies employed by hypnotised participants – including selective attention, imagery, and dissociation – could likewise play a role in accepting and maintaining other forms of irrational belief.

More broadly, the potential for social influence and 'top-down' cognitive strategies in altering belief can inform cognitive theories. Theories of delusions have historically emphasised 'bottom-up' processes, whereby anomalous sensory data can generate delusional hypotheses and beliefs (James 1890; Maher 1974; Coltheart et al. 2011). Hypnotic suggestions can be used to generate anomalous experiences and lead participants to infer delusional ideas in this way (Zimbardo et al. 1981; Connors et al. 2015). Hypnotic suggestions, however, can also be given for specific delusional beliefs directly without requiring such inference. In both cases, though particularly in the latter, the active involvement of hypnotised participants suggests a role for social influence and cognitive processes in modulating and maintaining belief. This is reflected in recent theories that have attempted to relate delusions to their social context (Bell et al. 2021; Williams, Chapter 35) and a more general cognitive model of belief (Connors and Halligan 2015; 2017; 2020; 2022).

Regardless of such theoretical issues, hypnotic models of delusions have a number of practical advantages. The use of hypnotic models avoids many of the challenges involved in studying clinical patients, including the relative rarity of some presentations; variable willingness to engage with research; ethical concerns about capacity to consent and challenging strongly-held beliefs; and frequent comorbidity that can confound findings. The analogue has the further key advantage of allowing researchers to experimentally manipulate variables of interest to determine their effect (Kihlstrom 1979; Oakley & Halligan 2009; Woody & Szechtman 2011; Connors 2012). While obviously not a substitute for studying clinical patients directly, such techniques could be used in future to test and refine theories for many different delusional beliefs. In addition, hypnotic models could be used for training purposes to recreate disorders with greater subjective verisimilitude than simulating actors (Oakley & Halligan 2009). In such various ways, hypnosis is likely to remain relevant to studying and understanding delusion.


## References


Attewell, J., Cox, R. E., Barnier, A. J. & Langdon, R. (2012). "A hypnotic analogue of erotomania". *International Journal of Clinical and Experimental Hypnosis, 60,* 1–31.

Barnier, A. J., Cox, R. E., Connors, M., Langdon, R. & Coltheart, M. (2011). "A stranger in the looking glass: Developing and challenging a hypnotic mirrored-self misidentification delusion". *International Journal of Clinical and Experimental Hypnosis, 59,* 1–26.

Barnier, A. J., Cox, R. E., O'Connor, A., Coltheart, M., Langdon, R., Breen, N. & Turner, M. (2008). "Developing hypnotic analogues of clinical delusions: Mirrored-self misidentification". *Cognitive Neuropsychiatry, 13,* 406–430.

Barnier, A. J. & McConkey, K. M. (1998). "Posthypnotic responding away from the hypnotic setting". *Psychological Science, 9,* 256–262.

Bell, V., Raihani, N. & Wilkinson, S. (2021). "Derationalizing delusions". *Clinical Psychological Science, 9,* 24–37.

Blakemore, S.-J., Oakley, D. A. & Frith, C. D. (2003). "Delusions of alien control in the normal brain". *Neuropsychologia, 41,* 1058–1067.

Bortolotti, L., Cox, R. & Barnier, A. (2012). "Can we recreate delusions in the laboratory?". *Philosophical Psychology, 25,* 109–131.

Bryant, R. A. & Mallard, D. (2003). "Seeing is believing: The reality of hypnotic hallucinations". *Consciousness and Cognition, 12,* 219–230.

Burn, C., Barnier, A. J. & McConkey, K. M. (2001). "Information processing during hypnotically suggested sex change". *International Journal of Clinical and Experimental Hypnosis*, 49, 231–242.

Coltheart, M., Langdon, R. & McKay, R. (2011). "Delusional belief". *Annual Review of Psychology*, 62, 271–298.

Connors, M. H. (2012). "Virtual patients in the hypnosis laboratory". *The Psychologist*, 25, 786–789.

Connors, M. H. (2015). "Hypnosis and belief: A review of hypnotic delusions". *Consciousness and Cognition*, 36, 27–43.

Connors, M. H., Barnier, A. J., Coltheart, M., Cox, R. E. & Langdon, R. (2012a). "Mirrored-self misidentification in the hypnosis laboratory: Recreating the delusion from its component factors". *Cognitive Neuropsychiatry*, 17, 151–176.

Connors, M. H., Barnier, A. J., Coltheart, M., Langdon, R., Cox, R. E., Rivolta, D. & Halligan, P. W. (2014a). "Using hypnosis to disrupt face processing: Mirrored-self misidentification delusion and different visual media". *Frontiers in Human Neuroscience*, 8, 361.

Connors, M. H., Barnier, A. J., Langdon, R. & Coltheart, M. (2015). "Hypnotic models of mirrored-self misidentification delusion: A review and an evaluation". *Psychology of Consciousness: Theory, Research, and Practice*, 2, 430–451.

Connors, M. H., Barnier, A. J., Langdon, R., Cox, R. E., Polito, V. & Coltheart, M. (2013). "A laboratory analogue of mirrored-self misidentification delusion: The role of hypnosis, suggestion, and demand characteristics". *Consciousness and Cognition*, 22, 1510–1522.

Connors, M. H., Barnier, A. J., Langdon, R., Cox, R. E., Polito, V. & Coltheart, M. (2014b). "Delusions in the hypnosis laboratory: Modeling different pathways to mirrored-self misidentification". *Psychology of Consciousness: Theory, Research, and Practice*, 1, 184–198.

Connors, M. H. & Coltheart, M. (2011). "On the behaviour of senile dementia patients vis-à-vis the mirror: Ajuriaguerra, Strejilevitch and Tissot (1963)". *Neuropsychologia*, 49, 1679–1692.

Connors, M. H., Cox, R. E., Barnier, A. J., Langdon, R. & Coltheart, M. (2012b). "Mirror agnosia and the mirrored-self misidentification delusion: A hypnotic analogue". *Cognitive Neuropsychiatry*, 17, 197–226.

Connors, M. H., Gibbs, J., Large, M. M., & Halligan, P. W. (2024). "Delusions in postpartum psychosis: Implications for cognitive theories". *Cortex*, 177, 194–208.

Connors, M. H. & Halligan, P. W. (2015). "A cognitive account of belief: A tentative roadmap". *Frontiers in Psychology*, 5, 1588.

Connors, M. H. & Halligan, P. W. (2017) "Belief and belief formation: Insights from delusions," in Angel, H.-F., Oviedo, L., Paloutzian, R. F., Runehov, A. L. C. & Seitz, R. J. (eds.), *Processes of Believing: The Acquisition, Maintenance, and Change in Creditions*, Cham: Springer International Publishing, pp. 153–165.

Connors, M. H. & Halligan, P. W. (2020). "Delusions and theories of belief". *Consciousness and Cognition*, 81, 102935.

Connors, M. H. & Halligan, P. W. (2022). "Revealing the cognitive neuroscience of belief". *Frontiers in Behavioral Neuroscience*, 16, 926742.

Connors, M. H., Halligan, P. W., Barnier, A. J., Langdon, R., Cox, R. E., Elliott, J., Polito, V. & Coltheart, M. (2014c). "Hypnotic analogues of delusions: The role of delusion proneness and schizotypy". *Personality and Individual Differences*, 57, 48–53.

Conway, M. A. (2005). "Memory and the self". *Journal of Memory and Language*, 53, 594–628.

Cox, R. E. & Barnier, A. J. (2009a). "Hypnotic illusions and clinical delusions: A hypnotic paradigm for investigating delusions of misidentification". *International Journal of Clinical and Experimental Hypnosis*, 57, 1–32.

Cox, R. E. & Barnier, A. J. (2009b). "Selective information processing in hypnotic identity delusion: The impact of time of encoding and retrieval". *Contemporary Hypnosis*, 26, 65–79.

Cox, R. E. & Barnier, A. J. (2010). "Hypnotic illusions and clinical delusions: Hypnosis as a research method". *Cognitive Neuropsychiatry*, 15, 202–232.

Cox, R. E., Barnier, A. J. & Scott, A. (2014). "An hypnotic analogue of alien control: Modeling the delusion and testing its impact on behavior and self and monitoring". *Psychology of Consciousness: Theory, Research, and Practice*, 1, 407–430.

Deeley, Q., Oakley, D. A., Walsh, E., Bell, V., Mehta, M. A. & Halligan, P. W. (2014). "Modelling psychiatric and cultural possession phenomena with suggestion and fMRI". *Cortex*, 53, 107–119.

Deeley, Q., Walsh, E., Oakley, D. A., Bell, V., Koppel, C., Mehta, M. A. & Halligan, P. W. (2013). "Using hypnotic suggestion to model loss of control and awareness of movements: An exploratory fMRI study". *PLoS ONE, 8*, e78324.

Elliott, J. M., Cox, R. E. & Barnier, A. J. (2016). "Using hypnosis to model Fregoli delusion and the impact of challenges on belief revision". *Consciousness and Cognition, 46*, 36–46.

Freeman, L. P., Cox, R. E. & Barnier, A. J. (2013). "Transmitting delusional beliefs in a hypnotic model of folie à deux". *Consciousness and Cognition, 22*, 1285–1297.

Hilgard, E. R. (1965) *Hypnotic susceptibility*, New York, NY, Harcourt, Brace & World.

Hilgard, E. R. (1977) *Divided consciousness: Multiple controls in human thought and action*, New York, NY, John Wiley & Sons.

Hill, Z., Hung, L. & Bryant, R. A. (2010). "A hypnotic paradigm for studying intrusive memories". *Journal of Behavior Therapy and Experimental Psychiatry, 41*, 433–437.

Hull, C. L. (1933) *Hypnosis and suggestibility: An experimental approach*, New York, NY, Appleton-Century Company.

James, W. (1890) *The principles of psychology*, New York, NY, Henry Holt and Company.

Kihlstrom, J. F. (1979). "Hypnosis and psychopathology: Retrospect and prospect". *Journal of Abnormal Psychology, 88*, 459–473.

Kihlstrom, J. F. (1985). "Hypnosis". *Annual Review of Psychology, 36*, 385–418.

Kihlstrom, J. F. (2002). "Demand characteristics in the laboratory and the clinic: Conversations and collaborations with subjects and patients". *Prevention and Treatment, 5*, 1–22.

Kihlstrom, J. F. (2007) "Consciousness in hypnosis," in P. D. Zelazo, Moscovitch, M. & Thompson, E. (eds.), *The Cambridge handbook of consciousness* New York, NY: Cambridge University Press, pp. 445–479.

Kihlstrom, J. F. (2008) "The domain of hypnosis, revisited," in Nash, M. R. & Barnier, A. J. (eds.), *The Oxford handbook of hypnosis: Theory, research and practice* Oxford, UK: Oxford University Press, pp. 21–52.

Kihlstrom, J. F. & Hoyt, I. P. (1988) "Hypnosis and the psychology of delusions," in Oltmanns, T. M. & Maher, B. A. (eds.), *Delusional beliefs*, New York, NY: John Wiley & Sons, pp. 66–109.

Laurence, J.-R., Beaulieu-Prévost, D. & Du Chéné, T. (2008) "Measuring and understanding individual differences in hypnotizability," in Nash, M. R. & Barnier, A. J. (eds.), *The Oxford Handbook of Hypnosis: Theory, Research, and Practice* Oxford, UK: Oxford University Press, pp. 225–253.

Maher, B. A. (1974). "Delusional thinking and perceptual disorder". *Journal of Individual Psychology, 30*, 98–113.

McConkey, K. M., Szeps, A. & Barnier, A. J. (2001). "Indexing the experience of sex change in hypnosis and imagination". *International Journal of Clinical and Experimental Hypnosis, 49*, 123–138.

Nash, M. (1987). "What, if anything, is regressed about hypnotic age regression? A review of the empirical literature". *Psychological Bulletin, 102*, 42–52.

Nash, M. R. (2005). "The importance of being earnest when crafting definitions: Science and scientism are not the same thing". *International Journal of Clinical and Experimental Hypnosis, 53*, 265–280.

Noble, J. & McConkey, K. M. (1995). "Hypnotic sex change: Creating and challenging a delusion in the laboratory". *Journal of Abnormal Psychology, 104*, 69–74.

Oakley, D. A. & Halligan, P. W. (2009). "Hypnotic suggestion and cognitive neuroscience". *Trends in Cognitive Sciences, 13*, 264–270.

Oakley, D. A. & Halligan, P. W. (2013). "Hypnotic suggestion: Opportunities for cognitive neuroscience". *Nature Reviews Neuroscience, 14*, 565–576.

Oakley, D. A., Walsh, E., Mehta, M. A., Halligan, P. W. & Deeley, Q. (2021). "Direct verbal suggestibility: Measurement and significance". *Consciousness and Cognition, 89*, 103036.

Orne, M. T. (1959). "The nature of hypnosis: Artifact and essence". *Journal of Abnormal and Social Psychology, 58*, 277–299.

Orne, M. T. (1979) "On the simulating subject as a quasi-control group in hypnosis research: What, why, and how," in Fromm, E. & Shor, R. E. (eds.), *Hypnosis: Developments in research and new perspectives*, New York, NY: Aldine Publishing Company, pp. 519–565.

Orne, M. T. & Evans, F. J. (1965). "Social control in the psychological experiment: Antisocial behavior and hypnosis". *Journal of Personality & Social Psychology, 1*, 189–200.

Parnas, J., Urfer-Parnas, A. & Stephensen, H. (2021). "Double bookkeeping and schizophrenia spectrum: Divided unified phenomenal consciousness". *European Archives of Psychiatry and Clinical Neuroscience, 271*, 1513–1523.

Peters, E., Joseph, S., Day, S. & Garety, P. (2004). "Measuring delusional ideation: The 21-item Peters et al. Delusions Inventory (PDI)". *Schizophrenia Bulletin, 30*, 1005–1022.

Piccione, C., Hilgard, E. R. & Zimbardo, P. G. (1989). "On the degree of stability of measured hypnotizability over a 25-year period". *Journal of Personality and Social Psychology, 56*, 289–295.

Rahmanovic, A., Barnier, A. J., Cox, R. E., Langdon, R. A. & Coltheart, M. (2012). "'That's not my arm': A hypnotic analogue of somatoparaphrenia". *Cognitive Neuropsychiatry, 17*, 36–63.

Roche, S. M. & McConkey, K. M. (1990). "Absorption: Nature, assessment, and correlates". *Journal of Personality and Social Psychology, 59*, 91–101.

Sutcliffe, J. P. (1961). "'Credulous' and 'skeptical' views of hypnotic phenomena: Experiments on esthesia, hallucination, and delusion". *Journal of Abnormal and Social Psychology, 62*, 189–200.

Walsh, E., Mehta, M. A., Oakley, D. A., Guilmette, D. N., Gabay, A., Halligan, P. W. & Deeley, Q. (2014). "Using suggestion to model different types of automatic writing". *Consciousness and Cognition, 26*, 24–36.

Walsh, E., Oakley, D. A., Halligan, P. W., Mehta, M. A. & Deeley, Q. (2015). "The functional anatomy and connectivity of thought insertion and alien control of movement". *Cortex, 64*, 380–393.

Woody, E. Z. & Barnier, A. J. (2008) "Hypnosis scales for the twenty-first century: What do we need and how should we use them?," in Nash, M. R. & Barnier, A. J. (eds.), *The Oxford handbook of hypnosis: Theory, research and practice*, Oxford, UK: Oxford University Press, pp. 255–281.

Woody, E. Z. & Szechtman, H. (2011). "Using hypnosis to develop and test models of psychopathology". *Journal of Mind-Body Regulation, 1*, 4–16.

Zimbardo, P. G., Andersen, S. M. & Kabat, L. G. (1981). "Induced hearing deficit generates experimental paranoia". *Science, 212*, 1529–1531.

# PART 6

# Responsibility, culture, and society

34

# DELUSION AND MORAL RESPONSIBILITY

*Matthé Scholten*

## 1.  Introduction

Delusions can occur in a wide variety of mental health conditions, notable examples of which are schizophrenia, bipolar disorder, and major depression. In 'Freedom and Resentment', his seminal essay on moral responsibility, P. F. Strawson treated schizophrenia and other mental health conditions involving delusions as paradigm examples of exemptions from moral responsibility. He argued that these mental health conditions require us to adopt toward the person concerned an attitude that is fundamentally different from the attitude we adopt in ordinary interpersonal relationships. This 'objective attitude', as Strawson called it, implies that our relations to people with delusions are void of a set of essential human social emotions and that we see people with delusions as something 'to be managed or handled or cured or trained' (Strawson 2008: 9).

Many responsibility theorists have followed Strawson since. R. Jay Wallace regards cases of 'insanity or mental illness' as 'accepted exemptions' (1994: 166) while emphasizing the role that delusions play in this. 'Delusion', Wallace claims, 'is a persisting condition, which [...] deprives the agent of the general powers of reflective self-control' (1994: 169, fn. 18). Benjamin Kozuch and Michael McKenna similarly consider 'extreme forms of schizophrenia' as 'clear cases' of mental health conditions that 'absolve the sufferer of any responsibility for her actions because the illness so thoroughly impairs a person that it undermines her having the capacities requisite for responsible agency' (2015: 92–93). Although calling for a nuanced approach to exemptions from moral responsibility, Matt King and Joshua May likewise use schizophrenia as a paradigm example of mental health conditions having 'global' and 'static' effects on agency (2018: 18).

A more nuanced picture emerges from a small literature that discusses the normative implications of findings from the debate on the nature and epistemic status of delusions (Broome et al. 2010; Bortolotti et al. 2014; Sullivan-Bissett et al. 2016). Analyzing a set of real-life cases on the premise that there is no categorical distinction between delusional other epistemically faulty beliefs, these authors argue that the presence of delusions is neither necessary nor sufficient for exemption from moral or criminal responsibility. It is still unclear, however, how this claim can be squared with the influential Strawsonian account of moral responsibility.

                    DOI: 10.4324/9781003296386-41

The question that I will address in this chapter is whether, why, and under which conditions people are absolved from moral responsibility for performing a morally impermissible action because of their delusional beliefs. Starting from a broadly Strawsonian account of moral responsibility, I radically depart from Strawson and other responsibility theorists in accounting for the exculpatory force of delusions. In contrast to Strawson and the responsibility theorists who followed him, I argue that people with delusions should be regarded as part of ordinary interpersonal relationships and the moral community. My contention is that we should judge people who act on delusions by the quality of their will and the attitudes and intentions that their actions manifest, much as we judge other people who act on false beliefs. In the course of the argument, I sketch the outlines of a new concept of exemption from epistemic responsibility.

The chapter is structured as follows. In Section 2, I define the key concepts of the chapter, delusions and moral responsibility, while devoting special attention to the intricacies related to the latter concept. In Section 3, I introduce and elucidate some essential distinctions in responsibility theory, namely the distinctions between justifications, excuses, and exemptions, and reconstruct Strawson's account of exemptions from moral responsibility in detail. I criticize this Strawsonian account and correct the associated picture of people with delusional disorders in Section 4. In Section 5, I present my account of the exculpatory force of delusions in the form of a Quality of Will Test for actions done from ignorance which applies to delusions and other false beliefs alike. I try to give more depth to my account by discussing real-life cases in Section 6 and sketch the outlines of a new concept of exemption from epistemic responsibility in the course of this discussion.

## 2. Defining delusions and moral responsibility

It would be helpful to start this chapter by defining the two key concepts. This Handbook discusses virtually all aspects of delusions, so there is no need to dwell too long on elucidating this concept. Since there are many different conceptions of the nature of delusions, however, and each of them is subject to debate, it would be helpful to make transparent which conception I assume in this chapter. The glossary of technical terms in the fifth edition of the *Diagnostic and Statistical Manual of Mental Disorders* (DSM-5) defines a delusion as 'a false belief based on incorrect inference about external reality that is firmly sustained despite what almost everyone else believes and despite what constitutes incontrovertible and obvious proof or evidence to the contrary' (DSM-5: 819). The glossary also provides a helpful taxonomy of delusions, distinguishing among others between persecutory, referential, grandiose, erotomanic, and bizarre delusions like thought broadcasting and thought insertion (DSM-5: 819–820). The *DSM* definition of delusions includes multiple elements, and it is useful to prize these apart for the sake of clarity: delusions are (a) beliefs, which are (b) false, (c) idiosyncratic, and (d) unresponsive to evidence to the contrary. Although each of these elements is debatable (Bortolotti 2022), I will stick to this definition in my analysis because it is accurate enough for the purposes of this chapter (for more on delusion and belief see Noordhof, Chapter 19, for more on delusion and evidence see Flores, Chapter 12).

The concept of moral responsibility might be less familiar to the reader of this Handbook, and it will thus be helpful to discuss this concept in somewhat greater detail. First consider this case:

Frances is a farmer, and her bull Sampson is the pride of her stock. Frances takes good care of Sampson and leads him out to pasture on a daily basis for fresh air and grass.

When building the fence around the pasture, she made sure that it was high enough to ensure that Sampson cannot escape, and she has kept the fences in a good state of thorough repair ever since. Careful as she is, Frances checks the fences every day as a matter of precaution before she lets Sampson out. One day Sampson is frightened by a thunderstorm, runs riot, breaks through the fence, and rams the car of the neighbor Alex.

The neighbors soon gather around the damaged car and get into a fierce disagreement about what happened. A heated conversation ensues:

ALEX:        'Frances is responsible for this!'
BETH:        'I totally disagree with you, Alex. Sampson is responsible!'
CHARLES:     'That's nonsense, Beth. I agree with Alex, Frances is responsible!'
DANA:        'Indeed, Frances is very responsible!'
EDWARD:      'I disagree with you all! Neither Frances nor Sampson is responsible for this.'

A brief discussion of H. L. A. Hart's dissection of the multiple meanings of the word 'responsibility' in his postscript to *Punishment and Responsibility* will help us to grasp what is going on here. Hart (2008) distinguishes between various senses of responsibility, among which are senses to which he refers as 'role responsibility', 'causal responsibility', and 'liability responsibility'.

Using the term 'responsibility' in the role-responsibility sense, people may say that a teacher is responsible for the progress of their students, a parent for the upbringing of their children, or a police officer for the safety of the town, to mention but a few examples. The role-responsibility sense of the expression '$X$ is responsible for $Y$', Hart explains, is interchangeable with the expression 'It is $X$'s duty to see to $Y$'. A 'responsible person', or one who 'acts responsibly', is a person who takes these duties to heart. When, by contrast, people use the term 'responsibility' in the causal-responsibility sense, they may for instance say that a low-pressure area is responsible for the bad weather, or that the ill-functioning mainspring was responsible for incorrect time indication of the clock. Hart makes clear that the causal-responsibility sense of the expression '$X$ was responsible for $Y$' can be substituted by the expression '$X$ caused $Y$'.

Liability responsibility must be distinguished from both role and causal responsibility and has a legal and moral counterpart. When people use the term 'responsibility' in the liability-responsibility sense in legal contexts, they may say, for instance, that the car seller was responsible for not delivering on the terms of contract, or that the local mobster was responsible for robbing the supermarket. The liability-responsibility sense of the expression '$X$ is responsible for $Y$' in legal contexts can thus be replaced by expressions like '$X$ is liable to pay compensation for $Y$' or '$X$ is liable to punishment for $Y$'.

The moral counterpart of liability responsibility is the topic of this chapter and can also be referred to as 'moral responsibility'. Whereas liability responsibility in legal contexts presupposes the breach of a legal duty and typically authorizes the state to ultimately use physical force (e.g., in carrying out punishment, or in enforcing payment of a monetary fine or compensation for damages), moral responsibility presupposes the breach of a moral duty and authorizes other individuals to morally blame the person who breached the moral duty. The moral liability-responsibility sense of the expression '$X$ is responsible for $Y$' is thus interchangeable with the expression '$X$ is morally blameworthy for $Y$'.

It remains to be determined what blaming a person entails. While there is by now a wide array of accounts of the nature of blame available,[1] I will in this chapter adopt P.F. Strawson's highly influential account. Strawson argues that blame should be understood in terms of what he calls the 'reactive attitudes'. Reactive attitudes are inextricably bound up with our human social relationships, and for Strawson, they include a relatively broad range of emotions and attitudes, including resentment, guilt, remorse, shame, moral indignation, gratitude, forgiveness, reciprocal love, and hurt feelings. 'Only by attending to this range of attitudes', he claims, 'can we recover from the facts as we know them a sense of what we mean, i.e. of *all* we mean, when, speaking the language of morals, we speak of [...] responsibility' (2008: 24).

Wallace (1994: 25–33) has argued that the class of reactive attitudes relevant to moral blame is narrower than Strawson assumed and restricted to the emotions of resentment, guilt, and moral indignation. We typically feel resentment when another has morally wronged us, guilt when we have morally wronged another, and moral indignation when another has morally wronged another. For both Strawson and Wallace, the 'self-reactive' attitude of guilt and the 'vicarious analogue' of moral indignation are derived from the primordial reactive attitude of resentment.

But what is exactly the nature of the relation between moral responsibility and the reactive emotions? It would seem that in order hold a person morally responsible, one need not actually feel resentment, guilt, or moral indignation, as there can be situations in which one for whatever reason cannot bring up these emotions, psychologically speaking.[2] I will therefore adopt Wallace's (1994: 91) 'normative interpretation', according to which saying that a person is morally responsible for a morally impermissible action (i.e., morally blameworthy) amounts to saying that it would be appropriate to feel resentment, guilt, or moral indignation toward the person for that action. This is the definition of moral responsibility to which I will adhere in this chapter.

In closing this section, let us return briefly to the case I described at the outset, and see whether we now have grasp of the nature of the neighbors' conversation. We can now see that due to the polysemy of the word 'responsible', it could very well be that none of the neighbors actually agreed or disagreed with any of the other neighbors. They might just have been talking about different things: Alex might have meant that Frances is liable to pay the damages of the car; Beth might have meant that Sampson rather than Frances caused the damage to the car; Charles might have meant that Frances had a duty to see to it that Sampson does not escape; Dana might have meant that Frances exercised due care in building, maintaining, and checking the fence; and Edward might have meant that neither Frances nor Sampson should be morally blamed for what happened. All the neighbors might thus have been right – although that by no means implies that they would be agreeing on anything. The take-home message is that if we use the words 'responsibility' or 'responsible', we must always make clear what exactly we mean, or else we are bound to talk at cross-purposes.


## 3. Justifications, excuses, and exemptions

Another piece of conceptual machinery is needed to be able to answer questions about whether a person is morally responsible for a morally impermissible action, and whether and under which conditions delusions absolve people from moral responsibility. These are the concepts of justification, excuse, and exemption.

A classic discussion of the distinction between justifications and excuses can be found in J. L. Austin's 'A Plea for Excuses'. Austin starts by drawing attention to the context in which justifications and excuses are offered: agents offer justifications or excuses when they have been accused of having done something morally impermissible and feel that these accusations are misplaced. Imagine that Grace is accused of hitting Henry in the face at the lockers in the hallway of high school. In that case, Grace can object to expressions of blame on the part of Henry or others in two different ways. The first way would be to concede from the outset that she hit Henry in the face yet contend that doing so was all things considered not morally impermissible. She could, for instance, claim that she hit Henry in the face in self-defense. In this case, Grace offers a *justification* for her action. The second way for Grace to object to being blamed would be to concede from the outset that hitting Henry in the face is morally wrong yet contend that she was not responsible for hitting Henry in the face. She could, for instance, claim that she was unaware of Henry standing behind her and that she inadvertently hit him in the face when putting on her jacket. In this case, Grace offers an *excuse*. Austin puts it as follows: 'In the one defence, we accept responsibility but deny that it was bad: in the other, we admit that it was bad but don't accept full, or even any, responsibility' (1956: 2).

Strawson distinguishes between two categories of excuses in the broad sense: excuses in the narrow sense and exemptions. I will henceforth refer to excuses in the narrow sense (i.e., non-exempting excuses) simply as 'excuses'. Both excuses and exemptions defeat the presumption that an agent is morally blameworthy for an action, albeit in different ways. Let us turn to excuses first. Strawson divides the category of excuses into two sub-categories. The first he illustrates with commonplaces like 'He didn't mean to', 'He hadn't realized', and 'He didn't know' (2008: 7), the second with commonplaces like 'He had to do it', 'It was the only way', and 'They left him no alternative' (2008: 7–8). The first subcategory of excuses can be referred to as 'the excuse of ignorance' and purports to show that the so-called 'epistemic condition' for moral responsibility is not fulfilled, while the second category can be referred to as 'the excuse of coercion or necessity' and purports to show that the so-called 'control condition' for moral responsibility is not fulfilled.

For the purposes of this chapter, it would be useful to describe the excuse of ignorance and the excuse of coercion and necessity in somewhat more detail. Wallace's typology of excuses (1994: 136–147) can be helpful here. Suppose that people hold a person morally responsible for a morally impermissible action or omission. A successful defense based on the excuse of ignorance shows that the action or omission was intentional under some description, yet not under the description under which it was morally impermissible (see Scholten 2023: 1707; Wallace 1994: 136–139). By way of illustration, consider a person who thinks she puts sugar in her partner's coffee, only to find out later that she poisoned him (because, unbeknownst to her and due to no fault of her own, the substance in the sugar bowl was arsenic). A successful defense based on the excuse of coercion and necessity, on the other hand, entails the acknowledgement that the action or omission was intentional under the description under which it was morally wrong, yet establishes that the person performed the morally impermissible action or omitted the morally obligatory action only to avoid great harm (see 2023: 1707; Wallace 1994: 143–147). A vivid demonstration of this is a government employee who gives away classified information to the enemy because the enemy threatens to kidnap her children; or a distribution company that fails to deliver goods on time because they called back their driver to prevent him from getting caught in tornado.

Strawson makes clear that offering and accepting excuses takes place against the back-drop of social and moral relationships characterized by the parties' susceptibility to the reactive attitudes (see 2008: 8). 'The offering and acceptance of such exculpatory pleas', he claims, 'in no way detracts in our eyes from the agent's status as a term of moral relation-ships. On the contrary, [...] it is an essential part of the life of such relationships' (2008: 17). Although there are more differences, this characteristic of excuses decisively sets them apart from exemptions in Strawson's view.

Strawson illustrates exemptions with 'commonplaces' like 'He's only a child', 'He's a hopeless schizophrenic', 'His mind has been systematically perverted', and 'That's purely compulsive behaviour on his part' (2008: 8). Since delusions are a definitory characteristic of mental health conditions within the schizophrenia spectrum (American Psychiatric Organization 2013: 87, see Grassi and Folesai, Chapter 6), it is primarily the 'commonplace' 'He's a hopeless schizophrenic' which interests us here. Strawson also illustrates the notion of exemptions with persons who are 'psychologically abnormal', 'warped or deranged' (2008: 9), or 'whose picture of the world is an insane delusion' (2008: 17). I will ignore the coarse and derogatory language for now and say something about it below, because it is necessary, for reasons that will become clear soon, first to make explicit the fundamental difference between excuses and exemptions on the Strawsonian account.

As said, both excuses and exemptions undermine attributions of moral blameworthiness but do so in different ways. Whereas excuses apply to *actions* and are offered against the backdrop of interpersonal relationships characterized by the parties' susceptibility to the reactive emotions, exemptions apply to *agents* and imply a fundamental change of perspec-tive from what Strawson calls 'the attitude of involvement or participation' to what he calls 'the objective attitude' (2008: 9). To adopt the attitude of involvement toward a person is to understand one's relationship to her as essentially interpersonal and characterized by the parties' susceptibility to the reactive attitudes. To adopt the objective attitude toward a person is an entirely different thing:

> To adopt the objective attitude to another human being is to see him, perhaps, as an object of social policy; as a subject for what, in a wide range of sense, might be called treatment; as something certainly to be taken account, perhaps precautionary account, of; to be managed or handled or cured or trained; perhaps simply to be avoided.
>
> *(2008: 9)*

Strawson makes clear that the objective attitude 'cannot include the range of reactive feelings and attitudes which belong to involvement or participation with others in inter-personal human relationships' (2008: 10). And since 'the making of the [moral] demand *is* the proneness to such attitudes' (2008: 23), we cannot hold the person to which we adopt the objective attitude to moral demands in the way we do with persons to whom we adopt the attitude of involvement. If we adopt the objective attitude toward a person, Strawson therefore claims, that person 'is not, to that extent, seen as a morally responsible agent, as a term of moral relationships, as a member of the moral community' (2008: 18).

I noticed before the coarse and derogatory language of the 'commonplaces' that Straw-son uses to illustrate his notion of exemptions, and we can see now that the same holds true for his characterization of the objective attitude. It would be my contention that by taking 'commonplaces' about people with mental health conditions as a starting point for his philosophical analysis, Strawson unconsciously incorporated societal mental health stigma into his philosophical theory of moral responsibility. Corroborating this claim with convincing evidence and argumentation, however, does not fall within the scope of this chapter.[3] The claim I want to make now is that we should not think of people who have delusions as being exempted from moral responsibility.

## 4.   Correcting the picture

Apart from referring to the abovementioned 'commonplaces', Strawson develops not much of an argument for his claim that people with schizophrenia and people who have delusions are exempted from moral responsibility. 'In the case of the abnormal', he writes, 'our adoption of the objective attitude is a consequence of our viewing the agent as *incapacitated* in some or all respects for ordinary inter-personal relationships' (2008: 13). Then he entertains the thought that a person with delusions is 'incapacitated [for ordinary inter-personal relationships], perhaps, by the fact that his picture of reality is pure fantasy, that he does not, in a sense, live in the real world at all' (2008: 13).

Wallace has tried to give more flesh to this notion of incapacitation. When persons are exempted from moral responsibility, in his view, they are exempted because they lack what he calls 'the powers of reflective self-control'. These consist of 'the power to grasp and apply moral reasons', and 'the power to control or regulate his behavior by the light of such reasons' (Wallace 1994: 157). Since the powers of reflective self-control are related to reasoning and rationality in relation to the discernment, application, and implementation of moral reasons, we may think of them as the abilities for moral reasoning and agency. Wallace emphasizes that even though these abilities come in degrees, there is nevertheless some threshold of these abilities that determines whether a person is exempted or not (1994: 160). People with delusions fall below this threshold in Wallace's view: 'delusion is a persisting condition, which [...] deprives the agent of the general powers of reflective self-control' (1994: 169, fn. 18).

Do people with delusions, or even people with psychosis, generally fail to meet the relevant threshold of abilities for moral reasoning and agency, as Strawson, Wallace, and other responsibility theorist seem to think? The answer, I think, is 'no'. Note that the question is empirical, at least if we assume a specific threshold for exemption. The question is difficult to answer because, to the best of my knowledge, there is no direct empirical evidence on the abilities for moral reasoning and agency in people with delusions. Having said that, some conclusions regarding this question can nevertheless be drawn based on the following set of considerations.

First, delusions often occur in the context of mental health conditions that are episodic rather than permanent, meaning that the symptoms of the condition, including delusions, manifest themselves in a relatively short period of time and then going into full or partial remission. Second, delusions are often not systemic or florid, affecting the person's total 'picture of reality', but rather monothematic and circumscribed, affecting only a subset of beliefs around a particular theme. Third, there are many different kinds of delusions, and each kind will likely have a different impact on the person's abilities for moral reasoning and agency, which implies that the subset of people who have delusions will show high internal heterogeneity in this regard. Fourth, in cases where a delusion absolves a person from moral responsibility for a morally impermissible action, it seems to do so precisely because it provides a rationale for understanding the action, which presupposes that the person who acted in the delusion acted rationally given her beliefs and hence that her formal reasoning abilities were sufficiently intact (for more on delusion and action see Tumulty, Chapter 18).

A fifth and final consideration is that although there is no direct empirical evidence on the abilities for moral reasoning and agency in people with delusions, indirect empirical evidence on the impairment of general cognition and decision-making capacity suggests that there is no reason to assume that people with schizophrenia or psychotic disorders would generally fail to meet any reasonable threshold of moral reasoning and agency. Empirical evidence on cognitive impairment in schizophrenia and psychosis shows that these conditions entail impairments in social cognition and reasoning (Gebreegziabhere et al. 2022), but the extent of these impairments is small in comparison to the impairment of abilities that would be required for an individual to fall below any reasonable threshold for having the powers of reflective self-control and the capacity for ordinary interpersonal relationships. Another area of empirical research that is relevant in this respect, though findings cannot be directly extrapolated without adequate interpretation, is research on the decision-making capacity of people with mental health conditions. Decision-making capacity in the health context denotes the ability of a person to make decisions about medical treatment or research based on their own values and convictions (Scholten forthcoming). Research shows that even if psychosis is a risk factor for impaired decision-making capacity, the group of people with psychosis is highly heterogeneous with regard to decision-making capacity, as a result of which incapacity cannot be inferred from the diagnosis (Kim 2010: 45). What is more, research shows that impairment of decision-making capacity is at most modestly correlated with positive symptoms of psychosis (including notably delusions) and that it is the presence of negative symptoms in the group of people with psychosis which distinguishes them from healthy controls regarding their level of decision-making capacity (Kim 2010: 46–47).

The conclusion that I draw from these considerations taken together is that there is no decisive reason to adopt the objective attitude to persons with delusions and hence that these persons should not be regarded as exempted from moral responsibility. This means, in other words, that persons with delusions are part of ordinary interpersonal relationships characterized by the parties' susceptibility to the reactive attitudes and full members of the moral community.

## 5.  Explaining the exculpatory force of delusions

The fact that people with delusions are full members of the moral community does not imply that delusions can play no role in explaining why a person is absolved from moral responsibility. Delusions can play such a role, albeit not by showing that the person is exempted from moral responsibility. My proposal rather is to treat the question under which conditions a person who acts on a delusion is absolved from moral responsibility much like the question under which conditions a person who acts on a regular false belief is absolved from moral responsibility.

Following this suggestion, I have developed a general Quality of Will Thesis and a Quality of Will Test for actions done from ignorance in earlier work (Scholten 2016b; 2023). McKenna formulates the idea of a Quality of Will Thesis as follows: 'Being morally responsible for an action is to be settled in terms of the moral quality of the will with which an agent acts' (2012: 58). The kernel of such a Quality of Will Thesis can already be found in *Freedom and Resentment*. 'The reactive attitudes', Strawson writes, 'are essentially reactions to the quality of others' wills towards us, as manifested in their behaviour: to their good or ill will or indifference or lack of concern' (2008: 15). The concept of 'the will' is a notoriously vague and is used mostly only in philosophical conversation. To avoid reification and unnecessary abstraction, we should specify what it stands for. Strawson drops a hint when he glosses the will of a person as her 'attitudes and intentions towards us or other human beings' (Strawson 2008: 5). The Quality of Will Thesis can thus be rephrased as saying that the question whether a person is morally blameworthy for an action should be settled in terms of whether that action manifests morally objectionable attitudes and intentions toward others on the part of the person.

Strawson provides an explanation of excuses based on the notion of quality of will when he writes that excuses function by showing that 'the fact of injury was quite consistent with the agent's attitude and intentions being just what we demand they should be' (2008: 8). As we have seen, however, Strawson provides a radically different explanation of why delusions can absolve a person from moral responsibility. My proposal, by contrast, would be to look for a comparable explanation in relation to delusions.

In earlier work, I have developed a Quality of Will Test for actions done from ignorance (Scholten 2016b; 2023), and I present it here with some modifications and improvements:

Agent $S$ is excused for performing a morally impermissible action $A$ if,
1  $S$ had false beliefs $B_{1-n}$ about the circumstances of $A$;
2  $B_{1-n}$ feature in a rationalizing explanation of $A$;
3  $S$ would not have performed $A$ if she had not had $B_{1-n}$;
4  $A$ would be morally permissible or excused if $B_{1-n}$ were true; and
5  $S$ is not culpable for having $B_{1-n}$

Condition (1) requires the agent is ignorant about the nature or circumstances of the action if she is to quality for the excuse of ignorance. To say that a set of beliefs features in a rationalizing explanation of an agent's action $A$ means that the agent took the set of beliefs as reason-giving and hence that the set of beliefs plays a prominent role in the answer to the question 'Why did the agent do $A$?'. Condition (2) thus ensures that agents who qualify for the excuse in question were not merely ignorant about the circumstances of action but also acted *from* ignorance. Condition (3) serves to rule out that agents qualify for the excuse of ignorance in cases where agents have a set of morally objectionable attitudes and intentions toward others which would also lead them to perform the morally impermissible action even in absence of the delusions; for in that case the action would still reflect morally objectionable attitudes and intentions toward others on the part of the agent. Condition (4) is the heart of the Quality of Will Test. It recognizes that our intentions and attitudes are necessarily formed not against the backdrop of what is the case but against the backdrop of what we *believe* is the case, and it operationalizes the fundamental insight that we should not judge people by their actions but rather by the quality of will which these actions manifest.[4] Condition (5) serves to rule out that culpably ignorant agents qualify for the excuse of ignorance.[5] In the case of ordinary false beliefs, an agent will typically not be culpable for having a false belief if holding the belief was justified based on the available evidence and the agent has taken the required inquisitive steps to gather additional evidence. The condition is added to the list because an agent who ignorantly performs a morally impermissible action due to her reluctance to take the required inquisitive step still manifests morally objectionable attitudes toward others. As will become apparent, the picture is different with delusions. In the following section, I will argue that another reason for judging that an agent is not culpable for having a false belief, namely the fact that the belief is not amenable to evidence.

It serves to note that this Quality of Will Test specifies conditions that are jointly sufficient but not independently necessary for a valid excuse. This is because there are other excuses besides the excuse of ignorance. That said, I do take the conditions to be independently necessary and jointly sufficient for a valid excuse of ignorance.

## 6.   An analysis of cases

We can give more depth to the proposed analysis of the exculpatory force of delusions and the associated Quality of Will Test by analyzing a set of cases. I purposely looked for cases that result in an action that is clearly morally impermissible yet not necessarily legally impermissible to ensure that assumptions about legal liability responsibility do not influence our intuitions about the cases.

The first case is adapted from a case report by Sulochana Joshi and colleagues (2021) and involves a Capgras delusion, a relatively rare kind of delusional misidentification syndrome that is characterized by the false the belief that a significant person in the patient's life has been replaced by an identical double (Berson 1983). The case has been shortened and modified to facilitate analysis.

> A 26-year-old Nepalese woman presented to the emergency services on her ninth postpartum day. She had undergone Caesarean Section for a transverse lie. She was doing well until her third postpartum day when she learned that her baby had developed jaundice. She started to change her clothes frequently, throw her own and the baby's clothes away, talk to herself, clench her fists, and stare at family members. This behavior continued until she was brought to the emergency room of the hospital. From day three on the psychiatric ward, she frequently expressed that her husband and the baby would be taken away by 'the witch'. After a few days, she started quarreling with her husband, claiming that he was an imposter. She was firm in her belief and became irritable when confronted. She did not elaborate much except claiming that she 'knew' he was not her husband. She would not talk to her husband or let him see the baby and would become angry when he approached.
>
> *(Adapted from Joshi et al. 2021)*

The action under consideration is the woman's denying her husband the opportunity to see his newborn child. I will assume that, absent good reasons, it is morally impermissible to prevent a father from seeing his newborn child. On this assumption, the woman behaves in a morally impermissible way. But is the woman also morally blameworthy for denying the father the opportunity to see the child? We can answer this question by determining whether the conditions of the Quality of Will Test are fulfilled.

Let us first turn to conditions (1) to (3). It seems clear that the woman had a false belief about the circumstances of her action (i.e., the belief that the man insisting on seeing her baby was an impostor) and acted on this belief when she denied her husband the opportunity to see their child. Based on the available evidence (i.e., the case report), there is no other belief, or set of beliefs, which could explain the woman's behavior, or could do so better than the delusional belief. Condition (3) seems fulfilled as well. It is plausible to assume that the woman would not have denied her husband the opportunity to see his child had she not believed that the man insisting on seeing the baby is an imposter, given that she did not prevent her husband from seeing the baby until after she reported the delusional belief.

Now turn to condition (4). This condition seems fulfilled as well. If the woman's delusional belief were true, the case would be one in which the woman would deny a stranger access to her newborn baby – and that would surely seem morally permissible. Note that condition (4) also allows for the action to be merely excused if the relevant false belief were true. Suppose, for example, that the woman had assaulted her husband with her fists when he was about to come into the hospital room. It is generally thought that people are morally permitted to use only the amount of force that is necessary to keep others from infringing on their rights. Assuming that there were other, less radical, means available to the woman to keep the man out (e.g., closing the door), physically assaulting a stranger who insists on seeing her child would not be morally permissible. Still, if the woman saw the imposter as a threat to her child, the case would arguably qualify for an excuse of necessity. An excuse of necessity, if successful, shows that a person performed a morally impermissible action only to avoid great harm, which in this case is the potential harm to the woman's newborn child. According to the proposed Quality of Will Test, the woman in this revised version of the case can thus still lay claim to the excuse of ignorance.

For this excuse to be successful in either of the two scenarios, however, condition (5) of the Quality of Will Test must be fulfilled as well. Although the woman's belief that her husband has been replaced by an identical double is consistent with the available empirical evidence (personal identity being a metaphysical property, and all empirical features of the doubles being exactly the same), it does not require argument to see that mere empirical possibility of a belief being true does not entail that the belief is justified. As for the inquisitive steps, it might not be immediately clear which inquisitive steps the woman could have taken to gather additional evidence on the identity on the man who insists on seeing her baby: having another look at the man or asking him some questions to which only her husband knows the answer would not help. Note, however, that the woman's belief that the man is an identical double is supported by her prior belief that her husband (whose place the imposter took) will be taken away by a witch. Accordingly, an inquisitive step that the woman could have taken, but did not take, to either corroborate or revise her belief in the existence of witches is, say, reading scientific literature about the topic. Had she done so, she would have learned that witches are socio-cultural constructs without any existence in the real world. But of course, all this is but a longwinded way of saying what we already knew: if the woman's delusion were an ordinary false belief, the woman would be culpable for her ignorance of the circumstances of her action, and condition (5) would not be fulfilled.

Yet I think we should not treat delusions entirely like ordinary false beliefs. Recall that following the *DSM-5* delusions are by definition not amenable to evidence.[6] Because the woman's delusional belief is not amenable to evidence, the practice of trying to refute the woman's belief by citing evidence to the contrary loses its point. This means that we have reason to change our attitude toward the woman regarding her delusional beliefs and regard her as exempted from epistemic responsibility those beliefs. Two qualifications must immediately be made. First, this exemption from epistemic responsibility applies only to the scope of her delusional beliefs and leaves our attitude toward the woman regarding other beliefs untouched. Second, the nature of this attitude differs in crucial respects from that of the objective attitude as described by Strawson.

Let me elaborate on the second qualification. What exactly does it involve to exempt the woman from epistemic responsibility in a particular belief domain? A concept of exemption from epistemic responsibility has not yet been developed in the literature, and I will therefore try to sketch the outlines of it. The concept of exemption I have in mind differs markedly from Strawson's account of exemption from moral responsibility. In particular, epistemic exemption as I understand it does not involve treating the woman and her delusional beliefs as something 'to be managed or handled or cured or trained'. Nor does it involve regarding the woman's statements in this domain as expressions of psychopathology, not taking them seriously, or simply discarding or ignoring them. We do take the woman's beliefs seriously if we revise our attitude to her in this respect; we merely approach them in a different way. When we exempt a person from epistemic responsibility for a set of beliefs, we regard these beliefs not as having truth value but rather as having existential value. In brief, we do not argue with this person about her beliefs; we talk with her about them.

It would be helpful to give a little more substance to this type of communication. The so-called Power Threat Meaning Framework (Johnstone & Boyle 2018) is one example of a framework that could provide a template for this epistemic attitude and type of communication. The framework has been developed as an alternative to the diagnostic model in psychiatry. It assumes that psychiatric symptoms are 'understandable responses to [...] adverse environments and that these responses [...] serve protective functions and demonstrate human capacity for meaning making and agency' (Johnstone & Boyle 2018: 1). In the present case, this would entail understanding the belief of the woman that her baby and husband will be taken away and that her husband has been replaced by an identical double as a meaningful response to the overwhelming experience of giving birth, potential feelings of loss of control due to the caesarian section, potential difficulties in coming to terms with new life and new responsibilities, and potential anxiety around the possibility that her newborn child will be harmed as a consequence of the jaundice.

It is crucial to note that the type of communication in which we regard a person's statements as having existential value is part and parcel of our ordinary interpersonal relationships. Regarding each other's statements as having truth value, stating our opinions, and exchanging arguments is but one aspect of communication within ordinary interpersonal relationships. Only a philosopher could think that this makes up the whole of interpersonal communication. This means that people are by no means excluded from ordinary interpersonal relationships because of their delusional beliefs. It also means that regarding another person's statements as having existential rather than truth value is not in any way disrespectful. More than that, I think it is much more respectful to the woman to regard her statements as having existential value than to try to argue with her, refute her beliefs, and convince her of the truth.

The aim of the analysis of this real-life case was to give more depth to the conditions of the Quality of Will Test for actions done from ignorance developed in the preceding section. While I hope that I have succeeded in doing so by means of the previous analysis, there is one final point I like to make about condition (4), the kernel of the test. I think this point can be made in a more convincing way by reflecting on another real-life example. Let us therefore, in closing, consider the following case involving persecutory delusions reported in a collection edited by Elizabeth Ventura (2017). Again, the case has been shortened and modified to facilitate analysis.

Tim is a 32-year-old software program developer who works freelance for large institutions. He bought a house with his high school sweetheart and owns and operates his own software development company. When a potentially break-through professional deal with a university falls through, Tim becomes suspicious of others and believes people are 'out to get him'. He believes the university is trying to steal his ideas and his software, stating that the university has bugged his home, his phone, and his computer. He furthermore reports that the university is sending him encrypted messages through the closed captioning on the TV and is trying to take pictures and make videos of him through his phone and computer. After Tim became suspicious, he refuses to work on a computer and eventually has to close down his business. He is now having difficulty securing gainful employment and has not worked in several months. His home is in foreclosure. His partner eventually becomes exasperated and moves out. Soon Tim begins stalking her because he wants to see her. When Tim unexpectedly shows up at her house, acting aggressively and threatening her, his former partner contacts the police.

*(Adapted from Ventura 2017)*

I will assume, quite plausibly, that it is morally impermissible to stalk and threaten a former partner. But is Tim morally blameworthy for doing so? Strawsonian accounts of exemptions from moral responsibility likely imply that Tim is not morally blameworthy for stalking and threatening his ex-partner. The reason is that these accounts yield that he is exempted from moral responsibility because of his delusions. Let us now check whether the Quality of Will Test for actions done from ignorance yields a different result.

Let us for the sake of the argument assume that conditions (1)–(3) and (5) of the test are fulfilled and focus exclusively on condition (4). Would Tim's actions be morally permissible or excused if his delusional beliefs were true? Obviously, the fact that a university tries to steal one's ideas by all kinds of objectionable technical means does not render stalking and threatening one's ex-partner morally permissible. Neither would Tim's actions qualify for an excuse of coercion or necessity under those conditions, for stalking and threatening his ex-partner are not a means to avoid the harm of having his ideas and software stolen by the university. In contrast to standard Strawsonian accounts of moral responsibility, the Quality of Will Test for actions done from ignorance thus yields that Tim is morally blameworthy for stalking and threatening his ex-partner. To be sure, we might want to be more lenient with Tim, and appease our moral indignation somewhat given the dire and stressful situations he is in; but that should not distract from the fact that we adopt an attitude of involvement to Tim and are hence susceptible to the full range of reactive emotions.[7]

## 7.  Conclusion

In contrast to what many Strawsonian responsibility theorists assume, I have argued that people with mental health conditions involving delusions are part of ordinary interpersonal relationships and the moral community. At the same time, I have provided an account of the exculpatory force of delusions by developing a Quality of Will Thesis for actions done from ignorance which applies to delusions and other false beliefs alike, and by sketching the outlines of a new concept of exemption from epistemic responsibility. Importantly, this concept of epistemic exemption is in line with the inclusion of people with delusions in ordinary interpersonal relationships. These theoretical innovations enable us to explain whether, why and under which conditions people with delusional beliefs are absolved from moral responsibility for performing a morally impermissible action.

## Notes

1 For an overview of alternative accounts of the nature of blame, see for example Tognazzini and Coates (2021).
2 See, for example, Wallace's example of a 'charming colleague' (1994: 76).
3 I develop this argument in Scholten (in preparation).
4 Broome et al. (2010), Bortolotti et al. (2014) and Sullivan-Bissett et al. (2016) also interpret the exculpatory force of delusions in terms of whether the agent's action would be permissible if the agent's action were true, though without developing a full account of moral responsibility for actions done from ignorance.
5 For an overview of debates on epistemic responsibility, see Chignell (2018) and Rudy-Hiller (2022).
6 This definition is widely endorsed, but Flores (2021) has recently argued against the claim that delusions are not amenable to evidence.
7 Compare the discussion of the case of Bill in Broome and colleagues (2010), Bortolotti and colleagues (2014), and Sullivan-Bissett and colleagues (2016). Bill attacks and harms a neighbor in response to auditory hallucinations about his neighbor constantly making a lot of noise. Quite in line with my approach, these authors argue that Bill is not absolved from moral responsibility for harming his neighbor because physically attacking his neighbor would not be morally permissible had the neighbor really constantly made a lot of noise.

## References

American Psychiatric Association (2013) *Diagnostic and Statistical Manual of Mental Disorders* (5th ed.). Arlington, VA: American Psychiatric Association.
Austin, J. L. (1956) "A Plea for Excuses." *Proceedings of the Aristotelian Society* 57: 1–30.
Berson, R. J. (1983) "Capgras' Syndrome." *American Journal of Psychiatry* 140(8): 969–978. https://doi.org/10.1176/ajp.140.8.969.
Bortolotti, L. (2022) "Delusion." *The Stanford Encyclopedia of Philosophy*. https://plato.stanford.edu/archives/sum2022/entries/delusion/.
Bortolotti, L. (2010) *Delusions and Other Irrational Beliefs*. Oxford: Oxford University Press.
Bortolotti, L., M. R. Broome, and M. Mameli (2014) "Delusions and Responsibility for Action: Insights from the Breivik Case." *Neuroethics* 7: 377–382.
Broome, M. R., L. Bortolotti, and M. Mameli (2010) "Moral Responsibility and Mental Illness: A Case Study." *Cambridge Quarterly of Healthcare Ethics* 19(2): 179–187. https://doi.org/10.1017/S0963180109990442.
Chignell, A. (2018) "The Ethics of Belief." *The Stanford Encyclopedia of Philosophy*. https://plato.stanford.edu/archives/spr2018/entries/ethics-belief/.
Flores, C. (2021) "Delusional Evidence-Responsiveness." *Synthese* 199(3): 6299–6330. https://doi.org/10.1007/s11229-021-03070-2.
Gebreegziabhere, Y., K. Habatmu, A. Mihretu, M. Cella, and A. Alem (2022) "Cognitive Impairment in People with Schizophrenia: An Umbrella Review." *European Archives of Psychiatry and Clinical Neuroscience* 272(7): 1139–1155. https://doi.org/10.1007/s00406-022-01416-6.
Hart, H. L. A. (2008) *Punishment and Responsibility: Essays in the Philosophy of Law*, 2nd ed. Oxford: Oxford University Press.
Johnstone, L., and M. Boyle. 2018. "The Power Threat Meaning Framework: An Alternative Non-diagnostic Conceptual System." *Journal of Humanistic Psychology*. https://doi.org/10.1177/0022167818793289
Joshi, S., M. Thapa, A. Manandhar, and R. Shakya (2021) "Capgras Delusion in Postpartum Psychosis: A Case Report." *Annals of General Psychiatry* 20(1): 21. https://doi.org/10.1186/s12991-021-00342-6.
Kim, S. Y. H. (2010) *Evaluation of Capacity to Consent to Treatment and Research*. New York: Oxford University Press.
King, M., and J. May (2018) "Moral Responsibility and Mental Illness: A Call for Nuance." *Neuroethics* 11(1): 11–22. https://doi.org/10.1007/s12152-017-9345-4.

Kozuch, B., and M. McKenna (2015) "Free Will, Moral Responsibility, and Mental Illness." In D. Moseley and G. Gala (eds) *Philosophy and Psychiatry*, pp. 105–129. New York: Routledge.

McKenna, M. (2012) *Conversation and Responsibility*. Oxford: Oxford University Press.

Rudy-Hiller, F. (2022) "The Epistemic Condition for Moral Responsibility." *The Stanford Encyclopedia of Philosophy*. https://plato.stanford.edu/archives/win2022/entries/moral-responsibility-epistemic/.

Scholten, M. (2016a) "Schizophrenia and Moral Responsibility: A Kantian Essay." *Philosophia* 44(1): 205–225. https://doi.org/10.1007/s11406-015-9685-4.

Scholten, M. (2016b) "Reminders of Duty: A Kantian Theory of Blame." PhD thesis, University of Amsterdam. http://hdl.handle.net/11245/1.539949.

Scholten, M. (2023) "A Kantian Quality of Will Account of Excuses." *Inquiry* 66(10): 1701–1727. https://doi.org/10.1080/0020174X.2020.1784784.

Scholten, M. (forthcoming) "Mental Capacity and Supported Decision-Making." In H. Helmchen, N. Sartorius and J. Gather (eds) *Ethics in Psychiatry: European Perspectives*. Berlin: Springer.

Scholten, M. (in preparation) "Responsibility Theory and Mental Health Stigma: Deconstructing Strawson's Theory of Exemptions in 'Freedom and Resentment'."

Scholten, M., J. Gather, and J. Vollmann (2021) "Equality in the Informed Consent Process: Competence to Consent, Substitute Decision-Making, and Discrimination of Persons with Mental Disorders." *The Journal of Medicine and Philosophy* 46(1): 108–136. https://doi.org/10.1093/jmp/jhaa030.

Strawson, P. F. (2008) "Freedom and Resentment." In *Freedom and Resentment and Other Essays*, pp. 1–28. London: Routledge.

Sullivan-Bissett, E., L. Bortolotti, M. Broome, and M. Mameli (2016) "Moral and Legal Implications of the Continuity between Delusional and Non-Delusional Beliefs." In G. Keil, L. Keuck and R. Hauswald (eds) *Vagueness in Psychiatry*, pp. 191–210. Oxford: Oxford University Press.

Tognazzini, N., and D. J. Coats (2021) "Blame." *The Stanford Encyclopedia of Philosophy*. https://plato.stanford.edu/archives/sum2021/entries/blame/.

Ventura, E. (2017) *Casebook for DSM-5: Diagnosis and Treatment Planning*. New York: Springer Publishing Company.

Wallace, R. J. (1994) *Responsibility and the Moral Sentiments*. Cambridge: Harvard University Press.

35

# THE SOCIAL TURN IN DELUSIONS RESEARCH

*Daniel Williams*

## 1. Introduction

Humans are intensely social animals. We are both fiercely competitive and extremely cooperative. We live in complex and differentiated groups, obsess about our reputation and status, and are completely dependent on the information, abilities, and support that we acquire from others. Most of the opportunities and challenges that we confront are social, and even our capacity to achieve non-social goals almost always depends on intricate social coordination, cooperation, and a massive cultural inheritance. It is this ultra-sociality and cultural nature that drove our lineage's unique evolutionary trajectory and that explains much of what is distinctive about the design and operation of the human mind (Raihani 2021; Richerson & Boyd 2005; Tomasello 2014).

Despite this, much research on clinical delusions is individualistic. As reviewed in several chapters in this anthology, research on the causes of clinical delusions typically appeals to anomalous experiences (see Bongiorno and Parrott, Chapter 26; Sullivan-Bissett, Chapter 28), abnormalities in domain-general inference (Ohlhorst, Chapter 27; Corlett, Chapter 30), or some combination of the two (Davies and Coltheart, Chapter 29; Bortolotti & Miyazono, 2015). Several theorists have recently pushed back against this individualistic paradigm. Drawing attention to various phenomena, including the social themes of delusions, their social risk factors, and the anomalous social behaviour of delusional individuals, such theorists propose that delusions are better understood in terms of disturbances to social cognition than in terms of non-social factors such as anomalous experiences or domain-general cognitive abnormalities (Bell et al. 2021; Gold 2017; Gold & Gold 2015; Raihani & Bell 2019; see Gold and Gold, Chapter 36).[1]

After reviewing some of the core ideas associated with this proposed social turn, this chapter has two aims. First, the controversy over the relevance of human sociality to clinical delusions is often framed in terms of whether delusions result from domain-specific sociocognitive dysfunction or domain-general cognitive dysfunction (Bell et al. 2021; Reed et al. 2020). It can be difficult to understand what is at stake in this dispute, however, or how evidence should be brought to bear on it. I will therefore clarify the claim that delusions result from domain-specific sociocognitive impairments and identify some problems for the

DOI: 10.4324/9781003296386-42

520

strongest versions of it. Second, I will argue that the social turn in delusions research should not be limited to hypotheses that link delusions to a localised sociocognitive dysfunction. There are many ways in which distinctive features of human social psychology and social life can be relevant to understanding delusions even if such hypotheses are mistaken.

Before this, however, three clarifications are important. First, my focus here is on clinical delusions of the sort that arise in conditions such as schizophrenia, bipolar disorder, delusional disorder, certain forms of brain damage, and so on. I will ignore a growing body of research that applies a social lens to understanding so-called extraordinary popular delusions (MacKay 1841; Bentall, Chapter 38) in the general population (Funkhouser 2017; Williams 2021a).

Second, the idea of a recent 'social turn' is potentially misleading. There has long been attention among both clinicians and researchers to various social dimensions of delusions. For example, delusions often come to medical attention precisely because of patients' social difficulties, and there is a long tradition of research focusing on the social determinants of delusions (see Freeman 2016). Thus, in writing of a 'social turn', I do not mean to imply that social phenomena relevant to delusions have only recently been noticed. Rather, I mean to identify a specific research programme according to which delusions result from dysfunctions in or disturbances to cognitive mechanisms with social functions.

Finally, some researchers argue that our species' unique susceptibility to psychotic disorders is a by-product of the complexity and organisation of our evolved social brains and associated capacities for language, mentalising, abstract reasoning, and more (Burns 2006). As interesting as such conjectures are, they are primarily addressed to the so-called schizophrenia paradox—that is, the puzzle of why a condition that is strongly heritable but evolutionarily maladaptive has not been selected out of human populations—and so have a different explanatory focus to the ideas that I will consider in this chapter.

I will proceed as follows. Section 2 describes the motivation for the social turn. Section 3 introduces some of the central ideas associated with it. Section 4 clarifies what it means to claim that clinical delusions emerge from domain-specific sociocognitive dysfunction and raises some problems for the claim. Section 5 then explores how human sociality might be integrated into our understanding of delusions without embracing any hypotheses concerning localised disorders to social cognition.

## 2. Motivating the social turn

Individuals with clinical delusions often appear to believe things that are not just false but at odds with easily accessible evidence (for more on delusion and evidence see Flores, Chapter 12). This can suggest that the primary task in delusions research is to explain this apparent 'loss of contact with reality', a phrase widely used in characterising delusions. From this perspective, common explanatory appeals to anomalous experiences and reasoning abnormalities are easy to understand: if delusional individuals are confronted with misleading experiences, or think and reason in abnormal or irrational ways, a loss of contact with reality is a predictable result.

This perspective on clinical delusions ignores certain important features of delusions and delusional individuals, however (see Bell et al. 2021; Gold & Gold 2015). First, delusions do not seem to range over all possible contents of thought but appear to focus on a relatively circumscribed set of themes (Gold & Gold 2015). Cross-culturally, the most common delusional theme involves persecution, the belief that other agents are intentionally attempting to harm or control the delusional individual (Freeman 2016). Other widespread delusional themes involve grandiosity (i.e., the belief that one has special powers or a special identity), erotomania (i.e., the belief that someone of high status is in love with one), and delusions of control (i.e., the belief that another agent is controlling one's mind or behaviour). In fact, most cross-cultural taxonomies typically list only 10 or 12 delusional themes, but even this might involve over-counting (see Gold 2017). For example, although persecutory delusions are often distinguished from delusions of control and delusions of jealousy, both also typically involve the thought that other agents are intentionally acting to harm the delusional individual. Similarly, although religious delusions are often distinguished from other delusions, many of them simply introduce supernatural elements into themes of persecution or grandiosity.

Observing this cross-cultural clustering of delusional themes, Joel Gold and Ian Gold (2015: 166) argue that there 'is a clear pattern in the phenomena of delusion, and any theory worth its salt is going to have to be able to explain why it is there'. Moreover, in line with others (Bell et al. 2021), they note that this relatively circumscribed focus of delusional belief typically revolves around the 'patient's place in *the social universe*' (Bentall et al. 1991:14). That is, delusions do not just focus on a surprisingly circumscribed set of domains; these domains are overwhelmingly social in nature.

Of course, not all delusions research ignores the contents of delusions. Most prominently, one tradition attempts to link the contents of specific delusions to specific anomalous experiences (Maher 1974; Noordhof & Sullivan-Bissett 2021). For example, an influential hypothesis concerning Capgras delusion—the delusion that a person (typically a loved one) has been replaced by an imposter—proposes that the content of the delusion results in some way from the absence of autonomic cues that typically accompany the recognition of people (Ellis & Young 1990). Similarly, delusions of control are widely thought to be linked to processes in which individuals lose the ability to predict the sensory consequences of their own behaviour, rendering self-generated actions surprising (Frith et al. 2000). It is not clear that such proposals address the issue of social themes, however. For one thing, experiences do not come pre-interpreted and explained, so even if specific experiences are relevant, there is still the question of why individuals interpret such experiences in social ways. For another, specific experiential abnormalities seem most relevant to monothematic delusions. It is more difficult to see what specific experiences are supposed to produce extremely common delusional themes such as persecution or grandiosity associated with polythematic delusions in conditions such as schizophrenia.

A second important feature of delusions that is sometimes overlooked concerns their irrationality. Specifically, although delusions often seem to be strikingly at odds with available evidence and pre-existing beliefs, this irrationality often seems highly localised. This is most obvious in monothematic delusions, where delusional beliefs are focused on just one highly specific topic. Even when it comes to polythematic delusions characteristic of psychotic disorders such as schizophrenia, however, individuals often seem to retain the capacity to think normally on topics unrelated to the delusions. To the extent that such delusions are elaborated, then, the elaboration appears to be largely confined to the relevant delusional themes and so falls short of wholly domain-general irrationality. It is plausibly for this reason that it has been difficult to identify global cognitive differences between delusional and non-delusional individuals that suffice to explain the striking departures from normality exhibited in delusions themselves. As Vaughan Bell and colleagues (2021: 25) put it, 'Most people with delusions appear not to have a generalized problem with rationality but a circumscribed irrationality by which conclusions are irrational solely in relation to the delusional content'.

Third, numerous aspects of social cognition and behaviour seem disturbed or abnormal in delusional individuals. Some aspects of this, such as difficulties with social interaction, are often consequences of delusions. In other cases, however, abnormal social cognition seems to be more closely implicated in the formation and maintenance of delusions themselves. For example, we are completely dependent on the information that we acquire from others, and we regulate our expressions of belief—as with our behaviour more generally—in response to social feedback (Williams 2021b). Individuals with clinical delusions seem highly resistant to both informational and reputational social influence, however. That is, they often discount the contrary testimony that they encounter on the topic of the relevant delusion, and they often express their delusional belief in the face of the clear incredulity—and often stigma—that it induces in other people (Bell et al. 2021; Miyazono & Salice 2021). This has suggested to some that ordinary processes of social influence are anomalous in many delusional individuals (Bell et al. 2021). In addition, some delusional individuals appear to exhibit other subtle differences in social cognition. For example, individuals with clinical paranoia are more likely than experimental controls to perceive neutral faces as expressing anger (Pinkham et al. 2011), they pay more attention than experimental controls to threat-related words and threat-related sentences (Green et al. 2003), and they are indistinguishable in their thoughts about social situations from those with social phobias (Newman Taylor & Stopa 2013) (for a review, see Gold 2017).

Finally, although there is a strong tendency in delusions research to attempt to explain delusions by looking to factors within the delusional individual, there are many important social risk factors for delusions. These include child abuse, being bullied, and being an immigrant, especially for immigrants living in neighbourhoods with a low proportion of people from their own ethnic group (Bell et al. 2021; Gold & Gold 2015; Hagen 2008).

## 3.  The social turn

According to proponents of the social turn in delusions research, the social aspects of delusions just outlined are best explained by the fact that clinical delusions result not—or at least not entirely (see Section 4)—from experiential or domain-general cognitive abnormalities but from dysfunction in certain aspects of social cognition. For example, Gold and Gold (2015: 293) propose that 'delusions are symptoms of a disorder in a mental capacity whose function is to navigate the threats of social living', a capacity grounded in a modular 'brain system' that they call 'the Suspicion System' (see also Gold 2016). Similarly, Bell and colleagues (2021: 25) propose that delusions result from 'socio-cognitive dysfunction' rather than problems with domain-general rationality, where they understand this socio-cognitive dysfunction to affect coalitional cognition, psychological 'processes involved in affiliation, group perception, and the strategic management of relationships'. Although there are important differences between these proposals, it will be helpful to mostly treat them together for the purposes of this chapter, only noting differences when relevant.

Both proposals are most usefully understood by starting with clinical paranoia and persecutory delusions, the most common form of delusion. Paranoia, the unfounded worry that other agents intend to harm you, seems to exist on a continuum in the general population, the extreme end of which involves persecutory delusions (Freeman 2016; Raihani & Bell 2019). It has long been argued that this propensity for paranoia is an adaptation—or a by-product of an adaptation—to the real problem of social threats that our ancestors confronted (Green & Phillips 2004). To understand this view, it is helpful to clarify the character of social threats and the design specifications for agents capable of managing and avoiding them.

First, social threats can be understood in terms of costs intentionally imposed by other agents. So described, social threats are an inevitable consequence of the intense sociality of our species and the fact that social life occurs among individuals with non-identical and often conflicting interests. Such threats range from outright violence and physical coercion to subtle forms of free riding on shared cooperative projects, and they have likely been the most consequential threat to individual fitness throughout our species' recent evolutionary history. Moreover, because social threats originate from agents with highly sophisticated capacities for deception, reasoning, planning, and social coordination, they are radically unlike other dangers that we must navigate. A viral disease might spread through a community. A predator might sneak up under cover of darkness. But neither a disease nor a predator will actively conceal intricate long-term plans coordinated with others to exploit, control, or eliminate you. Such threats are real. Recent histories of elite dominance, slavery, genocide, and so on are only the most extreme examples of such phenomena; social control, manipulation, and sophisticated deception are ancient and pervasive (Hayden 2018; Trivers 2011).

To manage a world of such threats effectively, human beings must have certain motivations and capacities. Most obviously, people must be vigilant. Because the costs of false positives are often lower than the costs of false negatives—that is, because it is often better to be safe than sorry in detecting social threats—individuals should typically err on the side of caution, at least if they have previously been exposed to significant social manipulation or inhabit an environment where such manipulation is prevalent. Moreover, such vigilance requires a capacity and willingness to attend to subtle and ambiguous cues of social threat—remember that people often go to great lengths to conceal the threat that they pose—and a motivation to ruminate on possible threat-related scenarios once the possibility of threat is raised (Williams & Montagnese 2020).

According to Gold and Gold (2015), these and other capacities pertaining to the avoidance of social threat are subserved by a modular brain system, the 'Suspicion System', and it is dysfunction in or damage to this system that underlies clinical delusions. Although there are subtleties in their account that I will ignore here, the main proposal is that such a dysfunction renders delusional individuals hypervigilant for social threat, producing constant false alarms. At first such hypervigilance might be reined in by more reflective processes that inhibit paranoid thoughts, perhaps corresponding to the prodromal phase of schizophrenia in which individuals retain some insight into the implausibility of delusional ideas. At some point, the imagined evidence becomes sufficiently strong, however, either because of an accumulation of false alarms or because of some kind of breakdown in the ability to inhibit such alarms (or both), that the individual begins to integrate the social threat into their broader worldview and develops a narrative to understand it.

Raihani and Bell's (2019) speculations about the causes of clinical paranoia are similar, although they argue that the relevant vigilance is against *coalitional* threats (i.e., threats posed by individuals coordinating in groups) and that this fact explains why persecutory delusions often focus on groups and illusory alliances. They also speculate that a dysfunction in cognitive processes underlying the representation of groups and group boundaries might be equally or even more important than hypervigilant threat detection itself in driving clinical paranoia.

Whatever the specific details, in broad outline, one can see how this framework might begin to address the phenomena detailed in Section 2. First, at least in the case of delusions focused on social threat, it explains their restriction to social themes. Second, because the proposed dysfunction specifically targets the capacity for social threat detection and not cognitive processes more broadly, it can illuminate the putatively localised nature of delusional irrationality. Third, it can accommodate some of the anomalous aspects of social cognition and behaviour in individuals with delusions. For example, it is not surprising why individuals who are hypervigilant for social threat would be resistant to accepting the claims made by others, and evidence for heightened social threat perception falls out naturally from this kind of proposal (Miyazono & Salice 2021; Raihani & Bell 2019). Finally, on this perspective many of the social risk factors for psychosis—for example, being isolated, victimised, and bullied—are precisely those that are likely to heighten the individual's vigilance for manipulation (Raihani 2021; Raihani & Bell 2019).

Of course, even if delusions oriented around social threat are the most common delusional theme, they are not the only theme (see Section 4 below). Nevertheless, proponents of this social turn speculate that other delusions might also result from disturbances to elements of social cognition. Gold and Gold (2015) propose that they all arise in different ways from a dysfunctional Suspicion System, whereas Bell and colleagues (2021) suggest that they result from disturbances to coalitional cognition. However, at present such proposals constitute highly speculative conjectures designed to spur future research, not well-developed theories.

## 4.   Evaluating the social turn

The social turn in delusions research is controversial. To evaluate this controversy, we must understand what it is committed to. As noted in Section 3, proponents of the social turn often frame their proposal in terms of the idea that delusions result from a disorder or dysfunction in cognitive mechanisms that are in some sense *domain-specific* or *modular*. Critics have targeted this aspect of the proposal, arguing that clinical paranoia and psychosis more broadly are associated with *domain-general* abnormalities in how individuals process information (Reed et al. 2020). To evaluate this disagreement, we therefore need to understand what it means to claim that delusions result from impairments to domain-specific sociocognitive mechanisms.

On the most straightforward interpretation, the social turn is committed to what I will call the *Localised Dysfunction Hypothesis*, according to which delusions emerge from a localised dysfunction or set of dysfunctions in cognitive mechanisms specialised for performing social tasks. This hypothesis can then be further disambiguated according to whether it claims that delusions result exclusively or just in part from localised sociocognitive dysfunction, and according to whether it is intended to apply to all delusions or just some of them.

Although the concept of dysfunction raises difficulties and complications of its own, the most controversial feature of the hypothesis is its commitment to *localised* dysfunction. Localised dysfunctions directly affect specialised cognitive mechanisms. For example, on one influential theory of prosopagnosia (impaired facial recognition), it results from a localised dysfunction in the fusiform gyrus, the part of the brain often held to subserve face recognition (McCarthy et al. 1997). Other aspects of vision and cognition often remain functional. Such localised dysfunctions must be sharply distinguished from systems or processes that are dysfunctional or disturbed only as a consequence of more global impairment. For example, Reed and colleagues (2020) propose that clinical paranoia results from a wholly domain-general aberration in how individuals weight uncertainty in probabilistic inference. If so, this aberration will affect social cognition only as an indirect effect of influencing cognitive processes across the board.

How plausible is the Localised Dysfunction Hypothesis? To begin with, it will be helpful to focus on its most ambitious form as a monofactorial theory applied to all delusions. Gold and Gold (2016) sometimes gesture at such a theory in their proposal that delusions result from a disordered Suspicion System, although they also suggest the possibility of views in which such disorders must interact with other dysfunctions, which I will return to at the end of the section.

First, the Localised Dysfunction Hypothesis rests on a controversial assumption about cognitive architecture: namely, that the mind can generally be divided into sub-systems performing specialised tasks that are susceptible to localised dysfunction. This is especially clear in Gold and Gold's (2016) analysis of the Suspicion System as a modular brain system. Some of what Bell and colleagues (2021) write about the nature of coalitional cognition also seems to suggest this picture of how the mind works, however. Although this is not the place to adjudicate controversies about cognitive architecture, it is important to note that the social turn does seem to make a relatively strong empirical bet here, opinions on which vary widely (for a critique of this bet, see Anderson 2014).

Second, although many delusions have broadly social themes, not all do. Consider, for example, delusional parasitosis, the belief that one's body is infected with parasites; or Cotard delusion, often chararactised as the belief that one has ceased existing (Gerrans 2023); or reduplicative paramnesia, a condition in which one believes that one's current setting (e.g., a hospital) has been duplicated or moved to another location. These and numerous other delusions are not obviously social in nature. Indeed, contra Gold (2017), one might worry that standard taxonomies of delusional themes undercount the prevalence of non-social delusions. As Gadsby (Chapter 8) notes, for example, psychiatrists typically resist use of the term 'delusion' to describe inaccurate beliefs about the body in anorexia nervosa, but the grounds for this terminological decision are very unclear.

It is not easy to see how a theory that links all delusions to localised sociocognitive dysfunction in the ways described above can explain non-social delusions of these kinds. In addressing this worry in the case of delusions centred on the body, Gold and Gold (2015: 291) argue that 'the foundation of the social self is the body', and suggest that 'somatic complaints are not merely expressions of the state of one's body but (among other things) invitations to be cared for'. Although this interesting conjecture deserves further exploration, to many, it will likely seem to be motivated more by the demands of their theory than by our current understanding of the nature and causes of such delusions (Gadsby, Chapter 8).

Third, even focusing just on delusions with clear social themes, existing formulations of the social turn are best suited to explaining persecutory delusions. It is not obvious how they could be extended to other common social themes such as grandiosity. Gold and Gold (2015:482) speculate that grandiose delusions result from 'the broken Suspicion System's disordered attempts to project social power and high status, with the aim of repelling (misperceived) social threats'. Once again, this is an interesting conjecture that deserves more exploration, but it is highly speculative at present and much less developed and intuitive than applications of the social turn to clinical paranoia.

Fourth, one might worry that proponents of the social turn exaggerate the circumscribed nature of cognitive differences between delusional and non-delusional individuals. The appearance of such circumscribed differences is most striking in monothematic delusions, but these are the delusions where a connection to a comparably circumscribed experiential abnormality seems most plausible (Noordhof & Sullivan-Bissett 2021). In polythematic delusions characteristic of psychotic disorders such as schizophrenia, in contrast, there often do appear to be relatively global aberrations in the relevant individual's experience and thought about the world, as well as correspondingly global neural differences as well (Giudice 2018; McCutcheon et al. 2020; Reed et al. 2020). Although proponents of the social turn argue that these relatively subtle differences are unable to explain the striking departures from normality often manifest in delusions (Bell et al. 2021; Gold & Gold 2015), it is not obvious why such departures at the level of delusions must be mirrored by comparably striking cognitive dysfunctions. Instead, one might think that delusions arise from an extended process in which subtle differences in experience and cognition accumulate and compound over time in interaction with a range of other affective, behavioural, and social factors, often in complex feedback loops (Freeman 2016).

Fifth, the Localised Dysfunction Hypothesis is at least superficially difficult to reconcile with what we know about the proximate physical causes of delusions. Delusions can notoriously arise from a vast range of different conditions, including diverse psychiatric and neurological disorders, brain damage of many different kinds, and numerous psychoactive substances (Bortolotti & Miyazono 2015). It is not impossible that all such conditions produce a localised dysfunction in or disturbance to the same sociocognitive mechanism, but, again, this is a risky empirical bet. Indeed, the radical heterogeneity in the causes of phenomena labelled 'delusions', and the profound diversity in their cognitive, affective, and behavioural manifestations, seems to be more consistent with the view that the very idea of a unified theory of delusions is misguided.

Fifth, existing evidence on the correlations between clinical delusions and social cognition do not seem to offer any clear support for the existence of an explanatorily relevant local sociocognitive dysfunction (Bliksted et al. 2017; Nelson et al. 2007; Ventura et al. 2013). Perhaps this existing research has not explored the right aspects of social cognition, or perhaps the relevant paradigms for identifying sociocognitive differences are inadequate (Bell et al. 2021). For example, existing studies that explore correlations between impaired social cognition and delusions do not directly explore either a hypothesised Suspicion System or coalitional cognition. Nevertheless, the current evidence in this area for the Localised Dysfunction Hypothesis seems to be quite weak.

Finally, it is not clear how existing proposals that link clinical delusions to localised sociocognitive dysfunction can explain what might be called the 'delusionality' of delusions. Although proponents of the social turn are correct that framing delusions solely as a loss of contact with reality ignores many of their important characteristics, the fact that delusions typically involve highly specific and often bizarre contents does require explanation. It is not clear that current social theories of delusions explain it. Consider three delusions expressed by the mathematician John Nash during his battle with schizophrenia, for example: that he was being persecuted by the Pope and the CIA, that he was the Emperor of Antartica, and that he was the left foot of God (Williams 2018). It is opaque how such specific and strange beliefs could emerge from hyperactive social threat detection, which seems more likely to produce chronic social anxiety, social withdrawal, and submissive behaviours (Raihani & Bell 2019). As noted above (Section 3), Raihani and Bell (2019) speculate that the important causal factor in persecutory delusions is not hyperactive threat detection itself but a dysfunction in the representation of coalitions and group boundaries. It is similarly unclear why a generic disturbance to this ability should manifest as specific and often bizarre delusions rather than as general confusion and cognitive difficulties, however.

Of course, none of these objections is decisive. Much more research—both theoretical and empirical—is needed. Nevertheless, they do raise several reasons for scepticism about the most ambitious version of the Localised Dysfunction Hypothesis. What about less ambitious versions? For example, one might maintain the commitment to a monofactorial theory in which localised sociocognitive dysfunction is sufficient for delusions but restrict its application to only some delusions. Thus, Bell and colleagues (2021: 31) suggest that a 'dysfunction to coalitional cognition may be sufficient, in itself, to account for some delusions'. Although this might address the worry that some delusions do not have social themes, however, it still confronts many of the same problems. For example, it continues to rest on controversial claims about cognitive architecture; it potentially exaggerates how localised the cognitive disturbances relevant to many delusions are; it is plausibly in tension with the diverse range of proximate causes of even paradigmatically social delusions such as persecutory and grandiose delusions; it is not well-supported by existing research on the associations between impaired social cognition and delusions; and it still confronts the challenge of explaining the delusionality of delusions.

Alternatively, one might embrace a multifactorial theory in which localised sociocognitive dysfunction must interact with other dysfunctions and disturbances to produce delusions. One could then apply this theory to all delusions, or claim that localised sociocognitive dysfunction is only a relevant factor in the case of some delusions. Without further details about which other factors are explanatorily relevant and how they interact, it is difficult to evaluate such a theory. Clearly it has the potential of addressing some of the worries just raised, although some still remain, including its controversial modular assumptions about cognitive architecture and the lack of strong evidence for the role of localised sociocognitive dysfunction in delusions. Moreover, once one weakens the commitments of the social turn in this way, it is unclear what the advantages of such a theory are over approaches that integrate human sociality into theories of delusions without positing localised sociocognitive dysfunction. I will conclude with a consideration of such approaches.

## 5.   Social factors without dysfunctional social modules

I began this chapter by describing the hyper-sociality of our species. The social turn has done an important service to the study of delusions by emphasising and exploring the relevance of this sociality to the themes, formation, and general characteristics of delusions. In much of the work developing and evaluating this social turn, the investigation has focused on the explanatory relevance of localised sociocognitive dysfunction. As I have noted, this is an important topic that demands more research. As I have also noted, however, hypotheses linking delusions to localised sociocognitive dysfunction face several theoretical and empirical objections. These objections are by no mean decisive. More research is needed. Nevertheless, they suggest at least some reasons for scepticism about current proposals associated with the social turn. They also motivate the search for ways of accommodating the importance of human sociality into our understanding of delusions without embracing the controversial hypothesis of localised sociocognitive dysfunction.

Such an approach is plainly possible. That is, the intense sociality of our species and distinctive features of the social world can be important for understanding delusions even if delusions do not result from any localised dysfunction to social cognition. This might be because socio-cognitive processes are not dysfunctional at all in delusions, or because socio-cognitive processes are dysfunctional only as a consequence of global dysfunction. As noted above (Section 4), for example, Reed and colleagues (2020) propose that clinical paranoia results from a global aberration in how individuals weight uncertainty in probabilistic inference. If so, the specific effects on social cognition might still be highly relevant to understanding delusions—the complexity and uncertainty associated with the social world might render the effects on social cognition uniquely challenging, for example (Sterzer et al. 2018)—even though social cognition is only indirectly affected by the factors that predispose people to becoming delusional.

I will conclude by highlighting two promising areas of research that illustrate this approach. First, consider again the fact that delusions often cluster around social themes such as persecution, surveillance, control, and status. As we have seen (Section 2), this pattern in delusions is not directly explained by influential frameworks that link delusions to anomalous experiences or domain-general cognitive abnormalities, and proponents of existing social theories identify this limitation as a reason for postulating localised socio-cognitive dysfunction. There are many ways in which human sociality might be relevant to explaining the social focus of delusions that do not involve localised dysfunction, however.

Consider persecutory delusions. Even if the only dysfunctions that predispose individuals to becoming delusional involve experiential abnormalities or domain-general information-processing disturbances, these disorders might interact with a wide range of additional social factors in ways that make themes such as persecution and surveillance likely magnets for delusional ideation. For example, social threats already constitute a strong focus of human anxiety; those individuals at risk for forming persecutory delusions are likely to be independently vigilant for manipulation and exploitation; and features of the social world itself—people's unique capacities for deception, concealment, and conspiracy—ensure that worries about persecution and surveillance are uniquely difficult to disconfirm once they have been seriously entertained (Williams & Montagnese 2020).

Similar lessons might apply to grandiose delusions. Independent of delusions, status constitutes a fundamental human motivation that shapes people's goals and experiences in profound ways, and people already have strong self-inflating tendencies by which they seek out and interpret evidence in ways conducive to achieving a socially desirable self-image (Williams 2021b). It is not difficult to see how such factors might explain why a general susceptibility to becoming delusional might often be channelled into themes of grandiosity, especially in the presence of other affective, psychological, and social factors that make status and social approval an independently salient domain for specific individuals.

Of course, such skeletal proposals require substantially more development and elaboration to even be considered, let alone taken seriously. Nevertheless, they illustrate the possibility of a fruitful research programme exploring how numerous facets of human sociality—sociocognitive processes, social motivations and emotions, social experiences, and the social world itself—might render the social world are common magnet for delusional belief even if localised sociocognitive dysfunction plays no role in making individuals susceptible to forming delusions in the first place.

Second, another relevant area of delusions research that looks especially promising and understudied concerns social learning. From the perspective of learning about the world, perception constitutes a radically different source of evidence to other people. Accurate vision might be undermined by bad lighting conditions or visual illusions, for example, but our perceptual systems evolved to serve our individual interests. In communication, in contrast, the source of information is other agents with potentially divergent interests who can often benefit from deception. Given this, we have evolved to scrutinise communicated information in ways that do not apply to the contents of our own perceptual experiences. Such scrutiny is underpinned by *epistemic vigilance*, cognitive processes that maximise the enormous benefits of social learning whilst minimising the risks of misinformation or intentional manipulation by other agents (Mercier 2020).

Theorists have recently begun to explore the relevance of epistemic vigilance to delusions (McKay & Mercier 2022; Miyazono & Salice 2021). This is a topic that deserves much greater attention. As several theorists have noted, individuals with delusions often seem to treat perceptual evidence differently from the social evidence that they receive from others via testimony and other sources. There is considerable scope for illuminating this asymmetry and other facets of delusions by appeal to the characteristics of epistemic vigilance and the ways in which it is modulated by different conditions and stressors. Crucially, this need not require the postulation of any localised sociocognitive dysfunction. For example, even if the only relevant dysfunctions implicated in delusions concern experience or domain-general cognitive abnormalities, the ways in which social learning is modulated by a range of factors in the aftermath of such dysfunctions might be highly relevant to explaining the tenacity of delusions, their resistance to social influence, their elaboration, and more.

In summary, there is significant scope for the possibility of integrating human sociality into our understanding of delusions without embracing the Localised Dysfunction Hypothesis. The social turn has done a great service in emphasising the importance of our social nature in delusions research, but we need not restrict this importance to the possibility of dysfunctional sociocognitive modules.

## Acknowledgements

For extremely helpful comments and suggestions, I would like to thank Carolina Flores, Ema Sullivan-Bissett, and Stephen Gadsby.

## Note

1 I use the term 'social cognition' throughout to refer to any cognitive processes implicated in dealing with the social world, not just the attribution of mental states.

## References

Anderson, M. L. (2014). *After phrenology*. Cambridge, MA: MIT Press.
Bell, V., Raihani, N., & Wilkinson, S. (2021). Derationalizing delusions. *Clinical Psychological Science*, 9(1), 24–37. https://doi.org/10.1177/2167702620951553
Bentall, R. P., Kaney, S., & Dewey, M. E. (1991). Paranoia and social reasoning: An attribution theory analysis. *British Journal of Clinical Psychology*, 30(1), 13–23. https://doi.org/10.1111/j.2044-8260.1991.tb00915.x
Bliksted, V., Videbech, P., Fagerlund, B., & Frith, C. (2017). The effect of positive symptoms on social cognition in first-episode schizophrenia is modified by the presence of negative symptoms. *Neuropsychology*, 31(2), 209–219. https://doi.org/10.1037/neu0000309

Bortolotti, L., & Miyazono, K. (2015). Recent work on the nature and development of delusions. *Philosophy Compass, 10*(9), 636–645. https://doi.org/10.1111/phc3.12249

Burns, J. K. (2006). Psychosis: A costly by-product of social brain evolution in Homo sapiens. *Progress in Neuro-Psychopharmacology and Biological Psychiatry, 30*(5), 797–814. https://doi.org/10.1016/j.pnpbp.2006.01.006

Ellis, H. D., & Young, A. W. (1990). Accounting for delusional misidentifications. *The British Journal of Psychiatry: The Journal of Mental Science, 157,* 239–248. https://doi.org/10.1192/bjp.157.2.239

Freeman, D. (2016). Persecutory delusions: A cognitive perspective on understanding and treatment. *The Lancet Psychiatry, 3*(7), 685–692. https://doi.org/10.1016/S2215-0366(16)00066-3

Frith, C. D., Blakemore, S., & Wolpert, D. M. (2000). Explaining the symptoms of schizophrenia: Abnormalities in the awareness of action. *Brain Research. Brain Research Reviews, 31*(2–3), 357–363. https://doi.org/10.1016/s0165-0173(99)00052-1

Funkhouser, E. (2017). Beliefs as signals: A new function for belief. *Philosophical Psychology, 30*(6), 809–831. https://doi.org/10.1080/09515089.2017.1291929

Gerrans, P. (2023). Cotard syndrome. The experience of inexistence. In Sullivan-Bissett (Ed.), *Belief, Imagination, and Delusion* (pp. 181–204). Oxford: Oxford University Press.

Giudice, M. D. (2018). *Evolutionary Psychopathology: A Unified Approach*. Oxford University Press.

Gold, I. (2017). Outline of a theory of delusion: Irrationality and pathological belief. In T.-W. Hung & T. J. Lane (Eds.), *Rationality* (pp. 95–119). Academic Press. https://doi.org/10.1016/B978-0-12-804600-5.00006-4

Gold, J., & Gold, I. (2015). *Suspicious Minds: How Culture Shapes Madness*. Simon and Schuster.

Green, M. J., & Phillips, M. L. (2004). Social threat perception and the evolution of paranoia. *Neuroscience and Biobehavioral Reviews, 28*(3), 333–342. https://doi.org/10.1016/j.neubiorev.2004.03.006

Green, M. J., Williams, L. M., & Davidson, D. (2003). Visual scanpaths to threat-related faces in deluded schizophrenia. *Psychiatry Research, 119*(3), 271–285. https://doi.org/10.1016/s0165-1781(03)00129-x

Hagen E. (2008). Nonbizarre delusions as strategic deception. In S. Elton & P. O'Higgins (Eds.), *Medicine and Evolution* (pp. 181–216). Boca Raton: CRC.

Hayden, B. (2018). *The Power of Ritual in Prehistory: Secret Societies and Origins of Social Complexity*. Cambridge University Press. https://doi.org/10.1017/9781108572071

MacKay, C. (1841). *Extraordinary Popular Delusions and the Madness of Crowds*. Simon and Schuster.

Maher, B. A. (1974). Delusional thinking and perceptual disorder. *Journal of Individual Psychology, 30,* 98–113.

McCarthy, G., Puce, A., Gore, J. C., & Allison, T. (1997). Face-specific processing in the human fusiform gyrus. *Journal of Cognitive Neuroscience, 9*(5), 605–610. https://doi.org/10.1162/jocn.1997.9.5.605

McCutcheon, R. A., Reis Marques, T., & Howes, O. D. (2020). Schizophrenia—An overview. *JAMA Psychiatry, 77*(2), 201–210. https://doi.org/10.1001/jamapsychiatry.2019.3360

McKay, R., & Mercier, H. (2022). Delusions as epistemic hypervigilance. *Current Directions in Psychological Science*. https://doi.org/10.1177/09637214221128320

Mercier, H. (2020). *Not Born Yesterday*. Princeton: Princeton University Press.

Miyazono, K., & Salice, A. (2021). Social epistemological conception of delusion. *Synthese, 199*(1), 1831–1851. https://doi.org/10.1007/s11229-020-02863-1

Nelson, A. L., Combs, D. R., Penn, D. L., & Basso, M. R. (2007). Subtypes of social perception deficits in schizophrenia. *Schizophrenia Research, 94*(1–3), 139–147. https://doi.org/10.1016/j.schres.2007.04.024

Newman Taylor, K., & Stopa, L. (2013). The fear of others: A pilot study of social anxiety processes in paranoia. *Behavioural and Cognitive Psychotherapy, 41*(1), 66–88. https://doi.org/10.1017/S1352465812000690

Noordhof, P., & Sullivan-Bissett, E. (2021). The clinical significance of anomalous experience in the explanation of monothematic delusions. *Synthese, 199*(3), 10277–10309. https://doi.org/10.1007/s11229-021-03245-x

Pinkham, A. E., Brensinger, C., Kohler, C., Gur, R. E., & Gur, R. C. (2011). Actively paranoid patients with schizophrenia over attribute anger to neutral faces. *Schizophrenia Research, 125*(2–3), 174–178. https://doi.org/10.1016/j.schres.2010.11.006

Raihani, N. (2021). *The Social Instinct*. Penguin UK. https://www.penguin.co.uk/books/440497/the-social-instinct-by-raihani-nichola/9781787332041

Raihani, N. J., & Bell, V. (2019). An evolutionary perspective on paranoia. *Nature Human Behaviour*, 3(2), Article 2. https://doi.org/10.1038/s41562-018-0495-0

Reed, E. J., Uddenberg, S., Suthaharan, P., Mathys, C. D., Taylor, J. R., Groman, S. M., & Corlett, P. R. (2020). Paranoia as a deficit in non-social belief updating. *ELife*, 9, e56345. https://doi.org/10.7554/eLife.56345

Richerson, P. J., & Boyd, R. (2005). *Not By Genes Alone: How Culture Transformed Human Evolution*. University of Chicago Press.

Sterzer, P., Adams, R. A., Fletcher, P., Frith, C., Lawrie, S. M., Muckli, L., ... & Corlett, P. R. (2018). The predictive coding account of psychosis. *Biological Psychiatry*, 84(9), 634–643.

Tomasello, M. (2014). *The ultra-social animal. European Journal of Social Psychology*, 44(3), 187–194. https://doi.org/10.1002/ejsp.2015

Trivers, R. (2011). *Deceit and Self-Deception: Fooling Yourself the Better to Fool Others*. Penguin UK.

Ventura, J., Wood, R. C., & Hellemann, G. S. (2013). Symptom domains and neurocognitive functioning can help differentiate social cognitive processes in schizophrenia: A meta-analysis. *Schizophrenia Bulletin*, 39(1), 102–111. https://doi.org/10.1093/schbul/sbr067

Williams, D. (2018). Hierarchical Bayesian models of delusion. *Consciousness and Cognition*, 61, 129–147. https://doi.org/10.1016/j.concog.2018.03.003

Williams, D. (2021a). Signalling, commitment, and strategic absurdities. *Mind & Language*. https://doi.org/10.1111/mila.12392

Williams, D. (2021b). Socially adaptive belief. *Mind & Language*, 36(3), 333–354. https://doi.org/10.1111/mila.12294

Williams, D., & Montagnese, M. (2020). *Bayesian Psychiatry and the Social Focus of Delusions* [Preprint]. http://philsci-archive.pitt.edu/18188/

# 36

# DELUSION AND CULTURE

*Ian Gold and Joel Gold*

## 1. Introduction

Sometime around 1800, James Tilly Matthews, a Welsh tea merchant, told his doctor that spies had been sent to England with machines called 'Air Looms' that made use of the chemistry of gases to send out waves of animal magnetism—the force that Anton Mesmer believed underpinned hypnosis. A group of seven villains, Matthews said, had one of these machines and was using it to torment him physically and psychologically. Matthews apparently knew the villains; they were Bill the King, Jack the Schoolmaster, Sir Archy (possibly a woman in men's clothing), the Middleman (the builder of the machine), August, Charlotte, and someone known only as the Glove Woman who wore cotton mittens to cover her scabies (Jay 2014). Around the same time in Germany, Friedrich Krauss, a travelling salesman, came to believe that he was also being physically tormented by animal magnetism but by a different group of people. He identified them as Janeke Simon-Thomas, van Asten, van Asten's daughter, and someone known only as the old magnetizer. They were watching him and reading his mind (Krauss 1967).

More than 100 years later, in 1919, a young philosophy student called Natalija also developed the view that she was being tormented by a machine that controlled her by means of telepathy. She conceived of the machine as a sort of electric voodoo doll with internal batteries. Whatever happened to it happened to her. The villain in this case was one of Natalija's former professors whom she had rejected (Tausk 1933).

In 1958, a middle-aged woman hospitalized at Mount Sinai in New York believed that a different electrical machine was being operated by her cardiologist and bringing about cardiac symptoms and sexual stimulation in her. This machine had radio tubes and wires and was like a robot or a cigar store Indian (Linn 1958). By the 21st century, the machines are more sophisticated. Victims believe that pornography is being broadcast to them by laser radiation; that they are being tracked by a computer chip implanted in their neck; or that Marilyn Manson is manipulating them by means of downloaded songs (Hirjak & Fuchs 2010).

Victor Tausk—a student of Freud and the psychiatrist who treated Natalija—coined the term 'influencing machine' for the delusions that run from Matthews to Marilyn Manson.

533

DOI: 10.4324/9781003296386-43

The machine envisaged by sufferers 'is operated by enemies', (p. 521) and its purpose is always the same—to persecute them, and manipulate their bodies and their thoughts. How the machine works, however, changes with history: 'with the progressive popularization of the sciences, all the forces known to technology are utilized to explain the functioning of the apparatus' (p. 520).

The influencing machine delusion provides a particularly good illustration of four important characteristics of delusions. First, the basic theme of persecution by means of technology remains unchanged despite the variations with each individual believer. In general, the themes of delusion—usually called 'forms'—tend to remain stable across culture and over history. When we examine these themes, we find that they are primarily concerned with the social world (see Williams, Chapter 35 on the social turn in delusion research). We'll call this characteristic of delusions *restricted themes*. The second characteristic is that the influencing machine delusion doesn't change randomly. The variations in the particular ideas expressed by the delusion—usually called its 'content'— reflect contemporary technology. The same is true of delusions more generally. Despite the stability of the forms of delusion, at least some delusions are highly sensitive to cultural context, and the details of delusional ideas vary as culture does. We'll call this characteristic *cultural sensitivity*. Third, the influencing machine delusion contains a good deal of fanciful and implausible detail, and many cases of delusion are similarly elaborate and far-fetched. We'll call this characteristic *elaborated content*. And fourth, the influencing machine delusion violates at least one of the standards of belief in being manifestly inconsistent with some of the believer's other commitments. Delusions in general famously defy some of the many norms of belief. Apart from frequent inconsistency with non-delusional beliefs, they are highly resistant to revision in the light of evidence (see Flores, Chapter 12) and do not always motivate behaviour in the presence of the appropriate desires (see Tumulty, Chapter 18). We'll call this characteristic *normative character*.

The purpose of this chapter is to explore these four features of the form and content of delusion. As we will see, culture will be central to a theory of delusion that takes them seriously.

## 2.   The forms of delusion: restricted themes

The aim of science, including the science of delusion, is to save the phenomena—that is, to explain the observables. Unfortunately, the phenomena of delusion are often dramatically under-described by psychiatry. *DSM-5* (*DSM-5-TR* 2022) characterizes delusions as 'fixed beliefs that are not amenable to change in light of conflicting evidence' (p. 101). While this is true of delusions, it is no less true of a wide range of other beliefs as well; conspiracy theories provide a conspicuous example (for more on delusion and conspiracy theories, see Pierre, Chapter 37). *DSM-IV* (*DSM-IV-TR* 2000) included a number of other conditions on the kind of belief that would count as a delusion—a 'false belief based on incorrect inference about external reality that is firmly sustained despite what almost everyone else believes and despite what constitutes incontrovertible and obvious proof or evidence to the contrary' (p. 821). Apart from the well-known difficulties associated with this definition (Coltheart 2007), it characterizes delusions by means of cognitive, epistemic, and semantic features and pays no attention to what delusions are actually about. In contrast, psychiatrists typically identify delusions by their forms, and there are only a few of them. For example, the delusions included in a widely used symptom checklist—the Scale for the Assessment of Positive Symptoms (SAPS; [Andreason 1984])—includes the following 12 types: persecutory delusions, delusions of jealousy, delusions of guilt or sin, grandiose delusions, religious delusions, somatic delusions, delusions of reference, delusions of being controlled, delusions of mind reading, thought broadcasting, thought insertion, and thought withdrawal. A handful of other forms are also found in the literature. These include nihilistic, erotomanic, and misidentification delusions. One also finds differences in delusional themes that depend on taxonomic choices—for example, whether one counts the delusion of being poisoned as a variant of persecution or an independent form. Nonetheless, of all the possible strange beliefs one might hold, there are only perhaps a dozen or two that psychiatry takes to be delusional.

The restricted nature of the forms of delusion would not be particularly significant if the themes of delusion were an artefact of 21st century (English-language) psychiatry. In addition to being restricted in the ideas they express, however, the forms of delusion appear to be stable across time and culture (Stompe et al. 2003). Consider time first. Grunfeld and colleagues (2022) investigated the rates of delusional forms in four cohorts of clients with first-episode psychosis treated in the same clinic between 2006 and 2017. With one exception (the delusion of guilt or sin), which is likely to be an artefact, the rates remained unchanged over that period (see Grunfeld and colleagues 200: 38).

The forms of delusion also appear to be stable across culture. Although there are variations in the delusions found in different countries, a cross-cultural comparison reveals considerable similarities (see Gold & Gold 2014: 64). For example, the theme of persecution is found everywhere and is typically the most common delusional form, often by a substantial margin. Grandiose delusions and delusions of reference are near-universal, as are religious delusions. Of the differences present, many are likely to be the result of taxonomic choice rather than variations in the psychiatric phenomena. More importantly, however, despite the variations, the forms of delusion are fundamentally about one subject: the social world, including the delusional person. The restricted nature of the themes of delusions thus appears to be a real phenomenon.

### 3.   Explaining the forms: a social threat model

Why are delusions restricted primarily to the social world? To answer this question we propose a social threat model of delusion (Gold & Gold 2014; Green & Phillips 2004; Zolotova & Brune 2006). According to the model, human beings possess a special-purpose cognitive system the function of which is to detect and respond to threats posed by others. When this system is disordered, delusions are the result.

The model draws on the specific themes of delusion, many of which are expressly concerned with threats from others. Apart from persecutory delusions themselves, religious delusions are often persecutory in nature. The same is true of some somatic delusions, as in Matthews's case. Delusional jealousy represents a fear of betrayal, and delusions of control, and of intrusion into one's mind (e.g. mindreading, thought insertion) also represent threats of manipulation. These are not fears of physical harm but rather of what could be called exploitation by others—behaviours that present a risk to one's human or material resources. In contrast, other delusions seem to represent a kind of social power. Grandiose delusions, including some religious delusions, represent the believer as at the top of a social hierarchy, with capacities or achievements that would give them control over others. Erotomania also appears to be a form of grandiosity insofar as it represents the sufferer as loved by someone of high social status (Enoch et al. 2021, chapter 2). The social threat model holds that these beliefs are expressions of an attempt to respond to social threat by means of assertions of social power.

A social threat system of this kind would be a highly adaptive form of cognition. Human beings live in large social groups and benefit enormously from cooperation with others (Enquist & Leimar 1993). A consequence of social living, however, is the risk of exploitation (e.g. free riding). When one is faced with the decision of whether to cooperate or compete with a member of one's social group, having the ability to detect the possibility of threat would enable one to benefit from cooperation while minimizing its risks. There is strong evidence that the primate brain evolved primarily under the pressure of coping with the complexities of the social world—an idea known as the social brain hypothesis (e.g., Dunbar 1998, 2010; Dunbar & Shultz 2007). On the assumption of the social brain hypothesis, the hypothesis of a social threat detection capacity is a relatively conservative one.

Jealousy provides a useful illustration of the model. Social living creates the threat of cheating by one's partner. The only way to completely eliminate the risk of cheating would be to opt out of social living altogether at the expense of the benefits of cooperation. Sensitivity to the signs of cheating makes it possible to act so as to prevent it and makes it possible to participate in social life while minimizing one of its risks. The feeling of jealousy is the conscious manifestation of one's having detected those signs, and because it is highly motivating, provides an impetus for acting to reduce the risk (e.g., by being more empathic; see Birnbaum et al. 2022). In this way, jealousy acts both to detect and respond to a social threat. If, however, one feels extreme and persistent jealousy in the absence of any evidence of cheating, then the jealousy is delusional.

### 3.1 *Modularity*

On our account, the social threat system is modular in the sense of Fodor (1983) who identified nine characteristic (but not necessary; see Coltheart 1999) features of this form of specialized cognition. For present purposes, we focus on three. First, modules are *domain specific*—they are responsive to a restricted range of input. Second, they *operate mandatorily*—they are always on and operate automatically. And, third, they are *informationally encapsulated*—the information that can enter a module from elsewhere in the mind is restricted. So, for example, the appearance of a visual illusion does not change even when one learns that the appearance is illusory because the visual system is modular.

The social threat system is domain specific in that it is responsive only to evidence of social threat. Faces that induce fear are a paradigm example of this sort of input, but more complex and abstract stimuli will also activate the system. When Iago tells Othello that Cassio has Desdemona's handkerchief, Othello comes to believe that Desdemona has been unfaithful. Moreover, the inference happens in a mandatory way: Othello does not have to decide to reflect on the significance of the handkerchief. Because the social threat system is always on, it automatically generates the thought that Othello is being threatened with infidelity.

The social threat system is informationally encapsulated to the extent that information about social threat from other sources cannot enter the module. However, the module itself *can* be activated or inhibited by the activity of other mental functions. Here is an analogy. There is something about the way we think about probabilities that disposes people to commit the base rate fallacy, and even when one learns about the fallacy, it is hard to resist the temptation to fall back into fallacious reasoning. With experience, however, the initial impulse to focus exclusively on features of the individual case is overridden by the knowledge that the features of the population are also relevant. The mistaken impulse, that is, is inhibited by acquired knowledge. We do not say that probabilistic reasoning is modular, but it is structurally parallel to the case of social threat detection. Suppose Othello had gone to therapy and developed a bit of insight into his jealous tendencies. When he sees Cassio with Desdemona's handkerchief, he immediately feels threatened by Desdemona's infidelity. But he reminds himself that he tends to be jealous and that Desdemona has never in fact cheated on him, and the jealousy subsides. It's not the case that the information about Desdemona's loyalty enters the social threat system. It is rather that Othello's reasoning inhibits the activity of the threat system.

If the social threat system generates the belief that Desdemona is unfaithful, and the social threat system is modular, then at least some beliefs about social threats are generated by a module. Fodor famously argued that belief fixation could not be modular (see Fodor 1983: 101ff. and Fodor 2001), roughly because the fixation of any particular belief is constrained by the content of any other (the property of being *isotropic*) and by the coherence of one's entire belief set (the property of being *Quinean*). Let that be the case. It is not inconsistent to suppose that, in addition to a belief fixation process that is isotropic and Quinean, there are redundant specialized modules that generate beliefs based on limited evidence that are sent to the belief system proper for evaluation. Before therapy, Othello's social threat system generates the belief that Desdemona is unfaithful, and the belief system proper adds that belief to Othello's belief set; after therapy the social threat system generates the same belief, but it is rejected by the belief system proper. According to the model, the social threat system generates threat-related beliefs which, in healthy functioning, are output to belief proper—the belief set that is isotropic and Quinean. In turn, belief proper, and the reasoning capacities that govern it, regulates the social threat module, accepting or rejecting social threat beliefs as it deems appropriate. We hypothesize that, in cases of delusion, the primary disorder is an absence of modulatory functions on the part of belief proper. As a result, the social threat system cannot be inhibited. We think it is also likely that, in some delusions, the output of the social threat system is also disordered (Figure 36.1).

We began by asking why the forms of delusion are restricted to the domain of the social world. The answer, according to our model, is that cognitive processes that generate delusions are functions of a module that is concerned exclusively with social threat. Although the details of delusional ideas vary from person to person, the basic themes of delusion remain the same over time and across culture because they are determined by the function of the social threat system which we presume to be universal. And because culture is, at least in part, a systematization of the behaviours, norms, and institutions of human societies, delusions are deeply connected to culture; culture is baked in because the function of the system which, when disordered, leads to delusions is to detect specific features of social organization.

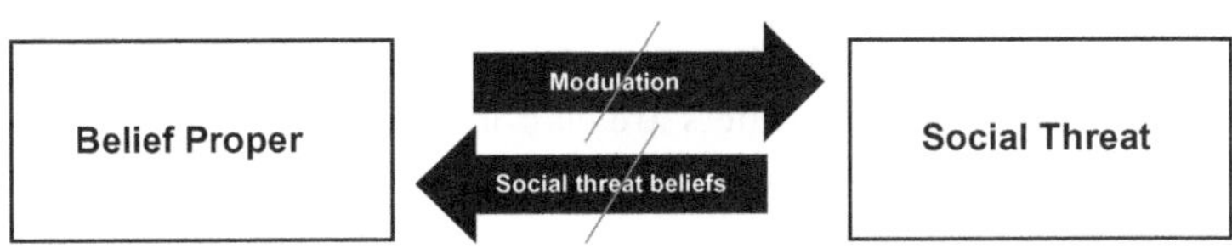


*Figure 36.1* The social threat module and belief proper.

### *3.2   Delusion formation and retention*

Because the social threat system operates in a mandatory fashion, we hypothesize that it continually generates threat narratives. It sees threats everywhere all the time. One can sometimes notice this happening. Two colleagues are whispering about something in the corridor before the meeting, and the thought pops into your head that they are planning to blame you for something they've done. The thought is easily dismissed as soon as you remind yourself that these are colleagues who have always been supportive. You might even wonder why such an improbable thought occurred to you in the first place. Because there is a probability, no matter how small, that even loyal colleagues might decide to betray you, the social threat system generates a narrative to that effect. Even if, all things considered, betrayal is very unlikely, it may, at least sometimes, be useful to have the thought of social threat cross your mind. On this account, then, delusions are formed by the same mechanisms that drive thoughts about social threat in healthy individuals. In some cases at least, the delusional thought is not in itself pathological. What distinguishes delusional from normal thought is that it is not inhibited. Where the healthy individual has a thought about betrayal that is immediately rejected, the same thought in the delusional individual remains in place.[1]

The question of delusion retention has proven difficult because the kinds of process that might explain it seem to be incompatible with the restricted nature of delusional thought. Suppose, for example, that one were to hypothesize that the Capgras thought is formed in the manner proposed by Ellis and Young (1990) and retained in virtue of a reasoning disorder like a jumping to conclusions bias (McLean et al. 2017). A bias of this kind is a domain-general reasoning style that would apply to many thoughts and would be expected to produce many other strange beliefs beyond the Capgras delusion. So far as we know, however, having many strange, but non-delusional, thoughts is not a characteristic of most patients with psychosis.

If the social threat system is a module, however, then it is informationally encapsulated. It can be turned on and off, but information from other systems cannot enter. We have suggested that in healthy individuals, inappropriately suspicious thoughts are suppressed, and this can happen if a cognitive process external to the social threat system inhibits it. If that modulatory connection is dysfunctional, however, then the social threat system remains on, and the delusion is not rejected. Beyond the disconnection of the social threat module, we do not have to posit any further cognitive disorder to explain the retention of delusions. As a result, there is no reason to expect to find that people suffering from delusions also hold many other strange beliefs.

Two qualifications are in order. First, while the suggestion we've made seems appropriate to some forms of delusion like persecution, it is not sufficient for others. While beliefs about thought insertion or reduplication are not utterly alien—they are, for example, perfectly comprehensible in fiction—they aren't the kinds of thought one is aware of. They are likely to be generated by additional disorders that remain to be explained. Second, there is a difference between the thought that your colleagues are plotting to betray you and the thought that you are being tormented by an Air Loom. Some delusions may be overly suspicious interpretations of real events; others are elaborate and cut out of whole cloth. This is one of the features of delusion retention, to which we turn next.

## 4.  The content of delusions

If there are only a few delusional forms, why is there such variety in the beliefs of people with delusions? Art provides a hint. There are apparently only a few basic plots in all of literature (Reagan et al. 2016): man falls into hole, man gets out of hole; boy meets girl, boy loses girl, boy gets girl; and so on (Vonnegut 2005). However, an author doesn't set out to write a story about a boy meeting a girl; they set out to write *Romeo and Juliet,* or *When Harry Met Sally.* Delusional ideas are also only concerned with a dozen or two basic plots, but they are also often complex narratives. Because of Maher's (1974) classic paper, it is widely believed that delusional narratives come about as responses to anomalous experience (see Bongiorno and Parrot, Chapter 26; see also Noordhof & Sullivan-Bissett, 2021 and Sullivan-Bissett, Chapter 28). For reasons that we will see, however, these narratives are not best characterized in this way but as products of the social threat system itself. When that system is functioning normally, it draws on the information it has about the social world to weave a plausible narrative about threat, and it is constrained by the belief system proper. When the system is disconnected from the rest of thought, the narrative is elaborated in ways that are unconstrained by the facts or by some of the norms of belief.

### 4.1  *Cultural sensitivity*

An American with a persecutory delusion might believe that the CIA is reading his email. Someone with a persecutory delusion in China, however, is unlikely to have the same fear because the CIA does not play the same cultural role in China as it does in the United States. If, as we have proposed, delusions are disorders of a system that evolved to detect social threats, that system would have to be sensitive to the facts about the world in which the delusional person lives—including facts about culture—because those facts determine where a threat may originate. A well-functioning social threat system will represent the fact that in the United States it is the CIA that one has to be concerned about and not, say, the Communist Party. Culture is thus 'pathoplastic' (Tseng 2001)—it shapes the manifestation of the symptom—because it is precisely the function of the social threat system to be sensitive to that part of the cultural world that may be threatening.

It is worth noting that cultural sensitivity presents a challenge to the standard model of delusion formation in which anomalous experience typically plays a central role. Suppose, for example, that one set out to account for persecutory delusions by hypothesizing the existence of an anomalous experience of extreme suspicion. The delusion would arise as an endorsement or explanation of this experience. How well would a traditional account of this kind fare? Notice, to begin with, that an endorsement account appears to be a nonstarter. In Ellis and Young's model, the structure of the hypothesized anomalous experience is both rich and specific; it purports to represent someone as both familiar in one way and unfamiliar in another. While there is some light between this content and the concept of a duplicate or imposter, it's not much (see Bongiorno 2020). In contrast, a model of persecutory delusions that begins with an anomalous experience of social threat cannot be endorsed in a way that leads to the belief in Air Looms. Most persecutory delusions are wildly underspecified by any sort of anomalous experience one can imagine.

Explanation accounts are more plausible. If one were to have a strange experience of extreme suspicion, one might naturally begin to engage in a process of trying to understand what might be happening to bring about that experience. One would then draw on whatever beliefs were ready to hand, and they are as variable as the life and times of the believer. Here again, the model of Capgras is attractive because it is not altogether implausible that an anomalous recognitional experience might be adequately explained by the duplicate hypothesis. In contrast, however, Matthews's putative explanation of his suspicion is poor by any standards. In Matthews's time, it might not have been unreasonable for him to hypothesize that someone was using animal magnetism to harm him. To suppose, however, that there were seven enemies including Bill the King, a woman wearing men's clothes, and someone who wears gloves because she has scabies is nothing like an explanation of Matthews's strange experiences for the obvious reason that most of what he believes adds no explanatory power to the hypothesis. Many delusions are like this. Someone with a persecutory delusions doesn't merely believe in a threat from others but that the British Labour Party is targeting them for murder (Kelly 1996); someone with a grandiose delusion does not only claim that she is important or powerful but that she has 2,082 law degrees (Gold & Gold 2014); and someone with a somatic delusion doesn't just believe that his body is being damaged but that his penis is being twisted off with a nerve probe (Schreber 2000). Explanations are supposed to save the phenomena in the simplest way possible. Delusions don't save the phenomena; they seem to improvise on the phenomena.

### 4.2  *Elaborated content and normative character*

The idea of delusion as improvisation is not meant to be a metaphor. The social threat system functions in a mandatory way, and when it is functioning normally, its outputs—beliefs about social threat—are delivered to the belief formation system proper—the system that is isotropic and Quinean. The belief formation system evaluates the output of the social threat system and modulates it appropriately. When the social threat system is disconnected from thought and is unmodulated, it continues to weave stories about social threats in a way that is unconstrained by the facts. Matthews's Air Loom delusions do not express Matthews's experience or provide an explanation of it. The delusions constitute an analogue of a story—complete with heroes, villains, and plot—that arises out of Matthews's imagination, but that is pathologically disconnected from the bulk of Matthews's other beliefs. Moreover, if the beliefs about social threat are not sent to belief proper, then they are not subject to the cognitive processes that implement the norms of belief—that beliefs should be plausible relative to one's background knowledge; responsive to the facts and revised if the evidence changes; that they be consistent; that, with the appropriate desire, they motivate action; and so on. These processes, as Fodor argues, cannot be implemented by modular cognition, so they do not govern social threat beliefs.

What emerges from the disconnected social threat system is therefore not unlike fictional belief in some respects.[2] Consider an illustration. David believes it to be true that Sherlock Holmes lived in Baker Street and that he liked to show off his mental powers (Lewis 1978: 37). These beliefs about Holmes have some of the features of ordinary beliefs. They can, for example, be used in reasoning: if one lives in Baker Street, and Baker Street is in London, then one lives in London; so Holmes lived in London. David's beliefs about Holmes are also like ordinary beliefs in being sensitive to evidence. When Holmes faces Moriarty at Reichenbach Falls, David (like Watson) believes that Holmes dies, and when

Holmes returns, David (and Watson) believe that their prior belief was false. David also has beliefs (or dispositions to believe) that derive from his general knowledge about Holmes's world. He is certain that Holmes never used Facebook; that he probably didn't bathe as often as Londoners now do; and that he could have seen *Macbeth* but not *Nixon in China*.

David's beliefs about Holmes don't, however, have some of the other features of ordinary belief. While David is quite happy to believe that an injection of monkey extract might give an old man renewed energy[3] in fiction, in most other contexts that would seem absurd. He is willing to believe both that Holmes knew nothing about literature[4] and that he could quote Goethe in the original.[5] He is not disposed in the least to revise his belief about Holmes's address even if the foremost authority on the history of London architecture assures him that there has never been a 221B Baker Street. And he's not going to look through the archives of the British Museum in the hopes of finding Holmes's unpublished letters. Beliefs in fiction can be manifestly false or absurd, contradictory, and unrevisable; and they do not motivate some types of action whatever one's desires. Ordinary beliefs are supposed to be none of these.

Fictional beliefs are instances of what Tamar Gendler (2008a, 2008b) calls 'aliefs'—mental states that have some of the properties of beliefs but not others. There are many ways to be an alief, and being a fictional belief is one of them. Fiction is possible because human beings have the cognitive capacity to entertain a narrative that has its own epistemic rules, some of which apply outside the narrative and some of which don't, and to understand that there is an important inferential boundary between the narrative and the real world.

Delusions are not fictional beliefs, but they have some of the same features. They are the outputs of a belief-formation module which becomes disconnected from other forms of thought and begins to generate a narrative that is unmoored from some of the constraints of thought. Delusional belief is isolated from other beliefs and not subject to evaluation for consistency. And because it is unconstrained by facts about the real world it can develop in all sorts of fanciful and implausible ways. Why is Matthews's tormentor called Bill the King? Well, why not? Matthews calls him Bill the King for the same reason we are asked to call the main character of *Moby Dick* Ishmael. No fact of the matter restricts the name of the delusional character any more than it does in fiction. The social threat system is, we have supposed, constantly telling stories about possible risks in the social environment. When the system is unconstrained by inputs from that world, it improvises.

## 5.  Conclusion: culture again

Psychosis is often characterized as a break with reality. In the case of delusions, this is, in one sense, quite inaccurate. Delusions are profoundly sensitive to the socio-cultural world in which the individual lives. We have argued that culture is central to delusions because the system that generates them is designed precisely to represent features of the social world—conspiracies, love triangles, social power—that are relevant to social threat. Moreover, the social threat system is a narrative capacity. It is always on the lookout for threats, and it represents those threats as narratives because social threats are best represented as stories about people, their malign intentions, and the actions they take to realize them. To ask why delusions often make reference to the culture of the believer, then, is analogous to asking why culture appears in fiction. All of fiction is constituted of stories about people, and so are delusions, even if the basic plots are different. Delusions are sensitive to culture because the delusional person is telling a story about their world, and that world is made up of the people in it and the culture they share.

## Notes

1 In locating the formation of some delusions in a failure to suppress a strange thought, our account is similar to the two-factor account (Davies et al. 2001).
2 The relation of delusions to fictional narratives is proposed by Currie and Jureidini (2014) for somewhat different reasons than those developed here.
3 'The Adventure of the Creeping Man'.
4 'A Study in Scarlet'.
5 'The Sign of the Four'.

## References

Andreasen, Nancy C. (1984). *The Scale for the Assessment of Positive Symptoms (SAPS)*. Iowa City: The University of Iowa.

Birnbaum, G., Bachar, T., Levy, G., Zholtack, K., & Reis, H. (2022). Put me in your shoes: Does perspective-taking inoculate against the appeal of alternative partners? *Journal of Sex Research, 2*, 1–10.

Bongiorno, F. (2020). Is the Capgras delusion an endorsement of experience? *Mind & Language, 35*, 293–312.

Coltheart, M. (1999). Modularity and cognition. *Trends in Cognitive Science, 3*(3), 115–120.

Coltheart, M. (2007). Cognitive neuropsychiatry and delusional belief (The 33rd Sir Frederick Bartlett Lecture). *The Quarterly Journal of Experimental Psychology, 60*(8), 1041–1062.

Currie, G., & Jureidini, J. (2014). Art and delusion. *The Monist, 86*(4), 556–578.

Davies, M., Coltheart, M., Langdon, R., & Breen, N. (2001). Monothematic delusions: Towards a two-factor account. *Philosophy, Psychiatry, and Psychology, 8*(2/3), 133–158.

DSM-5-TR. (2022). *Diagnostic and Statistical Manual of Mental Disorders* (5th ed.), Text Revision (DSM-5-TR). Washington, DC: American Psychiatric Publishing.

DSM-IV-TR. (2000). *Diagnostic and Statistical Manual of Mental Disorders-IV-TR*. Washington, DC: American Psychiatric Publishing.

Dunbar, R. (1998). The social brain hypothesis. *Evolutionary Anthropology, 6*(5), 178–190.

Dunbar, R. (2010). The social brain and its implications. In U. Frey, C. Störmer & K. Willführ (Eds.), (pp. 65–77). Berlin: Springer.

Dunbar, R., & Shultz, S. (2007). Evolution in the social brain. *Science, 317*, 1344–1347.

Ellis, H. D., & Young, A. W. (1990). Accounting for delusional misidentifications. *British Journal of Psychiatry, 157*, 239–248.

Enoch, M. D., Puri, B. K., & Ball, H. N. (2021). *Uncommon Psychiatric Syndromes* (5th ed.). London: Routledge.

Enquist, M., & Leimar, O. (1993). The evolution of cooperation in mobile organisms. *Animal Behaviour, 45*(4), 747–757.

Fodor, J. (1983). *The Modularity of Mind*. Cambridge: MIT Press.

Fodor, J. (2001). *The Mind Doesn't Work that Way*. Cambridge: MIT Press.

Gendler, T. S. (2008a). Alief and belief. *Journal of Philosophy, 105*(10), 634–663.

Gendler, T. S. (2008b). Alief in action (and reaction) *Mind & Language, 23*(5), 552–585.

Gold, J., & Gold, I. (2014). *Suspicious Minds: How Culture Shapes Madness*. New York: Free Press.

Green, M. J., & Phillips, M. L. (2004). Social threat perception and the evolution of paranoia. *Neuroscience and Biobehavioral Reviews, 28*(3), 333–342.

Grunfeld, G., Lemonde, A. C., Gold, I., Iyer, S. N., Malla, A., Lepage, M., Joober, R., Boksa, P., & Shah, J. (2023). "The more things change…"? Stability of delusional themes across 12 years of presentations to an early intervention service for psychosis. *Social Psychiatry and Psychiatric Epidemiology, 58*, 35–41.

Hirjak, D., & Fuchs, T. (2010). Delusions of technical alien control: A phenomenological description of three cases. *Psychopathology, 43*, 96–103.

Jay, M. (2014). *A Visionary Madness*. Berkeley: North Atlantic Books.

Kelly, C. (1996). Advertising, politicians, and delusions in the mentally vulnerable. *The Lancet, 348*(9038), 1385–1385.

Krauss, F. (1967). *Selbstschilderungen eines Geisteskranken: Nothschrei eines Magnetisch-Vergifteten (1852) und Nothgedrungene Fortsetzung meines Nothschrei (1867)*. Leverkusen: Bayer Pharmaceuticals.

Lewis, D. (1978). Truth in fiction. *American Philosophical Quarterly, 15*(1), 37–46.

Linn, L. (1958). Some comments on the origin of the influencing machine. *Journal of the American Psychoanalytic Association, 6*(2), 305–308.

Maher, B. (1974). Delusional thinking and perceptual disorder. *Journal of Individual Psychology, 30*(1), 98–113.

McLean, B. F., Mattiske, J. K., & Balzan, R. P. (2017). Association of the Jumping to Conclusions and Evidence Integration biases with delusions in psychosis: A detailed meta-analysis. *Schizophr Bull, 43*(2), 344–354.

Noordhof, P., & Sullivan-Bissett, E. (2021). The clinical significance of anomalous experience in the explanation of monothematic delusions. *Synthese, 199*(3), 10277–10309.

Reagan, A. J., Mitchell, L., Kiley, D., Danforth, C. M., & Dodds, P. S. (2016). The emotional arcs of stories are dominated by six basic shapes. *EPJ Data Science, 5*, 31 DOI:10.1140/epjds/s13688-016-0093-1.

Schreber, D. P. (2000). *Memoirs of My Nervous Illness*. New York: New York Review of Books.

Stompe, T., Ortwein-Swoboda, G., Ritter, K., & Schanda, H. (2003). Old wine in new bottles? Stability and plasticity of the contents of schizophrenic delusions. *Psychopathology, 36*(1), 6–12.

Tausk, V. (1933). On the origin of the "influencing machine" in schizophrenia. *Psychoanalytic Quarterly, 2*, 519–556.

Tseng, W.-S. (2001). *Handbook of Cultural Psychiatry*. San Diego: Academic Press.

Vonnegut, K. (2005). Here is a lesson in creative writing. In Daniel Simon (ed.), *A Man Without a Country* (pp. 23–38). New York: Random House.

Zolotova, J., & Brune, M. (2006). Persecutory delusions: reminiscence of ancestral hostile threats? *Evolution and Human Behavior, 27*, 185–192.

37

# DELUSION AND CONSPIRACY THEORIES

*Joseph M. Pierre*

Philosophical musings about delusions are inevitably complicated by the nagging challenges that always seem to thwart the easy definition of terms and plague the development of taxonomies and nosologies. To start with, defining terms relies on other terms, leaving definitions vulnerable to ambiguity. Just so, while delusions are often generally characterized as fixed and false beliefs, there is substantially less clarity and agreement about what a belief is (Bentall 2018; Pierre 2019). Meanwhile, some philosophers have advanced the 'argument against doxasticism' which claims that delusions should not be properly classified as beliefs at all (Berrios 1991; Currie 2000; for a refutation see Miyazono and Bortolotti (2014) and Bortolotti and Miyazono (2015), and for more on delusion and (non-)doxasticism see Noordhof, Chapters 19 and 20).

Definitions are also contextually dependent, so that words tend to take on different meanings according to where and by whom they are used. As a psychiatric term, delusions are formally defined in the *Diagnostic and Statistical Manual of Mental Disorders* (*DSM*), but that definition has been critiqued and revised many times over (Spitzer 1990; Feyaerts et al. 2021). In clinical practice, it is applied in the service of 'clinical utility' as an umbrella term to capture a wide range of phenomena with no presumption that there is any unitary pathophysiology for all delusional subtypes. Largely ignorant of prediction error theories (see Corlett, Chapter 30) and two-factor models (see Davies and Coltheart, Chapter 29) that attempt explanatory unification, psychiatry makes no claim that all delusions are created equally. On the contrary, delusions with persecutory, grandiose, nihilistic, jealous, somatic, and misidentification content often carry distinct diagnostic implications that may lead to different interventions.

Although a central goal of the *DSM* since its third edition has been to strengthen the reliability of the categorical diagnoses and clinical terms defined within its pages, a well-known limitation remains that the establishment of validity for those terms and disorders has proven elusive (Pierre 2010). Many have therefore disputed whether the manual adequately 'carves nature at its joints' so that it describes 'natural kinds' (Zachar 2015, for more on delusion and natural kinds see Samuels, Chapter 5). In that sense, just like so many other words and terms, delusions are only what we say they are and their definition may not always perfectly encompass the essential qualities of all the phenomena the term intends

DOI: 10.4324/9781003296386-44

544

to categorize. It should come as no surprise then that psychiatrists, psychologists, philosophers, and other academics interested in delusions continue to debate their ideal characterization while making arguments by exception. Meanwhile, in the media and in lay speech, the word 'delusion' is applied much more carelessly—and often pejoratively—to describe an even wider variety of strongly held beliefs that are either incredible or objectionable to the person applying the label.

As with many other terms attempting to describe natural kinds, delusions can be modeled not only as defined categorical constructs but also as continuous entities. Consequently, while 'caseness' is often relatively easy to recognize at the extreme, it is much harder to identify at the 'gray areas' where the borders that separate them from other related and normal phenomena are blurred (Pierre 2010, 2013). So it is that we have 'delusions'—already a wastebasket category of heterogeneous phenomena—and 'delusion-like beliefs' that make up an even larger wastebasket (Pierre 2020a).

Conspiracy theories offer an illustrative and timely example of delusion-like beliefs that might resemble delusions at first glance, but can be reliably disentangled upon more careful examination (Bortolotti et al. 2021; Pierre, 2021; Starcevic and Brakoulias 2021; Veling et al. 2021). With the aforementioned challenges of infallible definition and categorization in mind, this chapter adopts a phenomenological, experiential, and clinically pragmatic perspective to make the case that delusions and conspiracy theory beliefs (CTB) warrant distinction based on meaningful practical differences.

## 1. Definitions and dimensions

The *DSM-5* defines a delusion as:

> A false belief based on incorrect inference about external reality that is firmly held despite what almost everyone else believes and despite what constitutes incontrovertible and obvious proof or evidence to the contrary. The belief is not ordinarily accepted by other members of the person's culture or subculture (i.e., is not an article of religious faith). When a false belief involves a value judgment, it is regarded as a delusion only when the judgment is so extreme as to defy credibility.
>
> *(American Psychiatric Association 2013: 819)*

This more detailed expansion of a delusion beyond a mere fixed, false belief has its roots in the conceptualization of psychiatrist and philosopher Karl Jaspers who emphasized the subjective certainty (conviction), incorrigibility (resistance to counterargument), and impossible content of delusions (Spitzer 1990). In the spirit of Jaspers' further suggestion that delusions are 'un-understandable' (Walker 1991; Cermolacce et al. 2010; Kendler and Campbell 2014), the *DSM-5* definition acknowledges that delusions can be regarded as an 'extreme' of a continuum since they 'defy credibility' while also taking care to differentiate them from widely held—that is, normative—cultural beliefs that might otherwise meet the definition of a delusion such as religious doctrines, political ideologies, and childhood beliefs in Santa Claus or the Tooth Fairy (for more on delusion and culture see Gold and Gold, Chapter 36, and for more on delusion and the madness of crowds, see Bentall, Chapter 38).

Unlike the term 'delusion', there is no official definition of a conspiracy theory sanctioned by any specific academic discipline or professional organization. One definition from an authoritative cross-disciplinary review of the subject calls conspiracy theories 'attempts to explain the ultimate causes of significant social and political events and circumstances with claims of secret plots by two or more powerful actors' (Douglas et al. 2019: 4). Another definition, acknowledging that CTB typically include both a negation that 'official accounts are false' and an affirmation that 'malevolent groups are conspiring' (Douglas et al. 2019: 6), posits that 'conspiracy theories reject authoritative accounts of reality in favor of some plot involving a group of people with malevolent intent that is deliberately kept secret from the public' (Pierre 2020b: 617).

Superficially then, with content that references clandestine plots and malevolent motives, CTB have a decidedly paranoid quality so that it might be tempting to toss them into the delusion wastebasket. Indeed, several studies have found that paranoid ideation and schizotypy are associated with a greater propensity for conspiracist ideation, suggesting a link between CTB and delusional thinking (Darwin et al. 2011; Dagnall et al. 2015). However, it is likely that such correlations are at least partially tautological, touching upon different aspects of the same phenomenon.

Much like Jasper's original distinction between 'delusional mood' and 'delusions proper', it should also be recognized that there are both qualitative and quantitative differences between dimensional constructs like paranoia, schizotypy, and 'conspiracy mentality' that reflect *proclivities* to believe and categorical constructs like 'paranoid delusion' and CTB that reflect *actual* beliefs. In other words, there are substantive differences in conviction between beliefs about 'what could be' and 'what is' such that finding that those who believe in conspiracy theories have a quantifiably paranoid cognitive style does not warrant the conclusion that such individuals are delusional per se.

## 2. Prevalence and mental illness

Delusions are listed in the *DSM* as a psychotic symptom found in a variety of mental disorders including schizophrenia and acute mood states such as major depressive episodes and mania with psychotic features. They can also occur as a standalone symptom emblematic of delusional disorder. In the general population, the prevalence of clinically relevant or 'true' delusions (as measured by affirmative responses to questions like 'have you ever felt that your thoughts were being directly interfered with or controlled by another person?') varies from 0.1 to 13 per cent (Heilskov et al. 2020). In non-clinical samples, about 1–3 per cent report delusions of a severity level comparable to clinical populations with an additional 5–6 per cent who endorse delusions of lesser severity (Freeman 2006). By contrast, 'delusion-like beliefs' that fall short of 'true' delusions (based on affirmative responses to general questions like 'have your relatives or friends ever considered any of your beliefs strange or unusual?' or 'do you feel that you have sinned more than the average person?') are far more common, occurring in as much as 91 per cent of surveyed samples (Heilskov et al. 2020).

Such wide-ranging prevalences reflect differences in both sample populations and the wording of questionnaires, with greater rates of endorsement when asking about general delusional attitudes as opposed to specific delusional beliefs and lower rates of caseness when applying thresholds determined by clinicians. However, this differential gradient does not hold true for CTB where both generic 'conspiracy mentality' (based on endorsing statements like 'many very important things happen in the world which the public is never informed about') and belief in more specific conspiracy theories (e.g., 'there was a conspiracy behind the murder of JFK') have been found to be exceedingly common in the general population (Stojanov and Halberstadt 2019). For example, a 2019 YouGov survey found that some 67–91 per cent of respondents across the world endorsed belief in at least one specific conspiracy theory (YouGov 2019). The most commonly endorsed CTB, rated as true by 17–48 per cent of the sample by country, was 'members of Donald Trump's election team knowingly worked with the Russian Government to help him win the 2016 US Presidential election'.

Despite the media's occasional characterization of widespread CTB as indicative of 'mass delusion' or 'mass psychosis', these statistical findings make clear that unlike delusions, CTB are endorsed by the majority of the population so that they must be acknowledged as a normal phenomenon. This conclusion is in keeping with observations about conspiracy theories in the modern academic literature. For example, in his now classic 1964 essay on the emergence of pervasive conspiratorial thinking in the political sphere, *The Paranoid Style in American Politics*, the historian Richard Hofstadter's explained:

> I call it the paranoid style simply because no other word adequately evokes the sense of heated exaggeration, suspiciousness, and conspiratorial fantasy that I have in mind. In using the expression 'paranoid style' I am not speaking in a clinical sense, but borrowing a clinical term for other purposes. I have neither the competence nor the desire to classify any figures of the past or present as certifiable lunatics. In fact, the idea of the paranoid style as a force in politics would have little relevance or historical value if it were applied only to men with profoundly disturbed minds. It is the use of paranoid modes of expression by more or less normal people that makes the phenomenon significant.
>
> *(Hofstadter 1964: 77)*

Although psychology research over the past two decades has revealed a laundry list of psychological needs and cognitive quirks—like needs for closure, certainty, control, and uniqueness; attribution biases; bullshit receptivity; and lack of analytical thinking—associated with those who demonstrate a propensity for CTB (Douglas et al. 2019), these represent quantitative rather than qualitative differences and, in any case, do not constitute symptoms of mental illness (Pierre 2020b). Indeed, it has been noted that such findings have 'done much to humanize' conspiracy believers:

> Research has begun to make significant strides in shifting the conversation ever so slightly from the image of a foil-hat-wearing, conspiracy-theory-believing 'other people' to a more forgiving conception of conspiracy ideation arising in normal people exposed to the proper triggers—for example, circumstances that evoke feelings of vulnerability.
>
> *(Bost 2015)*

Unless we radically revise what it means to be mentally ill, it is therefore inappropriate to equate CTB with delusions or to claim they are indicative of mental disorder. Instead, CTB should be understood and more properly categorized as delusion-like beliefs with little direct relevance to psychiatric diagnosis.


## 3.   Falsity and fixity

Delusions are by definition 'false' and 'fixed', meaning that they are both 'wrong beliefs' as well as notoriously resistant to counterargument (Berrios 1991). However, there are inevitable exceptions to this rule, such as when delusions of jealousy are based on faulty reasoning or lack of evidence but turn out to be true anyway or when beliefs—like many with religious content—are not falsifiable. In such instances, it has been argued that caseness can be assessed by quantifying the cognitive dimensions of delusional belief including preoccupation, conviction, and distress (Pierre 2001, Peters et al. 2004).

With that in mind, a shortcoming of surveys about CTB is that they often force respondents into dichotomous answers without allowing them to quantify their belief conviction. And yet, since falsity and fixity are not defining elements of CTB, neither are requisites for caseness. Although delusions cease to be delusions when they are determined not to be 'wrong beliefs' or when they are no longer held with unassailable conviction, the same cannot be said of conspiracy theories. While conspiracy theories are often portrayed as improbable or based on flimsy evidence, they are—as conspiracy theory believers like to remind us—sometimes properly reasoned and occasionally turn out to be true. Just as when we sometimes refer to 'evolution' as 'evolutionary theory' however, we still often refer to conspiracies as conspiracies theories even when they are substantiated or factual.

In a similar fashion and in contrast to delusions, CTB remain CTB across a continuum of conviction. While they can be impassioned claims that are stereotypically resistant to counterevidence the way delusions are, they do not have to be. They are, after all, only beliefs about theories. Indeed, for those who identify as conspiracy theory believers, endorsed belief might reflect anything from a kind of dalliance to a signal of group or political affiliation (Lewandowsky 2021).

This point is aptly illustrated by a 2020 survey in which respondents endorsed support for the conspiracy theory-based political movement QAnon, but were often unaware of its more outrageous conspiratorial claims and nevertheless rated some of them as 'true' despite encountering them for the first time (Schaffner 2020). For example, 22 per cent of respondents believed that 'a global network tortures and sexually abuses children in Satanic rituals' and 18 per cent believed that 'Trump [was] secretly preparing a mass arrest of government officials and celebrities', but those percentages dropped to only 12 and 6 per cent respectively after subtracting out those who only encountered those claims for the first time through the survey. Unlike delusions then, endorsement of CTB may at times be more consistent with predispositions or attitudes than convicted beliefs. In that way, the argument against doxasticism applies much more to weakly held CTB than it does to delusions (Ichino and Räikkä 2021; Duetz 2022).

In other words, while delusions are fixed, false beliefs representing an extreme of unwarranted conviction, conspiracy theories refer to a much wider range of phenomena (Starcevic and Brakoulias 2021). Moving from one end of a continuum of conviction to the other, there is conspiracy mentality unassociated with any specific belief, conspiracy theories that are merely suppositions, CTB representing beliefs about theories held with variable conviction, and under certain circumstances discussed at the end of this chapter, delusional beliefs about conspiracy theories. The distinction between delusions and conspiracy theories would be less fraught with ambiguity if researchers, clinicians, and journalists alike took greater care to avoid the conflation of conspiratorial facts, suppositions, beliefs, and delusions.


## 4.  Shared beliefs and self-referentiality

Extending Jaspers' conceptualization that delusions are both impossible and un-understandable, it has been suggested that a defining feature of delusions is that they are also unshareable

(Pierre 2020a). Indeed, according to the *DSM* definition, when the falsity of beliefs—like those of a religious or political nature—cannot be determined, their exclusion from delusionality is instead judged based on a proxy of cultural or subcultural acceptance and sanctioning (Pierre 2001). Although cases of shared delusions (e.g., *folie á deux, folie impose*) have long been recognized in psychiatry as exceptions to this rule, this relatively rare phenomenon has generally been attributed to a dominant individual's ability to impose their delusional thinking on a susceptible subordinate (Shimizu et al. 2007). Shared delusions aside then, delusions are best characterized as idiosyncratic beliefs that are not typically shared by others.

As the prevalence data cited earlier clearly demonstrate however, that is hardly the case with CTB. While a conspiracy theory might be contrived and maintained by a single individual, more often they are widely shared to the point of being cultural memes.

Just what is it that makes CTB shareable, but delusions not? Historically, the unshareability of delusions has been linked to the improbability or impossibility of their 'bizarre' content, but the inter-rater reliability of bizarreness has since been found to be notoriously poor (Spitzer et al. 1993). Indeed, a cursory look at mainstream religious beliefs (e.g., Jesus Christ was the son of God) and CTB (e.g., the Earth is flat) alike readily demonstrates that impossible content is not a good predictor of shareability.

Instead, a more reliable determinant of the shareability of improbable or dubious beliefs relates to their self-referentiality. For example, while it is easy to find those who share the belief that there will be a second coming of Christ, that telekinesis is possible, that a microchip could be implanted in one's body for the purposes of tracking, or that alien abductions have occurred; it would be much harder to find confederates who share the belief that *you* are the Messiah, that *you* can move objects with your mind, that *you* have a microchip implanted in your brain, or that *you* were abducted by aliens.

When encountered in clinical practice, delusions are most commonly—if not always— self-referential beliefs. Paranoid patients worry that they are being followed, surveilled, or otherwise imperiled; grandiose delusions represent inflated attributions about one's self; somatic delusions relate to one's personal health, and even delusions of jealousy, erotomania, and misidentification that involve other people ultimately refer to how those people are interacting with the believer.

In contrast to delusions, CTB are almost never self-referential. Indeed, it has been said that while the 'paranoid person believes "they are out to get me"; the conspiracy theorist believes "they are out to get *us*"'(Stojanov and Halberstadt 2019: 216). Hofstadter made the same observation in the updated 1966 version of *The Paranoid Style in American Politics*:

> In the paranoid style, as I conceive it, the feeling of persecution is central, and it is indeed systematized in grandiose theories of conspiracy. But there is a vital difference between the paranoid spokesman in politics and the clinical paranoiac: although they both tend to be overheated, oversuspicious, overaggressive, grandiose, and apocalyptic in expression, the clinical paranoiac sees the hostile and conspiratorial world in which he feels himself to be living as directed specifically against him; whereas the spokesman of the paranoid style finds it directed against a nation, a culture, a way of life whose fate affects not himself alone but millions of others.
>
> *(Hofstadter 1966: 4)*

This distinction is supported by a study by Roland Imhoff and Pia Lamberty (2018) that explored correlations between measures of conspiracy mentality, CTB, paranoia, and spheres of control (e.g., personal, interpersonal, and sociopolitical) and found that while CTB and paranoia may be related constructs, CTB is associated with general sociopolitical concerns about powerful groups, whereas paranoia is linked to self-relevant beliefs related to concerns about interpersonal threats and control.

Such distinction based on self-referentiality—with delusions defined as fixed, false, and self-referential beliefs and CTB as improbable suppositions about world events—provides validation that delusions should remain a clinical term of psychiatry whose utility lies in its association with mental illness, whereas conspiracy theories should be considered to be a normative phenomenon of social psychology and political science unrelated to individual psychopathology.

## 5.    Rationale and evidence

Psychological research going back several decades has attempted to elucidate the cognitive underpinnings of delusional thinking. One of the most replicated findings from this research is that those with delusional beliefs tend to demonstrate a 'jumping to conclusions' (JTC) cognitive bias thought to reflect hasty decision-making based on inadequate evidence (Dudley et al. 2016). More recently, similar efforts have also detected evidence of the JTC bias among those who endorse conspiracy theories, suggesting a cognitive link between delusions and CTB (Pytik et al. 2020). Among those with CTB, the JTC bias has also been linked to a 'intuitive thinking'—a cognitive style or preferential way of thinking characterized by a reliance on intuition as opposed to analytical thinking or a need for evidence when forming factual beliefs (Garrett and Weeks 2017). A preference for intuitive thinking over analytical thinking appears to be a common unifying thread across several types of overconfident and 'epistemically suspect' misbeliefs, including delusional thinking, BCT, bullshit receptivity, and belief in 'fake news' (Bronstein et al. 2019; Binnendyk and Pennycook 2022).

Faith in intuition has been modeled as an automatic, gut-level, fast-reasoning heuristic that makes things seem true or feel true without bothering to second guess them. And yet, by itself, this cognitive style fails to account for the diversity of delusions and CTB and the differences between them so that we must look past common general cognitive mechanisms to more closely examine just what the 'things' are that feel true to believers. When assessing delusional thinking and CTB alike, we must therefore ask both *what* people believe and *why* they believe it—that is, what is the evidence to support a particular belief? (Pierre 2021).

When providing an account of delusions, patients often cite anomalous subjective experiences as the rationale for their self-referential beliefs (e.g. 'I believe that I'm Jesus Christ because I heard the voice of God tell me so and I can feel the Holy Spirit flowing through me') (Sakakibara 2019; Noordhof and Sullivan-Bissett 2021). Indeed, despite the *DSM*'s claim that delusions are 'false inferences about external reality', delusions are most often—if not always—beliefs about internal experiences and a kind of subjective reality. Following the tradition of Jaspers, this feature of delusional reasoning has been referred to as drawing from a 'private, quasi-solipsistic domain of experience' (Feyaerts et al. 2021: 239). While this perspective may be related to faith in intuition, it might be more appropriately described as 'faith in subjectivity'. A personal account based on lived experience with delusional thinking characterizes that subjectivity as a 'parallel or other reality that holds as much validity as the shared, ordinary world' or 'subjectivity outside subjectivity' (Jensen 2022: 1, 2).

It has been argued that in contrast to delusions, CTB are not based on subjective experience but instead arise from a combination from epistemic mistrust of authoritative sources of information and biased processing of misinformation (Pierre 2020b). According to this model, epistemic mistrust represents a lack of faith in mainstream accounts of events such that they are discounted and dismissed as unreliable. By itself, epistemic mistrust can lead to the kind of denialism that leaves an individual with a conspiracy mentality in the absence of any specific CTB per se. But such denialism can just as easily lead to actual CTB through an active search for information that is subject to normative processing biases like confirmation bias and motivated reasoning that leave us vulnerable to misinformation encountered when 'just asking questions' and 'looking for answers' (Klein et al. 2018). In this way, the formation of CTB is not so much a process of theorizing as it is one of gathering the evidence to support CTB by 'sifting through information, deciding what to believe and what to disregard' and 'crafting a narrative based on the synthesis of available information' (Pierre 2020b: 625). In other words, CTB 'do not arise *de novo*' the way that delusions do; 'they are already "out there", lying in wait' (Pierre 2020b: 625). For example, believing that the Earth is flat can be understood as a two-component process that involves both the premise that 'NASA is lying' and a justification that 'I did my own research on YouTube and found the *real* facts'.

Similar to shared delusions, CTB are therefore typically transmitted from one source to another. However, conspiracy theories rarely if ever originate with the delusion of someone with mental illness, but instead arise from unsubstantiated misinformation in the form of rumors and speculation, as well as deliberate disinformation disseminated by 'conspiracy entrepreneurs' in pursuit of profits that are both financial and political (Sunstein and Vermeule 2009). Indeed, conspiracy theories tend to spread much more widely than delusions, even in those cases when the latter are shared.

While the familiar aphorism, 'insanity is a sane response to an insane society' is overused and unjustified when referring to actual delusions that reflect mental illness, it is a reasonable way to characterize CTB that can be understood as byproducts of a 'sick society'. Accordingly, while the remedies for delusions involve individual mental health interventions like antipsychotic medication or cognitive behavioral therapy, the pervasiveness of CTB requires the remediation of both epistemic mistrust on a societal scale and the ubiquity and easy appeal of misinformation across today's media landscape (Pierre 2020b).

## 6.  Belief and action

In addition to symptomatic criteria, the *DSM* defines the caseness of mental disorders based upon the presence of distress and/or impairment of functioning. Just so, when delusions occurring in the context of disorders like schizophrenia are encountered in clinical practice, they are typically identified as complaints or sources of dysfunction even though they are associated with anosognosia or lack of insight. For example, while a patient does not recognize that he is suffering from paranoid delusions per se, he still laments that people are following him and that his life is in danger.

When delusions occur as a standalone symptom of delusional disorder, the *DSM-5* recognizes that 'functional impairment is usually more circumscribed than that seen with other psychiatric disorders' and specifies that 'apart from the impact of the delusion(s) or its ramifications, functioning is not markedly impaired, and behavior is not obviously bizarre or odd' (American Psychiatric Association 2013: 90, 93). However, it still notes that 'impairment may be substantial' including 'social, marital, and work problems', an 'irritable or dysphoric mood… as a reaction to… delusional beliefs', as well as anger, violence, and 'litigious or antagonistic behavior' (American Psychiatric Association 2013; 92, 93).

These sober clinical realities offer a refutation of arguments against doxasticism which claim that those with delusions do not act on their beliefs owing to a kind of 'double bookkeeping' (for more on double bookkeeping see Porcher, Chapter 13) or that delusions play a protective role so that they are 'epistemically innocent' in a fashion similar to 'positive illusions' (Bortolotti 2015; Sullivan-Bissett 2018). Of course, such a pathologizing perspective may reflect a clinical bias based on a selected sample of those who are seeking or are otherwise referred to psychiatric care. Certainly, there are some who prefer delusional beliefs over reality and can harbor delusional thinking without significant distress (Van Putten et al. 1976; Roberts 1991). And yet, clinical delusions more often involve content that is disturbing in some way or puts believers at odds with others—as in the case of grandiose and erotomanic delusions—so that they cause significant social disruption.

The dysfunctional reality of delusional beliefs is unsurprising when we consider that it is the characteristic self-referential nature of delusions that tends to motivate behavior. Conversely, the stereotypically non-self-referential nature of CTB means that they can be endorsed without any significant association with distress, dysfunction, or social impairment. After all, believing that the Earth is flat, that the moon landing was faked, or that 9/11 was an inside job does not demand action in the same way that passionate convictions about being in personal danger, or being the Messiah, or being the love object of a famous person do.

Still, much of the interest in conspiracy theories in recent years has stemmed from the fact that CTB are indeed sometimes associated with behaviors that are harmful and socially disruptive such as when anti-vaccine conspiracy theories lead to low vaccination rates that result in a loss of or failure to establish herd immunity against infectious disease or when political conspiracies lead to civil unrest and violent anti-government revolt. While anti-vaccine and political conspiracy theories may not refer to the believer per se, they do represent beliefs about personal vulnerability to global threats. In other words, behavior driven by CTB is not so much a result of self-referentiality as self-relevant consequentiality.

The 'two-pyramids model' of political radicalization and violent extremism that has been applied to both 'lone-wolf' terrorists and members of terrorist groups alike argues that ideological belief can be decoupled from action with differential forces that can escalate each separately (McCauley and Moskalenko 2014; McCauley and Moskalenko 2017). A similar, but integrative model relevant to CTB proposes that ideological affiliation can be usefully conceptualized along stages of belief conviction that include 'non-believers', 'fence-sitters', 'true believers', 'activists', and 'apostates' (Pierre 2023). At the activist stage, shared CTB have fused with a collective ideological identity so that challenges to beliefs are interpreted as existential threats that serve as a call to action in the name of self-defense or in order to fight for a cause.

While the case has been made for the epistemic innocence—that is, the potential benefit and adaptiveness—of delusions and CTB alike (Bortolotti 2015; Sullivan-Bissett 2018; Lancellotta and Bortolotti 2019; van Prooijen 2022), both can motivate dysfunctional and socially disruptive behavior in proportion to their respective self-referentiality and self-relevant consequentiality. If there is a practical commonality between these epistemic phenomena, it is that acting on false beliefs—whether delusions or CTB—always risks at least the potential for harm.

## 7.  Conclusion

This chapter makes the argument that delusions and CTB can be reliably distinguished based on phenomenological differences with practical relevance. However, as wastebasket terms, 'delusions' and 'conspiracy theories' encompass a wide range of misbeliefs that can be conceptualized according to both categorical definitions and continuous models with fuzzy boundaries. Attempts to reliably delineate them have therefore been fraught by inconsistency and imperfection with inevitable exceptions that point to the shortcomings of proposed definitional criteria, though this may be better thought of as a reflection of the underlying heterogeneity within a spectrum of phenomena than any broad definitional failure.

With such inevitable semantic limitations in mind, this chapter concludes by acknowledging that delusions and CTB are not always mutually exclusive—it is possible, as mentioned earlier, for individuals to have delusions about conspiracy theories. Consider the example of 'gang-stalking', a proposed phenomenon purporting that governments, law enforcement agencies, and other entities are secretly conducting mass surveillance, harassment, and mind-control of self-described 'targeted individuals' using the likes of electromagnetic field radiation and 'voice-to-skull' technology (Tait 2020; Pierre 2020a). With a significant volume of information available—much of it online—that claims that this is really happening and a cottage industry marketing electronic devices to protect consumers from gang-stalking such that it has become a widely shared belief about what is going on in the world, it qualifies as a conspiracy theory. And yet, targeted individuals also make self-referential claims about their personal experiences with gang-stalking that, when clinically assessed, have been found to be consistent with paranoid delusions (Sheridan and James 2015). In some cases, such paranoia—fueled by the shared CTB of like-minded individuals—has been linked to violence and mass shootings (Sarteschi 2018).

Gang-stalking lies at the intersection of conspiracy theory and paranoid delusions that have attained cultural or sub-cultural sanctioning as a purportedly global occurrence, with support groups that have emerged to validate the personal experiences of targeted individuals. That self-referential paranoid delusions that should, in theory, be unshareable can become shareable is testament to the complexity of social influences that impact delusions and CTB alike (Bell et al. 2020; Miyazono and Salice 2020), particularly in the internet era when misinformation and subjective experience masquerading as objective evidence can be easily found to support the most idiosyncratic beliefs. Such vexing examples will continue to challenge attempts to carve nature at its joints and develop a precise taxonomy of delusions and delusion-like beliefs.

## References


American Psychiatric Association. (2013) *Diagnostic and Statistical Manual of Mental Disorders*, Fifth Edition, American Psychiatric Association: Washington, DC.

Bell, V., Raihani, N. and Wilkinson, S. (2020) "Derationalizing Delusions," *Clinical Psychological Science* 9:24–37.

Bentall, R. (2018) "Delusions and Other Beliefs," in: L. Bortolotti (ed.) *Delusions in Context*, Palgrave Macmillan: Switzerland, pp. 67–95.

Berrios, G.E. (1991) "Delusions as 'Wrong Beliefs': A Conceptual History," *The British Journal of Psychiatry* 159 (Suppl 14):6–13.

Binnendyk, J. and Pennycook, G. (2022) "Intuition, Reason, and Conspiracy Beliefs," *Current Opinion in Psychology* 47:101387.

Bortolotti, L. (2015) "The Epistemic Innocence of Motivated Delusions," *Consciousness and Cognition* 33:490–499.

Bortolotti, L. and Miyazono, K. (2015) "Recent Work on the Nature and Development of Delusions," *Philosophy Compass* 10/9:636–645.

Bortolotti, L., Ichino, A. and Mameli, M. (2021) "Conspiracy Theories and Delusions," *Reti, Saperi, Linguaggi: Italian Journal of Cognitive Sciences* 8:183–200.

Bost, P. (2015) "Crazy Beliefs, Sane Believers: Toward a Cognitive Psychology of Conspiracy Ideation," *Skeptical Inquirer* 39, January/February.

Bronstein, M.V., Pennycook, G., Bear, A., Rand, D.G. and Cannon, T.D. (2019) "Belief in Fake News in Associated with Delusionality, Dogmatism, Religious Fundamentalism, and Reduced Analytical Thinking," *Journal of Applied Research in Memory and Cognition* 8:108–117.

Cermolacce, M., Sass, L. and Parnas, J. (2010) "What is Bizarre in Bizarre Delusions? A Critical Review," *Schizophrenia Bulletin* 36:667–679.

Currie, G. (2000) "Imagination, Delusion and Hallucinations," *Mind and Language* 15:168–183.

Dagnall, N., Drinkwater, K., Parker, A., Denovan, A. and Parton, M. (2015) "Conspiracy Theory and Cognitive Style: A Worldview," *Frontiers in Psychology* 6:206.

Darwin, H., Neave, N. and Holmes, J. (2011) "Belief in Conspiracy Theories. The Role of Paranormal Belief, Paranoid Ideation and Schizotypy," *Personality and Individual Differences* 50:1289–1293.

Douglas, K.M., Uscinski, J.E., Sutton, R.M., Cichocka, A., Nefes, T., Ang, C.S. and Deravi, F. (2019) "Understanding Conspiracy Theories," *Political Psychology* 40(Suppl 13–35):3–35.

Dudley, R., Taylor, P., Wickham, S. and Hutton, P. (2016) "Psychosis, Delusions and the 'Jumping to Conclusions' Reasoning Bias: A Systematic Review and Meta-analysis," *Schizophrenia Bulletin* 42:652–665.

Duetz, J.C.M. (2022) "Conspiracy Theories are Not Beliefs," *Erkenntinis*, September 20.

Feyaerts, J., Henriksen, M.G., Vanheule, S., Myin-Gerneys, I. and Sass, L.A. (2021) "Delusions Beyond Beliefs: A Critical Overview of Diagnostic, Aetiological, and Therapeutic Schizophrenia Research from a Clinical-Phenomenological Perspective," *Lancet Psychiatry*, 8:237–249.

Freeman, G. (2006). "Delusions in the Nonclinical Population." *Current Psychiatry Reports* 8: 191–204.

Garrett, R.K. and Weeks, B.E. (2017) "Epistemic Beliefs' Role in Promoting Misperceptions and Conspiracist Ideation," *PLoS ONE* 12(9):e0184733.

Heilskov, S.E.R., Urfer-Parnas, A. and Nordgaard, J. (2020) "Delusions in the General Population: A Systematic Review with Emphasis on Methodology," *Schizophrenia Research* 216:48–55.

Hofstadter, R. (1964) "The Paranoid Style in American Politics," *Harper's Magazine*, November, pp. 77–86.

Hofstadter, R. (1966) *The Paranoid Style in American Politics and Other Essays*, Cambridge MA: Harvard University Press.

Ichino, A. and Räikkä, J. (2021). "Non-doxastic Conspiracy Theories," *Argumenta* 7:247–263.

Imhoff, R. and Lamberty, P. (2018) "How Paranoid are Conspiracy Believers? Toward a More Fine-Grained Understanding of the Connect and Disconnect Between Paranoia and Belief in Conspiracy Theories," *European Journal of Social Psychology* 48:909–926.

Jensen, G. (2022). Delusion and Reason: An Argument for a Phenomenological Model of Understanding Schizophrenic Delusion. *Schizophrenia Bulletin* sbac185.

Kendler, K.S. and Campbell, J. (2014). "Expanding the Domain of the Understandable in Psychiatric Illness: An Updating of the Jasperian Framework of Explanation and Understanding," *Psychological Medicine* 44:1–7.

Klein, C., Clutton, P. and Polito, V. (2018) "Topic Modeling Reveals Distinct Interests Within an Online Conspiracy Forum," *Frontiers in Psychology* 9:189.

Lancellotta, E. and Bortolotti, L. (2019) "Are Clinical Delusions Adaptive?" *WIREs Cognitive Science* 10:e1502.

Lewandowsky, S. (2021) "Conspiracist Cognition: Chaos, Convenience, and Cause for Concern," *Journal for Cultural Research* 25:12–35.

McCauley, C. and Moskalenko, S. (2014) "Toward a Profile of Lone Wolf Terrorists: What Moves an Individual From Radical Opinion to Radical Action," *Terrorism and Political Violence* 26:69–85.

McCauley, C. and Moskalenko, S. (2017) "Understanding Political Radicalization: The Two-Pyramids Model," *American Psychologist* 72:205–216.

Miyazono, K. and Bortolotti, L. (2014). "The Causal Role Argument Against Doxasticism About Delusions," *AVANT* 5:30–50.

Miyazono, K. and Salice, A. (2020). "Social Epistemological Conception of Delusion," *Synthese* 199:1831–1851.

Noordhof, P. and Sullivan-Bissett, E. (2021) "The Clinical Significance of Anomalous Experience in the Explanation of Monothematic Delusions," *Synthese* 199:10277–10309.

Peters, E., Joseph, S., Day S. and Garety, P. (2004) "Measuring Delusional Ideation: The 21-item Peters et al. Delusions Inventory (PDI)," *Schizophrenia Bulletin* 30:1005–1022.

Pierre, J. (2001) "Faith or Delusion? At the Crossroads of Religion and Psychosis," *Journal of Psychiatric Practice* 7:163–172.

Pierre, J.M. (2010) "The Borders of Mental Disorder in Psychiatry and the DSM: Past, Present, and Future," *Journal of Psychiatric Practice* 16:375–386.

Pierre, J.M. (2013) "Overdiagnosis, Underdiagnosis, Synthesis: A Dialectic for Psychiatry and the DSM," in: J. Paris and J. Philips (eds) *Making the DSM-5: Concepts and Controversies*, Springer: New York, pp. 105–124.

Pierre, J.M. (2019) "Integrating Non-psychiatric Models of Delusion-like Beliefs into Forensic Psychiatric Assessment," *Journal of the American Academy of Psychiatry and the Law* 47:171–179.

Pierre, J.M. (2020a) "Forensic Psychiatry Versus the Variety of Delusion-like Beliefs," *Journal of the American Academy of Psychiatry and the Law* 48:327–334.

Pierre, J.M. (2020b) "Mistrust and Misinformation: A Two Component, Socio-epistemic Model of Belief in Conspiracy Theories," *Journal of Social and Political Psychology* 8:617–641.

Pierre, J.M. (2021) "Conspiracy Theory or Delusion? 3 Questions to Tell Them Apart," *Current Psychiatry* 20:44,60.

Pierre, J.M. (2023) "Down the Conspiracy Theory Rabbit Hole: How Does One Become a Follower of QAnon?" in: M. Miller (ed.) *The Social Science of QAnon*, Cambridge University Press: Cambridge.

Pytik, N., Soll, D. and Mehl, S. (2020) "Thinking Preferences and Conspiracy Belief: Intuitive Thinking and the Jumping to Conclusions-Bias as a Basis for the Belief in Conspiracy Theories," *Frontiers in Psychiatry* 11:568942.

Roberts, R. (1991) "Delusional Belief Systems and Meaning in Life: A Preferred Reality?" *British Journal of Psychiatry* 159 (Suppl 14):19–28.

Sakakibara, E. (2019) "Intensity of Experience: Maher's Theory of Schizophrenic Delusion Revisited," *Neuroethics* 12:171–182.

Sarteschi, C.M. (2018) "Mass Murder, Targeted Individuals, and Gang-Stalking: Exploring the Connection," *Violence and Gender* 5:45–54.

Schaffner, B. (2020) "QAnon and Conspiracy Beliefs," September 18–20. Available at: https://www.isdglobal.org/wp-content/uploads/2020/10/qanon-and-conspiracy-beliefs.pdf

Sheridan, L.P. and James, D.V. (2015) "Complaints of Group-Stalking ('Gang Stalking'): An Exploratory Study of Their Nature and Impact on Complainants," *The Journal of Forensic Psychiatry and Psychology* 26:601–623.

Shimizu, M., Kubota, Y., Toichi, M. and Baba, H. (2007) "Folie á deux and Shared Psychotic Disorder," *Current Psychiatry Reports* 9:200–205.

Spitzer, M. (1990) "On Defining Delusions," *Comprehensive Psychiatry* 31:377–397.

Spitzer, R.L., First, M.B., Kendler, K.S. and Stein, D.J. (1993) "The Reliability of Three Definitions of Bizarre Delusions," *American Journal of Psychiatry* 150:880–884.

Starcevic, V. and Brakoulias, V. (2021). "'Things Are Not What They Seem to Be': A Proposal for the Spectrum Approach to Conspiracy Beliefs," *Australasian Psychiatry* 29:535–539.

Stojanov, A. and Halberstadt, J. (2019) "The Conspiracy Mentality Scale," *Social Psychology* 50:215–232.

Sullivan-Bissett, E. (2018) "Monothematic Delusion: A Case of Innocence From Experience," *Philosophical Psychology* 31:920–947.

Sunstein, C. and Vermeule, A. (2009) "Conspiracy Theories: Causes and Cures," *The Jou]rnal of Political Philosophy* 17:202–237.

Tait, A. (2020) "'Am I Going Crazy or Am I being Stalked?' Inside the Disturbing Online World of Gangstalking," *MIT Technology Review*, August 7.

van Prooijen, J-W. (2022) "Psychological Benefits of Believing Conspiracy Theories," *Current Opinion in Psychology* 47:101352.

Van Putten, T., Crumpton, E. and Yale, C. (1976) "Drug Refusal in Schizophrenia and the Wish to Be Crazy," *Archives of General Psychiatry* 33:1443–1446.
Veling, W., Sizoo, B., van Buuren, J., van den Berg, C., Sewbalak, W., Pijnenborg, G.H.M., Boonstra, N., Castelein, S. and van der Meer, L. (2021) "Are Conspiracy Theories Psychotic? A Comparison Between Conspiracy Theories and Paranoid Delusions," *Tijdschrift Voor Psychiatrie* 63:775–881.
Walker, C. (1991) "Delusion: What Did Jaspers Really Say?" *British Journal of Psychiatry* 159 (Suppl 14):94–103.
YouGov. (2019) "Cambridge Globalism Project – Conspiracy Theories," YouGov; Fieldwork Dates 28th February to 26th March 2019. Available at: https://d25d2506sfb94s.cloudfront.net/cumulus_uploads/document/2c6lta5kbu/YouGov%20Cambridge%20Globalism%20Project%20-%20Conspiracy%20Theories.pdf
Zachar, P. (2015) "Psychiatric Disorders: Natural Kinds Made by the World or Practical Kinds Made by Us?" *World Psychiatry* 14:288–290.

# 38
# DELUSION AND THE UNREALISTIC COMPARATOR

*Richard Bentall*

In this chapter, I will attempt to achieve the following goals. First, by introducing some difficult cases and considering some contemporary definitions of delusions, I will highlight some of the challenges we encounter when attempting to distinguish between delusional and nondelusional beliefs. I will then proceed to discuss three research strategies that have been commonly employed with the aim of discovering the unique features of delusions. This will take me to my main point, namely that those attempting to discover the unique characteristics of delusions have very often used an unrealistic comparator (either mundane beliefs or an entirely hypothetical idea of what 'normal beliefs' look like). Although there will not be scope here to fully develop a more realistic account of beliefs, I will then point to three features of beliefs in general – that certainty is feeling rather than a judgement, that beliefs are organized, and that they are transmissible from one person to another – which have been overlooked by psychiatric researchers. These observations will lead me to a novel proposal about what makes beliefs delusional, namely that they are not generated or proliferated within a network of social relations.

## 1.   Difficult cases

Let us begin with the case of the celebrated modernist poet Ezra Pound, who was detained by American forces in the Italian village of Sant'Ambrogio as the Second World War in Europe was drawing to an end. After a period of interrogation in Italy, during which he was harshly treated by his captors, Pound, who was an American citizen but a long-time antisemite and supporter of fascism, was transported to Washington. There he was charged with treason on account of the propaganda broadcasts he had made during the war on behalf of the Italian government, which had insulted Churchill and Roosevelt and praised Hitler's genocidal policies ('Until England and America delouse, and get rid of her Jew gangs, there is no place for either England or the United States in the new world at all'). If found guilty, Pound faced the death penalty but, before his trial, he was referred for a psychiatric evaluation. After being examined by doctors who he later called 'kakiatrists' (most were Jewish), he spent 12 years as a patient at St Elizabeth's Hospital in Washington DC with a diagnosis of schizophrenia. During this period, he won the prestigious Bollingen

     DOI: 10.4324/9781003296386-45

Prize for his poetry, and he was eventually released following a campaign by friends and writers including the novelist Ernest Hemmingway and the poet Robert Frost (his lawyer had the treason indictment dismissed in 1958). To this day, a small industry of Pound scholars continues to debate whether the poet's attitude towards Jews and support for fascism disqualify him as a great artist, and whether they were evidence of a mental illness that long preceded his detention in hospital, or were simply expressions of his unpleasant character (Swift 2018).

Although psychiatric manuals do not include a category of political delusions, the rarely acknowledged difficulty of distinguishing between psychosis and extreme ideology has occasionally resurfaced more recently. During the 1970s, in the United States, the diagnosis of schizophrenia was often applied to black men involved in the violent protests of the civil rights movement (Metzel 2009) and some American psychiatrists proposed a new diagnosis of 'protest psychosis' characterized by 'delusional anti-whiteness' (Bromberg and Simon 1968). In the same period, political dissidents in the then Soviet Union found themselves at risk of detention on psychiatric wards with a diagnosis of 'sluggish schizophrenia', a practice that was not the result of organized political oppression but was, instead, the consequence of a very broad concept of schizophrenia developed by the Moscow School of Psychiatry (symptoms included 'contentiousness' and 'philosophical concerns') (Reich 1984). Even more recently, most readers will be familiar of the case of the Norwegian terrorist Anders Breivik, who justified his 2011 murder of 77 people (mostly teenage political activists) on the grounds that he was member of a secret organization fighting feminism and the Islamification of Europe. Breivik was initially diagnosed as suffering from paranoid schizophrenia, opening the possibility of an insanity defence, until protests by mental health professionals, by the general public and by Breivik himself led to the diagnosis being withdrawn (Melle 2013).

Religious ideologies similarly provide plenty of scope for blurring the distinction between delusions and nonpathological beliefs. When the Mormon fundamentalists Ron and Dan Lafferty murdered their brother's wife and infant daughter in 1983, American psychiatrists and psychologists were divided about whether Ron, who claimed he had been instructed to carry out the killings by Jesus Christ, was mentally ill (Krakauer 2003). Dan, who was tried separately after Ron made a suicide attempt, conducted his own defence and was not evaluated by mental health professionals. However, to this day he claims to be the Prophet Elijah who will one day walk free when the walls of his prison collapse. Meanwhile, empirical research has highlighted many similarities between people with strongly held religious beliefs and people with psychosis. For example, people with very strong religious beliefs sometimes score highly on measures of schizotypy and delusional ideation (Smith et al. 2009). They may also share with deluded patients an unusually strong desire for meaning in their lives (Roberts 1991) and some have a propensity for abnormal experiences (Jackson and Fulford 1997). Perhaps unsurprisingly, both mental health professionals and lay people struggle to decide whether some religious beliefs are delusional, especially when they are faced with the beliefs of minority religions (O'Connor and Vandenberg 2005, 2010). For example, followers of the Nation of Islam (an African-American religious movement founded in Detroit in the 1930s, which holds that the Earth is 76 trillion years old, black people were the original inhabitants, and that white people are a race of devils created 6,600 years-ago) are particularly at risk of being diagnosed as mentally ill.

Broadening our scope further, scholars and social commentators have noted that whole populations may succumb to what the Victorian journalist Charles MacKay (1841) termed 'the madness of crowds'. In the age of the internet, many beliefs of this kind have proliferated (Bentall 2023), including pseudosciences such as homeopathy and vaccine scepticism (Schermer 1997), conspiracy theories such as the idea that NASA faked the 1969 Moon landing (Brotherton 2015) and, most recently, QAnon (named after an alleged anonymous intelligence officer, 'Q'), a conspiracist ideology that holds that the former US President Donald Trump, aided by US intelligence agencies, is fighting a covert war against a gang of paedophiles and child murderers led by the Democratic Party politicians, and run out of a pizza parlour in New York (Rothschild 2021). (For more on delusion and conspiracy theories see Pierre, Chapter 37.)

## 2.   What do we mean when we talk about delusions?

In part stimulated by the obvious problems created by these difficult cases, scholars and clinicians have made considerable efforts to identify characteristics which they think distinguish psychotic delusions from ordinary beliefs. For pragmatic purposes, some of the resulting definitions have found their way into widely used diagnostic manuals.

For example, the current fifth edition of the American Psychiatric Association's *Diagnostic and Statistical Manual* (*DSM-5*; American Psychiatric Association 2013) says that delusions are

> fixed beliefs that are not amenable to change in light of conflicting evidence. Their content may include a variety of themes (e.g. persecutory, referential, somatic, religious, grandiose). [...] Delusions are deemed bizarre if they are clearly implausible and not understandable to same-culture peers and do not derive from ordinary life experiences.

Note that this definition emphasizes that delusions tend to follow particular themes. In a recent meta-analysis, my colleagues and I found remarkable consistency in these themes globally, with the most common being paranoid or persecutory delusions (pooled point estimate 64.5 per cent), followed by ideas of reference (39.7 per cent), grandiose delusions (28.2 per cent), delusions of control (21.6 per cent), and religious delusions (18.3 per cent) (Collin et al. 2023), apparently reflecting the core existential dilemmas of human existence. These dilemmas include deciding who we can trust, which events are significant for us, our place in the social order, our ability to control our own destiny, and the meaning of life. At a more fine-grain level, cultural variation in the content of delusions is, of course, observed, for example in the type of persecutor or the claimed attributes of grandiose patients (see, e.g., Azhar et al. 1995; Sendiony 1976; for more on delusion and culture, see Gold and Gold, Chapter 36).

The World Health Organization's International Classification of Disease, which is currently in its eleventh edition (ICD-11; World Health Organisation 2018), by contrast, contains a definition that is almost identical to that given in previous editions of the *DSM*:

> A belief that is demonstrably untrue or not shared by others, usually based on incorrect inference about external reality. The belief is firmly held with conviction and is not, or is only briefly, susceptible to modification by experience or evidence that contradicts it. The belief is not ordinarily accepted by other members or the person's culture or subculture (i.e., it is not an article of religious faith).

Both of these definitions emphasize the conviction with which delusions are held, and their apparent resistance to conflicting evidence, but these are characteristics that not only make the madnesses of crowds troubling but are also evident in socially consequential belief systems that are widely accepted as nonpathological. For example, in an early study, the British psychologist Robert Thouless (1935) found that, when he asked ordinary people how certain they were about their religious beliefs, most reported extreme certainty. More recently, when American political scientists asked people to rate their certainty about their political convictions on a 0–100 scale, the average score was 75.1 and a very large number (usually people who located themselves at either end of the left-right spectrum) reported holding their beliefs with 100 per cent certainty (Costello and Bowes 2023). Not surprisingly, beliefs held with a high level of certainty tend to also be held tenaciously (Tormala and Rucker, 2018). Political scientists, in particular, have explored the phenomenon of motivated reasoning, by which politically committed individuals tend to interpret evidence in terms of their partisan concerns and reject any evidence that seems to challenge their prejudices (Leeper and Slothuus 2014; Taber and Lodge 2013).

Without going into further detail here, other criteria proposed for identifying delusions face similar difficulties. For example, delusions have been described as bizarre which, in turn, has been defined in terms of deviation from culturally agreed norms (Kendler et al. 1983) or the violation of accepted ideas about what is possible (Mullen 2003). However, these criteria become problematic when comparing delusions to conspiracy theories or the beliefs of minority sects such as the Nation of Islam; in any case, clinicians find it hard to agree about which beliefs qualify as bizarre (Bell et al. 2006).

These challenges have led some philosophers to question the 'doxastic' status of delusions on the grounds that patients often show an absence of 'procedural rationality' (their delusions are not integrated with other beliefs), 'epistemic rationality' (they do not given reasons for their beliefs or adjust them in the light of evidence), or 'agential rationality' (they do not act in accordance with their beliefs) but, again, it has been pointed out that delusional beliefs are not unique in terms of these criteria (Bortolotti 2010). When patients are interviewed, they certainly seem to talk about their delusions as if they are beliefs, although they vary in the extent to which they can meet these criteria for rationality, sometimes but not always meeting all three (Green et al. 2018). (For more on delusion and doxasticism see Noordhof, Chapter 29.)

## 3.   Empirical approaches to defining delusions

Another way of addressing the distinction between delusions and nonpathological beliefs is to attack the problem empirically. Researchers have employed three main strategies for this purpose. The first is to argue that there is, in fact, no dividing line and that, instead, there exists a continuum running from those beliefs that are mundane to those that are obviously pathological. One type of evidence often cited to support this contention is the apparently high prevalence of delusion-like beliefs recorded in epidemiological studies. For example, in the Dutch NEMISIS study, 3.3 per cent of the 7,000 people interviewed were judged to have true delusions and 8.7 per cent were judged to have delusion-like ideas that were not a cause of distress (van Os et al. 2000). However, a recent systematic review of 17 studies of this kind found that the reported prevalence rates for delusions varied considerably, possibly because many used self-report questionnaires rather than clinical interviews (Heilskof et al. 2020).

More compelling support for the continuum idea has emerged from psychometric studies focusing specifically on paranoid beliefs. Freeman and colleagues (2005) have proposed that these beliefs vary in severity from the kind of self-consciousness that most of us experience when surrounded by strangers, through mistrustfulness and suspiciousness, to extreme beliefs about imminent harm. Using a large dataset that included both ordinary people and psychiatric patients, my colleagues and I were able to use 'taxometric' statistical methods designed to detect 'taxons' of people with distinct characteristics (Elahi et al. 2017). We found no evidence of separate paranoid and nonparanoid taxons and, instead, found that paranoia was best understood as a continuum.

The second approach to pinning down the nature of delusions has involved trying to discover psychological characteristics that are uniquely associated with them, either by comparing patients and nonpatients or by comparing ordinary people differing on questionnaire measures of delusional belief. This work has spawned a vast literature and there is only space here to consider a few highlights. One widely cited phenomenon is the apparent tendency of people with delusions to 'jump to conclusions' when making decisions about sequentially presented information, for example when deciding whether a sequence of green and red beads has been drawn from a bag containing mostly green beads or mostly red beads (referred to as the jumping to conclusions or JTC bias) (Huq et al. 1988). Another is the tendency for deluded patients to be biased against accepting disconfirmatory evidence (BADE) once they have formed a hypothesis (Woodward et al. 2006). Both of these cognitive abnormalities have been apparently supported by meta-analyses of the relevant studies (Dudley et al. 2016; McLean et al. 2016; Zhu et al. 2018) but both measures are vulnerable to the effects of inattention, which causes people to respond in a much more 'delusional' way (Sulik et al. 2023). There is evidence that the JTC can be accounted for almost entirely by random responding (Moutoussis et al. 2011) and, in the case of the BADE, it has been found that patients only demonstrate the effect when considering evidence that contradicts beliefs that they already hold strongly (Speechley et al. 2012). The BADE effect has also been found in people with strong political ideologies (Bronstein et al. 2017) which should surprise nobody because, as we have already seen, motivated reasoning about political beliefs is a phenomenon that has been extensively documented by political scientists (Leeper and Slothuus 2014; Taber and Lodge, 2013). Hence, it is not clear whether these reasoning abnormalities are really delusion-specific or, on the contrary, evident when anyone deliberates about a topic that is personally significant (for more on delusion and abnormal reasoning see Sullivan-Bissett, Chapter 28, and Davies and Coltheart, Chapter 29).

A final approach, pioneered by the philosopher psychiatrist Karl Jaspers (1913/1963), has involved using phenomenological interviews to identify experiential features of delusions that are not evident in other kinds of beliefs (Feyaerts et al. 2021). Jaspers held that true delusions, in contrast to 'delusion-like' or 'over-valued' ideas, are 'ununderstandable' in the sense that they cannot be understood in terms of the patient's personality or life history. Later researchers working within this tradition have focused on both the period before the onset of delusions and also subtle abnormalities in the way that deluded people experience themselves in the world. An example of the former approach is the work of Klaus Conrad (1958/2012) who identified three stages in the development of delusions: *das trema* (sometimes called delusional mood), in which the patient experiences a profound sense of tension and that 'something is in the air'; *apophany,* (revelation) in which the delusion appears suddenly as an 'ah ha' experience; and finally *anastrophe* (turning back) in which the patient feels the passive focus of the delusional world. Investigators who have considered the deluded patient's more global experience of being in the world have proposed that there is a fragmentation of the basis sense of the self as a locus of thought, feeling, and action (Henriksen et al. 2021). Another idea is that patients can be simultaneously in their grip of their delusions while, at the same time, aware that their beliefs are inconsistent with reality, a process known as 'double book-keeping' (Stephensen et al. 2023). According to some, this sense of simultaneously existing in two unresolvable realities creates a subjective sense of solipsism, in which truths about the delusional world cannot be tested (Sass 1994).

However, it is unclear whether these kinds of experiences are unique to delusions. Psychotic experiences are in many ways similar to the mystical states associated with extreme religiosity (Parnas and Henriksen 2016), which were famously described by the psychologist-philosopher William James (1902) as 'ineffable' (by which he meant that they are difficult to describe and can only be fully appreciated first-hand). In the 1970s, accounts of these states were collected by the biologist Sir Alistair (Hardy 1979) and, as already noted, later, careful examination of his archive revealed that they are often difficult to distinguish from the experiences of patients with severe mental illness (Jackson and Fulford 1997).

## 4.   The unrealistic comparator

The attempts to define delusions considered earlier, and also the three empirical approaches that I have just reviewed, are all undermined by a common limitation. In various ways, they have all involved contrasting delusions with an unrealistic comparator. This comparator has usually been mundane beliefs of no particular significance (the majority of psychological studies), or an entirely hypothetical conception of a 'normal' belief drawn from folk psychology (the continuum approach, the phenomenological approach, some philosophical analyses). In making this claim, I am not simply arguing that it would be more informative to contrast pathological beliefs with ideological beliefs and the madness of crowds (although this would surely be an advance) but that researchers have almost always underappreciated the complexity of even mundane beliefs. Mapping this complexity is a task that is well beyond the scope of this essay but, in what follows, I will outline three features of *a realistic account of beliefs* that point towards an entirely different way of thinking about why some beliefs are pathological.

## 5.   Outline of a realistic account of beliefs

We can start with the Oxford English Dictionary definition of belief as, 'A proposition or set of propositions held to be true', with the corresponding verb, 'believe', meaning, 'To have confidence in the truth or accuracy of (a statement, doctrine, etc.)'. The *Stanford Encyclopedia of Philosophy* (Schwitzgebel 2015) similarly states:

> Contemporary analytic philosophers of mind generally use the term 'belief' to refer to the attitude we have, roughly, whenever we take something to be the case or regard it as true.

An important feature of these definitions is that they imply that every belief is an amalgam of two components: a proposition and some kind of estimation that the proposition is true (sometimes called a propositional attitude). The first of these components is a product of the human ability to use language, about which much can be said, although not within the space allotted to this essay (see Bentall 2023). Suffice it to say here that human beings, in contrast to nonanimal species, have the capacity to reason using language-based propositional rules, but retain also the associative mechanisms that are responsible for the often complex behaviour of animals.

Note also that there are many other words in the English language that convey roughly the same idea, for example, 'attitude', 'theory', 'expectation', 'value'. Although each of these words has generated a considerable volume of scholarship, it is unlikely that any human language accurately reflects the taxonomy of the human mind, and therefore it is probably best not to be too preoccupied by the distinctions implied by these terms. Here I am making the assumption that a common set of social and psychological processes is involved in all of these activities. By 'believing' I therefore mean any activity that involves generating any kind of proposition about the world that is held to be (possibly) true.

## 5.1   Certainty is a feeling

As noted earlier, a feature of delusions that have attracted considerable attention is the certainty with which they are held but this is also a feature of many religious and political ideologies (Costello and Bowes 2023; Thouless 1935). Indeed, there is evidence that, within the general population, there are individual differences in the general disposition to experience certainty so that, for example, people who feel very certain in their attitudes towards, say, government policies, are also likely to feel very certain about their attitudes towards paper plates (DeMarree et al. 2020).

Research into certainty has been conducted by cognitive psychologists focusing on the recall of factual information (Koriat 2012), and by social and consumer psychologists interested in attitudes and the way people make judgements about commercial products (Tormala and Rucker 2018), but their findings have rarely been applied to psychopathology. In ordinary life, the feeling of certainty usually comes to us automatically and belongs to a class of epistemic feelings which include the pleasant sense of curiosity and the very aversive sense of extreme uncertainty. Unsurprisingly, the feeling of certainty is usually greatest when we base or beliefs on direct experience, rather than on second hand information (Smith et al. 2008). More importantly, when retrieving knowledge from memory, or when expressing attitudes, certainty is related to ease of recall and hence decision time – the faster the judgement, the greater the certainty (Alter and Oppenheimer 2009; Koriat 1993). However, this does not mean that we simply 'read off' our feeling of certainty from our response times. William James (1893) first noticed that we can sometimes feel that we know something without being able to fully recall it (a phenomenon which later became known as the 'tip-of-the-tongue phenomenon'; Brown and McNeill 1966). What seems to be happening, both in the tip-of-the-tongue phenomenon and when expressing ordinary beliefs and opinions, is that our certainty is determined not just by the swiftness of our response but by the totality of the associations linked to the belief (including, in a general knowledge test, associations provoked by the question itself). In other words, whereas it is our ability to formulate statements in sentences that determines the content of our beliefs, associative processes determine the conviction with which they are held.

These findings may help to explain some of the features of delusions that have long puzzled psychopathologists. For example, it would be interesting to consider how the tip-of-the- tongue phenomenon (the feeling of knowing something that cannot, for the moment, be recalled) relates to Conrad (1958/2012)'s state of das trema that precedes the onset of delusions (the feeling of being about to know something but not knowing what it is). Consider also double book-keeping (see Porcher, Chapter 13). This phenomenon seems paradoxical only because it appears to involve feeling certain about two incompatible types of propositions – those that are delusional and those that pertain to the real world. However, if the feeling of certainty is a product of the kinds of associative processes that underlie animal cognition, there is no requirement for these feelings to be logically consistent. Indeed, I suspect that the feeling of being 'in two minds' is a common experience when wrestling with personal or existential dilemmas (e.g., when agnostics attempts to juggle a sense of the spiritual world with a commitment to the scientific world view).

## 5.2 *Beliefs are organized*

An important difference between, on the one hand, mundane beliefs (my train will leave the station at noon) and, on the other, the kinds of beliefs that are socially significant (religious and political ideologies, conspiracy theories, and so on) is that the latter, as it where, go around in families so that, just by knowing someone's attitudes in one domain (there should be more spending on the armed forces; Jesus was the son of God) it is usually possible to make fairly accurate predictions about his or her beliefs in another (e.g., about the virtues of free-market economics or the sanctity of marriage).

In 1964, the American political scientist Philip Converse (1964/2006) published a theoretical analysis of belief systems that focused on political ideologies, but which he claimed could be applied to any beliefs of 'mass publics'. His fundamental observation was that beliefs that are important to us are often organized into systems or networks of inter-connected beliefs, and that the degree to which this is the case varies from person to person. In the political arena, people who are 'ideologues', he argued, will have spent many years debating and refining their belief systems, and all the elements will therefore be closely connected. These connections are sometimes logical or propositional so that, for example, if you believe in a small state, you must want to reduce spending on social security benefits. However, they can also be associative. For example, there is no logical connection between social and economic conservativism, but they have been paired in the same 'cultural package' in most countries and hence have become highly correlated. In the countries of Eastern Europe, however, the former communist regimes were very socially conservative so, in these countries, social conservativism is associated with left-wing economic beliefs (Malka et al. 2019). An important implication of this model, noted by Converse, was that the strength of the interconnections between beliefs should determine the certainty with which they are held, their resistance to counterargument and their persistence because in a highly interconnected belief system, changing one belief will require changing many others. Note that this prediction is entirely consistent with the account given in the previous section, where we saw that the feeling of certainty is determined by the totality of associations related to a belief.

A wrinkle in this model not considered by Converse is that strong connections between beliefs can also sometimes be explained by hidden psychological factors. This idea is consistent with many non-Conversian attempts to understand belief systems which seek to identify 'core' 'primal', or 'fundamental' beliefs that explain their covariation. Models of this kind include, for example, Jonathan Haidt's (2013) theory that political ideologies can be explained in terms of variations in five 'moral foundations' and a recent, ambitious attempt by Clifton and colleagues (2019) to identify a hierarchy of 'primal beliefs' that are organized into three main groups: the belief that the world is safe vs dangerous; that it is enticing vs dull; and that it is alive vs mechanistic.

The idea of core beliefs is sometimes evoked to explain psychological phenomena that seem otherwise perplexing. For example, the observation that people who endorse one conspiracy theory (that Princess Diana faked her own death) will often endorse others with which they are incompatible (she was killed by the British secret service) (Wood et al. 2012) becomes understandable when we realize that both ideas could be expressions of the core belief that official explanations for events cannot be trusted. An obvious difficulty raised by this kind of account, however, is that it invites an infinite regression. As Wittgenstein (1969) argued, there ultimately has to be a nonpropositional bedrock on which our propositions about the world can be anchored. Indeed, the idea that fundamental beliefs are 'beliefs' may be an illusion created by the fact that we can only express them in words. For example, the 'big three' primal beliefs described by Clifton and colleagues (2019) seem to reflect sensitivity to threat (the world is assumed to be safe vs dangerous), sensitivity to reward (the world is enticing vs dull) and specifically human cognitive processes that have evolved to allow us to understand the behaviour of other human beings (the world is alive vs mechanistic), all processes that likely operate at the associative level.

Statistical methods that allow us to test network models of belief have only recently become available, more than 50 years after Converse proposed his account. Using *network psychometrics*, it is now possible to represent belief networks in the form of graphical diagrams, in which beliefs are 'nodes' and the connections between them are represented by 'edges'. Various additional statistical methods are available to test how the belief networks of various populations differ, but these need not detain us here. A number of researchers have begun to apply this approach to political beliefs. As Converse predicted, more tightly interconnected belief networks are better predictors of future voting behaviour than loosely connected networks (Dalege and colleagues 2017), and network connectivity predicts the persistence of beliefs over time (Dalege and colleagues 2019).

In my own recent work, I have compared the network structure of UK citizens who self-identify as 'left', 'centre' or 'right' on the political spectrum (Bentall et al. 2023, in submission). The nodes were 18 political constructs which people were asked to state their attitude towards, for example 'more money for the armed forces' and 'Brexit'. A striking finding was that, although those on the left and right had polar opposite beliefs (they rated each of the constructs very differently) their network structures were similar and very different to the networks of the centrists. In particular, compared to the centrists, those who described themselves as strongly left- or right-wing had networks that were highly interconnected.

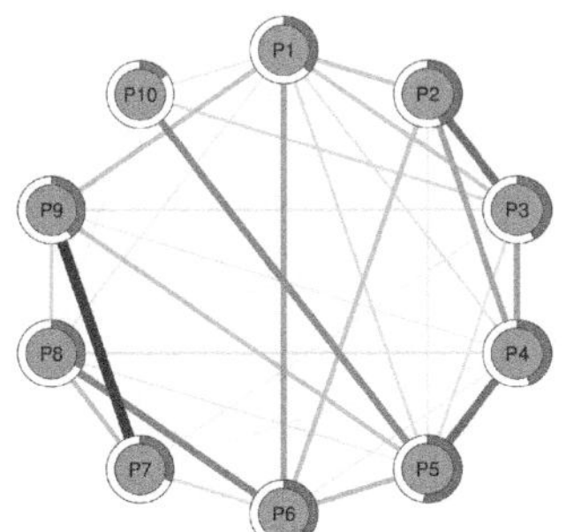

Do you agree with:
P1: Others plotting against me
P2: Others have negative ideas of me
P3: Friends often tell me to relax
P4: Bad rumours of me
P5: Suspicious of others
P6: People talking critically about me
P7: People think I am a bad person
P8: People almost certainly lie to me
P9: People want to hurt me deliberately
P10: You should only trust yourself

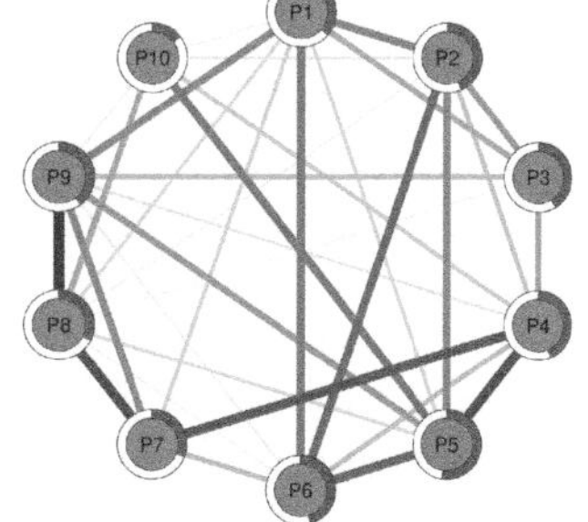

An implication of this analysis is that network connectivity might explain the persistence and incorrigibility of delusional beliefs. Recently, with colleagues, I was able to conduct a preliminary test of this hypothesis using data from a questionnaire measure of paranoia which had been given to over 2,000 ordinary people and about 600 psychiatric patients (Zavlis et al. 2023). Comparing the interconnectivity between responses to each of the items between clinical participants and matched nonclinical participants, as expected we found that connectivity was much greater for the former, as shown in the figure.

## 5.3   Beliefs are transmissible

A final property of beliefs that has implications for delusions is that they usually move from one person to another, which, of course, is a consequence of the way that we express them in language. This property has sustained every important social and scientific advance made by our species. Cultures emerge when a large number of people, usually but not always in the same geographical area, begin to share sets of beliefs and the practices surrounding them. To a great extent, therefore, a culture is defined by the epidemiology of beliefs (Sperber 1996). During cultural evolution, the words that humans have used to describe the world have undergone parallel changes that have enlarged the concepts available to our species, and facilitated profound transformations which have been mapped by archaeologists, historians, and anthropologists. Although detailed historical examples cannot be discussed here for reasons of space, the emergence of religious beliefs from animism (Peoples et al. 2016) and the later invention of monotheism amongst the polytheistic Canaanites (Finkelstein and Silberman 2002) are obvious examples. Another is the further transformation of 'religion' into a universal category that encompasses culturally diverse beliefs, which occurred at the time of the Protestant Reformation (Nongbri 2013; Shagan 2018). This was soon followed by the Scientific Revolution, in which the modern concepts of 'discovery' and 'fact' were employed for the first time (Wootton 2015).

The mechanisms of belief propagation are complex. A well-known metaphor, suggested by the biologist Richard Dawkins (1999) involves likening the spread of beliefs, or 'memes', to the natural selection of biological traits. Although briefly popular (Blackmore 1999), this model has not survived well (ironically, the *Journal of Mimetics* closed down after seven years because of a lack of interest in the academic community). Amongst its many limitations, it failed to specify the conditions in which beliefs move efficiently from one person to another, and could not capture the creativity with which they are edited and revised as they are passed on (Atran 2001). Importantly, unlike genetic transmission, belief propagation does not involve replication. Instead, beliefs are usually melded so that, when one person passes a belief to another, the resultant belief is often some kind of amalgam of the belief of the speaker and the pre-existing beliefs of the listener (Sperber 1996).

A metaphor which I think is more fruitful (although still a metaphor) was first suggested in the early twentieth century by Ronald Ross, the physician who discovered the disease vector responsible for malaria (Kucharski 2020). Ross noted that ideas spread in much the same way as diseases. Elaborating Ross's model, we can see that the spread of beliefs depends on both their origin and the vectors through which they are transmitted. Some people – Mohamed, Martin Luther, and Karl Marx come to mind – are effective belief entrepreneurs, and have been skilled at exploiting the vectors available to them so that, for example, the availability of the printing press played a crucial role in the Protestant

Reformation (Pettegree 2015), and the mysterious 'Q' could not have achieved his malign influence without access to the internet (Rothschild 2021).

As the sociologist Max Weber (1905/2002) was one of the first to recognize, beliefs are not equally embraced by everyone who encounters them. Borrowing a metaphor from the chemistry of his day, Weber argued that there are 'elective affinities' between certain kinds of beliefs and certain kinds of people (McKinnon 2010), an insight that has been embraced by modern political scientists (Jost 2009). The characteristics that make certain people vulnerable to being infected by certain kinds of beliefs are, of course, very likely the very same underlying psychological traits that explain why some beliefs coalesce into networks or systems.

## 6.   Why delusions are different

My main argument in this chapter has been that we need to compare delusions with realistic comparators and stop comparing them to a hypothetical idea of belief drawn from folk psychology. To this end, I have tried to sketch three important but neglected features of beliefs, making occasional reference to rich research literatures on political ideologies, religions and conspiracy theories.

These features help to explain features of delusions that have long puzzled psychopathologists. For example, I have pointed to how research on the feeling of certainty might help to explain delusional mood and double bookkeeping. With respect to the organization of beliefs, I used network models to show that delusional systems appear to be structured similarly to political ideologies, and argued that this structure helps to account for the tenacity with which they are held.

However, it is the third property of transmissibility that I think has the most promise for explaining why delusions may, after all, be different from other kinds of beliefs. A feature of delusions that seems to distinguish them from the other types of beliefs considered here is that they are idiosyncratic, which is to say nontransmissible. With the rare exception of folie à deux (which typically occurs in people who are very close to each other but are otherwise socially isolated; Arnone et al. 2006) delusions are believed by only one person. They do not seem to come from anywhere – the patient does not hear them from someone else – and they do not go anywhere – patients may talk about their delusions when distressed or when asked to do so by a clinician but they do not gather in the corners of psychiatric wards to decide between themselves which theories of persecution are the correct ones, and they do not go out into the world to proselytize their paranoia.

The madnesses of crowds catalogued by MacKay (1841) and the political and religious ideologies with which I began this essay are transmissible; that is why MacKay described them as madnesses *of crowds*. Ezra Pound did not develop his antisemitic obsessions in isolation; he lived in a Europe in which these ideas were spread by a cacophony of voices, with genocidal consequences. As Krakauer (2003) documented, the Lafferty brothers absorbed Mormon theological doctrines that had evolved and been argued over for more than a century; their ideas were then further shaped by the extremist Mormon cults they encountered in their travels. Anders Breivik is, perhaps, a more difficult case to adjudicate; he was raised by a psychologically disturbed mother, suffered mental health difficulties from childhood, and became socially isolated as an adult (Borchgrevink 2013), and yet his extremist views echoed a culture of far-right extremism propagated throughout Europe by social media.

This analysis highlights a crucial property of beliefs that I have not sufficiently emphasized thus far: they are social phenomena. In everyday life we rarely decide what to believe on our own. Instead, we meld new information with what we have already learned from other people; we share gossip with our friends; we build coalitions of like-minded people with whom we can debate and refine our ideas; we have arguments with those we disagree with and try and resolve our disputes about the causes of events that are mutually important. In other words, in nearly all domains of everyday life, we coordinate our beliefs with those around us and, moreover, we do this systematically with groups we identify with because they belong to the same family, profession, church, political organization, neighbourhood, sports team, supporters' club, book club, or any other kind of formal or informal social organization. Delusional patients, by contrast are influenced by the surrounding culture only in the sense that the culture provides them with concepts with which they can fashion their beliefs. Delusions are not part of the life of a culture and, in this sense, can be described as acultural (cf. Gold and Gold, Chapter 36).

Past research has shown that paranoia is associated with a failure to identify with social groups (Elahi et al. 2018; McIntyre et al. 2018) and that paranoid people tend to be isolated (Butter et al. 2017) and lonely (Chau et al. 2019). These are, of course, circumstances in which it may be difficult for people to test their beliefs by sharing and coordinating them with others. However, we know very little about how even mentally well people build belief sharing coalitions, or about the social and cognitive skills required to achieve this (although see Cikara 2021). Focusing on these processes should provide new avenues for understanding the psychological difficulties that lead to psychosis, and will hopefully point to new therapies for patients and strategies for improving the wellbeing of whole populations.

# References


Alter, A. L., & Oppenheimer, D. M. (2009). Uniting the tribes of fluency to form a metacognitive nation. *Personality and Social Psychology Review, 13*(3), 219–235. https://doi.org/10.1177/1088868309341564

American Psychiatric Association. (2013). *Diagnostic and statistical manual for mental disorders*. 5th edition. Author.

Arnone, D., Patel, A., & Tan, G. M.-Y. (2006). The nosological significance of Folie à Deux: A review of the literature. *Annals of General Psychiatry, 5*(1), 11. https://doi.org/10.1186/1744-859X-5-11

Atran, S. (2001). The trouble with memes. *Human Nature, 12*, 351–381. https://doi.org/10.1007/s12110-001-1003-0

Azhar, M. Z., Varma, S. L., & Hakim, H. R. (1995). Phenomenological differences of delusions between schizophrenic patients of two cultures of Malaysia. *Singapore Medical Journal, 36*, 273–275.

Bell, V., Halligan, P. W., & Ellis, H. D. (2006). Diagnosing delusions: A review of inter-rater reliability. *Schizophrenia Research, 86*(1–3), 76–79. https://doi.org/10.1016/j.schres.2006.06.025

Bentall, R. P. (2023). Delusional beliefs and the madness of crowds. In K. Hardy & D. Turkington (Eds.), *Decoding delusions: A clinician's guide to working with delusions and other extreme beliefs* (pp. 3–46). American Psychiatric Association.

Bentall, R. P., Zavlis, O., Hyland, P., McBride, O., Bennett, K. M., & Hartman, T. K. (in submission). The structure of mass political belief systems: A network approach to understanding the left-right spectrum.

Blackmore, S. (1999). *The meme machine*. Oxford University Press.

Borchgrevink, A. (2013). *A Norwegian tragedy: Anders Behring Reivik and the massacre on Utoya* (G. Puzey, Trans.). Polity Press.

Bortolotti, L. (2010). *Delusions and other irrational beliefs*. Oxford University Press.

Bromberg, W., & Simon, F. (1968). The 'protest psychosis': A new form of reactive psychosis. *Archives of General Psychiatry*, *19*, 155–160.

Bronstein, M. V., Dovidio, J. F., & Cannon, T. D. (2017). Both bias against disconfirmatory evidence and political orientation partially explain the relationship between dogmatism and racial prejudice. *Personality and Individual Differences*, *105*, 89–94. https://doi.org/10.1016/j.paid.2016.09.036

Brotherton, R. (2015). *Suspicious minds: Why we believe conspiracy theories*. Bloomsbury.

Brown, R., & McNeill, D. (1966). The "tip of the tongue" phenomenon. *Journal of Verbal Learning and Verbal Behavior*, *5*(4), 325–337. https://doi.org/10.1016/S0022-5371(66)80040-3

Butter, S., Murphy, J., Shevlin, M., & Houston, J. (2017). Social isolation and psychosis-like experiences: A UK general population analysis. *Psychosis*, *9*, 291–300.

Chau, A. K. C., Zhu, C., & So, S. H.-W. (2019). Loneliness and the psychosis continuum: A meta-analysis on positive psychotic experiences and a meta-analysis on negative psychotic experiences. *International Review of Psychiatry*, *31*(5–6), 471–490. https://doi.org/10.1080/09540261.2019.1636005

Cikara, M. (2021). Causes and consequences of coalitional cognition. In B. Gawronski (Ed.), *Advances in Experimental Social Psychology* (Vol. 64, pp. 65–128). Academic Press. https://doi.org/10.1016/bs.aesp.2021.04.002

Clifton, J. D. W., Baker, J. D., Park, C. L., Yaden, D. B., Clifton, A. B. W., Terni, P., Miller, J., Zeng, G., Giorgi, S., Schwartz, H. A., & Seligman, M. E. P. (2019). Primal world beliefs. *Psychological Assessment*, *31*(1), 82–99. https://doi.org/0.1037/pas0000639

Collin, S., Rowse, G., Martinez, A., & Bentall, R. P. (2023). Delusions and the dilemmas of life: A systematic review and meta-analyses of the global literature on the prevalence of delusional themes in clinical groups. *Clinical Psychology Review*, *104*, 102303

Conrad, K. (1958/2012). Beginning schizophrenia: Attempt for a Gestalt-analysis of delusion. In M. R. Broome, R. Harland, G. S. Owen, & A. Stringaris (Eds.), *The Maudsley reader in phenomenological psychiatry* (pp. 176–193). Cambridge University Press.

Converse, P. (1964/2006). The nature of belief systems in mass publics. *Critical Review*, *18*, 1–74. https://doi.org/10.1080/08913810608443650

Costello, T. H., & Bowes, S. M. (2023). Absolute certainty and political Ideology: A systematic test of curvilinearity. *Social Psychological and Personality Science*, *14*(1), 93–102. https://doi.org/10.1177/19485506211070410

Dalege, J., Borsboom, D., van Harreveld, F., & van der Maas, H. L. J. (2019). A network perspective on attitude strength: Testing the connectivity hypothesis. *Social Psychological and Personality Science*, *10*(6), 746–756. https://doi.org/10.1177/1948550618781062

Dalege, J., Borsboom, D., van Harreveld, F., Waldorp, L. J., & van der Maas, H. L. J. (2017). Network structure explains the impact of attitudes on voting decisions. *Scientific Reports*, *7*, 4909. https://doi.org/10.1038/s41598-017-05048-y

Dawkins, R. (1999, April 11). The selfish meme. *Time*. http://content.time.com/time/magazine/article/0,9171,22988-2,00.html

DeMarree, K. G., Petty, R. E., Briñol, P., & Xia, J. (2020). Documenting individual differences in the propensity to hold attitudes with certainty. *Journal of Personality and Social Psychology*, *119*(6), 1239.

Dudley, R., Taylor, P., Wickham, S., & Hutton, P. (2016). Psychosis, delusions and the 'jumping to conclusions' reasoning bias: A systematic review and meta-analysis. *Schizophrenia Bulletin*, *42*, 652–665. https://doi.org/10.1093/schbul/sbv150

Elahi, A., McIntyre, J. C., Hampson, C., Bodycote, H., Sitko, K., & Bentall, R. P. (2018). Home is where you hang your hat: Host town identity, but not hometown identity, protects against mental health symptoms associated with financial stress. *Journal of Social and Clinical Psychology*, *37*, 159–181. https://doi.org/10.1521/jscp.2018.37.3.159

Elahi, A., Perez Algorta, G., Varese, F., McIntyre, J. C., & Bentall, R. P. (2017). Do paranoid delusions exist on a continuum with subclinical paranoia? A multi-method taxometric study. *Schizophrenia Research*, *190*, 77–81. https://doi.org/10.1016/j.schres.2017.03.022

Feyaerts, J., Henricksen, M. G., Vanheule, S., Myin-Germeys, I., & Saas, L. A. (2021). Delusions beyond beliefs: A critical overview of diagnostic, aetiological, and therapeutic schizophrenia research from a clinical-phenomenological perspective. *Lancet Psychiatry*, *8*, 237–249. https://doi.org/10.1016/S2215-0366(20)30460-0

Finkelstein, I., & Silberman, N. A. (2002). *The Bible unearthed: Archaeology's new vision of Ancient Israel and the origin of sacred texts*. Simon and Schuster.

Freeman, D., Garety, P. A., Bebbington, P. E., Smith, B., Rollinson, R., Fowler, D., Kuipers, E., Ray, K., & Dunn, G. (2005). Psychological investigation of the structure of paranoia in a non-clinical population. *British Journal of Psychiatry, 186*, 427–435. https://doi.org/10.1192/bjp.186.5.42

Green, H., Hauser, L., & Troyakov, V. (2018). Are delusions beliefs? A qualitative examination of the doxastic features of delusions. *Psychosis, 10*(4), 319–328. https://doi.org/10.1080/17522439.2018.1528298

Haidt, J. (2013). *The righteous mind: Why good people are divided by politics and religion*. Allen Lane: The Penguin Press.

Hardy, A. (1979). *The spiritual nature of man: Study of contemporary religious experience*. Oxford University Press.

Heilskof, S. E. R., Urfer-Parnas, A., & Norgaard, J. (2020). Delusions in the general population: A systematic review with emphasis on methodology. *Schizophrenia Research, 216*, 48–55. https://doi.org/10.1016/j.schres.2019.10.043

Henriksen, M. G., Raballo, A., & Nordgaard, J. (2021). Self-disorders and psychopathology: A systematic review. *The Lancet Psychiatry, 8*(11), 1001–1012. https://doi.org/10.1016/S2215-0366(21)00097-3

Huq, S. F., Garety, P. A., & Hemsley, D. R. (1988). Probabilistic judgements in deluded and nondeluded subjects. *Quarterly Journal of Experimental Psychology, 40A*, 801–812.

Jackson, M., & Fulford, K. W. M. (1997). Spiritual experience and psychopathology. *Philosophy, Psychiatry and Psychology, 4*(1), 41–65.

James, W. (1893). *Principles of psychology*. Volume 1. Holt.

James, W. (1902). *The varieties of religious experience*. Penguin Press.

Jaspers, K. (1913/1963). *General psychopathology* (J. Hoenig & M. W. Hamilton, Trans.). Manchester University Press.

Jost, J. T. (2009). "Elective affinities": On the psychological bases of left–right differences. *Psychological Inquiry, 20*, 129–141.

Kendler, K. S., Glazer, W., & Morgenstern, H. (1983). Dimensions of delusional experience. *American Journal of Psychiatry, 140*, 466–469.

Koriat, A. (1993). How do we know that we know? The accessibility model of the feeling of knowing. *Psychological Review, 100*(4), 609–639.

Koriat, A. (2012). The self-consistency model of subjective confidence. *Psychological Review, 119*(1), 80–113. https://doi.org/10.1037/a0025648

Krakauer, J. (2003). *Under the banner of heaven: A story of violent faith*. Doubleday.

Kucharski, A. (2020). *The rules of contagion: Why things spread and why they stop*. Profile Books.

Leeper, T. J., & Slothuus, R. (2014). Political parties, motivated reasoning, and public opinion formation. *Political Psychology, 35*(S1), 129–156. https://doi.org/10.1111/pops.12164

MacKay, C. (1841). *Memoirs of extraordinary popular delusions and the madness of crowds: A study in crowd psychology*. Volumes 1–3. Richard Bentley.

Malka, A., Lelkes, Y., & Soto, C. J. (2019). Are cultural and economic conservatism positively correlated? A large-scale cross-national test. *British Journal of Political Science, 49*(3), 1045–1069. https://doi.org/10.1017/S0007123417000072

McIntyre, J. C., Wickham, S., Barr, B., & Bentall, R. P. (2018). Social identity and psychosis: Associations and psychological mechanisms. *Schizophrenia Bulletin, 44*, 681–690. https://doi.org/10.1093/schbul/sbx110

McKinnon, A. M. (2010). Elective affinities of the Protestant ethic: Weber and the chemistry of capitalism. *Sociological Theory, 28*(1), 108–126. https://doi.org/10.1111/j.1467-9558.2009.01367.x

McLean, B. F., Mattiske, J. K., & Balzan, R. P. (2016). Association of the jumping to conclusions and evidence integration biases with delusions in psychosis: A detailed meta-analysis. *Schizophrenia Bulletin, 43*(2), 344–354. https://doi.org/10.1093/schbul/sbw056

Melle, I. (2013). The Breivik case and what psychiatrists can learn from it. *World Psychiatry, 12*, 16–21.

Metzel, J. M. (2009). *The protest psychosis: How schizophrenia became a black disease*. Beacon Press.

Moutoussis, M., Bentall, R. P., El-Deredy, W., & Dayan, P. (2011). Bayesian modeling of Jumping-to-Conclusions Bias in delusional patients. *Cognitive Neuropsychiatry, 16*, 422–447.

Mullen, R. (2003). The problem of bizarre delusions. *Journal of Nervous & Mental Disease, 191*(8), 546–548. https://doi.org/10.1097/01.nmd.0000082184.39788.de

Nongbri, B. (2013). *Before religion: A history of a modern concept.* Yale University Press.

O'Connor, S., & Vandenberg, B. (2005). Psychosis or faith? Clinicians' assessment of religious beliefs. *Journal of Consulting and Clinical Psychology, 73*, 610–616. https://doi.org/10.1037/0022-006X.73.4.610

O'Connor, S., & Vandenberg, B. (2010). Differentiating psychosis and faith: The role of social norms and religious fundamentalism. *Mental Health, Religion & Culture, 13*, 171–186. https://doi.org/10.1080/13674670903277984

Parnas, J., & Henriksen, M. G. (2016). Mysticism and schizophrenia: A phenomenological exploration of the structure of consciousness in the schizophrenia spectrum disorders. *Consciousness and Cognition, 43*, 75–88. /https://doi.org/10.1016/j.concog.2016.05.010

Peoples, H. C., Duda, P., & Marlowe, F. W. (2016). Hunter-gatherers and the origins of religion. *Human Nature, 27*, 261–282.

Pettegree, A. (2015). *Brand Luther: How an unheralded monk turned his small town into a centre of publishing, made himself the most famous man in Europe – and started the Protestant Reformation.* Penguin.

Reich, W. (1984). Psychiatric diagnosis as an ethical problem. In S. Bloch & P. Chodoff (Eds.), *Psychiatric ethics* (pp. 61–88). Oxford University Press.

Roberts, G. (1991). Delusional belief systems and meaning in life: A preferred reality? *British Journal of Psychiatry, 159*(Supplement 14), 19–28.

Rothschild, M. (2021). *The storm is upon us: How QAnon became a movement, a cult, and a conspiracy theory of everything.* Monoray.

Sass, L. A. (1994). *The paradoxes of delusion: Wittgenstein, Schreber and the schizophrenic mind.* Cornell University Press.

Schermer, M. (1997). *Why people believe wierd things: Pseudoscience, superstition and other confusions of our time.* W.H. Freeman.

Schwitzgebel, E. (2015). Belief. *Stanford Encyclopedia of Philosophy.* https://plato.stanford.edu/archives/sum2015/entries/belief/

Sendiony, M. F. (1976). Cultural aspects of delusions: A psychiatric study of Egypt. *Australian and New Zealand Journal of Psychiatry, 10*, 201–207.

Shagan, E. H. (2018). *The birth of modern belief.* Princeton University Press.

Smith, L., Riley, S., & Peters, E. R. (2009). Schizotypy, delusional ideation and well-being in an American new religious movement population. *Clinical Psychology & Psychotherapy, 16*(6), 479–484. /https://doi.org/10.1002/cpp.645

Smith, S. M., Fabrigar, L. R., MacDougall, B. L., & Wiesenthal, N. L. (2008). The role of amount, cognitive elaboration, and structural consistency of attitude-relevant knowledge in the formation of attitude certainty. *European Journal of Social Psychology, 38*(2), 280–295. https://doi.org/10.1002/ejsp.447

Speechley, W. J., Ngan, E. T.-C., Moritz, S., & Woodward, T. S. (2012). Impaired evidence integration and delusions in schizophrenia. *Journal of Experimental Psychopathology, 3*(4), 688–701. https://doi.org/10.5127/jep.018411

Sperber, D. (1996). *Explaining culture: A naturalistic approach.* Blackwell.

Stephensen, H., Urfer-Parnas, A., & Parnas, J. (2023). Double bookkeeping in schizophrenia spectrum disorder: An empirical-phenomenological study. *European Archives of Psychiatry and Clinical Neuroscience.* https://doi.org/10.1007/s00406-023-01609-7

Sulik, J., Ross, R. M., Balzan, R., & McKay, R. (2023). Delusion-like beliefs and data quality: Are classic cognitive biases artifacts of carelessness? *Journal of Psychopathology and Clinical Science, 132*(6), 749–760. https://doi.org/10.1037/abn0000844

Swift, D. (2018). *The bughouse: The poetry, politics and madness of Ezra Pound.* Vintage.

Taber, C. S., & Lodge, M. (2013). *The rationalizing voter.* Cambridge University Press.

Thouless, R. H. (1935). The tendency to certainty in religious belief. *British Journal of Psychology, 26*(1), 16–31.

Tormala, Z. L., & Rucker, D. D. (2018). Attitude certainty: Antecedents, consequences, and new direction. *Consumer Psychology Review*, *1*, 72–89. https://doi.org/10.1002/arcp.100

van Os, J., Hanssen, M., Bijl, R. V., & Ravelli, A. (2000). Strauss (1969) revisited: A psychosis continuum in the normal population? *Schizophrenia Research*, *45*, 11–20.

Weber, M. (1905/2002). *The Protestant ethic and the 'spirit' of capitalism and other writings* (B. P. & G. C. Wells, Trans.). Penguin.

Wittgenstein, L. (1969). *On certainty* (D. Paul & G. E. M. Anscombe, Trans.). Blackwell.

Wood, M. J., Douglas, K. M., & Sutton, R. M. (2012). Dead and alive: Beliefs in contradictory conspiracy theories. *Social Psychological and Personality Science*, *3*, 767–773.

Woodward, T. S., Moritz, S., Cuttler, C., & Whitman, J. C. (2006). The contribution of a cognitive bias against disconfirmatory evidence (BADE) to delusions in schizophrenia. *Journal of Clinical and Experimental Neuropsychology*, *28*(4), 605–617. https://doi.org/10.1080/13803390590949511

Wootton, D. (2015). *The invention of science: A new history of the scientific revolution*. Allen Lane.

World Health Organisation. (2018). *International classification of disease*. 11th edition. WHO.

Zavlis, O., Elahi, A., Alba, C., Valiente, C. M., Hartman, T. K., & Richard, B. P. (2023). Increased network connectivity among paranoid beliefs characterizes the clinical end of the schizophrenia-spectrum: A Conversian systems perspective. *Schizophrenia Research*, *258*, 55–57. https://doi.org/10.1016/j.schres.2023.07.016

Zhu, C., Sun, X. J., & So, S. H. (2018). Associations between belief inflexibility and dimensions of delusions: A meta-analytic review of two approaches to assessing belief flexibility. *British Journal of Clinical Psychology*, *57*, 59–81. https://doi.org/10.1111/bjc.12154

# INDEX



abductive inference 363, 391, 418, 434, 435, 436, 440

aberrant salience theory 127, 451, 464, 467, 468, 473; Fletcher/Frith/Corlett modification 469–470; origins of 466–467; reference and misinterpretation 467; strengths and weaknesses 468–469; testing 470–473

abnormal data 223, 224, 417

abnormality 83, 161, 196, 197, 218, 224, 350, 358n2, 383, 415, 417, 424, 426n3, 427, 444, 465, 466, 470, 527, functional 416, 427n4; statistical 416, 427n4

acceptances 16, 308, 310, 319–321, 361

action 277–287; affordance and 165; beliefs and 13, 35, 78, 143, 203, 204–206, 216, 277, 280, 296, 298, 299, 327, 329, 332, 540, 541, 551–552; compulsive 150, 151, 152, 153, 154, 155n3; delusion and 15, 22, 35, 55, 57, 74, 204–206, 212, 216, 246, 247, 249, 277–289, 300, 303–304, 314, 320, 321, 325, 332, 333, 339, 377, 481, 483–484, 493, 506, 508, 511–512, 513–517, 518n4, 522; defensive 372; emotion and 38, 39, 40, 41, 43n4; guidance 15, 35, 204–206, 212, 246, 247, 279–280, 282–284, 314; imagination and 16, 25n5, 280, 309, 327, 330, 332, 374; monitoring 147, 151–152; overvalued ideas and 138

adaptive misbeliefs 79

adaptiveness 8, 42, 62–70, 81; clinical practice and conclusions 68–70, 283; of delusions 8, 9, 23, 34, 37, 42, 43, 47, 48, 49, 62–70, 79, 80, 81, 123, 128–129, 153, 341, 552; insight paradox 63–64

affectivity 11, 38, 39, 41, 43n4, 49, 50, 55, 106, 111, 112, 122, 151, 153, 159, 162, 164, 165, 166–170, 176, 177, 178, 181, 193, 203, 204, 205, 219, 220, 222, 223, 224, 248, 267, 268, 302, 309, 318, 327, 332, 333, 347, 349, 350, 351, 352, 353, 355, 356, 358, 364, 368, 370, 371, 373, 381, 391, 395, 397, 416, 417, 421, 427n10, 455, 458, 463, 477, 479, 480–481, 482, 527, 529

affordance 55, 130, 165

alien abduction 426, 443, 445, 446

AlphaGo 483, 484, 488n3

altered self-agency 495

Alternative Uses paradigm 437, 438

Alzheimer's disease 179, 180, 182, 289n10, 348

anomalous experiences 8, 12, 13, 15, 17, 18, 19, 20, 21, 25n8, 33, 51, 52, 53, 54, 55, 56, 66, 79, 94, 115, 127, 128, 139, 161, 162, 163, 166, 191, 192, 193, 194, 196, 197, 198n5, 199n6, 202, 206, 207, 208, 209, 211, 219, 220, 221, 222, 223, 231, 245, 246, 247, 248, 249, 250, 251, 252, 253, 254, 264, 267, 268, 269, 301–302, 310, 311, 313, 315, 340–342, 343, 349, 350, 352, 356, 361, 366, 370, 373, 377, 390–399, 402, 403, 405, 410, 411, 412n2, 414, 416–425, 427n6, 427n9, 427n10, 438, 445, 455, 456, 463, 464–465, 467, 468, 477, 478, 494, 495, 496, 498, 520, 521, 522, 529, 539, 540, 550, 558, 561, 562; *see also* hallucination

anorexia nervosa (AN) 10, 11, 12, 135–143;
American tradition 135, 143; body size
beliefs 136–139; Brown Assessment of Beliefs
Scale 140–143; continuum delusionality
140–143; European tradition 135, 136,
137–138, 139, 140, 143
anosognosia 17, 252, 295, 319, 441–443, 495,
551; mirror anosognosia 248
antipsychotics 63, 112, 115, 131, 174, 175,
178, 180, 181, 450, 466, 470
Anton-Babinski syndrome (ABS) 246, 251–252,
255n1
anxiety 37, 43n4, 49, 57, 65, 67, 74, 80, 110,
123, 130, 149, 151, 153, 174, 181, 192,
289n9, 293, 299, 309, 319, 341, 370, 377,
516, 527, 529
artificial systems 480, 481–485, 487
autobiographical memory 363, 437, 438
autonomic nervous system 95, 96, 399n1, 432
autotrophy 112, 116n1–117n1
basal cognition 21, 481–485, 486, 487

Bayesian inference 224, 399n2, 453
Bayesian rationality 82, 125, 269, 271n6
Bayne, T. 15, 17, 25n8, 76, 124, 136, 137, 205,
216, 222, 223, 252, 281, 292, 298, 316,
331–332, 334n12, 350, 390, 405–408
Beck, A. T. 65, 160, 161, 169
Beck Depression Inventory 48
belief 4, 5, 6, 7, 10, 14, 15, 16, 18, 19, 22,
25n5, 34, 35, 36–38, 78, 203, 204, 205,
206, 279, 293–300, 377–378, 383, 562–567;
biological-functional approaches 8–9, 73–83,
294–295; degrees of 125; dispositional
approaches 15, 279, 296–300, 318;
fictional 540–541; functional approaches
78, 90, 204, 292, 296–300; and identity
239–240; motivational role 16, 24n5, 234,
277, 279–281, 282–284, 288n4, 298–299,
300–301, 303–304, 314, 327, 329, 551–552;
normative-interpretive approaches 295–296;
norms of 6, 23, 35, 36, 37, 41, 76, 124,
155n3, 199n11, 217, 230, 235, 280, 296,
363, 367, 534, 539, 540; phenomenological
approaches 293–294; representationalist
approaches 294; shared 106, 548–550;
Spinozan theories of 25n1, 310, 311, 312,
320, 392, 393, 439; unconscious 64; *see also*
rationality, belief; and irrationality, belief
Bell, V. 23, 127, 287, 397, 426n4, 520, 522,
523, 524–528
Bentall, R. 24, 522, 559, 563, 565
Berrios, G. E. 47, 170n4, 330
bimagination 16, 76, 208, 317, 332, 333
bizarreness 131, 147, 148, 149, 150, 152,
155n1, 163, 170n5, 173, 176, 182, 222, 223,

224, 231, 237, 238, 247, 248–249, 250, 261,
265, 311, 324, 344n1, 361, 366–367, 368,
370, 390, 396, 398, 404, 406, 410, 418–419,
426, 456, 464, 473, 485, 506, 527–528, 549,
551, 559, 560
blameworthiness 285, 338, 342, 344n2, 507,
508, 509, 513, 514, 517
Bleuler, E. 175, 202, 205, 468
bodily aspect 39, 40
bodily preoccupation 108
body mass index (BMI) 136, 143n2
body size beliefs 136–139
Bongiorno, F. 13, 19, 24–25n1, 95, 192, 223,
310, 350, 399n6, 427n7
borderline personality disorder 87
Bortolotti, L. 3, 5, 6, 7, 8, 15, 23, 33–38, 40,
42, 43n3, 47, 65, 67, 74, 75, 80–82, 83n2,
128, 153, 159, 160–162, 170, 205, 216,
217, 235–237, 238–239, 240, 243n6, 288n3,
288n5, 296, 300, 377, 411, 412n1, 412n3,
420, 518n4, 518n7
Boyd, R. 9, 88, 91, 92–94, 96, 99n11, 99n12
Boyer, P. 18, 382, 384
Broome, M. R. 131, 412n3, 518n4, 518n7
Brown Assessment of Beliefs Scale (BABS)
140–143
bulimia nervosa 137, 143n1

Cahill, C. 422, 423
Campbell, J. 19–20, 219, 221, 249, 389, 390,
394–397, 399, 402–412; *see also* rationalism
cannabis 456
Capgras delusion 1–2, 14, 18, 21, 25n2, 37, 87,
95, 96, 109, 128, 152, 164, 179, 180–181,
190–191, 192, 194, 210, 215, 216, 217,
219–220, 222, 223, 224, 248, 267, 268, 279,
281, 285, 289n10, 292, 295, 301, 302, 303,
304, 311, 316, 319, 320, 321, 324, 329, 330,
334n10, 338–339, 341, 345n9, 347–358,
390–391, 392, 393, 395, 396, 398, 399, 404,
406, 407, 416, 420, 421, 427n6, 427n10,
431, 432, 440, 455, 456, 457, 514, 515, 522,
538, 539, 540; *see also* recognition, facial
'Cassandra's Curse' 261
catatonia 438
central executive network (CEN) 367, 370
certainty in belief 24, 51, 106, 124, 125, 137,
206, 208, 354, 406, 545, 557, 560, 563–564,
567
Charles-Bonnet syndrome 251
childhood trauma 130
Churchland, P. M. 380, 381
Churchland, P. S. 251
civil rights movement 558
Clinician-Rated Dimensions of Psychosis
Symptom Severity 108

coalitional cognition 23, 127, 455, 523, 525, 526, 527, 528
coalitional threats 524
cognitive behavioural therapy 112, 243n5, 301, 459
cognitive biases 17, 33, 64, 111, 126–127, 249, 267, 418, 441, 550
cognitive feelings 16, 320–321
cognitive loading 221
cognitive neuropsychiatry 231, 433, 450–451, 458
cognitive trash 361–366
Coliva, A. 404, 411
collective human agents 485–487
collective intelligence 482, 485
colonization process 41
Coltheart, M. 5, 20, 21, 191, 223–224, 229, 245, 269, 325, 334n4, 352, 391, 399n1, 417, 418, 419, 421, 426, 426n1, 433, 437, 440, 444
compulsions 152
computational approaches, psychosis 125–126
computational neuroscience 451
computational psychiatry 126, 459
confabulation 17, 18, 25n7, 217, 254, 255n1, 286, 324, 347
conscious deliberation 21, 478, 479, 480
consciousness 49, 57, 164, 176, 287, 293, 361, 362, 366, 469
conspiracy theories 37, 42, 113, 238, 463, 465, 529, 541, 544–553; belief in 5, 23, 24, 41, 116, 238, 286, 398, 419, 420, 426, 534, 544–553, 559, 564, 565; definitions of 545–546; and delusion 23, 24, 41, 116, 238, 286, 398, 419, 420, 426, 534, 544–553, 560, 567–568; and evidence 5, 238, 534, 548; falsity and fixity 547–548; and harm 37; mental illness 546–547; prevalence 546–547
context-binding 366
Continuity Thesis (CT) 33, 35, 36
Corlett, P. R. 20, 21, 66, 95, 152, 220, 427n7, 469–470, 473
Cotard delusion 2, 109, 128, 160, 165, 166, 167, 168, 170, 182, 193, 195, 205, 215, 216, 218, 279, 302, 304, 319, 324, 331, 394, 403, 404, 406, 407, 416, 431, 438, 455, 526
Cotard, J. 170n4, 181
COVID-19 pandemic 149, 454; conspiracy beliefs 116; denialism 116
Craver, C. F. 96, 97
credibility 3, 139, 229, 545; epistemic 14, 259, 261–262, 265–266; interpreter 239; prejudicial 258, 260
culture 378–379, 381, 382, 533–541; diagnostic clause 2–3, 5–6, 89, 90, 107, 147, 155n1, 170n5, 204, 210, 229, 238, 288n2, 344n1,

384; content of delusions 23, 124, 485, 534–535, 537, 539–541
Currie, G. 16, 75, 83n5, 315–316, 325, 328, 330, 334n9

das trema 561, 564
David, A. S. 141, 230
Davidson, D. 35, 288n3, 295, 392, 396, 399n10, 408
Davies, M. 4, 17, 20, 192–193, 222, 223, 391, 414, 415, 418–419, 421, 422, 423, 424, 426, 426n2, 427n11, 437, 440, 444
daydreaming 325, 328, 333, 366, 368, 371
decision making 126, 154, 160, 281, 363, 365, 381, 420, 482, 484, 512, 536; clinical 62; biased 93, 269, 465, 550, 561, 563
Deep Dream network 365
Deep Meaning 50
default mode network (DMN) 18, 362, 363, 364, 365, 366, 367, 368, 369, 370, 371, 373, 374
delirium (acute confusion) 122, 178, 182
delusion attribution 14, 15, 228–243, 282; criteria tracked by 237–240; descriptivism 228–232, 236; epistemic approaches 230–231; expressivism 14, 232–236; and folk psychology 18, 383–384; hybrid approach 236–240; issues and future directions 241–243; psychiatric approaches: 229–230; social turn and informational ecology 242–243
delusional atmosphere 51, 115, 207, 208, 209, 478, 484
delusional disorders 9–12, 105–117, 178, 285, 289n8, 406, 463, 465, 546, 551; biopsychosocial factors 108–112, 110; eponyms related to 109; neurobiological basis of 108–110; prognosis of 112; psychiatric nosological systems 107–108; psychiatry 105–106; responsibility 284; socio-demographic correlates 111; social isolation 286
delusions of control 2, 5, 23, 68, 163, 170, 177, 203, 210, 324, 431, 432, 451–452, 493, 495, 521–522, 529, 535, 559
delusions of persecution 2, 3, 10, 11, 23, 55, 80, 87, 106, 108, 111, 112, 115, 116, 122, 127, 128, 130, 150, 160, 177, 178, 179, 181, 182, 248, 279, 284, 285, 286, 289n7, 337, 407, 457, 463, 465, 468, 473, 485, 506, 516, 521–522, 523–524, 526, 528, 529, 534, 535, 538, 539, 540, 544, 559
dementia 176, 178, 180, 286, 347, 389; delirium and 178–181; frontotemporal 182; Lewy body 182, 285, 289n8, 289n10, 486; praecox 106, 175, 202; prevalence of 179; testimonial injustice 271n1, vascular 181

demoralisation 62, 64, 66, 68, 69

Dennett, D. C. 67, 79, 81, 295

depersonalization 222, 370, **431, 432,** 455

depression 7, 11, 37, 48, 64, 65, 69, 106,
158–170, 179, 209, 218, 444, 473; affectivity
162, 166–170, 181–182; cognitive account
of 161–162; delusions 11, 12, 37, 47, 49, 62,
66, 68, 69, 107–108, **109,** 112, 124, 128,
158–170, 175, 192, 205, 218, 302, 303,
406, 444, 450, 505, 546; manic 106, 482,
487; phenomenological perspective 164–170;
post-psychotic 63, 64; psychotic 109, 128,
158, 159, 160, 170n1, 170n2, 182, 334n10;
remission from delusion 7, 62, 64, 66, 68,
69; unipolar 11, 159, 160

deprivation 130

derealization **431,** 455

desire 139, 152, 153, 167, 169, 233, 281, 286,
295, 298, 309, 319, 340, 343, 381; and
action 298, 304, 381, 540; and anorexia
nervosa 135; and delusion 295, 319; and
imagination 298, 309; for meaning 558;
and OCD 153; pathological 135; and
self-deception 17, 295, 344n4

despair 47, 63, 66, 260, 283

Dewey, J. 34, 38–41, 43n3

*Diagnostic and Statistical Manual of Mental
Disorders III (DSM-III)* 107, 115, 544

*Diagnostic and Statistical Manual of Mental
Disorders IV (DSM-IV)* 2; delusion 2–6, 21,
89, 98n5, 107, 124, 245, 377, 384, 534;
delusional disorders 107; doxasticism 6, 124;
evidence 4–5; paraphrenia 11; psychosis 122;
*see also* culture; diagnostic clause

*Diagnostic and Statistical Manual of Mental
Disorders 5 (DSM-5)* 2, conspiracy theory
545; delusional disorders 107; delusional
value-based beliefs 139; descriptivism 229;
delusion 3–6, 15, 21, 35, 43n2, 83n1, 89,
98n5, 124, 147, 155n1, 160, 161, 170n5,
189, 204, 229, 245, 265, 325, 329, 330,
334n4, 337, 339, 344n1, 376, 377, 384,
430, 506, 515, 534, 545, 549, 550, 551,
559; delusional disorders 107, 108, 110;
doxasticism 6, 124, 216, 324, 325, 329,
337, 384; evidence 5, 12, 35, 83n1, 148,
189, 265, 271n2, 288n2, 324, 330, 337,
376, 430, 515, 550; overvalued ideas 10, 12,
140; paraphrenia 11; psychosis 126; *see also*
culture; diagnostic clause

diagnostic overshadowing 260

discharge 43n4

disembodiment 55, 455

disorders of old age 173–183; affective
181–182; delirium and dementia 178–181;
delusional 178; late-onset schizophrenia

177–178; late paraphrenia 175–176; very
late-onset schizophrenia 177–178; vignettes
174–175, 180, 181; *see also* Alzheimer's
disease

disorders of the self 163

dissociation, objection from 219–220, 421–425,
432–433, 438–439, 456, 457, 464–465; deny
421–423, 427n10; embrace 423–425

divergent hinges 404, 405, 410

dogmatism 223, 399n3

dopamine 108, 110, **371,** 371, 451, 456, 471,
483; salience 20, 127, 372, 451, 466, 467–
468, 470, schizophrenia 130–131, 450, 467;
system 21, 93, 372

dorsolateral prefrontal cortex (DLPFC) 367,
373, 457; left 433; right 433, 442, 443, 446

Dotson, K. 259, 261

double bookkeeping 13, 56, 202–212, 407, 552,
562, 567; behavioural inertia 205; belief and
action 204–206; belief and experience
206–208; phenomenology 208–211

doxasticism 6, 12, 13, 15, 16, 33, 34, 36, 38,
41, 74–75, 83n4, 123, 124, 126, 161, 204,
205–206, 215–216, 278, 279–284, 287,
288n2, 288n3, 289n9, 292–305, 308, 313,
414; Spinozan 16, 25n1; malfunction 73,
76–78, 80, 83; weak 292, 300, 303, 305

dreaming 361–374; AIM model 364, 368–373;
beliefs 373–374; cognitive trash 361–366; as
delusions 373–374; as mindwandering
366–368; as states of imagination 373–374

Drury, M. O'C. 173, 174, 183

dry-functionalism 78

Dub, R. 24n1, 320–321

echo chambers 415, 486

Egan, A. 75, 76, 208, 223, 317, 332–333

egodystonicity 150

egosyntonicity 150

Eilan, N. 409, 410

eliminativism, belief 380, dreams 364, 365;
natural kinds 87

Ellis, H. D. 349, 352, 355, 390–391, 538, 539

Emergence Model of Delusions 49, 129

emotions 8, 13, 17–18, 24n1, 34, 37, 38,
39–40, 41, 43n3, 47, 52, 53, 54, 56, 57, 67,
69, 106, 111, 114, 127, 128, 151, 165, 166,
167, 169, 192, 196, 197, 203, 204, 205, 219,
233, 234, 235, 242, 279, 293, 298, 302, 303,
309, 316, 317, 318, 327, 329, 340, 341, 343,
348, 352, 369, 370, 373, 381, 402, 410, 416,
486, 495, 496, 505, 508, 510, 517, 529;
Darwinian picture of 38; *qua* mental states
43n4; *qua* psychological states 39; trauma 55

empiricism 19, 20, 25n8, 79, 219, 389–399,
414; causal 392–393; content 393–394;

endorsement 13, 25n8, 192, 222, 223, 246, 249, 250, 251, 252, 253, 255, 350, 352, 391, 399n3, 539; exhaustiveness and exclusivity 397–398; explanationist 13, 25n8, 192, 222, 249, 250, 350, 352, 391, 539; normative 390–392; one-factor versions 414; rationalism and reasons 394–397
endocrine disturbance 122
epistemic bubbles 37, 415, 486
epistemic injustice 14, 258–270; disputing false stereotypes 266–270; ethical and epistemic implications 260–261; hermeneutical 14, 258–259, 260, 262–264, 270; testimonial 8, 258, 259, 260, 261–262, 265, 266, 271n1
epistemic innocence 67, 217, 552
epistemic vigilance 530
euthymia 64
evidence 189–190; and belief 6, 16, 35, 41, 66, 67, 74, 155n3, 216, 217, 230, 238, 265, 266–267, 288n4, 294, 295, 296, 309, 327, 330, 332, 376, 398, 480, 540; and body size beliefs 137, 138, 140–141, 142; and delusion 1, 2, 3, 4–5, 10, 12, 14, 17–18, 23, 74, 78, 114, 189–199, 216, 217, 222, 223, 231, 235, 246, 247, 248, 249, 254, 265, 279, 299–302, 303, 311–314, 318–319, 320, 330, 331, 332, 333, 337, 339, 341, 344n1, 348, 376–377, 389, 390, 391, 406, 417, 418, 419, 420, 426, 427n5, 427n8, 430, 432, 445, 467–468, 484, 496, 506, 515, 518n6, 521, 522, 524, 525, 534, 560; externalism 12, 190, 192, 193, 195, 196, 198n4; factivity 190, 192, 193, 194, 198n1, 199n9; internalism 12, 189–190, 192, 193, 194, 195–196, 198, 199n13; and OCD 147, 148, 149, 150–151, 154, 155n2; perceptual 21, 190, 191, 192, 480, 530; phenomenal conception 190; sensory 126, 362, 477, 483, social sources of 22, 485, 530; *see also Diagnostic and Statistical Manual of Mental Disorders IV (DSM-IV), and evidence; Diagnostic and Statistical Manual of Mental Disorders 5 (DSM-5), and evidence; rationality, and evidence*
evolutionary gradualism 481, 483, 487
excusing conditions 15, 282, 285, 286, 298, 299, 301–302, 303, 304, 314, 317, 318, 321, 322
excusing behaviour 22, 281, 285, 508–511, 513–514, 515, 517
exemptions 505–506, 508–511
existential feelings 52, 58n2, 167, 168, 169
explanationism 13, 25n8, 192, 222, 391
explanatory pluralism 129–130
explanatory unavailability 420
expressivism 13–14, 232–236; deep disagreement 234; disjunctive norm pluralism 235; evaluation and evaluative discourse 232; heterogeneity 234–235; intrinsic motivation 234; intuitive folk norms 235–236; moral 14; non-factualist and non-cognitivist alternatives 241–242; parsimony 233–234
externalism 190, 193

factors 12, 20, 21, 47; and abnormality 415–416, 426n2; neuropsychological damage 426n3, 446; *see also* one-factor theory; two-factor theory
fake delusion 3
false belief test 378
feature binding 18, 366, 373
fecundity 91, 99n9
fictional beliefs 540, 541
figurative language 13, 53, 57, 206
fixity 547–548; in delusion 3, 5, 35, 106, 147, 161, 181, 216, 245, 271n2, 334n1, 337, 376, 411, 430, 450, 454, 534, 544, 545, 550, 559
Fletcher, P. C. 152, 469–470, 473
Flores, C. 5, 12, 15, 197, 198, 312–313
Fodor, J. 379, 536, 537
*folie à deux* 23, 89, 106, 107, 108, 443–444, 446, 484, 486, 493, 547, 549, 567
*folie communiquée* 106
folk psychology 16, 17, 18, 19, 208, 280, 362, 365, 374, 378–382, 562; delusion and 1, 15, 18–19, 204, 208, 212, 363, 374, 382–384, 567; skeptics 380
fortune-telling 486
fragmentation 127, 225n5, 295, 396, 399n10, 562
framework propositions 20, 221, 292, 395, 408
Frankish, K. 319–320
Freeman, D. 561
Fregoli delusion **109**, 128, 303, 304, 324, 431, 432, 493, 496
French, C. C. 445
Freud, S. 34, 38–39, 40, 41, 43n3, 43n4, 47, 69, 110
Fricker, M. 14, 258, 259, 260, 261–263, 265, 270
Friston, K. J. 453, 469
Frith, C. D. 469–470, 473
functional dopamine excess 467, 468, 470
functionalism 78, 90, 204, 292, 297
functional magnetic imaging (fMRI) 253, 443, 458, 470
functional neuroimaging data 452
function debate 77–78

GABA 131
Gallagher, S. 16, 164, 209–211, 325, 328–329, 377
Garety, P. 268, 465

Garson, J. 42, 47, 69
Gendler, T. S. 325, 541
Gerrans, P. 18, 203, 269–270, 377, 406, 416,
    424–425
Gilbert, D. T. 439
Gold, I. 5, 23, 522, 523, 524–526
Gold, J. 5, 23, 522, 523, 524–526
Goldman, A. 381
Grahame, P. S. 176
grandiose delusions 3, 17, 23, 48–49, 74, 75,
    76, 80, 83n3, 96, 106, 108, 127, 128, 150,
    177, 181, 182, 194, 337, 342, 463, 467, 506,
    522, 526, 528, 529, 535, 540, 544, 549,
    552, 559
grief 55, 329
Griffiths, P. 94, 381
guilt 57, 124, 159, 170n3, 175, 508; delusions
    of 128, 160, 168, 169, 181, 535

Haidt, J. 564
Halligan, P. W. 252, 434
hallucinations 10, 63, 106, 107, 117n3, 122,
    128, 130, 158, 159, 176, 177, 178, 181, 190,
    193, 202, 206, 208, 246, 247, 248, 249, 250,
    251, 254, 334n8, 365, 368, 412n6, 416, 422,
    445, 450, 453, 454, 456, 457, 458–459, 464,
    465, 471, 492, 493, 518n7
harmful dysfunction analysis (HDA) 80, 82,
    83n9
Heidegger, M. 52, 58n1, 167
Henriksen, M. G. 52, 208, 412n5
hermeneutical injustice 14, 258, 259, 260,
    262–264, 270
heterogeneity 23, 176, 117n4; of belief 140,
    142, 553; of delusion 1, 10, 11, 206, 232,
    234–235, 236, 264, 511, 527
Hierarchical Taxonomy of Psychopathology
    (HiTOP) 115, 117n4
higher-order evidence 191, 198n2
higher-stakes attributions 284–285
hinges 41, 221, 404–412
Hirstein, W. 349, 351–353, 356, 357, 358n3
Hobson, J. A. 364, 370, 373
Hofstadter, R. 547, 549
Hohwy, J. 410, 411, 427n7
homeopathy 559
homeostatic property cluster account (HPC) 9,
    88, 92–98, 99n10, 99n11, 99n12; challenges
    93–96; continuity objections 94; delusion
    93–96; unity problem 94–96
Honey, G. D. 152
hopelessness 62, 64, 205
Hume, D. 362, 393
Huq, S. F. 82
Husserl, E. 52, 209
hydraulic model 43n4

hypervigilance 40, 524
hypnosis 253, 491–498, 533; delusion
    21, 491–498; evaluation 496–
    497; hypnosis-as-procedure 491;
    hypnosis-as-product 491; hypnotic
    suggestion 433, 494; implications 497–498;
    modelling underlying processes 494–496
hypochondriacal delusion 89, 106, **109**, 128,
    182, 464
hypothesis generation 196, 418, 427n7, 431,
    433, 435, 436; individual differences
    437–438, 445

Ichino, A. 288n4, 299
identity-prejudicial credibility deficit 258–260
illusions 43n1, 67, 108, 320, 393, 442, 565; of
    control 267; positive 65, 79, 552; visual 192,
    223, 393, 530, 536
imagination 16, 25n5, 54, 55, 68, 151, 193,
    202, 208, 251, 252, 253, 254, 281, 288n4,
    297, 298–299, 301, 309, 325–327, 363, 364,
    367, 370, 381, 410, 486, 492, 524; delusion
    as 16, 19, 33, 43n1, 74, 75–76, 83n3, 83n5,
    205, 207–208, 217, 225n2, 229, 280, 302,
    308–310, 314–317, 324–334, 373–374, 377;
    *see also* bimagination
implausibility 3, 4, 12, 22, 47, 52, 69, 89, 114,
    115, 136, 140, 147, 155n1, 170n5, 222, 224,
    237–238, 239, 240, 337, 340, 341, 344n1,
    418, 419, 441, 524, 534, 541, 559
incoherence 74, 78, 370; internal 13, 35;
    narrative 373
incomprehensibility 136, 137, 139, 147, 148,
    150, 163, 209, 211, 238, 261, 265, 394,
    477, 485
incorrigibility 14, 66, 67, 106, 115, 136, 137,
    140, 174, 208, 211, 246, 254, 545, 566
inference 21, 63, 216, 224, 231, 254, 354,
    362–363, 364, 366, 368, 369, 370, 371,
    373, 377, 379, 380, 384, 391, 392, 399n2,
    418, 434–435, 436, 440, 451, 453, 454,
    465, 477–487, 520, 526, 529, 536; active
    362–363, 364, 365, 366, 368, 369, 370, 371,
    371, 482, 483; artificial systems 481–485;
    basal cognition 481–485; collective human
    agents 485–487; definition of 478; (non)
    epistemic 478–481; non-human systems
    481–485; (non)propositional 478–481; (un)
    conscious 478–481
inferential promiscuity 311, 315
influencing machine delusion 533, 534
inner speech 53, 379, 450, 452; non-literal 53
innocence defence 67
insight 10, 51, 52, 53, 57, 62, 122, 140, 141,
    142, 147, 211, 316, 317, 494, 497, 524, 537,
    551; paradox 8, 62, 63–64, 65–66, 68, 69–70

intention 66, 97, 278, 279, 282, 283, 285, 286, 287, 288n1, 289n12, 455, 465, 506, 513, 541; and action 2, 18, 285, 287, 368, 458, 509, 513; to deceive 17; and self-deception 17, 340, 342, 343, 344
intentional content 90, 289n12, 364
intentionalism 340
intentionality 90, 168, 488n2; bodily 52
intentionality bias 415
intentional object 149, 168
Interpretative Phenomenological Analysis 51
introspection 14, 63, 190, 191, 192, 193, 196, 207, 245–255, 379, 419; Anton-Babinski syndrome 14, 246, 250, 251–252, 254, 255; introspective delusions 14, 247–255; mistakes 14, 246–247; supernumerary limb delusion 252; thought insertion 250–251, 264
intuitive folk norms 235–236
intuitive thinking 550
ion channel permeability 482
irrationality 7, 13, 36, 125, 149, 207, 235, 237, 261, 278, 343, 403, 484, 485; abnormal 14, 215, 217–218, 222, 261; beliefs 33, 35–36, 41, 42, 67, 74–75, 76–77, 80, 141, 216, 288n3, 299, 374, 383, 498; delusion 8, 13, 35–36, 37, 38, 41, 69, 74–75, 76–77, 80, 124, 126–127, 128, 217–218, 222–224, 225n2, 230–231, 248, 261, 262, 265–270, 271n4, 279, 336, 343–344, 362, 390, 391, 392, 396, 397, 412n1, 416, 419, 424–425, 477, 521, 522–523, 525; inaccurate attribution 258, 266–270; normal range 13, 20, 22, 35–36, 219–222, 230, 243n4, 271n3, 416, 419, 424–425; self-deception 25n6, 243n3, 336, 343–344

James, W. 209, 417, 430, 439, 562, 563
Jaspers, K. 51–52, 106, 128, 137, 208, 210, 225n1, 263, 394, 410, 412n7, 474, 545, 546, 548, 550, 561
jealousy 179, 410, 536, 537; delusions of 105, 106, 108, 112, 116, 178, 262, 410, 522, 535, 536, 544, 548, 549
Jeppsson, S. 58n3, 411
jumping to conclusions (JTC) bias 82, 93, 110, 111, 126, 199n12, 268, 269, 271n5, 465, 468, 477, 485, 538, 550, 561
Jureidini, J. 315
justification 19, 40, 189–190, 195, 197, 218, 249, 278, 281–282, 286, 289n13, 348, 354, 361, 381, 383, 390, 391, 392, 393, 395, 399n4, 427n6, 506, 508–511, 513, 515, 551

Kamin blocking effect 452
Kant, I. 203
Kapur, S. 20–21, 451, 467–470

Khalidi, M. A. 88, 96, 99n17
Kind, A. 16, 288–289n6, 317, 333, 334n13
Klee, R. 410, 411
Kraepelin, E. 11, 106, 107, 175, 205, 468
Kyratsous, M. 261, 262, 265

Lancellotta, E. 81, 128
Langdon, R. 136–137, 245, 252, 255n1, 352, 443, 444
language 49, 53, 54, 241, 378, 379, 403, 404, 480, 492, 521, 563, 566; body 463; constitutive function 409; figurative 13, 53, 57, 206; medical 263, 264; metaphorical 13, 54, 55, 56, 123, 206; philosophy of 354, 380, 408; of thought 318
learning 152, 155, 365, 451, 452–453, 455, 459, 466–467, 469, 478, 482, 484; automated 66, 67; cultural 6; reinforcement 453, 483; resumption of 66–67; reversal learning tasks 154, 454; reward-based 453, 466, 469; social 529–530
Littlemore, J. 54, 55
Localised Dysfunction Hypothesis 525, 526, 527, 528, 530
Locke, J. 327, 393
loss of sensibility 165

MacKay, C. 486, 558, 567
madness of crowds 486, 545, 559, 560, 562, 567
Maher, B. A. 3, 13, 192, 219–222, 231, 390, 417–418, 420–425, 427n9, 430, 452, 464, 465, 539
major depressive disorder 181
malfunction 73–83, 294, 356, 455; approach 8; of belief 8–9, 19, 20, 47, 73, 80–83, 139, 221, 249–250, 294, 334n8, 395, 405; doxasticism 73, 76–78; dreams 366; function and 77–78; harmfulness thesis 80–81; memory 347, 356; nature and pathology 74–76; thesis 81–83
manic depression 482, 487
Martha Mitchell Effect 3
McDowell, J. 296, 399n5, 408
McGinn, C. 328, 334n8
McKay, R. 67, 79, 81, 198n5, 218, 352, 415
McNally, R. J. 445
meanings 20, 3, 8, 40, 46–58, 209, 211, 241, 247, 292, 380, 393, 403, 404, 405, 407, 409, 453, 463, 474, 477, 483, 516, 558, 559, 562; delusion and 7–8, 9, 34, 42, 46–58, 68, 115, 123, 124–125, 127, 128–129, 131, 158, 163, 208, 216–217, 249, 264, 266, 268, 285–287, 341–342, 394, 417, 424, 467; experience as source of 19, 393; generative effect 53; metaphorical 46, 55, 56

memory 54, 154, 254, 300, 347–358, 380, 437, 457, 480, 482, 496, 563; affective responsiveness hypothesis 349; archival view 356; autobiographical 363, 437–438; Capgras delusion 347–358; constructive view 356; delusion and 17–18, 19, 193, 347–358; episodic 357, 358, 437; long term 296; semantic 357, 437; updating account 355–358; working memory 110, 367, 370
mental files 351, 352, 353, 354–355, 356, 357
mental time travel 364, 371
Merleau-Ponty, M. 52
mesolimbic dopamine system 21
meta-cognition 83n5, 93, 151, 152, 153, 192, 205, 316, 361, 364, 366, 372, 373
metaphorical thinking 13, 53, 54, 55–57
metaphor 46, 53–55, 58n4, 123, 206, 220, 453; and meaning 46, 53–57
methodological naturalism 91
metonymy 56, 57
Millikan, R. G. 77–78
mindreading 351, 353–354, 357, 358n3, 378, 535
mindwandering 362, 366–368, 371
misidentification 107, 328, 348, 456; delusion of 10, 18, 109, 128, 177, 180, 205, 235, 279, 304, 348, 354, 357, 358n3, 358n7, 390, 456, 514, 535, 544, 549; mirrored-self 324, 421, 431, 493, 494, 496; see also Capgras; Fregoli
Miyazono, K. 8–9, 25n1, 33, 83n10, 194, 345n7, 485
modularity 381, 458, 523, 524, 525, 526, 528, 536–537, 537, 540
monetary incentive delay task 472
monothematic delusion 9, 19–21, 87, 178, 191, 193, 215, 216, 220, 221, 222, 225n1, 245, 267, 269, 271n5, 279, 289n10, 292, 300, 314, 319, 321, 399, 404, 407, 414, 417, 422, 426, 427n11, 430, 431, 446, 455, 511, 522, 527
mood 52, 56, 58n1, 58n2, 162, 283, 284, 285, 289n8, 381, 477, 546; congruent delusions 11, 159, 160, 181; delusional 51, 127, 458, 463, 464, 467, 468, 470, 473, 474, 546, 561, 567; disorders 107, 135, 162; incongruent delusions 159; low 62, 64, 65, 67; phenomenological account 166–167
moral psychology 278, 382
moral responsibility 286, 289n11, 289n13, 505–517; definition of 506–508; and delusion 1, 22, 24, 160, 189, 278, 284, 285, 289n10, 342, 344n5, 505–518; epistemic condition 509; excuses 508–511; exemptions 508–511; justifications 508–511
morphogenesis 483

Moscow School of Psychiatry 558
motivation 7, 19, 65, 67, 524, 536; belief 38, 193, 230, 235, 241, 247, 343, 419; confabulation 17; delusion 17, 23, 152–155, 193, 195, 199n7, 205, 249, 252, 254, 302, 313, 319, 320, 341, 343–344, 419–420, 443, 444, 445, 529; self-deception 17, 23, 313, 339, 340, 341, 342, 343–344, 427n8; see also belief, motivational role
motivational unavailability 419–420
motivated delusions 67, 217
mourning 69
Moyal-Sharrock, D. 404, 407, 411
multiple realities 204, 209, 210, 211, 328, 329
Murphy, D. 6, 18–19, 43n2, 243n2
Nash, J. 207, 397, 464, 527
natural kind essentialism (NKE) 88–90; individuation condition 88–89; reasons to reject 91–92, 98
natural kinds 9, 87–98, 544; delusions as 9, 97–98; dominant assumptions 90–91; fecundity 91, 99n9; individuation 88, 89, 90, 92, 94, 96, 97; inductive potential 91, 99n9; intrinsicality 88, 90, 91, 98n3; paradigmatic candidates of 87; simple causal theory 96–98; stickiness 91, 99n9; see also natural kind essentialism (NKE); homeostatic property cluster account
negative identity prejudice 259
negative stereotyping 259
neo-Kraepelinianism 107
network psychometrics 565
network theory 115, 117n4
neurodegeneration 289n10, 348, 380
neuropsychological impairment 421, 423, 426n3, 431, 433, 442, 443, 446, 497; absence of 443–445; Alzheimer's disease 179; erotomania 21
neuroscience 33, 130, 380, 450, 451, 459
neurotransmission 108
neuro-vulnerabilities 129
Nielssen, O. 443, 444
nihilistic delusions 109, 128, 159, 160, 167, 182, 337, 535, 544
non-cognitivism 241–242
non-doxasticism 6, 16, 19, 73, 75, 78, 83n3, 206, 217, 279–282, 292, 293, 294, 295, 300–304, 308–322; acceptances 310; arguments 311–314; cognitive imaginings 19, 308–309; hybrid first-order states 317–319; meta-cognitive states 314–317; suppositions 309; two level accounts of cognition 319–321; weak 292, 304, 308, 311, 314
non-monotonicity 125
non-neuropsychological somatic delusion 444

non-rapid eye movement (NREM) 370, **371,** 372, 373
Noordhof, P. 16, 25n6, 193, 220, 243n3, 267, 419, 427n5
norepinephrine system 372
normality 13, 116, 117n4, 176, 423, 479, 522, 527; functional 416; statistical 416
Nozick, R. 80, 235

object memory 357
obsessions 40, 137, 147, 148, 149–150, 154, 377
obsessive-compulsive disorder (OCD) 11, 12, 147–155, 198, 377, 441; action monitoring dysfunction 151–152; cognitive profile of 148–151; *see also* overvalued ideas
Ohlhorst, J. 411, 412n4
one-factor theory 13, 20, 79, 81, 161, 164, 197, 220, 243n4, 249, 267–268, 269, 271n4, 340–341, 342, 350, 358n2, 414–426, 452; delusions as explanations of experience 416–417; delusions as normal explanations for experience 13, 220, 267, 417–420; delusions as poor explanations 418–420; delusions as rational 13, 427n9; experience as sufficient for delusion 412n2, 421, 422, 423–424; prediction error 454, 456; *see also* dissociation, objection from; factors
optimism 65, 342; bias 65, 74, 266, 267
organic malfunction 19, 20, 221, 249, 395, 405
Other Specified Feeding and Eating Disorder (OSFED) 143n1
overt recognition 349
overvalued ideas 10–11, 12, 25n3, 135–140, 141, 142, 143

Pace-Schott, E. F. 18, 373
Pacherie, E. 15, 216, 223, 331, 332, 334n12, 350, 405–408
Pandis, C. 348, 354
panic attack 39, 40, 41
paranoia 66, 105, 111, 112, 116–117n1, 129, 175, 176, 194, 248, 251, 253, 454, 455, 456, 457, 459, 467, 494, 523, 524, 525, 526, 529, 546, 547, 549–550, 553, 561, 566, 567, 568; psychiatric nosological systems 107–108; in psychiatry 105–106
paranoid delusions 22, 110, 175, 176, 177, 179, 181, 410, 463, 465, 546, 551, 553, 559
paraphrenia 11, 106, 175; late onset 11, 174, 175–177, 182
parasitosis **109,** 178, 181, 398
Parnas, J. 163, 166, 208, 209
Parrott, M. 13, 19, 196, 225n6, 400n12, 418, 427n7
parsimony 14, 233–234

partial insanity 106
pathology 7, 34, 38–41, 74, 76, 80, 94, 114, 243n4, 403; belief 8, 33, 34, 36, 37, 40–43, 52, 135–136, 140, 254, 383, 560, 562; delusion 1, 6–7, 9, 33–43, 47, 50, 66, 69, 73–77, 80, 83, 83n2, 83n5, 94, 106, 107, 122, 124, 140, 215, 220, 222, 229–230, 246, 247, 248, 286, 342–343, 345n7, 373–374, 376, 378, 384, 409, 410, 425, 538, 558; desire 135–136; emotion 34, 39–40, 41; memory 17; neuro 182, 444, 465; question 9, 33, 34, 36, 37, 38, 41, 73–77, 83n3; self-deception 342–343, 345n6
pedestrian delusions 410–411
Peircean pathway model 433–437, *436,* 438, 439, 440, 442, 445, 446n2
Peirce, C. S. 434–437, 439–440
perceptual knowledge 52
perfectionism 139, 148; beliefs 148, 151
performance failure 20, 267, 268, 269, 270, 341, 414
perplexity 21, 40, 51, 399, 463, 565
persecutory delusions 2, 3, 10, 11, 23, 55, 63, 65, 68, 80, 87, 106, 108, 111, 112, 115, 116, 122, 127, 128, 130, 150, 160, 175, 177, 178, 179, 181, 182, 248, 279, 284, 285, 286, 289n7, 337, 407, 457, 463, 465, 468, 473, 485, 506, 516, 521, 522, 523, 524, 526, 527–528, 529, 534, 535, 538, 539, 540, 544, 559, 567
person-centered adaptiveness 128–129
personification 57
Petrolini, V. 7, 40, 43n3, 83n4
phantom border delusion **179,** 180, 181
phantom limb 252, 253, 464; pain 252, 253
phenomenology 47, 50, 52, 54, 55, 56, 57, 58n2, 116, 123, 124, 127, 130, 131, 138, 158, 159, 160–161, 162–167, 168, 169, 170, 173, 192, 197–198, 204, 208–211, 212, 252, 270, 362, 365, 368, **371,** 374, 459, 474, 477, 545, 562; belief 16, 204, 206, 208, 293–294; clinical context 8; delusions and 13, 46, 50–51, 115, 162–164, 183, 204, 208, 254, 398, 450, 451, 468, 553, 561; memory 17; obsessive-compulsive disorder 153; psychopathology 158, 162, 163; social 455; social cognition 380, 455; *see also* Interpretative Phenomenological Analysis
phobias 40, 43n4, 250, 320, 321, 523
Piaget's model 161
Plato 182
polythematic delusions 87, 215, 245, 404, 422, 426n1, 522, 527
positron emission tomography (PET) 130
posthypnotic suggestion 492, 494
post-psychotic depression 64
postsynaptic dopamine D2 receptors 466

post-traumatic stress disorder 112
powerlessness 47
Power Threat Meaning Framework 516
praecox feeling 115
pragmatic rationality 270
pragmatism 34, 38, 41
predictive processing 8, 20, 66, 95, 191,
    450–459, 466–474; and delusion 8, 20,
    66–67, 95–96, 110, 123, 126, 129, 131, 152,
    248–249, 340, 341, 342, 397, 400n12, 418,
    427n7, 450–459, 467–470, 473–474, 481;
    hierarchy 453–454; and OCD 147, 148, 152,
    153–155; model fitting 453; and two-factor
    approach 82–83, 430
prefrontal cortex 442, 451, 453, 458;
    dorsolateral (DLPFC) 367, 370, 373, 433,
    443, 446, 455, 457, 473; ventromedial 369,
    373, 416, 421, 470, 473
preoccupation 74, 138, 143, 497, 548
procedural rationality 35, 249, 270, 367, 560
prosopagnosia 349, **431**, 525
psychiatry 33, 46, 47, 55, 74, 87, 90, 105, 106,
    114, 115, 138, 173, 203, 211, 212, 221,
    243n5, 258–260, 270, 336, 343, 408, 409,
    481, 487, 516, 534, 535, 544, 549, 550;
    computational 116, 125, 126, 399, 450, 451,
    459; folk 381; old age 176; philosophy of
    158, 212, 215
psychoanalysis 34, 38, 41
psychodynamic theories 37, 64, 345n9, 364
psychoeducation 69
psychosis 10, 11, 20, 47, 51, 53, 55, 56, 57,
    58n4, 63, 64, 66, 69, 70, 106, 110, 111,
    112, 122–131, 135, 138, 160, 170n1,
    178, 182, 205, 209, 341, 361, 364, 367,
    368, 369, 451, 452–453, 454, 456, 459,
    463, 511, 512, 525, 535, 538, 541, 558;
    affective 176; arteriosclerotic 176; biological
    factors 130–131; bio-pheno-social model
    129–130; delusions in 3, 9, 10, 11, 20,
    47, 53, 66, 94, 122–131, 135, 341, 451,
    464, 535; epistemic injustice and 262, 264;
    rationality and computational approaches
    125–126; salience 452–453; senile 175;
    socio-developmental factors 130
psychotherapy 63, 69, 70, 112
psychotic depression **109**, 159, 160, 170,
    170n1, 170n2, 181, 182, 334n10
psychotomimetic drugs 456
Purpose in Life Test 48

Quality of Will Test 506, 512–515
Quality of Will Thesis 512, 513, 517

radicalization 277, 552
Radden, J. 25n1, 98n4, 203, 231, 376

Radua, J. 471, 472
Raihani, N. J. 524, 527–528
Ramachandran, V. S. 348, 355
rapid eye movement (REM) sleep 368, 370,
    372, 373
Ratcliffe, M. 52, 58n1, 58n2, 165, 167–169,
    209, 380–381, 398
rationalism 19, 221, 248, 389–390, 394–395,
    397, 398, 399n9, 402–412; developments of
    410–412; Wittgensteinian criticisms
    408–409; *see also* hinges
rationality 13, 18, 19, 33, 37, 125–126,
    215–224, 225n3, 240, 248, 403, 404,
    480, 511, 523; agential 36, 128; and belief
    6, 19, 24, 33, 35, 124, 198n2, 239, 265,
    281, 288n3, 295–296, 363, 377, 383–384,
    402–403, 478; and delusion 12, 13, 19, 20,
    23, 47, 89, 90, 126–127, 189, 195–198,
    199n9, 215–225, 231, 247, 301–302, 361,
    367, 390, 392, 393, 395, 396, 400n13, 403,
    405, 427n9, 464, 477–478, 511, 560; and
    evidence 5, 12, 14, 17, 137, 140–141, 142,
    189–190, 195–198, 217, 247, 296, 311,
    312–314, 377; norms of 33, 35, 36, 37, 41,
    43n3, 217, 362, 363, 367, 384; and OCD
    11, 149, 152, 154; practical 230, 279, 281,
    282, 284, 286; *see also* epistemic innocence;
    irrationality
Ravenscroft, I. 330
reactive attitudes 240, 242, 508, 510, 512
reality testing 18, 203, 206, 361, **371, 432**, 494
recognition 52, 140, 300, 349, 356, 358, 522;
    covert 349; facial 18, 95, 96, 191, 349, 350,
    352, 355, 391, 525, 540; overt 349; self 496
reduplicative paramnesia 18, 210, 357, 358n7,
    526
Reed, E. J. 526, 529
Reed, G. 424
referential delusions 108, 337, 464, 465, 466,
    468, 470, 473
region of interest (ROI) approach 471
religious beliefs 3, 4, 6, 24, 35, 37, 38, 40, 41,
    43n2, 79, 107, 137, 204, 229, 300, 301, 304,
    485, 486, 545, 548, 549, 558, 559, 560, 563,
    564, 566, 567
religious delusion 3, 128, 337, 420, 522, 535,
    558, 559
repetitive transcranial magnetic stimulation
    (rTMS) 433
Rescorla and Wagner model 466
responsibility 148, 151, 152; epistemic 197,
    242, 518n5; *see also* moral responsibility;
    moral responsibility and delusion
retrosplenial cortex 457
reverse Othello 17, 37, 42, 67, 68, 218, 235,
    238, 342, 420

Revonsuo, A. 366, 370
Rhodes, J. 57, 411
riddle task 442, **443**
Ritunnano, R. 7–8, 10, 47, 49, 123, 127, 264
Roth, M. 175, 176, 178, 182
Ryan, L. 113, 117n2

sadness 53, 64, 135
Saks, E. R. 203, 253
Salice, A. 25n1, 194, 485
salience 20–21, 40, 66, 127, 129, 130, 198,
    209, 248–249, 251, 341, 361, 362, 363,
    364, 372, 373, 451–452, 453, 455, 457,
    463–474; erotomania 20; network 367; *see
    also* aberrant salience theory
salience network (SN) 367, 368, 370
Sanati, A. 261, 262, 265
Sartre, J. P. 52, 344n4
Sass, L. 129, 163, 166, 202, 203, 206, 207, 209,
    210, 225n1, 302
Scale for the Assessment of Positive Symptoms
    (SAPS) 534–535
schizophrenia 10, 18, 47, 48, 50, 51, 55, 56, 65,
    87, 106, 107, 111, 112, 116, 122, 127, 128,
    130, 131, 152, 159, 160, 162, 163, 175, 180,
    192, 193, 202, 203, 205, 206, 208, 209, 211,
    215, 221, 225n1, 229, 245, 250–251, 254,
    289n8, 302, 324, 328, 334n9, 334n10, 348,
    368, 389, 396–397, 399, 406, 410, 411, 417,
    422, 427n11, 450, 454, 458, 463, 464, 465,
    468, 471, 472, 473, 474, 483, 487, 505, 510,
    511, 512, 522, 524, 527, 546, 551, 557, 558;
    bodily experience 166; diagnosis 115, 158,
    175–176, 181, 558; dopamine hypothesis
    466, 467, 468, 470; late-onset 177–178;
    late paraphrenia 176; overinclusiveness 11;
    paradox 521; reasoning 65, 126, 194–195,
    199n10, 271n5, 440–441, 443, 454, 459,
    465; senile paraphrenia 176; very late-onset
    177–178
Schneider, K. 175, 208, 464
Schreber, D. P. 110, 206–207
Schultz, W. 451, 466, 467
Schütz, A. 209, 210
Schwitzgebel, E. 246, 288n2, 297, 298, 318
SCR *see* skin conductance response (SCR)
seeing of meaning 51, 52
selectivity problem 352–353, 354, 355, 357,
    358, 358n5
self-administered psychometric scales 48
self-deception 17, 23, 296, 336–344, 399n10;
    *vs.* delusion 17, 24, 25n6, 295–296, 336,
    338–343; motivation 17, 23, 313, 339, 340,
    341, 342, 343–344, 427n8
self-esteem 17, 62, 64, 68, 70, 74, 111, 128,
    169, 170, 217, 283, 284, 342

self-hypnosis 492
self-referentiality 548–550
Seligman, M. 65
Sellars, W. 378–379
semantic memory 357, 437, 438
senile paraphrenia 176
senile psychosis 175, 176
sense of coherence (SOC) 7, 47, 128
serotonin (5HT) 108, 369, 372, 373
sleep paralysis 368, 445
SOC *see* sense of coherence (SOC)
social, alliances 8; anxiety 370, 527; cognition
    22, 127, 278, 363, 368, 381, 458, 485, 486,
    497, 512, 520, 521, 523–530, 527, 530n1,
    568; delusional contents 22, 23, 127, 455,
    522, 526, 528, 529, 534, 539–541; incentives
    243, influence 23, 397–398, 400n13,
    497–498, 523, 530; isolation 37, 49, 111,
    112, 130, 260, 284, 286, 287, 341, 485;
    media 567; norms 285, 480–481, 485, 486;
    psychology 266, 382, 425, 521, 550; psychotic
    symptoms 454–455; risk factors 520, 523,
    525; sanctioned belief 24, 419, 479; scaffolds
    287, 289n13; social brain hypothesis 536;
    social threat model 535–538; threats 524–525,
    526, 527, 529; transmission 24, 446, 557,
    566–567; value 66; *see also folie à deux*
social turn 22, 242–243, 397–398, 400n13,
    498, 520–530; evaluation of 525–528; ideas
    associated with 523–525; motivation
    521–523; social factors without
    dysfunctional social modules 528–530
somatic delusions 3, 10, 112, 115, 160, 178,
    181, 337, 443, 444, 446, 526, 535, 540, 544,
    549, 559
somatoparaphrenia 215, 217, 431, **432**, 456,
    493, 495
spectrum of mistrust-related phenomena 23
Spencer, L. 259, 271n1
Spinozan theories of belief 25n1, 310, 311, 312,
    320, 392, 393, 439; *see also* doxasticism,
    Spinozan
Staton, R. D. 18, 347, 354–358
Steinglass, J. E. 141, 142
Strawsonian account of moral responsibility
    505, 506, 508, 509, 501, 511, 512, 513, 517
Strawson, P. F. 242, 505, 508–513, 515, 516
strict unavailability 419
structural rationality 13, 218, 225n3
structural testimonial injustice 259
substantive irrationality 218, 225n3
Sullivan-Bissett, E. 25n6, 83n7, 193, 220,
    243n3, 243n4, 267, 377, 419, 427n5, 445,
    518n4, 518n7
supernumerary limb delusion 246, 250, 252,
    253, 254

supposition 37, 308, 309, 310, 326, 548, 550
Suspicion System 523–526, 527

teleo-functionalism 73, 78, 79, 83n8
testimonial injustice 8, 258, 259, 260, 261–262,
    265, 266, 271n1
testimony 12, 24, 25n1, 137, 190, 193, 194,
    195, 196, 224, 258, 259, 260, 261–262,
    265–266, 267, 269, 270, 302, 303, 311, 312,
    320, 321, 350, 367, 409, 485; abnormalities
    485, 523, 530; smothering 259, 263; *see also*
    testimonial injustice
theory of mind *110*, 351, 378, 381, 382, 468;
    impairment 111, 465
Thornton, T. 407–409
thought/action fusion 149, 151
thought insertion 128, 170n5, 177, 229, 346,
    250–251, 254, 410, 495, 506, 535, 538
thought/reality fusion 148, 149
tip-of-the-tongue phenomenon 563
trade-off view 65–66
Tranel, D. 219, 220, 421, 442
true delusion 3, 230, 271n2
Trump, D. 4, 42, 220, 547, 548, 559
Turner, S. 54, 55
two-factor theory 20, 79, 81, 82, 83n10, 161,
    164, 197, 215, 222–224, 249, 267, 268, 269,
    340, 341, 342, 343, 345n8, 350, 358n2,
    412n2, 414, 415, 417, 418, 419, 421, 422,
    430–446, 450, 455–456, 457, 458, 494,
    542n1, 544; bias against disconfirmatory
    evidence (BADE) 301, 440–441, **441**, 442,
    444, 445, 446, 561; bias versions 267, 268,
    269, 341, 418; belief evaluation deficit
    20, 222, 249, 267, 268, 269, 341, 345n8,
    414, 415, 441, 455, 494; bias towards
    observational adequacy 81–82, 345n8;
    failure of hypothesis evaluation 440–441;
    hypothesis generation 431, 433, 435,
    436, 437–438, 445; neuropsychological
    impairment 431, 442, 443–445, 446;
    Peircean pathway model 433–437, *436*; 438,

439, 440, 442, 445, 446n2; performance
    error 20, 267, 269–270, 341, 414; prediction
    error 20, 82, 430, 435, *436*, 454; rationalist
    403, 411
two-pyramids model 552

understandability 147, 155, 170, 210, 235,
    344n1, 403, 404, 405, 409, 410, 412n3, 545,
    548, 559, 561
unipolar depression 11, 159, 160
Unity Problem 94–97, 98
unshakeability 58, 108, 151, 174, 206, 237,
    238–239, 240
un-understandability 3, 147, 155n1, 170n5,
    344n1, 403, 404, 405, 410, 412n3, 545, 548,
    559, 561

value-based beliefs 136, 139, 142, 143
Van Leeuwen, N. 288n4, 304
ventral tegmental area (VTA) 451, 458
visual processing 191, 219, 364–365, 458
visual trash 365
volatility 454, 455–456, 459

Wakefield, J. C. 80, 82, 229
Wallace, R. J. 505, 508, 509, 511, 518n2
Wanderer, J. 259
what-it-is-likeness 53
Wilkinson, S. 14, 53, 220, 240, 242, 351–354,
    356, 357, 358n4, 421
Wisconsin Card Sorting Task 442
Wittgenstein, L. 20, 173, 174, 221, 395, 404,
    408–409, 410, 412, 565
World Health Organization International
    Classification of Disease (ICD) 89, 107, 108,
    110, 115, 117n4, 559

Xenobots 484

Young, A. W. 331, 349, 352, 355, 415, 538, 539

Zoja, L. 112, 116n1–117n1